Advances in the Management of Cardiovascular Disease

Advances in the Management of Cardiovascular Disease

Editors

Michał Ciurzyński
Justyna Domienik-Karłowicz

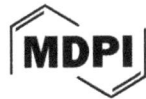

Basel • Beijing • Wuhan • Barcelona • Belgrade • Novi Sad • Cluj • Manchester

Editors
Michał Ciurzyński
Department of Internal
Medicine and Cardiology
Medical University
of Warsaw
Warsaw, Poland

Justyna Domienik-Karłowicz
Department of Internal
Medicine and Cardiology
Medical University
of Warsaw
Warsaw, Poland

Editorial Office
MDPI
St. Alban-Anlage 66
4052 Basel, Switzerland

This is a reprint of articles from the Special Issue published online in the open access journal *Journal of Clinical Medicine* (ISSN 2077-0383) (available at: https://www.mdpi.com/journal/jcm/special_issues/Advances_Management_Cardiovascular_Disease).

For citation purposes, cite each article independently as indicated on the article page online and as indicated below:

Lastname, A.A.; Lastname, B.B. Article Title. *Journal Name* **Year**, *Volume Number*, Page Range.

ISBN 978-3-0365-8874-2 (Hbk)
ISBN 978-3-0365-8875-9 (PDF)
doi.org/10.3390/books978-3-0365-8875-9

© 2023 by the authors. Articles in this book are Open Access and distributed under the Creative Commons Attribution (CC BY) license. The book as a whole is distributed by MDPI under the terms and conditions of the Creative Commons Attribution-NonCommercial-NoDerivs (CC BY-NC-ND) license.

Contents

Justyna Domienik-Karlowicz and Michał Ciurzynski
Forging Ahead in Cardiovascular Disease Management
Reprinted from: *J. Clin. Med.* **2023**, *12*, 5739, doi:10.3390/jcm12175739 1

Olga Dzikowska-Diduch, Katarzyna Kurnicka, Barbara Lichodziejewska, Iwona Dudzik-Niewiadomska, Michał Machowski, Marek Roik, et al.
Electrocardiogram, Echocardiogram and NT-proBNP in Screening for Thromboembolism Pulmonary Hypertension in Patients after Pulmonary Embolism
Reprinted from: *J. Clin. Med.* **2022**, *11*, 7369, doi:10.3390/jcm11247369 3

Aleksandra Justyna, Olga Dzikowska-Diduch, Szymon Pacho, Michał Ciurzyński, Marta Skowrońska, Anna Wyzgał-Chojecka, et al.
Decreased Haemoglobin Level Measured at Admission Predicts Long Term Mortality after the First Episode of Acute Pulmonary Embolism
Reprinted from: *J. Clin. Med.* **2022**, *11*, 7100, doi:10.3390/jcm11237100 13

Przemysław Seweryn Kasiak, Barbara Buchalska, Weronika Kowalczyk, Krzysztof Wyszomirski, Bartosz Krzowski, Marcin Grabowski and Paweł Balsam
The Path of a Cardiac Patient—From the First Symptoms to Diagnosis to Treatment: Experiences from the Tertiary Care Center in Poland
Reprinted from: *J. Clin. Med.* **2022**, *11*, 5276, doi:10.3390/jcm11185276 23

Anna Rulkiewicz, Iwona Pilchowska, Wojciech Lisik, Piotr Pruszczyk and Justyna Domienik-Karłowicz
Prevalence of Cigarette Smoking among Professionally Active Adult Population in Poland and Its Strong Relationship with Cardiovascular Co-Morbidities-POL-O-CARIA 2021 Study
Reprinted from: *J. Clin. Med.* **2022**, *11*, 4111, doi:10.3390/jcm11144111 33

Anna Rulkiewicz, Iwona Pilchowska, Wojciech Lisik, Piotr Pruszczyk, Michał Ciurzyński and Justyna Domienik-Karłowicz
Prevalence of Obesity and Severe Obesity among Professionally Active Adult Population in Poland and Its Strong Relationship with Cardiovascular Co-Morbidities-POL-O-CARIA 2016–2020 Study
Reprinted from: *J. Clin. Med.* **2022**, *11*, 3720, doi:10.3390/jcm11133720 47

Andreas Rukosujew, Arash Motekallemi, Konrad Wisniewski, Raluca Weber, Fernando De Torres-Alba, Abdulhakim Ibrahim, et al.
Transversal Arch Clamping for Complete Resection of Aneurysms of the Distal Ascending Aorta without Open Anastomosis
Reprinted from: *J. Clin. Med.* **2022**, *11*, 2698, doi:10.3390/jcm11102698 61

Robert Irzmański, Renata Glowczynska, Maciej Banach, Dominika Szalewska, Ryszard Piotrowicz, Ilona Kowalik, et al.
Prognostic Impact of Hybrid Comprehensive Telerehabilitation Regarding Diastolic Dysfunction in Patients with Heart Failure with Reduced Ejection Fraction—Subanalysis of the TELEREH-HF Randomized Clinical Trial
Reprinted from: *J. Clin. Med.* **2022**, *11*, 1844, doi:10.3390/jcm11071844 69

Tomasz Fabiszak, Michał Kasprzak, Marek Koziński and Jacek Kubica
Assessment of Selected Baseline and Post-PCI Electrocardiographic Parameters as Predictors of Left Ventricular Systolic Dysfunction after a First ST-Segment Elevation Myocardial Infarction
Reprinted from: *J. Clin. Med.* **2021**, *10*, 5445, doi:10.3390/jcm10225445 83

Miriam Freundt, Philipp Kolat, Christine Friedrich, Mohamed Salem, Matthias Gruenewald, Gunnar Elke, et al.
Preoperative Predictors of Adverse Clinical Outcome in Emergent Repair of Acute Type A Aortic Dissection in 15 Year Follow Up
Reprinted from: *J. Clin. Med.* **2021**, *10*, 5370, doi:10.3390/jcm10225370 . . . . **101**

Łukasz Kuźma, Anna Tomaszuk-Kazberuk, Anna Kurasz, Sławomir Dobrzycki, Marek Koziński, Bożena Sobkowicz and Gregory Y. H. Lip
Predicting Mortality in Patients with Atrial Fibrillation and Obstructive Chronic Coronary Syndrome: The Bialystok Coronary Project
Reprinted from: *J. Clin. Med.* **2021**, *10*, 4949, doi:10.3390/jcm10214949 . . . . **111**

Justine M. Ravaux, Michele Di Mauro, Kevin Vernooy, Silvia Mariani, Daniele Ronco, Jorik Simons, et al.
Impact of Bundle Branch Block on Permanent Pacemaker Implantation after Transcatheter Aortic Valve Implantation: A Meta-Analysis
Reprinted from: *J. Clin. Med.* **2021**, *10*, 2719, doi:10.3390/jcm10122719 . . . . **127**

Jarosław Hiczkiewicz, Paweł Burchardt, Jan Budzianowski, Konrad Pieszko, Dariusz Hiczkiewicz, Bogdan Musielak, et al.
Patients with Non-Obstructive Coronary Artery Disease Require Strict Control of All Cardiovascular Risk Factors: Results from the Polish Local Population Medical Records
Reprinted from: *J. Clin. Med.* **2021**, *10*, 2704, doi:10.3390/jcm10122704 . . . . **147**

Jan Budzianowski, Jarosław Hiczkiewicz, Katarzyna Łojewska, Edyta Kawka, Rafał Rutkowski and Katarzyna Korybalska
Predictors of Early-Recurrence Atrial Fibrillation after Catheter Ablation in Women and Men with Abnormal Body Weight
Reprinted from: *J. Clin. Med.* **2021**, *10*, 2694, doi:10.3390/jcm10122694 . . . . **159**

Piotr Bienias, Zuzanna Rymarczyk, Justyna Domienik-Karłowicz, Wojciech Lisik, Piotr Sobieraj, Piotr Pruszczyk and Michał Ciurzyński
Holter-Derived Autonomic Function, Arrhythmias and Carbohydrate Metabolism in Patients with Class III Obesity Treated with Laparoscopic Sleeve Gastrectomy
Reprinted from: *J. Clin. Med.* **2021**, *10*, 2140, doi:10.3390/jcm10102140 . . . . **175**

Emil Julian Dąbrowski, Marcin Kożuch and Sławomir Dobrzycki
Left Main Coronary Artery Disease—Current Management and Future Perspectives
Reprinted from: *J. Clin. Med.* **2022**, *11*, 5745, doi:10.3390/jcm11195745 . . . . **185**

Valentina Buda, Andreea Prelipcean, Dragos Cozma, Dana Emilia Man, Simona Negres, Alexandra Scurtu, et al.
An Up-to-Date Article Regarding Particularities of Drug Treatment in Patients with Chronic Heart Failure
Reprinted from: *J. Clin. Med.* **2022**, *11*, 2020, doi:10.3390/jcm11072020 . . . . **205**

Teruhiko Imamura, Nikhil Narang and Koichiro Kinugawa
Adaptive Servo-Ventilation as a Novel Therapeutic Strategy for Chronic Heart Failure
Reprinted from: *J. Clin. Med.* **2022**, *11*, 539, doi:10.3390/jcm11030539 . . . . **237**

Domenico Acanfora, Marco Matteo Ciccone, Valentina Carlomagno, Pietro Scicchitano, Chiara Acanfora, Alessandro Santo Bortone, et al.
A Systematic Review of the Efficacy and Safety of Direct Oral Anticoagulants in Atrial Fibrillation Patients with Diabetes Using a Risk Index
Reprinted from: *J. Clin. Med.* **2021**, *10*, 2924, doi:10.3390/jcm10132924 . . . . **245**

Dominika Siwik, Magdalena Gajewska, Katarzyna Karoń, Kinga Pluta,
Mateusz Wondołkowski, Radosław Wilimski, et al.
Pleiotropic Effects of Acetylsalicylic Acid after Coronary Artery Bypass Grafting—Beyond Platelet Inhibition
Reprinted from: *J. Clin. Med.* **2021**, *10*, 2317, doi:10.3390/jcm10112317 . . . . **259**

Annette M. Maznyczka, Connor J. Matthews, Jonathan M. Blaxill, John P. Greenwood, Abdul M. Mozid, Jennifer A. Rossington, et al.
Fractional Flow Reserve versus Angiography–Guided Management of Coronary Artery Disease: A Meta–Analysis of Contemporary Randomised Controlled Trials
Reprinted from: *J. Clin. Med.* **2022**, *11*, 7092, doi:10.3390/jcm11237092 . . . . **275**

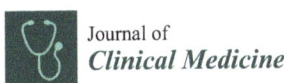
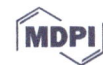

Editorial

Forging Ahead in Cardiovascular Disease Management

Justyna Domienik-Karlowicz * and Michał Ciurzynski

Department of Internal Medicine and Cardiology, Medical University of Warsaw, 02-005 Warsaw, Poland
* Correspondence: justyna.domienik@wum.edu.pl

The common threat of cardiovascular diseases (CVDs) constantly holds a dominant position among the leading causes of global mortality.

These diseases are everywhere and, combined with many risks, make studying heart problems both challenging and very important. Just like in other areas of medicine, continuous questions and new ideas help us to make progress. The way we understand and handle heart issues shows how far we have come and what the milestones yet to be achieved are. Against this background, this Special Issue of the *Journal of Clinical Medicine* (JCM), titled "Advances in the Management of Cardiovascular Diseases", stands out as a leading light with new discoveries and methods that aim to change the way we currently deal with heart problems.

A standout contribution from this issue, by Dobrzycki et al. [1], provides a comprehensive review of state-of-the-art diagnostic and treatment methods of left main coronary artery (LMCA) disease, focusing on percutaneous methods. While there is no one-size-fits-all approach for LMCAD, a team-based approach offers the best care. It is key to note that percutaneous coronary intervention and coronary artery bypass grafting methods complement each other, aiming for the best results in different situations. As we look ahead, more research on LMCA treatments will emerge, but finding the absolute best approach will remain an ongoing journey. In the next article, the authors [2] explore the various effects of acetylsalicylic acid (ASA) following CABG and offer a deeper understanding of how ASA helps beyond just inhibiting platelets. While some of ASA's effects appear to heighten bleeding risks, this raises questions about whether intensifying ASA treatment post-CABG is advantageous for these patients.

The value of ECG has been re-evaluated by Kubica et al. Their innovative approach seeks to confirm certain initial and post-PCI ECG indicators to predict left ventricular systolic dysfunction following an initial ST-segment elevation heart attack [3].

Further, the exploration of cardiovascular implications of other systemic diseases finds resonance in the insightful study by Pruszczyk et al. [4,5]. Their work on pulmonary embolism and its impact on cardiovascular health provides pivotal insights, reshaping our strategies for this disease management.

In this Special Issue, readers will find invaluable contributions, notably the detailed epidemiological research conducted by Rulkiewicz and her team [6,7]. Their studies shed light on the escalating concerns associated with obesity and smoking, offering a comprehensive exploration into these pressing health challenges.

Navigating through the myriad contributions in this Special Issue, it is palpable that the frontier of CVD management is expansive and ripe for revolutionary breakthroughs. As the Guest Editors, we want to thank our reviewers for their helpful feedback and the JCM team for their hard work. A big thanks to the authors who shared their knowledge in this Special Issue. Together, we hope to make progress in fighting cardiovascular diseases.

Author Contributions: Conceptualization, J.D.-K. and M.C.; writing J.D.-K. and M.C. All authors have read and agreed to the published version of the manuscript.

Funding: This research received no external funding.

Conflicts of Interest: The authors declare no conflict of interest.

Citation: Domienik-Karlowicz, J.;
Ciurzynski, M. Forging Ahead in
Cardiovascular Disease Management.
J. Clin. Med. **2023**, *12*, 5739.
https://doi.org/10.3390/
jcm12175739

Received: 24 August 2023
Accepted: 1 September 2023
Published: 3 September 2023

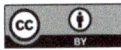

Copyright: © 2023 by the authors.
Licensee MDPI, Basel, Switzerland.
This article is an open access article distributed under the terms and conditions of the Creative Commons Attribution (CC BY) license (https://creativecommons.org/licenses/by/4.0/).

References

1. Dąbrowski, E.J.; Kożuch, M.; Dobrzycki, S. Left Main Coronary Artery Disease—Current Management and Future Perspectives. *J. Clin. Med.* **2022**, *11*, 5745. [CrossRef] [PubMed]
2. Siwik, D.; Gajewska, M.; Karoń, K.; Pluta, K.; Wondołkowski, M.; Wilimski, R.; Szarpak, Ł.; Filipiak, K.J.; Gąsecka, A. Pleiotropic Effects of Acetylsalicylic Acid after Coronary Artery Bypass Grafting—Beyond Platelet Inhibition. *J. Clin. Med.* **2021**, *10*, 2317. [CrossRef] [PubMed]
3. Fabiszak, T.; Kasprzak, M.; Koziński, M.; Kubica, J. Assessment of Selected Baseline and Post-PCI Electrocardiographic Parameters as Predictors of Left Ventricular Systolic Dysfunction after a First ST-Segment Elevation Myocardial Infarction. *J. Clin. Med.* **2021**, *10*, 5445. [CrossRef] [PubMed]
4. Dzikowska-Diduch, O.; Kurnicka, K.; Lichodziejewska, B.; Dudzik-Niewiadomska, I.; Machowski, M.; Roik, M.; Wiśniewska, M.; Siwiec, J.; Staniszewska, I.M.; Pruszczyk, P. Electrocardiogram, Echocardiogram and NT-proBNP in Screening for Thromboembolism Pulmonary Hypertension in Patients after Pulmonary Embolism. *J. Clin. Med.* **2022**, *11*, 7369. [CrossRef] [PubMed]
5. Justyna, A.; Dzikowska-Diduch, O.; Pacho, S.; Ciurzyński, M.; Skowrońska, M.; Wyzgał-Chojecka, A.; Piotrowska-Kownacka, D.; Pruszczyk, K.; Pucyło, S.; Sikora, A.; et al. Decreased Haemoglobin Level Measured at Admission Predicts Long Term Mortality after the First Episode of Acute Pulmonary Embolism. *J. Clin. Med.* **2022**, *11*, 7100. [CrossRef] [PubMed]
6. Rulkiewicz, A.; Pilchowska, I.; Lisik, W.; Pruszczyk, P.; Ciurzyński, M.; Domienik-Karłowicz, J. Prevalence of Obesity and Severe Obesity among Professionally Active Adult Population in Poland and Its Strong Relationship with Cardiovascular Co-Morbidities-POL-O-CARIA 2016–2020 Study. *J. Clin. Med.* **2022**, *11*, 3720. [CrossRef] [PubMed]
7. Rulkiewicz, A.; Pilchowska, I.; Lisik, W.; Pruszczyk, P.; Domienik-Karłowicz, J. Prevalence of Cigarette Smoking among Professionally Active Adult Population in Poland and Its Strong Relationship with Cardiovascular Co-Morbidities-POL-O-CARIA 2021 Study. *J. Clin. Med.* **2022**, *11*, 4111. [CrossRef] [PubMed]

Disclaimer/Publisher's Note: The statements, opinions and data contained in all publications are solely those of the individual author(s) and contributor(s) and not of MDPI and/or the editor(s). MDPI and/or the editor(s) disclaim responsibility for any injury to people or property resulting from any ideas, methods, instructions or products referred to in the content.

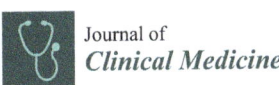

Article

Electrocardiogram, Echocardiogram and NT-proBNP in Screening for Thromboembolism Pulmonary Hypertension in Patients after Pulmonary Embolism

Olga Dzikowska-Diduch [1,*], Katarzyna Kurnicka [1], Barbara Lichodziejewska [1], Iwona Dudzik-Niewiadomska [1], Michał Machowski [1], Marek Roik [1], Małgorzata Wiśniewska [2], Jan Siwiec [1], Izabela Magdalena Staniszewska [1] and Piotr Pruszczyk [1]

[1] Department of Internal Medicine & Cardiology, Medical University of Warsaw, Lindleya 4, 02-005 Warsaw, Poland
[2] 1st Department of Radiology, Medical University of Warsaw, Lindleya 4, 02-005 Warsaw, Poland
* Correspondence: olga.dzikowska-diduch@wum.edu.pl; Tel.: +48-22-502-11-44; Fax: +48-22-502-21-42

Abstract: Background: The annual mortality of patients with untreated chronic thromboembolism pulmonary hypertension (CTEPH) is approximately 50% unless a timely diagnosis is followed by adequate treatment. In pulmonary embolism (PE) survivors with functional limitation, the diagnostic work-up starts with echocardiography. It is followed by lung scintigraphy and right heart catheterization. However, noninvasive tests providing diagnostic clues to CTEPH, or ascertaining this diagnosis as very unlikely, would be extremely useful since the majority of post PE functional limitations are caused by deconditioning. Methods: Patients after acute PE underwent a structured clinical evaluation with electrocardiogram, routine laboratory tests including NT-proBNP and echocardiography. The aim of this study was to verify whether the parameters from echocardiographic or perhaps electrocardiographic examination and NT-proBNP concentration best determine the risk of CTEPH. Results: Out of the total number of patients (n = 261, male n = 123) after PE who were included in the study, in the group of 155 patients (59.4%) with reported functional impairment, 13 patients (8.4%) had CTEPH and 7 PE survivors had chronic thromboembolic pulmonary disease (CTEPD) (4.5%). Echo parameters differed significantly between CTEPH/CTEPD cases and other symptomatic PE survivors. Patients with CTEPH/CTEPD also had higher levels of NT-proBNP (p = 0.022) but concentration of NT-proBNP above 125 pg/mL did not differentiate patients with CTEPH/CTEPD (p > 0.05). Additionally, the proportion of patients with right bundle brunch block registered in ECG was higher in the CTEPH/CTED group (23.5% vs. 5.8%, p = 0.034) but there were no differences between the other ECG characteristics of right ventricle overload. Conclusions: Screening for CTEPH/CTEPD should be performed in patients with reduced exercise tolerance compared to the pre PE period. It is not effective in asymptomatic PE survivors. Patients with CTEPH/CTED predominantly had abnormalities indicating chronic thromboembolism in the echocardiographic assessment. NT-proBNP and electrocardiographic characteristics of right ventricle overload proved to be insufficient in predicting CTEPH/CTEPD development.

Keywords: screening after pulmonary embolism; chronic thromboembolic pulmonary disease; chronic thromboembolic pulmonary hypertension; diagnostic work-up of post-pulmonary syndrome

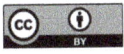

1. Introduction

Chronic thromboembolism pulmonary hypertension (CTEPH) is a rare disease but, unlike other forms of pulmonary hypertension, is curable [1]. Untreated CTEPH significantly affects the patient's prognosis [2]. The annual mortality in patients with untreated pulmonary hypertension is approximately 50% unless a timely diagnosis is followed by adequate treatment [3]. Early diagnosis of CTEPH is nonetheless essential but continues to be a huge challenge because there are no specific signs or symptoms of CTEPH. Moreover, symptoms of pulmonary hypertension develop slowly and are usually explained by more common causes. It has been estimated that the majority of CTEPH diagnoses nowadays still have a diagnostic delay by well over 1 year [4]. Chronic thromboembolic pulmonary disease (CTEPD) describes patients with chronic thromboembolic occlusions of pulmonary arteries but without PH at rest; however, change in the definition of PH with a decrease in the threshold mean pulmonary artery pressure from 25 to 21 mmHg may influence the designation of former CTEPD as CTEPH patients. Moreover, PE survivors with CTEPD benefit from the same treatment, including pulmonary endarterectomy, balloon pulmonary angioplasty and lifelong anticoagulation. Most cases of CTEPD/CTEPH occur in patients with a history of pulmonary embolism (PE) or/and deep vein thrombosis; therefore, screening for pulmonary hypertension seems reasonable in these patients.

In PE survivors with functional limitation, the diagnostic work-up starts with echocardiography, followed by ventilation/perfusion lung scintigraphy and right heart catheterization (RHC) with pulmonary angiography [5]. RHC is the gold standard for the diagnosis of pulmonary hypertension [2]; however, noninvasive tests providing diagnostic clues to confirm CTEPH or ascertain this diagnosis as very unlikely would be extremely useful, since the majority of post PE functional limitations are caused by deconditioning.

The European Society of Cardiology (ESC) guidelines propose echocardiography at rest as an initial examination, when CTEPH is suspected based on patient's clinical presentation [2,5]. Echo evaluations include estimating peak velocity of tricuspid valve regurgitation, calculation of atrioventricular pressure gradients and detection of indirect signs of pulmonary hypertension which should aim to estimate a level of probability of pulmonary hypertension. However, the accuracy of echocardiography that provides clues to the presence or absence of CTEPH is quite high (sensitivity of 70–100% and specificity of 72–89%) but echocardiography, performed according to the European Association of Cardiovascular Imaging (EACVI) guidelines, is not widely available and is associated with overdiagnosis and cost-ineffectiveness [6]. N-terminal pro-brain natriuretic peptide (NT-proBNP) levels correlate with myocardial dysfunction and can be elevated in case of almost any heart disease. NT-proBNP has been evaluated to stratify risk in patients with acute PE and remains the only biomarker that seems to be a strong predictor of prognosis and therefore is widely used in the routine practice in PH centers [2]. Its sensitivity and specificity in the diagnosis of CTEPH are around 82% and 70%, respectively [7]. Electrocardiogram (ECG) abnormalities including P pulmonale, right axis deviation (RAD), right ventricle (RV) hypertrophy and right bundle branch block (RBBB) are more common in severe PH than in the mild elevation of pulmonary pressure [2]. Normal ECG does not exclude the diagnosis of PH. Klok et al. showed in two independent cohort studies that the combination of a normal NT-proBNP level and the absence of specific ECG characteristics of RV overload accurately differentiates patients after PE with PH from those without PH with a sensitivity of 94–100% [7,8]. Moreover, the InShape II study showed that an algorithm including clinical probability of CTEPH, ECG and NT-proBNP levels can accurately exclude CTEPH, without the need for echocardiography (Boon InShape II) [8].

The aim of our study was to verify whether the parameters from echocardiographic or perhaps electrocardiographic examination and NT-proBNP concentration best determine the risk of CTEPH.

2. Methods

This is a post hoc analysis of a prospectively followed cohort of patients after pulmonary embolism. Patients were eligible for inclusion if aged 18 years or older and had a computed tomography pulmonary angiography proving diagnosis of symptomatic acute PE, and had been treated with therapeutically dosed anticoagulant therapy for at least 3 months according to current guidelines. After the discharge, all patients underwent, as previously reported, standard outpatient follow-up for at least 6 months following the acute PE event and were anticoagulated for at least 6 months. Briefly, we included all consecutive patients after acute PE with the exception of subjects with comorbidities significantly limiting survival or mobility (patients with advanced cancer or bed ridden subjects). At follow-up, all subjects underwent a structured clinical examination focused on their functional limitation. All patients were evaluated for the presence of exertional dyspnea, effort angina, exercise-limiting palpitations and a reduced exercise tolerance. In all patients ECG and routine laboratory tests were analyzed including hemoglobin, estimated glomerular filtration rate and NT-proBNP. All patients underwent a structured evaluation with echocardiography, which were performed by an experienced cardiologist according to the current EACVI recommendations [9]. Subjects with at least intermediate echocardiographic probability of PH according to the ESC guidelines [2] were referred to the detailed complete work-up for CTEPH.

2.1. Echocardiography

All echocardiograms were performed with Philips IE33 or Epic 7 according to the predefined standardized protocol by an experienced cardiologist, and focused on echocardiographic criteria for suspected PH (increased systolic peak tricuspid regurgitation velocity, dilated right ventricle, flattened interventricular septum, distended inferior vena cava with diminished inspiratory collapsibility or enlarged right atrial area) according to the 2015 ESC guidelines [2]. However, detailed evaluation of left ventricular (LV) morphology and function was also performed. The examinations were digitally recorded, and reviewed, when necessary. Patients were examined in the left lateral position. The dimensions of the right and left ventricles were measured in the parasternal long-axis view and apical four chamber view (4C) at the level of the mitral and tricuspid valve tips in late diastole defined by the R wave of continuous ECG tracing [10]. Tricuspid valve regurgitation was qualitatively assessed with color Doppler and peak gradient (tricuspid regurgitation peak gradient—TRPG) was calculated by simplified Bernoulli's formula after using tricuspid regurgitant flow peak velocity. The examination was completed by the measurement of the inferior vena cava (IVC) at late expiration. In the parasternal short axis view flattening of the interventricular septum was assessed qualitatively, and acceleration time (AcT) of pulmonary ejection was measured in the RV outflow tract, just below the pulmonary valve. Measurements were averaged over 3 consecutive heart cycles. In M-mode presentation, RV function was assessed by tricuspid annular plane systolic excursion (TAPSE) measurement. We measured the distance (mm) of systolic excursion of the RV annular segment along its longitudinal plane, from a standard apical 4-chamber view. The left ventricular ejection fraction was calculated according to Simpson's formula employing a two-dimensional image of the LV chamber during systole and diastole in the four and two chamber apical views.

2.2. Electrocardiogram

Conventional 12-lead ECGs will be recorded with the patient in supine position for a 10-s period using the standard 12-lead electrode configuration at a conventional speed (25 mm/s) and sensitivity (1 mV/10 mm). Sinus rhythm or arrhythmias and heart rate were registered. ECGs were also evaluated for the presence or absence of the following criteria that had been reported to occur more commonly in PH: right axis deviation (RAD defined as dominant S wave lead I with dominant R wave leads II and III), right bundle branch block (RBBB defined as QRS duration >120 ms with rSR pattern V1–V3), S1Q3T3 pattern (the presence of S waves in lead I and Q waves in lead III, each with amplitudes > 1.5 mm in association with negative T waves in lead III).

2.3. NT-proBNP

NT-proBNP levels were determined with the use of a quantitative immunoassay. Age- and gender-dependent thresholds for normal values as determined by the respective manufacturers were used.

2.4. Diagnoses

CTEPH was diagnosed when the invasive right heart catheterization showed that the mean pulmonary artery pressure was ≥25 mmHg at rest, pulmonary wedge pressure was ≤ 15 mmHg and abnormal imaging findings on the ventilation/perfusion lung scan, while CTEPD was diagnosed as CTEPH when mean pulmonary artery pressure, was< 25 mmHg [2].

2.5. Statisitcal Analysis

Statistical analysis was carried out in R software, version 4.0.5. Normality of distribution was verified using Shapiro–Wilk test and based on skewness and kurtosis values as well as visual assessment of histograms. Groups' comparison was conducted with chi-squared test or Fisher's exact test (nominal data) and with Welch *t*-test or Mann–Whitney U test (quantitative data), as appropriate. Additionally, we calculated odds ratio (OR) or mean/median differences (MD) between groups, including 95% confidence intervals.

In order to identify optimal cut-off points for each parameter as discriminator of CTEPH/CTED vs. healthy patients with symptoms, receiver operating characteristic (ROC) curves were created. Cut-off point calculation was based on Youden index, including measures of sensitivity, specificity, accuracy, negative predictive value (NPV) and positive predictive value (PPV).

3. Results

Out of the total number of patients (n = 261, male n = 123) after PE who were included in the study, 155 patients (59.4%) were with symptoms (mainly functional impairment) and 106 patients (40.6%) were without any symptoms. No significant differences were confirmed between both groups in sex, while age was significantly different—patients with symptoms were older than patients without symptoms, MD = 11.32 CI95 [7.41,6.21], p < 0.001.

In the group of patients with symptoms, 13 patients (8.4%) had CTEPH and 7 were survivors of CTEPD (4.5%) vs. no cases of CTEPH/CTEPD in the group without symptoms, p < 0.001. Chronic heart failure was recognized in about 50% of patients as the major cause of reduced exercise tolerance. Most of them presented a preserved ejection fraction. Other causes of functional limitation in the studied group included valve heart disease (6%), coronary artery diseases (6%), chronic obstructive pulmonary diseases (6%) and newly diagnosed permanent or paroxysmal atrial fibrillation in 6.4% of patients. Noncardiopulmonary pathologies including severe obesity in patients, newly diagnosed neoplasms or anemia contributed to decreased functional capacity in approximately 10% of symptomatic patients.

Echocardiogram, ECG and NT-proBNP were assessed 6 ± 0.97 months after PE.

Patients with symptoms had a significantly higher level of diameter of inferior vena cava (IVC) (p = 0.008), RV in 4 chamber view (RV4ch) (p = 0.002), elevated RV to LV ratio in 4 chamber view (p = 0.006), right atrium area (RAA) (p < 0.001), TRPG (p = 0.001), and left atrium area (LAA) (p < 0.001), than patients without functional impairment after PE. Indeed, there was a significant difference in LV EF% between the symptomatic and asymptomatic groups: 60.77 ± 5.43% vs. 62.91 ± 3.22%; p < 0.001. The LAA differed significantly between groups and was significantly elevated in symptomatic patients, which indicates that persistent dyspnea on exertion was also caused by the disease of the left heart, mainly left ventricular diastolic dysfunction. The AcT of pulmonary output average level was significantly lower (p = 0.001) in patients with functional limitation.

NT-proBNP concentrations were significantly higher in symptomatic patients than in the group without symptoms (p < 0.001). Additionally, the proportion of patients with NT-proBNP above norm was higher in symptomatic PE survivors (43.9% vs. 18.9% in group without symptoms), OR = 3.35 CI95 [1.82,6.34], p < 0.001. Interestingly, every fifth patient after PE without any deterioration of exercise tolerance had an increased concentration of NT-proBNP.

PE survivors with exercise intolerance had a higher level of d-dimer compared to patients who fully recovered functionally (p = 0.049) despite ongoing anticoagulation and no significant difference in drug taken.

Heart rhythm was also significantly different between both groups ($p = 0.005$). Patients with symptoms more often had atrial fibrillation (6.5% of cases vs. no cases in patients without symptoms) and less frequently had sinus rhythm (92.7% vs. 99.1%). No significant differences between both groups for drugs taken, echocardiographic LV4ch, TAPSE and ECG parameters (HR, RAD, RBBB, S1Q3T3) (Table 1.) were found.

Table 1. Comparison of patients after pulmonary embolism with and without symptoms.

Characteristics	n	Patients with Symptoms	n	Patients without Symptoms	MD/OR (95% CI)	p
n	155		106			
Sex, female, n (%)	155	85 (54.8)	106	53 (50.0)	1.21 (0.72,2.05)	0.52
Age, years, mean ± SD	155	61.07 ± 17.10	106	49.75 ± 18.36	11.32 (7.4,16.21)	<0.001 [2]
CTEPH/CTED, n (%)	155	20 (12.9)	106	0 (0.0)	-	<0.001 [1]
Drug, n (%)						
Acenocumarol		52 (34.2)		37 (43.0)		
Dabigatran		10 (6.6)		4 (4.7)		
Dalteparin		1 (0.7)		1 (1.2)		
Enoxaparin	152	8 (5.3)	86	5 (5.8)	-	0.0651
Nadroparin		2 (1.3)		0 (0.0)		
Riwaroxaban		64 (42.1)		22 (25.6)		
Warfarin		15 (9.9)		17 (19.8)		
IVC, mean ± SD	151	15.36 ± 4.60	104	13.96 ± 3.76	1.40 (0.37,2.44)	0.0082
LV4ch, mean ± SD	131	45.67 ± 5.50	73	43.50 ± 4.24	2.17 (−1.23,1.87)	0.6832
RV4ch, mean ± SD	130	33.50 ± 6.60	74	31.88 ± 2.59	1.63 (0.85,3.86)	0.0022
RV/LV, mean ± SD	130	0.80 ± 0.12	73	0.75 ± 0.12	0.04 (0.01,0.08)	0.0062
LV EF, mean ± SD	155	60.77 ± 5.43	106	62.91 ± 3.22	−2.14 (−3.19,01.07)	<0.001 [2]
LAA, cm^2, mean ± SD	140	19.89 ± 4.07	81	16.96 ± 3.31	2.92 (1.89,3.88)	<0.001 [2]
RAA, cm^2, mean ± SD	138	18.12 ± 4.14	78	15.42 ± 3.28	2.71 (1.67,3.68)	<0.001 [2]
Heart rhythm, n (%)						
Atrial fibrillation		10 (6.5)		0 (0.0)		
Stimulation	154	1 (0.6)	106	0 (0.0)	-	0.0051
Tachycardia		0 (0.0)		1 (0.9)		
Sinus rhythm		143 (92.7)		105 (99.1)		
TRPG, median (Q1,Q3)	150	25.50 (20.00,32.75)	103	23.00 (17.00,27.50)	2.50 (1.00,6.00)	0.0013
RVSP, median (Q1,Q3)	146	31.00 (25.00,40.75)	102	28.00 (23.00,33.75)	3.00 (2.00,7.00)	0.0013
AcT, mean ± SD	148	112.08 ± 28.07	101	123.70 ± 24.03	−11.62 (−18.17,−5.07)	0.0012
TAPSE, mean ± SD	134	23.34 ± 3.79	80	23.66 ± 3.21	−0.33 (−1.29,0.63)	0.5032
HR, mean ± SD	137	70.58 ± 10.66	58	69.45 ± 9.71	1.14 (−1.97,4.24)	0.4702
RAD, n (%)	131	4 (3.1)	57	0 (0.0)	-	0.3161
RBBB, n (%)	121	10 (8.3)	53	1 (1.9)	4.65 (0.63,206.97)	0.1761
S1Q3T3, n (%)	117	26 (22.2)	53	7 (13.2)	1.87 (0.72,5.50)	0.243
NTproBNP, median (Q1,Q3) (pg/mL)	155	108.00 (45.00,339.50)	106	29.00 (20.00,96.25)	79.00 (31.00,85.00)	<0.001 [3]
NTproBNP > 125 pg/mL, n (%)	155	68 (43.9)	106	20 (18.9)	3.35 (1.82,6.34)	<0.001
D-dimer,(ng/mL) median (Q1,Q3)	95	300.00 (205.50,488.50)	95	239.00 (170.00,420.00)	61.00 (0.01,93.00)	0.0493

AcT—acceleration time of pulmonary ejection, CTEPD—chronic thromboembolic pulmonary disease, CTEPH—chronic thromboembolic pulmonary hypertension, HR—heart rate, LV—left ventricle, 4ch—four chamber view, NT-proBNP: N-terminal pro-brain natriuretic peptide, RAD—right axis deviation, RBBB—right heart catheterization, RV—right ventricle, TRPG—tricuspid regurgitation peak gradient, TAPSE—tricuspid annular plane systolic excursion, RVSP—right ventricle systolic pressure, MD—mean/median difference between groups calculated as patients with symptoms minus patients without symptoms with 95% confidence interval, OR—odds ratio between both groups, with 95% confidence interval. Groups compared with chi-square test or Fisher exact test [1] for nominal data with t-test [2] or Mann–Whitney U test [3] for continuous data.

As a second step, in the 155 patients with symptoms, patients with and without CTEPH/CTEPD were compared. Patients with CTEPH/CTEPD had a significantly higher level of: RV4ch ($p = 0.003$), RAA ($p = 0.004$), TRPG ($p < 0.001$) and NTproBNP ($p = 0.022$) than patients without CTEPH/CTEPD. For AcT of pulmonary ejection average level was significantly lower ($p = 0.008$) in patients with CTEPH/CTEPD. Additionally, the proportion of patients with RBBB was higher in the group with CTEPH/CTEPD (23.5% vs. 5.8% in the group without CTEPH/CTED), OR = 4.92 CI95 [1.90,24.18], $p = 0.034$. No differences between patients with and without CTEPH/CTEPD were confirmed for LAA, the proportion of RAD and S1Q3T3 in ECG and NTproBNP> 125 pg/mL ($p > 0.05$ in all cases) (Tables 2 and 3).

Table 2. Comparison of patients after pulmonary embolism with and without CTEPH/CTED among symptomatic patients.

Characteristics.	n	Patients with Symptoms with CTEPH/CTEPD	n	Patients with Symptoms without CTEPH/CTEPD	MD/OR (95% CI)	p
n	20		135			
RV4ch, mean ± SD	20	36.50 ± 7.78	110	32.00 ± 6.58	4.50 (1.61,6.99)	0.003 [2]
LAA, cm^2, mean ± SD	19	21.58 ± 4.68	121	19.62 ± 3.93	1.96 (−0.39,4.31)	0.097 [2]
RAA, cm^2, mean ± SD	19	21.53 ± 5.08	119	17.58 ± 3.71	3.95 (1.42,6.47)	0.004 [2]
TRPG, median (Q1,Q3)	20	45.00 (30.75,62.00)	130	24.00 (20.00,30.00)	21.00 (13.00,33.00)	<0.001 [3]
AcT, mean ± SD	19	88.42 ± 39.21	129	115.57 ± 24.36	−27.15 (−46.43,−7.86)	0.008 [2]
RAD, n (%)	19	1 (5.3)	112	3 (2.7)	2.01 (0.04,26.60)	0.469 [1]
RBBB, n (%)	17	4 (23.5)	104	6 (5.8)	4.92 (1.90,24.18)	0.034 [1]
S1Q3T3, n (%)	16	6 (37.5)	101	20 (19.8)	2.41 (0.64,8.40)	0.191
NTproBNP, median (Q1,Q3)	20	151.00 (85.25,843.00)	135	99.00 (43.00,300.50)	52.00 (12.00,372.00)	0.022 [3]
NTproBNP > 125, n (%)	20	12 (60.0)	135	56 (41.5)	2.11 (0.74,6.36)	0.149

AcT: acceleration time of pulmonary ejection, CTEPD: chronic thromboembolic pulmonary disease, CTEPH: chronic thromboembolic pulmonary hypertension, LAA—left atrium area, NT-proBNP: N-terminal pro-brain natriuretic peptide, RAA—right atrium area, RAD—right axis deviation, RBBB—right heart catheterization, RV4ch—right ventricle 4 chamber view, TRPG—tricuspid regurgitation peak gradient, MD—mean/median difference between groups calculated as patients with CTEPH/CTED minus patients without CTEPH/CTED with 95% confidence interval, OR—odds ratio between both groups, with 95% confidence interval. Groups compared with chi-square test or Fisher exact test [1] for nominal data, with t-test [2] or Mann–Whitney U test [3] for continuous data.

Table 3. Comparison of patients after pulmonary embolism with CTEPH and CTED among symptomatic patients.

Characteristics	n	Patients with CTEPH	n	Patients with CTED	MD / OR (95% CI)	p
n	13		7			
RV4ch, mean ± SD	13	42.00 (42.00,42.00)	7	31.00 (31.00,31.00)	11.00 (−4.00,18.00)	0.249 [3]
LAA, cm^2, mean ± SD	13	21.92 ± 4.70	6	20.83 ± 5.00	1.09 (−4.36,6.54)	0.663 [2]
RAA, cm^2, mean ± SD	13	22.77 ± 4.90	6	18.83 ± 4.75	3.94 (−1.33,9.21)	0.127 [2]
TRPG, median (Q1,Q3)	13	59.23 ±23.81	7	34.71 ± 12.66	24.52 (7.39,41.65)	0.008 [2]
AcT, mean ± SD	12	78.50 (67.50,86.25)	7	106.00 (78.50,140.00)	−27.50 (−72.00,10.00)	0.162 [3]
RAD, n (%)	12	1 (8.3)	7	0 (0.0)	-	>0.999 [1]
RBBB, n (%)	10	3 (30.0)	7	1 (14.3)	2.44 (0.15,156.95)	0.603 [1]
S1Q3T3, n (%)	10	3 (30.0)	6	3 (50.0)	0.45 (0.03,5.51)	0.607 [1]
NTproBNP, median (Q1,Q3)	13	435.00 (132.00,1494.00)	7	107.00 (76.50,313.50)	328.00 (−33.00,1387.00)	0.115 [3]
NTproBNP > 125, n (%)	13	10 (76.9)	7	2 (28.6)	7.32 (0.74,117.26)	0.062 [1]

AcT: acceleration time of pulmonary ejection, CTEPD: chronic thromboembolic pulmonary disease, CTEPH: chronic thromboembolic pulmonary hypertension, LAA—left atrium area, NT-proBNP: N-terminal pro-brain natriuretic peptide, RAA—right atrium area, RAD-right axis deviation, RBBB-right heart catheterization, RV4ch—right ventricle 4 chamber view, TRPG-tricuspid regurgitation peak gradient, MD—mean/median difference between groups calculated as patients with CTEPH minus patients without CTEPD with 95% confidence interval, OR—odds ratio between both groups, with 95% confidence interval. Groups compared with Fisher exact test [1] for nominal data, with t-test [2] or Mann–Whitney U test [3] for continuous data.

Receiver operating characteristic curves as discrimination of CTEPH/CTEPD vs. symptomatic but without CTEPH/CTED were significant for RV4ch ($p = 0.002$), RAA ($p = 0.001$), TRPG ($p < 0.001$) and AcT ($p = 0.001$) with satisfactory or very good level of area under the curve (AUC); from AUC = 0.723 CI95 [0.591,0.855] for RV4ch to AUC = 0.868 CI95 [0.785,0.952] for TRPG. The level of optimal cut-off points for particular parameters with corresponding sensitivity and specificity is summarized in Table 4.

Table 4. Results for measurement of different parameters in the diagnosis of CTEPH/CTEPD in symptomatic pulmonary embolism survivors.

Characteristics	AUC (95% CI)	Cut-off Point	Sensitivity	Specificity	Accuracy	NPV	PPV	p
RV4ch	0.723 (0.591,0.855)	37.5	0.7	0.72	0.72	0.93	0.31	0.002
LAA, cm^2	0.617 (0.464,0.771)	23.5	0.42	0.86	0.8	0.9	0.32	0.056
RAA, cm^2	0.734 (0.589,0.879)	19.5	0.68	0.78	0.77	0.94	0.33	0.001
TRPG	0.868 (0.785,0.952)	29.5	0.85	0.72	0.73	0.97	0.31	<0.001
AcT	0.763 (0.611,0.914)	86	0.63	0.89	0.86	0.94	0.46	0.001
NTproBNP	0.659 (0.528,0.789)	434.5	0.45	0.85	0.8	0.91	0.31	0.297

AcT: acceleration time of pulmonary ejection, AUC—area under the curve with 95% confidence interval (CI), CTEPD—chronic thromboembolic pulmonary disease, CTEPH—chronic thromboembolic pulmonary hypertension, LAA—left atrium area, NPV—negative predictive value, NT-proBNP—N-terminal pro-brain natriuretic peptide, PPV—positive predictive value, RAA—right atrium area, TRPG—tricuspid regurgitation peak gradient.

4. Discussion

Our analysis showed that screening for CTEPH should be given to symptomatic patients after PE. Although ECG, echo and NT-proBNP screening was performed in all of 261 patients included in our study, CTEPH and CTEPD was diagnosed only in group of patients with dyspnea on exertion. PE survivors who completely recovered functionally had no significant abnormalities in the echo, ECG and laboratory test. This is consistent with the observations of Held et al. who suggested focusing diagnostic procedures on only symptomatic patients [11]. Habib and Torbicki also said in 2010 that echocardiographic screening for CTEPH is not effective in asymptomatic patients [12].

The echocardiographic estimation of the likelihood of PH is among the key elements in the decision-making process by identifying patients for whom RHC is warranted, facilitating earlier diagnosis and earlier medical management [13]. A meta-analysis calculated the accuracy of echocardiography vs. RHC for PH diagnosis and found a sensitivity of 83% (95% CI, 73–90%) and specificity of 72% (95% CI, 53–85%) and that echocardiography has been shown to miss PH in as many as 10–31% of cases [14]. Indeed, in our analysis, significant echocardiographic abnormalities were assessed in CTEPH/CTEPD group, but the diagnosis of chronic thromboembolic pulmonary artery occlusion explaining exercise intolerance was made in only 20 of 155 patients who complained of functional limitation. It cannot be ruled out that some cases of CTEPH/CTEPD had been missed. Patients with CTEPH/CTEPD had typical echocardiographic signs of pulmonary hypertension included enlargement of the right atrium and right ventricle, elevated RV to LV ratio in the four chamber view and significant elevated TRPG, IVC diameter and RVSP. Our findings are consistent with previous observations of Habib, Torbicki and Surinder Janda et al. [12,14]. In our study, the AcT of pulmonary output was significantly lower in patients with CTEPH/CTEPD compared to other symptomatic PE survivors, as in the analysis of Kitabatake et al. [15]. Moreover, our echocardiographic assessment after PE revealed a significant elevated left atrium area in patients suffering from dyspnea on exertion, which suggests that the functional limitation is also due to left heart disease, mainly diastolic dysfunction [16]. Chronic heart failure with preserved systolic function, which is much more common than chronic pulmonary artery occlusion, may explain elevated concentrations of NT-proBNP in symptomatic patients after PE [17,18]. Survivors with symptoms were also much older and more likely to have fibrillation than asymptomatic patients, which also explains the increased concentration of BNP [19]. Obviously, mean concentrations of BNP were higher in CTEPH/CTEPD but levels above 125 pg/mL were exceeded similarly frequently in symptomatic patients with and without chronic thromboembolism. NT-proBNP allows for only sufficient differentiation of patients with CTEPH/CTEPD (AUC 0.659, Figure 1). In general, conventional ECG criteria had low diagnostic accuracy for the presence of increased RV afterload [20,21]. In our study, the proportion of patients with RBBB was higher in groups with CTEPH/CTEPD (23.5% vs. 5.8%), p = 0.034, but there were no significant differences in ECG characteristics of right ventricle overload as RAD and S1Q3T3. The combination of ECG and NT-proBNP in the Leiden CTEPH rule-out criteria may be useful in diagnostic after PE but in in the group of 261 patients we studied, they did not allow to safely and effectively exclude PH or indicate patients for further invasive work-up [22]. Meaningful screening programs should be simple, widely available and non-invasive. However, diagnostic tests should quickly and clearly indicate which patient will benefit from further work-up [23,24]. Since symptoms initially in CTEPH appear during exercise, the tests performed at rest, including electrocardiogram, echocardiogram or RHC, may lack sensitivity. Although prospective evaluation of larger cohorts is still lacking, functional tests are a promising complementary diagnostic tool for functional evaluation of patients with chronic pulmonary vascular disease [7,25].

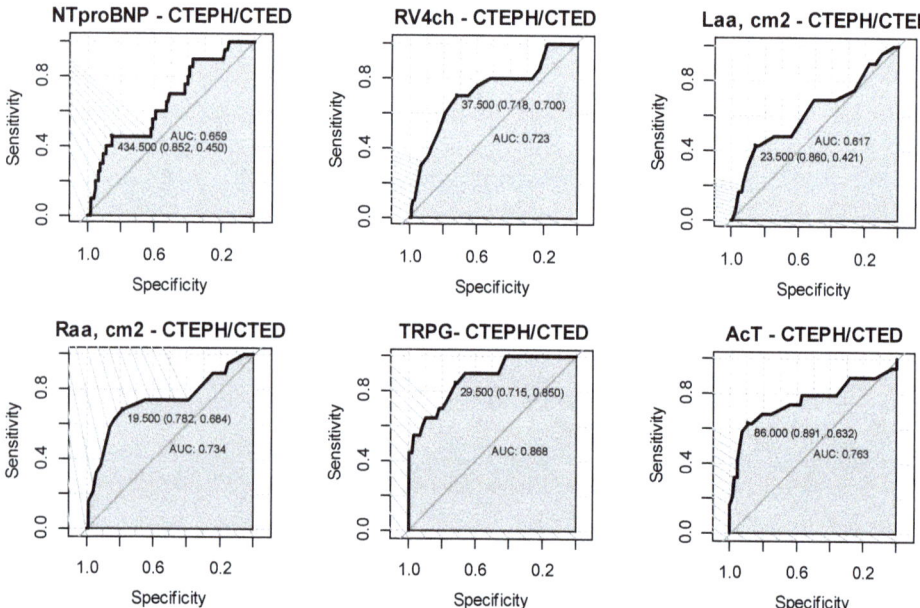

Figure 1. ROC curves for particular parameters as diagnostic test for CTEPH/CTEPD vs. patients with symptoms but without CTEPH/CTEPD (numbers of each chart include AUC value as well as optimal cut-off point with specificity and sensitivity values).

5. Conclusions

Screening for CTEPH/CTEPD should be performed in patients with reduced exercise tolerance compared to the pre PE period, and it is not effective in asymptomatic PE survivors. Patients with CTEPH/CTED had presented predominantly abnormalities indicating chronic thromboembolism in the echocardiographic assessment. NT-proBNP and electrocardiographic characteristics of right ventricle overload proved to be insufficient in predicting CTEPH/CTEPD development.

Author Contributions: Investigation, K.K., B.L. and M.W.; Data curation, M.R., J.S. and I.M.S.; Writing—original draft, O.D.-D.; Writing—review & editing, M.M.; Supervision, P.P.; Project administration, I.D.-N. All authors have read and agreed to the published version of the manuscript.

Funding: This research received no external funding.

Institutional Review Board Statement: The study was conducted in accordance with the Declaration of Helsinki, and approved by the Bioethics Committee at the Medical University of Warsaw. Ethics approval number is KB 88/2008.

Informed Consent Statement: Informed consent was obtained from all subjects involved in the study.

Data Availability Statement: The study did not report any data.

Conflicts of Interest: The authors declare no conflict of interest.

Abbreviations

AcT	acceleration time of pulmonary ejection
AUC	area under the ROC curve
CTEPD	chronic thromboembolic pulmonary disease
CTEPH	chronic thromboembolic pulmonary hypertension
EACVI	European Association of Cardiovascular Imaging
ECG	electrocardiogram
ESC	European Society of Cardiology
HR	heart rate
IVC	inferior vena cava
LAA	left atrium area
LV	left ventricle
4ch	four chamber view
MD	mean/median differences
NPV	negative predictive value
NT-proBNP	N-terminal pro-brain natriuretic peptide
OR	odds ratio
PE	pulmonary embolism
PH	pulmonary hypertension
PPV	positive predictive value
RAA	right atrium area
RAD	right axis deviation
RBBB	right bundle branch block
RHC	right heart catheterization
ROC	receiver operating characteristic
RV	right ventricle
RVSP	right ventricle systolic pressure
TRPG	tricuspid regurgitation peak gradient
TAPSE	tricuspid annular plane systolic excursion

References

1. Ende-Verhaar, Y.M.; Cannegieter, S.C.; Vonk Noordegraaf, A.; Delcroix, M.; Pruszczyk, P.; Mairuhu, A.T.; Huisman, M.V.; Klok, F.A. Incidence of chronic thromboembolic pulmonary hypertension after acute pulmonary embolism: A contempo-rary view of the published literature. *Eur. Respir. J.* **2017**, *49*, 1601792. [CrossRef] [PubMed]
2. Galiè, N.; Humbert, M.; Vachiéry, J.-L.; Gibbs, S.; Lang, I.; Torbicki, A.; Simonneau, G.; Peacock, A.; Vonk-Noordegraaf, A.; Beghetti, M.; et al. 2015 ESC/ERS Guidelines for the diagnosis and treatment of pulmo-nary hypertension: The Joint Task Force for the Diagnosis and Treatment of Pulmonary Hypertension of the European Society of Cardiology (ESC) and the European Respiratory Society (ERS): Endorsed by: Association for European Paediatric and Congenital Cardiology (AEPC), International Society for Heart and Lung Transplanta-tion (ISHLT). *Eur. Respir. J.* **2015**, *46*, 903–975. [PubMed]
3. Lewczuk, J.; Piszko, P.; Jagas, J.; Porada, A.; Sobkowicz, B.; Wrabec, K.; Wójciak, S. Prognostic Factors in Medically Treated Patients With Chronic Pulmonary Embolism. *Chest* **2001**, *119*, 818–823. [CrossRef] [PubMed]
4. Klok, F.A.; Barco, S.; Konstantinides, S.; Dartevelle, P.; Fadel, E.; Jenkins, D.; Kim, N.H.; Madani, M.; Matsubara, H.; Mayer, E.; et al. Determinants of diagnostic delay in chronic thromboembolic pulmonary hypertension: Results from the European CTEPH Registry. *Eur. Respir. J.* **2018**, *52*, 1801687. [CrossRef]

5. Konstantinides, S.V.; Meyer, G.; Becattini, C.; Bueno, H.; Geersing, G.-J.; Harjola, V.-P.; Huisman, M.V.; Humbert, M.; Jennings, C.S.; Jimenez, D.; et al. The Task Force for the diagnosis and management of acute pulmonary em-bolism of the European Society of Cardiology (ESC). 2019 ESC Guidelines for the diagnosis and management of acute pulmonary embolism developed in collaboration with the European Respiratory Society (ERS): The Task Force for the diagnosis and management of acute pulmonary embolism of the European Society of Cardiology (ESC). *Eur. Respir. J.* **2019**, *54*, 543–603.
6. Gopalan, D.; Delcroix, M.; Held, M. Diagnosis of chronic thromboembolic pulmonary hypertension. *Eur. Respir. Rev.* **2017**, *26*, 160108. [CrossRef]
7. Delcroix, M.; Torbicki, A.; Gopalan, D.; Sitbon, O.; Klok, F.A.; Lang, I.; Jenkins, D.; Kim, N.H.; Humbert, M.; Jais, X.; et al. ERS statement on chronic thromboembolic pulmonary hypertension. *Eur. Respir. J.* **2020**, *57*, 2002828. [CrossRef]
8. Boon, G.J.A.M.; Ende-Verhaar, Y.M.; Bavalia, R.; El Bouazzaoui, L.H.; Delcroix, M.; Dzikowska-Diduch, O.; Huisman, M.V.; Kurnicka, K.; Mairuhu, A.T.A.; Middeldorp, S.; et al. Non-invasive early exclusion of chronic thromboembolic pulmonary hypertension after acute pulmonary embolism: The InShape II study. *Thorax* **2021**, *76*, 1002–1009. [CrossRef]
9. Galderisi, M.; Cosyns, B.; Edvardsen, T.; Cardim, N.; Delgado, V.; di Salvo, G.; Donal, E.; Sade, L.E.; Ernande, L.; Garbi, M.; et al. Standardization of adult transthoracic echocardiography reporting in agreement with recent chamber quantification, diastolic function, and heart valve disease recommendations:an expert consen-sus document of the European Association of Cardiovascular Imaging. *Eur. Heart J. Cardiovasc. Imaging* **2017**, *18*, 1301–1310.
10. Lang, R.M.; Badano, L.P.; Mor-Avi, V.; Afilalo, J.; Armstrong, A.; Ernande, L.; Flachskampf, F.A.; Foster, E.; Gold-stein, S.A.; Kuznetsova, T.; et al. Recommendations for cardiac chamber quantification by echocardiography in adults: An update from the American Society of Echocardiography and the European Association of Cardiovascular Im-aging. *Eur. Heart J. Cardiovasc. Imaging* **2015**, *16*, 233–271. [CrossRef]
11. Held, M.; Hesse, A. A symptom-related monitoring program following pulmonary embolism for the early detection of CTEPH: A prospective observational registry study. *BMC Pulm. Med.* **2014**, *14*, 141.
12. Habib, G.; Torbicki, A. The role of echocardiography in the diagnosis and management of patients with pulmo-nary hypertension. *Eur. Respir. Rev. Eur. Respir. Soc.* **2010**, *19*, 288–299. [CrossRef] [PubMed]
13. Dunlap, B.; Weyer, G. Pulmonary Hypertension: Diagnosis and Treatment. *Am. Fam. Physician* **2016**, *94*, 463–469.
14. Janda, S.; Shahidi, N.; Gin, K.; Swiston, J. Diagnostic accuracy of echocardiography for pulmonary hypertension: A systematic review and meta-analysis. *Heart* **2011**, *97*, 612–622. [CrossRef] [PubMed]
15. Kitabatake, A.; Inoue, M.; Asao, M.; Masuyama, T.; Tanouchi, J.; Morita, T.; Mishima, M.; Uematsu, M.; Shimazu, T.; Hori, M.; et al. Noninvasive evaluation of pulmonary hypertension by a pulsed Doppler technique. *Circulation* **1983**, *68*, 302–309. [CrossRef] [PubMed]
16. Dzikowska-Diduch, O.; Kostrubiec, M.; Kurnicka, K.; Lichodziejewska, B.; Pacho, S.; Miroszewska, A.; Bródka, K.; Skowrońska, M.; Łabyk, A.; Roik, M.; et al. The post-pulmonary syndrome-results of echocardiographic driven follow up after acute pulmonary embolism. *Thromb. Res.* **2019**, *186*, 30–35. [CrossRef]
17. McDonagh, T.A.; Metra, M.; Adamo, M.; Gardner, R.S.; Baumbach, A.; Böhm, M.; Burri, H.; Butler, J.; Čelutkienė, J.; Chioncel, O.; et al. 2021 ESC Guidelines for the diagnosis and treatment of acute and chronic heart failure. *Eur. Heart J.* **2021**, *42*, 3599–3726. [CrossRef]
18. Nagueh, S.F.; Smiseth, O.A.; Appleton, C.P.; Byrd BF 3rd Dokainish, H.; Edvardsen, T.; Flachskampf, F.A.; Gil-lebert, T.C.; Klein, A.L.; Lancellotti, P.; Marino, P.; et al. Recommendations for the Evaluation of Left Ventricular Diastolic Function by Echocardiography: An Update from the American Society of Echocardiography and the European Association of Cardiovascular Imaging. *J. Am. Soc. Echocardiogr.* **2016**, *29*, 277–314. [CrossRef]
19. Kerr, B.; Brandon, L. Atrial Fibrillation, thromboembolic risk, and the potential role of the natriuretic peptides, a focus on BNP and NT-proBNP–A narrative review. *IJC Heart Vasc.* **2022**, *43*, 101132. [CrossRef]
20. Henkens, I.R.; Mouchaers, K.T.B.; Vonk-Noordegraaf, A.; Boonstra, A.; Swenne, C.A.; Maan, A.C.; Man, S.-C.; Twisk, J.W.R.; Van Der Wall, E.E.; Schalij, M.J.; et al. Improved ECG detection of presence and severity of right ventricular pressure load validated with cardiac magnetic resonance imaging. *Am. J. Physiol. Circ. Physiol.* **2008**, *294*, H2150–H2157. [CrossRef]
21. Thomson, D.; Kourounis, G.; Trenear, R.; Messow, C.-M.; Hrobar, P.; Mackay, A.; Isles, C. ECG in suspected pulmonary embolism. *Postgrad. Med. J.* **2019**, *95*, 12–17. [CrossRef] [PubMed]
22. Klok, F.A.; van Kralingen, K.W.; van Dijk, A.P.; Heyning, F.H.; Vliegen, H.W. Prospective cardiopulmonary screening program to detect chronic thromboembolic pulmonary hypertension in patients after acute pulmonary embolism. *Haematologica* **2010**, *95*, 970–975. [CrossRef] [PubMed]
23. Coquoz, N.; Weilenmann, D.; Stolz, D.; Popov, V.; Azzola, A.; Fellrath, J.-M.; Stricker, H.; Pagnamenta, A.; Ott, S.; Ulrich, S.; et al. Multicentre observational screening survey for the detection of CTEPH following pulmonary embolism. *Eur. Respir. J.* **2018**, *51*, 1702505. [CrossRef]
24. Surie, S.; Gibson, N.S.; Gerdes, V.E.; Bouma, B.J.; Smit, B.L.V.E.; Buller, H.R.; Bresser, P. Active search for chronic thromboembolic pulmonary hypertension does not appear indicated after acute pulmonary embolism. *Thromb. Res.* **2010**, *125*, e202–e205. [CrossRef]
25. Caravita, S.; Faini, A.; Deboeck, G.; Bondue, A.; Naeije, R.; Parati, G.; Vachiéry, J.-L. Pulmonary hypertension and ventilation during exercise: Role of the pre-capillary component. *J. Heart Lung Transplant.* **2017**, *36*, 754–762. [CrossRef] [PubMed]

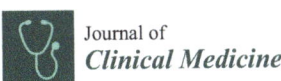

Article

Decreased Haemoglobin Level Measured at Admission Predicts Long Term Mortality after the First Episode of Acute Pulmonary Embolism

Aleksandra Justyna [1], Olga Dzikowska-Diduch [1,*], Szymon Pacho [1], Michał Ciurzyński [1], Marta Skowrońska [1], Anna Wyzgał-Chojecka [1], Dorota Piotrowska-Kownacka [2], Katarzyna Pruszczyk [3], Szymon Pucyło [1], Aleksandra Sikora [1] and Piotr Pruszczyk [1]

[1] Department of Internal Medicine & Cardiology, Medical University of Warsaw, 02-091 Warsaw, Poland
[2] 1st Department of Radiology, Medical University of Warsaw, 02-091 Warsaw, Poland
[3] Department of Hematology, Institute of Hematology and Transfusion Medicine, 02-776 Warsaw, Poland
* Correspondence: olga.dzikowska-diduch@wum.edu.pl

Abstract: Background: Decreased hemoglobin concentration was reported to predict long term prognosis in patients various cardiovascular diseases including congestive heart failure and coronary artery disease. We hypothesized that hemoglobin levels may be useful for post discharge prognostication after the first episode of acute pulmonary embolism. Therefore, the aim of the current study was to evaluate a potential prognostic value of a decreased hemoglobin levels measured at admission due to the first episode of acute PE for post discharge all cause mortality during at least 2 years follow up. Methods: This was a prospective, single-center, follow-up, observational, cohort study of consecutive survivors of the first PE episode. Patients were managed according to ESC current guidelines. After the discharge, all PE survivors were followed for at least 24 months in our outpatient clinic. Results: During 2 years follow-up from the group of 402 consecutive PE survivors 29 (7.2%) patients died. Non-survivors were older than survivors 81 years (40–93) vs. 63 years (18–97) $p < 0.001$ presented higher sPESI 2 (0–4) vs. 1 (0–5), $p < 0.001$ driven by a higher frequency of neoplasms (37.9% vs. 16.6%, $p < 0.001$); and had lower hemoglobin (Hb) level at admission 11.7 g/dL (6–14.8) vs. 13.1 g/dL (3.1–19.3), $p < 0.001$. Multivariable analysis showed that only Hb and age significantly predicted all cause post-discharge mortality. ROC analysis for all cause mortality showed AUC for hemoglobin 0.688 (95% CI 0.782–0.594), $p < 0.001$; and for age 0.735 (95% CI 0.651–0.819) $p < 0.001$. A group of 59 subjects with hemoglobin < 10.5 g/dL showed mortality rate of 16.9% (OR for mortality 4.19 (95% CI 1.82–9.65), p-value < 0.00, while among 79 patients with Hb > 14.3 g/dL only one death was detected. Interestingly, patients in age > 64 years hemoglobin levels < 13.2 g/dL compared to patients in the same age but with >13.2 g/dL showed OR 3.6 with 95% CI 1.3–10.1 $p = 0.012$ for death after the discharge. Conclusions: Lower haemoglobin measured in the acute phase especially in patients in age above 64 years showed significant impact on the prognosis and clinical outcomes in PE survivors.

Keywords: pulmonary embolism; follow-up after pulmonary embolism; long term mortality after pulmonary embolism; predictors of survival after pulmonary embolism

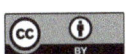

1. Introduction

Acute pulmonary embolism (PE) is not only life-threatening disease in the acute phase but also affects long term prognosis of PE survivors. PE patients may also experience serious adverse events at long term, in particular in the first years after PE diagnosis especially recurrent venous thromboembolism (VTE) and chronic thromboembolic pulmonary hypertension (CTEPH) [1]. Importantly PE survivors have an increased all-cause mortality risk [2]. Therefore, in order to optimize patients follow-up after acute PE it is recommended to ensure an integrated patient care after PE which should include interdisciplinary standardized management and treatment [1,3]. Clinical indices including pulmonary embolism severity index assessed in the acute phase were reported to predict accurately long-term mortality [4]. Notably, widely available biomarkers such as NT-proBNP and hemoglobin concentration were reported to predict long term prognosis not only in patients after congestive heart failure [5,6] or coronary artery disease [7], but also after exacerbation of chronic obstructive pulmonary disease or even pneumonia [8,9]. We hypothesized that hemoglobin levels may be useful for post discharge prognostication after the first episode of acute pulmonary embolism. Therefore, the aim of the current study was to evaluate a potential prognostic value of a decreased hemoglobin levels measured at admission due to the first episode of acute PE for post discharge all cause mortality during at least 2 years follow up.

2. Material and Methods

This was a prospective, single-center, follow-up, observational, cohort study of consecutive survivors of the first PE episode, managed in a single reference centre as part of the "PE-aWARE" registry (NCT03916302). The PE-aWARE (Pulmonary Embolism WArsaw REgistry) is an on-going single-centre prospective observational study of consecutive patients with confirmed acute pulmonary embolism. Its main objective is to collect and provide information on patients' characteristics, management and outcome including short and long term survival, the frequency of chronic thromboembolic pulmonary hypertension and recurrences. The diagnosis of PE was objectively confirmed using contrast-enhanced computed tomography pulmonary angiogram when thromboembolic were visualized in at least segmental or more proximal pulmonary artery. At the admission due to acute PE transthoracic echocardiography routine laboratory tests including high-sensitivity troponin and NT-proBNP were performed. Echocardiographic examination was performed with a Philips iE 33 system (Philips Medical System, Andover, MA, USA) with 2.5–3.5 MHz transducers, within the first 24 h after admission. The dimensions of the right and left ventricles were measured in the four chamber RV focused view and R view at the level of the mitral and tricuspid valve tips in late diastole, as defined by the R wave of the continuous ECG tracing. Moreover, during hospitalization of PE index episode information was collected on PE severity according to ESC risk stratification model which included hemodynamic stability, right ventricular dysfunction detected at echocardiography or CTPA, and signs of myocardial injury assessed with elevated troponin plasma levels, and comorbidities [3] (congestive heart failure, coronary artery disease, chronic lung diseases, neoplasms). The simplified Pulmonary Embolism Severity Index (sPESI) with 1 point for each of the following: age > 80 years, history of cancer, chronic cardiopulmonary disease, pulse $\geq$ 110 beats/min, systolic blood pressure < 100 mmHg, oxygen saturation < 90% was calculated for every patient [10]. Patients were managed according to ESC's current guidelines [3]. After the discharge, all PE survivors excluding moribund patients were followed for at least 24 months in our outpatient clinic. Bed ridden patients with advanced, end stage generalized cancer, requiring nursing care were regarded as moribund patients. After the acute PE phase they were transferred from our department to nursing facilities.

All patients were anticoagulated for at least 6 months. The decision to extend anticoagulation was based on the current ESC recommendations [1,3]. Briefly, anticoagulation was terminated only in patients with transient major VTE risk factor, while in subjects with unprovoked PE or when major or intermediate risk factors persisted such as active cancer, anticoagulation by default was continued undetermined unless high bleeding risk was present. During the index hospitalization or within 30 days after the discharge all patients were subjected to a routine age and gender specific screening for neoplasms. Control visits were performed in a standardized way by one of the coauthors (ODD, SP, AWC). During the first visit not only clinical status was assessed but it was also focused on results of age and sex specific cancer screening. During every control visit taking place every 6–9 months routine diagnostic laboratory tests were performed. After 6 month of anticoagulation patients reporting persistent or new onset functional limitations were referred for echocardiography. Subsequent detailed diagnostic workup was planned by managing physician.

At the end of the follow-up patients underwent a control visit or at least were interviewed by phone. Ninety patients who discontinued outpatient care in our outpatient clinic mostly due to distant residence or limitation in mobility could not be reached by phone. In this group information on clinical status, the cause and date of potential death was obtained from record of National Health Insurance which collects health records of all citizens of Poland. We recorded all-cause mortality, objectively confirmed VTE recurrences, CTEPH diagnosed according to ESC criteria [3], severe bleedings according to ISTH criteria [11], and neoplasm diagnosed during the follow-up.

3. Statistics

Baseline characteristics of patients are presented as parameters or median followed by interquartile range. The Shapiro–Wilk test was used to identify continuous variables with a skewed distribution which were then compared using the Mann–Whitney U test or Chi-square test. All tests were two-sided. For all performed tests p-values of <0.05 were considered significant. Receiver operating characteristic (ROC) analysis was used to determine the area under the curve (AUC) and the corresponding 95% confidence intervals (CIs). The prognostic relevance of analyzed parameters was assessed using univariable analysis, subsequently multivariable analysis was performed with use of logistic regression, including factors statistically important in univariate analysis Odds ratio (OR) was calculated for cutoff values identified with Youden index in ROC analysis. All analyses were performed using the STATISTICA13 data analysis software system (Dell Software, USA) or the MedCalc data analysis software system (MedCalc Software, Ostend, Belgium).

4. Results

Patients Characteristics and Management

In the current study, we included 402 PE survivors after the first PE episode diagnosed and managed in our department (216 women and 186 men (aged 62.6 ± 19.51 years) and subsequently followed in our outpatient clinic for at least 2 years (Table 1). Additional 19 patients with acute PE managed in our department died during the hospital stay or were moribund patients who after the acute PE phase were transferred from our department to nursing homes and died shortly after. All those 19 patients were not included into the current study. At PE diagnosis 53% of all analyzed 402 patients had significant VTE risk factor: preexisting active neoplasm or diagnosed during the index hospitalization (18.2% patients), major trauma or surgery (34% patients). At admission intermediate risk PE was diagnosed in 74.4% of studied patients, while low risk PE and high risk in 21.4% and 4.2%, respectively. After the discharge, all patients were managed in our outpatient clinic with regular control visits. During the follow-up, new neoplasms were diagnosed in additional 13 (3.2%) patients.

All patients with detected decreased hemoglobin level below 10 g/dL on admission, underwent diagnostic work up for its causes during the index hospitalization or within 30 days after the discharge. Eventually, in 12 patients active chronic or acute bleeding was detected (6 gastro intestinal, 3 urinary tract, 3 central nervous system), while in 21 others anemia was related to chronic diseases such as chronic kidney disease or hematological disorders. During the index hospitalization, blood was transfused in order to discharge them with hemoglobin level above 9 g/dL.

After the discharge, 10% of all patients with transient major risk factors for VTE were anticoagulated for 6 months only. Moreover, in additional 3.5% subjects anticoagulation was stopped due to significant bleedings that occurred during follow-up or high bleeding risk. Additionally, 6 patients (1.5%) decided to stop anticoagulation despite physician advice. The remaining patients were anticoagulated in the long term.

In 90 patients who could not be reached by phone, clinical status was assessed with data from records of national health insurance. Due to clinically assessed very compromised prognosis based on clinical data and lack of follow-up data including type of anticoagulation they were not included in the analysis.

Table 1. Clinical characteristics and all-cause mortality during follow-up of 402 consecutive PE survivors.

		All Patients n = 402	Survivors n = 373	Nonsurvivors n = 29	p-Value
Female/Male, n		216/186	197/176	19/10	0.19
Age, years		57.5 (18–97)	63 (18–97)	81 (40–93)	<0.001
Chronic heart failure, n (%)		71 (17.7%)	63 (16.9%)	8 (27.5%)	0.15
Coronary artery disease, n (%)		23 (5.7%)	20 (5.4%)	3 (10.4%)	0.25
Chronic lung disease, n (%)		45 (11.2%)	40 (10.7%)	5 (17.3%)	0.28
Active neoplasm at PE diagnosis, n (%)		73 (18.2%)	62 (16.6%)	11 (37.9%)	0.004
Neoplasm diagnosed during follow-up, n (%)		13 (3.2%)	9 (2.4%)	4 (13.8%)	<0.001
Unprovoked PE, n (%)		190 (47%)	180 (48%)	10 (34%)	0.21
Major surgery, n (%)		35 (8.7%)	33 (8.8%)	2 (6.9%)	Ns
sPESI, points		1.5 (0–5)	1 (0–5)	2 (0–4)	<0.001
PE severity, n (%)	Low	86 (21.4%)	84 (22.5%)	2 (6.9%)	0.13
	Intermediate	299 (74.4%)	273 (73.2%)	26 (89.7%)	
	High	17 (4.2%)	16 (4.3%)	1 (3.4%)	
right to left ventricular ratio > 1 in echo 4 chamber view, n (%)		101 (32.4%)	94 (32.7%)	7 (29.2%)	0.72
LV EF (%)		60 (15–70)	60 (15–70)	60 (20–65)	0.08
Troponin (µg/L)		0.0175 (0.003–1.59)	0.038 (0.003–1.59)	0.074 (0.01–0.8)	0.17
NT-proBNP (pg/mL)		3710.5 (2–28,879)	344.5 (5–28,879)	1440 (74–12,330)	0.004
D-dimer (µg/L)		19,050 (2–111,459)	4558 (2–111,459)	4613 (580–26,945)	0.79
Hemoglobin at admission (g/dL)		10 (3.1–19.3)	13.1 (3.1–19.3)	11.7 (6–14.8)	<0.001
Plasma creatinine (mg/dL)		1.04 (0.33–6.5)	0.9 (0.33–5.4)	1 (0.48–6.5)	0.36
estimated glomerular filtration rate (CockroftGault, mL/min)		89.18 (9.2 ≥ 100)	80.11 (10.9 ≥ 100)	59.52 (9.2 ≥ 100)	0.03

PE—pulmonary embolism, sPESI simplified Pulmonary Embolism Severity Index.

During a 2-year follow-up from the group of 402 consecutive PE survivors, 29 (7.2%) patients died. There were an additional 19 in-hospital deaths (all-cause 2 years mortality in 432 "all comers" was 11.4%). The latter group was not included in the analysis. Causes of 29 deaths included: severe infection or sepsis (13 cases), fatal bleeding (4 cases), progression of advanced neoplastic disease (3 cases), congestive heart failure (8 cases), and 1 case of recurrent VTE. The median time from discharge to death was 239 days varying from 14 to 1901 days. Subjects who died were older than survivors and had higher sPESI driven especially by a higher frequency of active neoplasms (37.9% vs. 16.6%, $p < 0.001$). Interestingly, elevated NT-proBNP level at admission, decreased eGFR and lower hemoglobin level characterized patients who died during the follow-up. Notably, PE severity in the acute phase assessed by ESC risk stratification model did not influence survival after the discharge. Multivariable analysis showed that only older age ($p < 0.01$) and lower hemoglobin level at admission ($p < 0.01$) were relevant for survival during the follow-up, while neoplasms were not.

We performed receiver operating characteristics analysis for hemoglobin concertation and for age in the prediction of all-cause mortality after the discharge. For hemoglobin AUC was 0.688 (95% CI 0.782–0.594), *p*-value < 0.001; Youden index based on ROC curve analysis was 13.2 g/dL. AUC for age was 0.735 (95% CI 0.651–0.819), *p*-value < 0.001 and age of 64 years was identified with Youden Index (Figure 1).

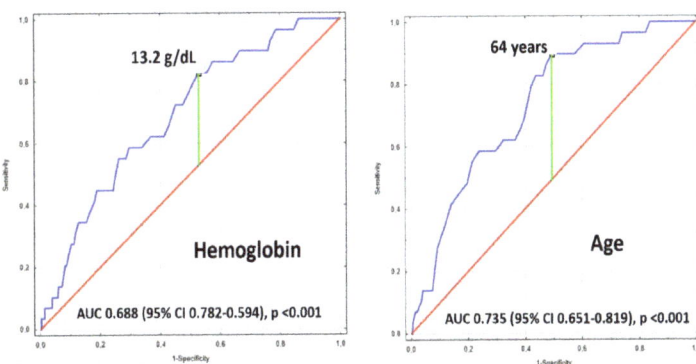

Figure 1. Receiver Operator Characteristics of haemoglobin concentration at admission and age of 2 year mortality in 402 PE survivors. AUC Area under the curve, CI—confidence interval.

Using ROC curve we selected 2 cut-off point values of hemoglobin level. A group of 59 subjects with hemoglobin at admission below 10.5 g/dL included 10 post-discharge deaths (mortality rate 16.9%). Thus, this hemoglobin level predicted post-hospital 2-year mortality with the sensitivity 34.5% (95% CI 17.9% to 54.3%) and specificity 86.7% (95% CI 83.01–90.12%), PPV of 16.95% (95% CI 9.82–27.66%) and NPV of 5.62% (3.91–8.03%). Moreover, hemoglobin below 10.5 g/dL increased post-discharge mortality risk with OR of 4.19 (95% CI 1.82–9.65), *p*-value < 0.001. Another cut of value, hemoglobin level above 14.3 g/dL indicated low post-discharge mortality. Among 79 patients with hemoglobin level > 14.3 g/dL only one death was detected (mortality rate 1.26%). Thus, this cut off value showed high NPV of 98.73% (95% CI 91.84–99.82%), and low PPV of 8.81% (95% CI 8.13–9.53%).

Using age and hemoglobin cut off values defined by Youden index in the ROC analyses we assessed OR of all cause mortality in 4 groups. The group of patients in age ≥ 64 years hemoglobin levels < 13.2 g/dL compared to patients in the same age but with >13.2 g/dL showed OR 3.6 with 95% CI 1.3–10.1 *p* = 0.012 for death after the discharge. Moreover, when patients with age < 64 years and Hb ≥ 13.2 g/dL s were used as reference only patients in age ≥ 64 years hemoglobin levels < 13.2 g/dL showed significant OR for increased mortality (Table 2).

Table 2. Prognostic value of age and hemoglobin levels in PE survivors.

	n	Deaths	Mortality	OR	OR When Group with Age < 64 Years and Hb > 13.2 g/dL as Reference
Age < 64 years and Hb > 13.2 g/dL	97	1	1.03%	2.1 95% CI 0.2–23.7, *p* = 0.54	1 as reference
Age < 64 years and Hb < 13.2 g/dL	93	2	2.15%		2.1 95% CI 0.2–23.7, *p* = 0.54
Age > 64 years and Hb > 13.2 g/dL	89	5	5.62%	3.6 95% CI 1.3–10.1 *p* = 0.012	5.7 95% CI 0.7–49.9, *p* = 0.11
Age > 64 years and Hb < 13.2 g/dL	118	21	17.80%		20.8 95% CI 2.7–157.6, *p* = 0.003

5. Discussion

The major findings of our study can be summarized as follows. During at least 2 years of follow-up of a group of 402 consecutive PE survivors 29 (7.2%) patients died. There were 19 additional in hospital deaths. All-caused 2 years mortality in 432 "all comers" was 11.4%. It should be underlined that this group of patients who died during hospital stay or were moribund and were transferred to nursing facilities was not included in further analysis. In the group discharged home hemoglobin level below 10.5 g/dL assessed at the admission identifies subjects at risk of increased mortality in long term after the discharge due to the first PE episode with OR of 4.19 (95% CI 1.82–9.65), p-value < 0.001. Whereas hemoglobin levels above 14.3 g/dL indicate a benign clinical course during follow-up. Moreover, since increased age and decreased hemoglobin levels were found to be significant in multivariable analysis we especially patients in advanced age with low haemoglobin level are at risk of post discharge mortality. The group of patients in age ≥ 64 years hemoglobin levels < 13.2 g/dL compared to patients in the same age but with >13.2 g/dL showed OR 3.6 with 95% CI 1.3–10.1 p = 0.012 for death after the discharge. We suggest that specially elderly PE survivors with decreased hemoglobin levels should be carefully supervised and followed. Austin Chin Chwan Ng et al. showed that lower serum hemoglobin and elevated troponin-T ≥ 0.1 µg/L at the time of PE are independent predictors of long-term mortality post PE [12].

It was reported that anemia, with hemoglobin levels < 13.0 g/dL in male adults and <12.0 g/dL in female adults, is an independent predictor of reduced exercise capacity, quality of life, and recurrent hospitalizations [13]. Moreover, anemia has been shown to be associated with increased mortality in both acute and chronic heart failure [14–16]. McCullough et al. reported that anemia in patients with heart failure is independently associated with an excess hazard for all-cause mortality and all-cause hospitalization [17]. Chronic and acute anemia lead also to poor outcomes in myocardial infarction and is a marker of an increased risk in one-year cardiovascular mortality in patients with ST elevation myocardial infarction [18,19]. In our study, patients with hemoglobin levels at hospital admission below 10.5 g/dL had the most severe prognosis, and among those whose concentration was above 14.3 g/dL, the prognosis was definitely better. There was only one death among 79 patients with hemoglobin levels above 14.3 g/dL.

NT-proBNP has been evaluated to stratify risk in patients with acute PE and remains the only biomarker that seems to be a strong predictor of 30-day prognosis [20]. Effects on short-term survival of troponin and creatinine concentrations have also been reported [21]. However, NT-proBNP was reported to be a good risk stratification marker in identifying low-risk patients who could be treated in an outpatient setting [22]. Despite the fact that NT-proBNP levels are predictors for adverse long-term outcomes in patients with known heart failure or pulmonary arterial hypertension [23], Bassan et al. showed that BNP measured at hospital admission in patients with non ST elevation acute coronary syndrome is a strong, independent predictor of very long-term all-cause mortality [24]. There is a lack of data on the effect of NT-proBNP on admission on distant complications after pulmonary embolism.

There are few reports of a post-pulmonary embolism follow-up [25,26], and there are hardly any that link data from the acute period of the disease to distant sequelae. Prognostic factors such as biomarker levels contribute to long-term morbidity after pulmonary embolism and are not fully elucidated. Although several studies have reported that among the survivors of an acute PE there is an ongoing increased risk of death long-term [27,28], current guidelines from ESC provide the same recommendation for follow-up after PE regardless of the expected survival and long-term outcome [3]. Identifying acute PE predictors of long-term mortality would allow to develop a detailed plan of care for PE patients with the worst prognosis.

In our study, nearly 400 PE patients were followed for at least 24 months. Elevated NT-proBNP and lower hemoglobin levels in the acute phase showed a significant impact on the prognosis and clinical outcomes in PE survivors.

6. Limitations of the Current Study

This is a single center study performed in a referral center focused on the management of venous thromboembolism both in the acute phase and in outpatient care. Causes of deaths were extracted from data of health insurance and were not adjudicated. Therefore, the results of the current study should be interpreted with caution.

7. Conclusions

Lower haemoglobin measured in the acute phase especially in patients in age above 64 years showed significant impact on the prognosis and clinical outcomes in PE survivors.

Author Contributions: Conceptualization, A.J.; Formal analysis, K.P.; Investigation, S.P. (Szymon Pacho), A.W.-C. and M.S.; Data curation, D.P.-K., S.P. (Szymon Pucyło) and A.S.; Writing–original draft, O.D.-D.; Writing–review & editing, M.C.; Supervision, P.P. All authors have read and agreed to the published version of the manuscript.

Funding: This research received no external funding.

Institutional Review Board Statement: Not applicable.

Informed Consent Statement: Not applicable.

Data Availability Statement: Not applicable.

Conflicts of Interest: The authors declare no conflict of interest.

Abbreviations

AUC	area under the ROC curve
CTEPH	chronic thromboembolic pulmonary hypertension
CI	confidence intervals
ESC	European Society of Cardiology
HR	heart rate
ISTH	International Society on Thrombosis and Haemostasis
MD	mean/median differences
NPV	negative predictive value
NT-proBNP	N-terminal pro-brain natriuretic peptide
OR	odds ratio
PE	pulmonary embolism
PH	pulmonary hypertension
PPV	positive predictive value
RHC	right heart catheterisation
sPESI	simplified Pulmonary Embolism Severity Index
ROC	receiver operating characteristic
VTE	venous thromboembolism

References

1. Klok, F.A.; Ageno, W.; Ay, C.; Bäck, M.; Barco, S.; Bertoletti, L.; Becattini, C.; Carlsen, J.; Delcroix, M.; van Es, N.; et al. Optimal follow-up after acute pulmonary embolism: A position paper of the European Society of Cardiology Working Group on Pulmonary Circulation and Right Ventricular Function, in collaboration with the European Society of Cardiology Working Group on Atherosclerosis and Vascular Biology, endorsed by the European Respiratory Society. *Eur. Heart J.* **2021**, *43*, 183–189. [CrossRef]
2. Carson, J.L.; Kelley, M.A.; Duff, A.; Weg, J.G.; Fulkerson, W.J.; Palevsky, H.I.; Schwartz, J.S.; Thompson, B.T.; Popovich, J.; Hobbins, T.E.; et al. The Clinical Course of Pulmonary Embolism. *N. Engl. J. Med.* **1992**, *326*, 1240–1245. [CrossRef] [PubMed]
3. Konstantinides, S.V.; Meyer, G.; Becattini, C.; Bueno, H.; Geersing, G.J.; Harjola, V.P.; Huisman, M.V.; Humbert, M.; Jennings, C.S.; Jiménez, D.; et al. 2019 ESC Guidelines for the diagnosis and management of acute pulmonary embolism developed in collaboration with the European Respiratory Society (ERS). *Eur. Heart J.* **2020**, *41*, 543–603. [CrossRef] [PubMed]
4. Dentali, F.; Riva, N.; Turato, S.; Grazioli, S.; Squizzato, A.; Steidl, L.; Guasti, L.; Grandi, A.M.; Ageno, W. Pulmonary embolism severity index accurately predicts long-term mortality rate in patients hospitalized for acute pulmonary embolism. *J. Thromb. Haemost.* **2013**, *11*, 2103–2110. [CrossRef]

5. Buchan, T.A.; Ching, C.; Foroutan, F.; Malik, A.; Daza, J.F.; Hing, N.N.F.; Siemieniuk, R.; Evaniew, N.; Orchanian-Cheff, A.; Ross, H.J.; et al. Prognostic value of natriuretic peptides in heart failure: Systematic review and meta-analysis. *Heart Fail. Rev.* **2021**, *27*, 645–654. [CrossRef]
6. Gardner, R.S.; Özalp, F.; Murday, A.J.; Robb, S.D.; McDonagh, T.A. N-terminal pro-brain natriuretic peptide A new gold standard in predicting mortality in patients with advanced heart failure. *Eur. Heart J.* **2003**, *24*, 1735–1743. [CrossRef]
7. Bibbins-Domingo, K.; Gupta, R.; Na, B.; Wu, A.H.; Schiller, N.B.; Whooley, M.A. N-terminal fragment of the prohormone brain-type natriuretic peptide (NT-proBNP), cardiovascular events, and mortality in patients with stable coronary heart disease. *JAMA* **2007**, *297*, 169–176. [CrossRef]
8. Hoiseth, A.D.; Omland, T.; Hagve, T.A.; Brekke, P.H.; Soyseth, V. NT-proBNP independently predicts long term mortality after acute exacerbation of COPD—A prospective cohort study. *Respir. Res.* **2012**, *13*, 97. [CrossRef]
9. Malezieux-Picard, A.; Azurmendi, L.; Pagano, S.; Vuilleumier, N.; Sanchez, J.C.; Zekry, D.; Reny, J.L.; Stirnemann, J.; Garin, N.; Prendki, V. Role of Clinical Characteristics and Biomarkers at Admission to Predict One-Year Mor-tality in Elderly Patients with Pneumonia. *J. Clin. Med.* **2021**, *11*, 105. [CrossRef]
10. Jiménez, D.; Aujesky, D.; Moores, L.; Gómez, V.; Lobo, J.L.; Uresandi, F.; Otero, R.; Monreal, M.; Muriel, A.; Yusen, R.D. Simplification of the Pulmonary Embolism Severity Index for Prognostication in Patients with Acute Symptomatic Pulmonary Embolism. *Arch. Intern. Med.* **2010**, *170*, 1383–1389. [CrossRef]
11. Kaatz, S.; Ahmad, D.; Spyropoulos, A.C.; Schulman, S. Subcommittee on Control of Anticoagulation. Definition of clinically relevant non-major bleeding in studies of anticoagulants in atrial fibrillation and venous thromboembolic disease in non-surgical patients: Communication from the SSC of the ISTH. *J. Thromb. Haemost.* **2015**, *13*, 2119–2126. [CrossRef]
12. Ng, A.C.C.; Yong, A.S.C.; Chow, V.; Chung, T.; Freedman, S.B.; Kritharides, L. Cardiac troponin-T and the prediction of acute and long-term mortality after acute pulmonary embolism. *Int. J. Cardiol.* **2013**, *165*, 126–133. [CrossRef]
13. Nutritional Anaemias. Report of a WHO Scientific Group. Geneva, World Health Organization. 1968. (WHO Technical Report Series, No. 405). Available online: http://whqlibdoc.who.int/trs/WHO_TRS_405.pdf (accessed on 3 September 2022).
14. Chopra, V.K.; Anker, S.D. Anaemia, iron deficiency and heart failure in 2020: Facts and numbers. *ESC Heart Fail.* **2020**, *7*, 2007–2011. [CrossRef]
15. Komajda, M.; Anker, S.D.; Charlesworth, A.; Okonko, D.; Metra, M.; Di Lenarda, A.; Remme, W.; Moullet, C.; Swedberg, K.; Cleland, J.G.; et al. The impact of new onset anaemia on morbidity and mortality in chronic heart failure: Results from COMET. *Eur. Heart J.* **2006**, *27*, 1440–1446. [CrossRef]
16. Von Haehling, S.; Schefold, J.C.; Hodoscek, L.M.; Doehner, W.; Mannaa, M.; Anker, S.D.; Lainscak, M. Anaemia is an independent predictor of death in patients hospitalized for acute heart failure. *Clin. Res. Cardiol.* **2010**, *99*, 107–113. [CrossRef]
17. McCullough, P.A.; Barnard, D.; Clare, R.; Ellis, S.J.; Fleg, J.L.; Fonarow, G.C.; Franklin, B.A.; Kilpatrick, R.D.; Kitzman, D.W.; O'Connor, C.M.; et al. Anemia and Associated Clinical Outcomes in Patients with Heart Failure Due to Reduced Left Ventricular Systolic Function. *Clin. Cardiol.* **2013**, *36*, 611–620. [CrossRef]
18. Padda, J.; Khalid, K.; Hitawala, G.; Batra, N.; Pokhriyal, S.; Mohan, A.; Cooper, A.C.; Jean-Charles, G. Acute Anemia and Myocardial Infarction. *Cureus* **2021**, *13*, e17096. [CrossRef]
19. Lee, W.-C.; Fang, H.-Y.; Chen, H.-C.; Chen, C.-J.; Yang, C.-H.; Hang, C.-L.; Wu, C.-J.; Fang, C.-Y. Anemia: A significant cardiovascular mortality risk after ST-segment elevation myocardial infarction complicated by the comorbidities of hypertension and kidney disease. *PLoS ONE* **2017**, *12*, e0180165. [CrossRef]
20. Akgüllü, Ç.; Ömürlü, I.K.; Eryılmaz, U.; Avcil, M.; Dağtekin, E.; Akdeniz, M.; Güngör, H.; Zencir, C. Predictors of early death in patients with acute pulmonary embolism. *Am. J. Emerg. Med.* **2015**, *33*, 214–221. [CrossRef]
21. Vuilleumier, N.; Le Gal, G.; Verschuren, F.; Perrier, A.; Bounameaux, H.; Turck, N.; Sanchez, J.-C.; Mensi, N.; Perneger, T.; Hochstrasser, D.; et al. Cardiac biomarkers for risk stratification in non-massive pulmonary embolism: A multicenter prospective study. *J. Thromb. Haemost.* **2009**, *7*, 391–398. [CrossRef]
22. Hendricks, S.; Dykun, I.; Balcer, B.; Totzeck, M.; Rassaf, T.; Mahabadi, A.A. Higher BNP/NT-pro BNP levels stratify prognosis equally well in patients with and without heart failure: A meta-analysis. *ESC Heart Fail.* **2022**, [CrossRef] [PubMed]
23. Boucly, A.; Weatherald, J.; Savale, L.; Jaïs, X.; Cottin, V.; Prevot, G.; Picard, F.; de Groote, P.; Jevnikar, M.; Bergot, E.; et al. Risk assessment, prognosis and guideline implementation in pulmonary arterial hypertension. *Eur. Respir. J.* **2017**, *50*, 1700889. [CrossRef] [PubMed]
24. Bassan, F.; Bassan, R.; Esporcatte, R.; Santos, B.; Tura, B. Very Long-Term Prognostic Role of Admission BNP in Non-ST Segment Elevation Acute Coronary Syndrome. *Arq. Bras. Cardiol.* **2016**, *106*, 218–225. [CrossRef] [PubMed]
25. Kahn, S.R.; Houweling, A.H.; Granton, J.; Rudski, L.; Dennie, C.; Hirsch, A. Long-term outcomes after pulmonary embolism: Current knowledge and future research. *Blood Coagul. Fibrinolysis Int. J. Haemost. Thromb.* **2014**, *25*, 407–415. [CrossRef] [PubMed]
26. Konstantinides, S.V.; Barco, S.; Rosenkranz, S.; Lankeit, M.; Held, M.; Gerhardt, F.; Bruch, L.; Ewert, R.; Faehling, M.; Freise, J.; et al. Late outcomes after acute pulmonary embolism: Rationale and design of FOCUS, a prospective observational multicenter cohort study. *J. Thromb. Thrombolysis* **2016**, *42*, 600–609. [CrossRef]

27. Heit, J.A.; Silverstein, M.D.; Mohr, D.N.; Petterson, T.M.; O'Fallon, W.M.; Melton, L.J., III. Predictors of survival after deep vein thrombosis and pulmonary embolism: A population-based, cohort study. *Arch. Intern. Med.* **1999**, *159*, 445–453. [CrossRef]
28. Klok, F.; Zondag, W.; Van Kralingen, K. Patient Outcomes after Acute Pulmonary Embolism: A Pooled Survival Analysis of Different Adverse Events. *Am. J. Respir. Crit. Care Med.* **2010**, *181*, 501–506. [CrossRef]

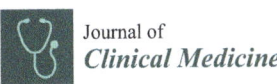

Article

The Path of a Cardiac Patient—From the First Symptoms to Diagnosis to Treatment: Experiences from the Tertiary Care Center in Poland

Przemysław Seweryn Kasiak *,†, Barbara Buchalska †, Weronika Kowalczyk ‡, Krzysztof Wyszomirski ‡, Bartosz Krzowski, Marcin Grabowski and Paweł Balsam

1st Chair and Department of Cardiology, Medical University of Warsaw, Banacha 1A, 02-097 Warsaw, Poland
* Correspondence: przemyslaw.kasiak1@gmail.com; Tel.: +48-501-168-103
† These authors contributed equally to this work.
‡ These authors contributed equally to this work.

Abstract: Cardiovascular diseases (CVDs) are major concerns in the healthcare system. An individual diagnostic approach and personalized therapy are key areas of an effective therapeutic process. The major aims of this study were: (1) to assess leading patient problems related to symptoms, diagnosis, and treatment of CVDs, (2) to examine patients' opinions about the healthcare system in Poland, and (3) to provide a proposal of practical solutions. The 27-point author's questionnaire was distributed in the Cardiology Department of the Tertiary Care Centre between 2nd September–13th November 2021. A total of 132 patients were recruited, and 82 (62.12%; n_{male} = 37, 45.12%; n_{female} = 45, 54.88%) was finally included. The most common CVDs were arrhythmias and hypertension (both n = 43, 52.44%). 23 (28.05%) patients had an online appointment. Of the patients, 66 (80.49%) positively assessed and obtained treatment, while 11 (13.41%) patients declared they received a missed therapy. The participants identified: (1) waiting time (n = 31; 37.80%), (2) diagnostic process (n = 18; 21.95%), and (3) high price with limited availability of drugs (n = 12; 14.63%) as the areas that needed the strongest improvement. Younger patients more often negatively assessed doctor visits (30–40 yr.; p = 0.02) and hospital interventions (40–50 yr.; p = 0.008). Older patients (50–60 years old) less often negatively assessed the therapeutic process (p = 0.01). The knowledge of the factors determining patient adherence to treatment and satisfaction by Medical Professionals is crucial in providing effective treatment. Areas that require the strongest improvement are: (1) waiting time for an appointment and diagnosis, (2) limited availability and price of drugs, and (3) prolonged, complicated diagnostic process. Providing practical solutions is a crucial aspect of improving CVDs therapy.

Keywords: cardiologic care; cardiovascular disease; diagnosis; quality of care; treatment

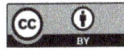

1. Introduction

Cardiovascular diseases (CVDs), primarily ischemic heart disease and stroke, are one of the leading causes of death worldwide [1,2]. Despite numerous efforts, the prevalence and incidence of CVDs are still rising, especially in low- and middle-income countries [1]. Hence, it is of the highest importance to develop new, effective methods of treatment and implement them in health care systems [3]. If the introduced changes should be effective and respond to the patient's needs, it is crucial to acknowledge physicians with the current requirements and the areas that need improvement [3]. As part of the patients' involvement, it is also worth knowing what they pay attention to during their hospitalization and appointments. It will further facilitate physicians' cooperation with patients and provide more personalized therapy.

Individualized treatment and diagnostic approaches are essential elements of effective therapy [2,4]. It is especially important in CVD management, as CVDs affect all ages and social groups, and numerous diseases could be treated in outpatient circumstances [1,5]. A correctly implemented treatment protocol facilitates the development of patient compliance, which remains the main pillar of the cardiological care [4,5]. Developing the patient's voluntary rigor (i.e., regularity in taking medications, measuring the blood pressure, heart rate, and other vital functions, as implementing proper lifestyle changes) and compliance with medical recommendations reduces the overload on particular hospital departments [5].

Currently, many variables are described as negatively affecting adherence to recommendations provided by medical professionals [6]. The main predictors are lack of understanding of the treatment protocol and goals of the therapy, insufficient patient health education, and factors related to the limited availability of drugs, their high price, and long waiting times for appointments [7]. However, the problem with developing unified compliance recommendations is the constantly changing attitude of patients, their expectations, and areas of healthcare where improvement is required [8,9]. Hence, providing comprehensive reports and collecting therapy outcomes in hospitals of all levels of specialty (including primary, secondary, and tertiary care Centers) is a crucial element in increasing the effectiveness of the health care system.

We assume that the improvement of the effectiveness of the health care system, and in particular the field of cardiology, will increase patient satisfaction with the therapy and have a positive impact on their compliance.

The aims of this study were: (1) to assess patients' opinions about the recommendations they receive from their attending physicians, (2) to recognize the steps the patients are taking to obtain a diagnosis of their symptoms, and (3) to identify the main ways of knowledge that patients use for self-education about their CVDs, (4) to point out major areas that require improvement, and (5) provide the direction of potential changes in the healthcare sector.

2. Materials and Methods

2.1. General Study Design and Data Collection Process

The questionnaire was fulfilled by 132 patients from the cardiology department at the tertiary care diagnostic center (University Clinical Center of the Medical University of Warsaw; https://uckwum.pl/, accessed on 17 July 2022). Data were collected at (1) the Clinical Department of General Cardiology, and (2) the Department of Intensive Cardiac Care. The clinic consists of 4 sub-departments and offers a wide spectrum of diagnostics and treatment, from basic procedures (Echocardiography), through more specialized (Cardiac ablation) to highly advanced (TricValve®; P+F Products & Features GMBH, Wessling, Germany). The inclusion criteria were: (1) admission to the hospital at the cardiology department, (2) answering all questions (no empty fields). In order to maximize the credibility of the analyzed data and to exclude people with unviable and lacking answers (with a high risk of misunderstanding the survey and study assumptions), the data-cleaning process was applied. All participants met criterion number 1. Patients who did not meet criterion number 2 were excluded from further analysis (n = 50; 37.88%). A total of 82 patients (62.12%) met all inclusion criteria. Data were collected from 2 September 2021 to 13 November 2021. The patient's name and the room they were staying in the clinic were noted during hospital admission (only clinicians know the patients' data). This enabled verification of patients and ensured that no one completed the questionnaire more than once, but also that all patients fulfilled the form. The questionnaire did not include the question for name or surname; therefore, it was fully anonymous. Patients received a questionnaire during their hospital admission. Data were obtained via in-person meetings with the usage of the paper survey or via the online form. The participant could receive a link to an interactive questionnaire and complete it during the hospital stay from any device at any time. The terms of participation in the study and data anonymity regulations were described at the beginning of the form. By completing the survey, participants gave their informed consent to participate in the study. Participation in the study was fully voluntary. Patients did not receive any financial or material benefits for completing the questionnaire. According to the regulations of the Bioethics Committee of the Medical University of Warsaw, the study did not require registration and further consent.

2.2. Construction of the Questionnaire

The 27-point questionnaire was prepared and jointly agreed upon by experts and physicians from the hospital's cardiology clinic. The survey consisted of the author's original questions related to (1) demographic data of participants, (2) past medical history, (3) diagnostic process, (4) current medical conditions and therapeutic process, (5) personal thoughts about the disease and health care sector. The survey consisted of two types of questions—(1) closed ($n = 17$) and (2) open ($n = 10$)—in which patients could provide their own answers. In the last two questions, participants could express their own thoughts about the disease and feelings related to the therapeutic process or health care system functioning in Poland. The original questionnaire form is available in the printed English version at the Supplementary Material (S1—Questionnaire form) and in the Polish online version via the link (https://docs.google.com/forms/d/e/1FAIpQLSf97PdpxCVIraD_ZWgNMabAR8kRbDPacouAbqO3zUoxuRqtKg/formResponse; accessed on 17 July 2022).

2.3. Data Analysis

The data were exported to the Excel spreadsheet (Microsoft Corporation, Redmond, WA, USA). Statistical analysis was performed in the STATISTICA software (version 13.3, StatSoft Polska Sp. z o.o., Kraków, Poland) and SPSS software (version 28; IBM SPSS, Chicago, IL, USA). Basic calculations were made, and categorical data were calculated as numbers (n) with percentages (%). General linear models and one-way ANOVA [10,11] were applied to assess correlations between clinical and demographic variables and were presented in accordance with the unified APA guidelines [12]. The results were additionally presented with the usage of 95% confidence intervals (CI). The borderline for statistically significant results was defined as p-value = 0.05. Graphical abstract was created with BioRender.com (https://biorender.com/, accessed on 26 July 2022; BioRender, Toronto, ON, Canada).

3. Results

3.1. Study Group Characteristic

We collected surveys from 82 patients. Of the patients, 37 (45.12%) were females and 45 (54.88%) were males. The majority of the patients ($n = 57$; 69.51%) were above 60 years old, while 13 (15.85%) patients were between 50–60 years old, 7 (8.54%) were 40–50 years old, and 5 (6.10%) individuals were 30–40 years old. The most common conditions and complexes the patients were diagnosed with depending on their age are presented in Table 1. Briefly, the most frequent were arrhythmias ($n = 43$; 52.44%) and hypertension ($n = 43$; 52.44%). Table 2 presents the symptoms experienced by the patients stratified by age. The most frequently reported symptom was dyspnea ($n = 26$; 31.71%). A total of 38 (46.34%) patients were reading about their symptoms on the Internet. A total of 62 (75.61%) patients had diagnostic tests. The diagnostic tests were reimbursed to the majority of the patients ($n = 63$; 76.83%), and 17 (20.73%) of them had private health insurance. A total of 61 (74.39%) patients had an attending physician. The first step in the diagnostic investigation was an examination by the physician ($n = 45$; 54.88%) as presented in Table 3. Most of the patients had control appointments, which usually occurred every 3 months ($n = 38$; 46.34%). Only 23 (28.05%) patients had an online appointment with a cardiologist ($n = 6$; 7.32% had a paid fee for an online appointment). The majority of patients ($n = 66$; 80.49%) felt "taken care of" at the hospital. In total, 33 (40.24%) patients reported that cardiac disease negatively affects their daily living. Only 11 (13.41%) patients said that the therapies they received were missed. The most frustrating elements in the diagnostic process were the appointments with the doctors ($n = 31$; 37.81%), medical tests ($n = 18$; 21.95%), and the purchase of medications ($n = 12$; 14.63%). Figure 1 shows duration of the diagnostic investigations.

Table 1. Conditions and complexes which the patients were diagnosed with. Data are additionally stratified by age and presented as the number of patients with a percentage of the whole population or a particular subgroup.

Condition/Complex	Whole Population		30–40 Years		40–50 Years		50–60 Years		>60 Years	
	n of Patients	% of the Group	n of Patients	% of the Subgroup	n of Patients	% of the Subgroup	n of Patients	% of the Subgroup	n of Patients	% of the Subgroup
Arrythmias	43	(52.44%)	3	(6.98%)	4	(9.30%)	5	(11.63%)	31	(72.09%)
Hypertension	43	(52.44%)	3	(6.98%)	4	(9.30%)	8	(18.60%)	28	(65.12%)
Overweight	25	(30.49%)	1	(4.00%)	4	(16.00%)	6	(24.00%)	14	(56.00%)
Type 2 diabetes mellitus	24	(29.27%)	1	(4.17%)	2	(8.33%)	6	(25.00%)	15	(62.50%)
Coronary artery disease	23	(28.05%)	0	(0.00%)	0	(0.00%)	5	(21.74%)	18	(78.26%)
Heart failure	17	(20.73%)	2	(11.76%)	1	(5.88%)	3	(17.65%)	11	(64.71%)
Hypercholesterolemia	14	(17.07%)	0	(0.00%)	3	(21.43%)	2	(14.29%)	9	(64.29%)
Chronic pulmonary disease	13	(15.85%)	0	(0.00%)	2	(15.38%)	1	−7.69%	10	−76.92%
Hypothyroidism	13	(15.85%)	0	(0.00%)	3	(23.08%)	2	(15.38%)	8	(61.54%)
Depression	10	(12.20%)	2	(20.00%)	1	(10.00%)	2	(20.00%)	5	(50.00%)
Atherosclerosis	9	(10.98%)	0	(0.00%)	0	(0.00%)	0	(0.00%)	9	(100.00%)
Valvular heart disease	5	(6.10%)	0	(0.00%)	2	(40.00%)	1	(20.00%)	2	(40.00%)

Table 2. Symptoms reported by the patients during the diagnostic process. Data are additionally stratified by age and presented as the number of patients with a percentage of the whole population or a particular subgroup.

Symptom	Whole Population		30–40 Years		40–50 Years		50–60 Years		>60 Years	
	n of Patients	% of the Group	n of Patients	% of the Subgroup	n of Patients	% of the Subgroup	n of Patients	% of the Subgroup	n of Patients	% of the Subgroup
Dyspnea	26	(31.71%)	2	(7.69%)	2	(7.69%)	5	(19.23%)	17	(65.38%)
Pain in the chest	20	(24.39%)	1	(5.00%)	2	(10.00%)	2	(10.00%)	15	(75.00%)
Exertion fatigue	20	(23.17%)	3	(15.00%)	2	(10.00%)	2	(10.00%)	13	(65.00%)
Palpitations	19	(20.73%)	2	(10.53%)	1	(5.26%)	2	(10.53%)	14	(73.68%)
Tiredness	17	(9.76%)	1	(5.88%)	1	(5.88%)	2	(11.76%)	13	(76.47%)
Fainting	8	(3.66%)	1	(12.50%)	2	(25.00%)	2	(25.00%)	3	(37.50%)
Edema	3	(3.66%)	0	(0.00%)	2	(66.67%)	0	(0.00%)	1	(33.33%)
Cough	3	(31.71%)	1	(33.33%)	0	(0.00%)	0	(0.00%)	2	(66.67%)

Table 3. The first step in the diagnostic process. Data are additionally stratified by age and presented as the number of patients who declared a particular step as the first during the diagnostic process and the percentage of the whole population or a particular subgroup. Abbreviations: GP, general practitioner.

First Diagnostic Step	Whole Population		30–40 Years		40–50 Years		50–60 Years		>60 Years	
	n of Patients	% of the Group	n of Patients	% of the Subgroup	n of Patients	% of the Subgroup	n of Patients	% of the Subgroup	n of Patients	% of the Subgroup
Reimbursed examination by the GP	45	(54.88%)	3	(6.67%)	5	(11.11%)	6	(13.33%)	31	(68.89%)
Examination by the cardiologist	18	(21.95%)	2	(11.11%)	2	(11.11%)	2	(11.11%)	12	(66.67%)
Calling an ambulance	9	(10.98%)	0	(0.00%)	0	(0.00%)	2	(22.22%)	7	(77.78%)
Appointment at the hospital	6	(7.32%)	0	(0.00%)	1	(16.67%)	1	(16.67%)	4	(66.67%)
Paid examination by the GP	4	(4.88%)	0	(0.00%)	0	(0.00%)	1	(25.00%)	3	(75.00%)

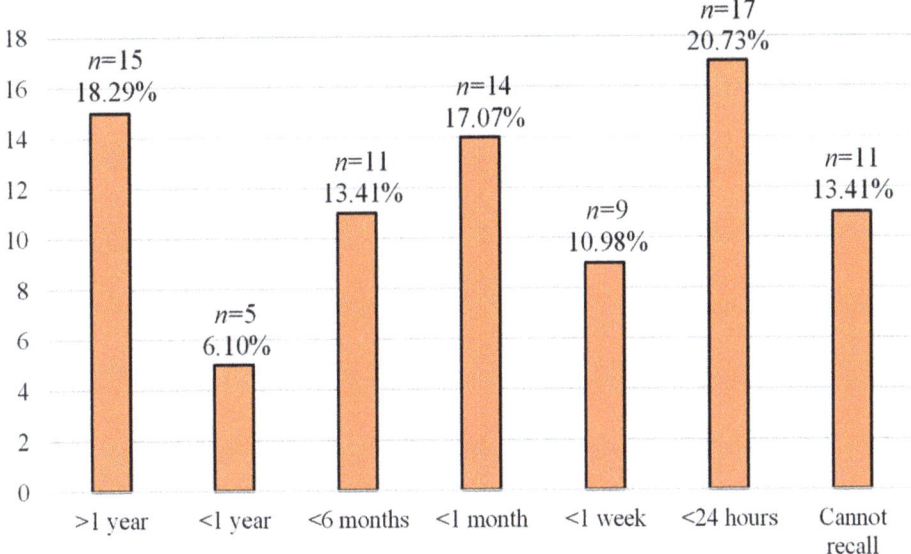

Figure 1. The time in which the patients obtained definitive diagnosis. Data are presented as the number of patients and the percentage of the whole population.

3.2. Clinical Characteristic

The females more commonly received the diagnosis of hypothyroidism ($p = 0.02$, $F[1, 63] = 5.49$), and males more frequently received the diagnosis of valvular heart disease ($p = 0.04$, $F[1, 63] = 4.35$). Younger patients (30–40 years old) pointed out that the appointments with the doctor were the most frustrating elements in the diagnostic process ($p = 0.02$, $F[1, 61] = 5.83$). Furthermore, they more often bought the drugs on the Internet or did not buy any drugs at all, rather than buying drugs at the pharmacy ($p = 0.04$, $F[1, 61] = 4.38$). Patients aged 40–50 years rated the hospital interventions as the most frustrating ($p = 0.008$, $F[1, 61] = 7.54$). Patients aged 50–60 years less frequently had atherosclerosis than other conditions ($p = 0.03$, $F[1, 62] = 5.06$). However, the oldest patients (above 60 years of age) more commonly were diagnosed with atherosclerosis than with other conditions ($p = 0.0007$, $F[1, 62] = 12.68$), and rated the medical tests less frustrating ($p = 0.01$, $F[1, 61] = 7.08$). For further analysis related to the clinical characteristics of participants see Figure 2.

3.3. Open Questions

The questionnaire also contained open questions numbers 26 and 27. Patients could express their own opinions and add commentaries about CVD-related lifestyle restrictions and online appointments. Descriptive responses acquired from each patient are presented in Supplementary material (S2—Answers in open questions). Briefly, participants mostly reported the negative impact of their CVD on numerous lifestyle areas, indicating worsening workability, and a decrease in physical fitness. Individuals also declared that daily activities such as shopping or household chores are more difficult for them. Patients underlined that they prefer stationary visits to online methods. They indicated the possibility of performing a wider spectrum of diagnostic tests and direct contact with their attending physician as a major advantage of in-person appointments. Respondents expressed their negative thoughts about the medical care system in Poland, pointing out its ineffectiveness, long waiting times, and lack of receiving proper treatment recommendations. The answers varied in characteristics and length, from single comments to multi-sentence statements. A minority of the respondents claimed a positive outcome, mostly expressing gratitude to medical professionals for their work.

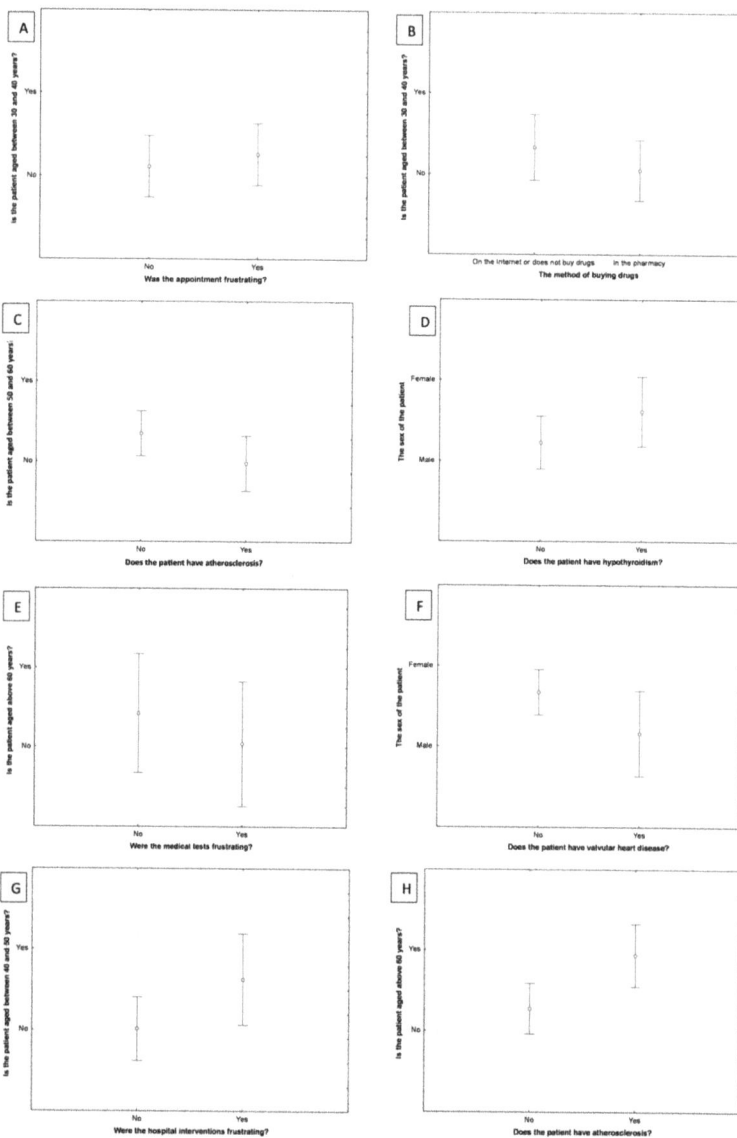

Figure 2. The results of general linear models. (**A**) The frustration of the appointment at the doctor in the group of patients aged between 30 and 40 years. (**B**) The method of buying the drugs in the group of patients aged between 30 and 40 years. (**C**) The occurrence of atherosclerosis in the group of patients aged between 50 and 60 years. (**D**) The occurrence of hypothyroidism in males and females. (**E**) The frustration of the medical tests in the group of patients aged above 60 years. (**F**) The occurrence of valvular heart disease in males and females. (**G**) The frustration of the hospital interventions in the group of patients aged between 40 and 50 years. (**H**) The occurrence of atherosclerosis in the group of patients aged above 60 years. Panels show box-and-whiskers plots. The panels present the statistical relationship between particular variables at the X and Y axes. The longer the whiskers are and the more centrally the median point is located between variables, the weaker correlation between the two variables presented at the X and Y axes.

4. Discussion

In this study, we present the variable opinions of patients from a highly specialized cardiology clinic at a tertiary care center in Poland. The unquestionable advantage of this study is the protocol of data collection. All questionnaires were obtained from registered and other individuals. Data were provided during in-person meetings or in an online-based controlled setting, which maximized the credibility of the received responses. It allowed for reliable conclusions, and the data collected in this way provide valuable material for the preparation of practical solutions and recommendations.

The novelty of this study is also its comprehensive approach because our survey covers various stages of cardiac care, from the occurrence of the earliest symptoms, by obtaining a definitive diagnosis, to the undergoing full treatment process. We also examined additional patients' opinions on medical education, their sources of health knowledge, attitudes to attending physicians, etc.

Finally, we prepared a set of practical recommendations and solutions, the implementation of which should increase the effectiveness of cardiological care, and thus positively impact the patient's compliance.

The study population was mostly the elderly, above 60 years of age, which is commonly seen in the case of CVDs [13]. This implies that diagnostic investigations should be specifically accustomed to older patients so that they will receive the proper treatment.

The majority declared they felt "taken care of", which is one of the indicators of receiving good healthcare and proper diagnostic procedures [14]. Our results are in line with those provided by Deaton et al., because in other hospitals CVD patients also are satisfied with the amount of care they receive [15].

However, as much as 40% of our patients reported that they have a decreased quality of life due to CVD, which negatively affected their daily living. Unfortunately, a decreased quality of life is commonly seen in people with CVDs [16,17]. Thus, we explored one of the areas where special efforts have to be made in improving the well-being of the patients. Perhaps that could be achieved by additional psychological and social care [18], as CVD is associated with numerous limitations in variable lifestyle areas such as occupational abilities [19], and these restrictions strongly affect mental health as well.

As the most frequently reported constraints were worsening workability, and a decrease in physical fitness, the patients should receive the appropriate rehabilitation after the treatment to overcome the inconveniences [20,21]. We propose simple solutions that could be considered by employers to include: (1) modification of the work mode, e.g., by limiting night or unbroken shifts, and (2) extending the number of vacation/rest days for patients with CVD. There is also a wide field for the application of medical rehabilitation and fitness training [21,22]. During visits and at discharge from the hospital, patients should receive personalized recommendations from their attending physicians regarding physical activity, its amount (i.e., number of sessions per week), form (i.e., strength or cardio training, yoga, etc.), and intensity (based on "speech test", percentage of maximal heart rate, oxygen uptake, or subjective feeling) [23]. A similar solution has already been introduced at the University Clinical Center of the Medical University of Warsaw, referred to as Managed Care after Acute Myocardial Infarction ("KOS-zawal"). Wita et al. found that cardiac post-infarction rehabilitation can reduce mortality by as much as 45%. Moreover, the data suggest that patients are satisfied with such a treatment protocol despite it being implemented only as part of outpatient hospital care [24].

The patients also highlighted the negatives associated with healthcare in Poland such as ineffectiveness, long waiting times, and lack of receiving proper treatment recommendations. This may be due to a lack of human resources, shortened appointment time spent for discussing and explaining doubts, as well as the lack of funding for the hospital sector [25,26]. Government investments [27] in medical education (e.g., by increasing the number of universities, places of internships, and improving the current education environment) would allow not only an increase in the number of graduates but also primarily increase the number of specialist doctors [28,29]. The general practitioner is responsible for screening tests and long-term monitoring of a CVD patient [30,31], whereas the specialist is responsible for definitive diagnosis and prescribing advanced, patient-centered, and individualized treatment [32,33]. In an effective cardiac care scheme, the role of both specialists—general practitioners and specialists, and their collaboration is crucial. What is more, general practitioners in Poland are overworked. Hence, it is difficult for them to conduct effective screening tests, and therefore patients are later admitted to a specialized diagnostic center. Thus, they are presented with more advanced conditions [34].

To summarize, all these factors contribute to the lengthened time needed to make a proper diagnosis and, perhaps, could provide missed therapies. Consequently, the above-described variables lower the patient's compliance, their tendency to trust the medical professionals, and let them provide and control a comprehensive therapeutic process [6,35]. Moreover, those factors favor the patient's search for alternative and faster methods of treatment which often are not supported by evidence-based medicine and derive from beliefs and subjective feelings [35].

4.1. Further Studies Directions

As this study was the first use of the questionnaire, it has not yet been externally validated in other populations. To improve the precision and accuracy of the quality of life assessment for cardiologic patients, we recommend further studies which apply our questionnaire for varied populations (both healthy and clinical), and perhaps pair it with other well-studied, validated quality of life questionnaires (i.e., WHOQOL-100 [36] and the WHOQOL-BREF [37]).

As our study was conducted at a tertiary care hospital in Poland and this study is single-center experience, the results will be most valuable locally and regionally to improve the quality of care provided in Poland. We recommend that further studies should compare our questionnaire and similar forms (i.e., CMS-mandated HCAHPS survey [38]) to investigate its transferability.

4.2. Limitations

Some limitations should be mentioned when analyzing the results. The study group is primarily small, and further populational studies on wider samples should be conducted (perhaps including patients from local hospitals to enrich sample variability). The incidence of certain diseases (e.g., arrhythmias) may differ from the general characteristics due to the specialization profile of the hospital. Moreover, the declared diseases of the patients have not been verified with the actually diagnosed ones in their medical documentation. Hence, a few inaccuracies may occur as patients are not always able to accurately define their condition [39]. We did not ask patients about their economic status and individuals with higher salaries could describe the treatment and particular procedures as expensive in other conditions than those with lower income. Thus, our outcomes have to be interpreted carefully. Due to the data's self-reported characteristics, they could be subjective. To minimize the impact of the above-mentioned limitations, we applied an additional data cleaning protocol and provided precise instructions for each part of the questionnaire. Moreover, we recommend further studies of similar protocols on variable and wide populations at all levels of cardiac care.

5. Conclusions

CVD patients assessed the effectiveness of the cardiac care system in Poland as moderate with numerous areas requiring improvement. Despite, the majority being declared "taken care of", younger participants often reported negative outcomes. The areas that were most commonly indicated as needed improvement were the availability and price of drugs, as well as waiting time for and the quality of medical appointments. Knowledge about the current situation and patient opinions provides valuable information for medical professionals and should be used in the development of long-term programs to increase the effectiveness of healthcare systems.

Supplementary Materials: The following supporting information can be downloaded at: https://www.mdpi.com/article/10.3390/jcm11185276/s1, Supplementary material S1: Questionnaire form. Supplementary material S2: Answers in open questions.

Author Contributions: Conceptualization, P.S.K., P.B. and M.G.; methodology, P.S.K.; software, P.B.; validation, P.S.K., B.K. and P.B.; formal analysis, B.B. and P.B.; investigation, P.S.K., B.B., W.K., K.W. and B.K.; resources, P.S.K. and P.B.; data curation, B.B., W.K., K.W. and P.B.; writing—original draft preparation, P.S.K. and B.B.; writing—review and editing, P.S.K., B.B., W.K., K.W. and B.K.; visualization, P.S.K., B.B. and P.B.; supervision, P.S.K., B.K., P.B. and M.G.; project administration, P.S.K., B.K., P.B. and M.G.; funding acquisition, P.B. All authors have read and agreed to the published version of the manuscript.

Funding: This research received no external funding.

Institutional Review Board Statement: Not applicable.

Informed Consent Statement: Informed consent was obtained from all subjects involved in the study.

Data Availability Statement: The data presented in this study are available on request from the corresponding author. The data are not publicly available due to not obtaining consent from respondents to publish the data.

Conflicts of Interest: The authors declare no conflict of interest.

References

1. Roth, G.A.; Mensah, G.A.; Johnson, C.O.; Addolorato, G.; Ammirati, E.; Baddour, L.M.; Barengo, N.C.; Beaton, A.Z.; Benjamin, E.J.; Benziger, C.P.; et al. Global Burden of Cardiovascular Diseases and Risk Factors, 1990–2019 Update From the GBD 2019 Study. *J. Am. Coll. Cardiol.* **2020**, *76*, 2982–3021. [CrossRef] [PubMed]
2. Deaton, C.; Froelicher, E.S.; Wu, L.H.; Ho, C.; Shishani, K.; Jaarsma, T. The Global Burden of Cardiovascular Disease. *Eur. J. Cardiovasc. Nurs.* **2011**, *10*, S5–S13. [CrossRef]
3. Nieuwlaat, R.; Schwalm, J.-D.; Khatib, R.; Yusuf, S. Why are we failing to implement effective therapies in cardiovascular disease? *Eur. Heart J.* **2013**, *34*, 1262–1269. [CrossRef] [PubMed]
4. Morris, L.S.; Schulz, R.M. Patient Compliance—An Overview. *J. Clin. Pharm. Ther.* **1992**, *17*, 283–295. [CrossRef] [PubMed]
5. Khera, A.; Baum, S.; Gluckman, T.J.; Gulati, M.; Martin, S.S.; Michos, E.D.; Navar, A.M.; Taub, P.R.; Toth, P.P.; Virani, S.S.; et al. Continuity of care and outpatient management for patients with and at high risk for cardiovascular disease during the COVID-19 pandemic: A scientific statement from the American Society for Preventive Cardiology. *Am. J. Prev. Cardiol.* **2020**, *1*, 100009. [CrossRef]
6. Eraker, S.A.; Kirscht, J.P.; Becker, M.H. Understanding and Improving Patient Compliance. *Ann. Intern. Med.* **1984**, *100*, 258–268. [CrossRef] [PubMed]
7. Cameron, C. Patient compliance: Recognition of factors involved and suggestions for promoting compliance with therapeutic regimens. *J. Adv. Nurs.* **1996**, *24*, 244–250. [CrossRef] [PubMed]
8. El-Haddad, C.; Hegazi, I.; Hu, W. Understanding Patient Expectations of Health Care: A Qualitative Study. *J. Patient Exp.* **2020**, *7*, 1724–1731. [CrossRef] [PubMed]
9. Hoffmann, T.C.; Del Mar, C. Patients' Expectations of the Benefits and Harms of Treatments, Screening, and Tests A Systematic Review. *JAMA Intern. Med.* **2015**, *175*, 274–286. [CrossRef] [PubMed]
10. Casals, M.; Girabent-Farres, M.; Carrasco, J.L. Methodological Quality and Reporting of Generalized Linear Mixed Models in Clinical Medicine (2000–2012): A Systematic Review. *PLoS ONE* **2014**, *9*, e112653. [CrossRef] [PubMed]
11. Christensen, R. *Plane Answers to Complex Questions: The Theory of Linear Models*, 4th ed.; Springer: New York, NY, USA, 2011; pp. 1–482. [CrossRef]
12. Weissgerber, T.L.; Garcia-Valencia, O.; Garovic, V.D.; Milic, N.M.; Winham, S.J. Why we need to report more than 'Data were Analyzed by *t*-tests of ANOVA'. *eLife* **2018**, *7*, e36163. [CrossRef]
13. O'Neill, D.E.; Forman, D.E. Cardiovascular care of older adults. *BMJ* **2021**, *374*, n1593. [CrossRef]
14. Ballard, D.J. Indicators to improve clinical quality across an integrated health care system. *Int. J. Qual. Health Care* **2003**, *15*, I13–I23. [CrossRef] [PubMed]
15. Koning, C.; Lock, A.; Bushe, J.; Guo, C. Patient Satisfaction with Heart Health Clinics in Fraser Health, Canada. *J. Patient Exp.* **2021**, *8*, 2374373520981475. [CrossRef]
16. Soleimani, M.A.; Zarabadi-Pour, S.; Motalebi, S.A.; Allen, K.A. Predictors of Quality of Life in Patients with Heart Disease. *J. Relig. Health* **2020**, *59*, 2135–2148. [CrossRef] [PubMed]
17. Chatzinikolaou, A.; Tzikas, S.; Lavdaniti, M. Assessment of Quality of Life in Patients with Cardiovascular Disease Using the SF-36, MacNew, and EQ-5D-5L Questionnaires. *Cureus* **2021**, *13*, e17982. [CrossRef]

18. Reblin, M.; Uchino, B.N. Social and emotional support and its implication for health. *Curr. Opin. Psychiatry* **2008**, *21*, 201–205. [CrossRef]
19. Pinckard, K.; Baskin, K.K.; Stanford, K.I. Effects of Exercise to Improve Cardiovascular Health. *Front. Cardiovasc. Med.* **2019**, *6*, 69. [CrossRef]
20. Price, K.J.; Gordon, B.A.; Bird, S.R.; Benson, A.C. A review of guidelines for cardiac rehabilitation exercise programmes: Is there an international consensus? *Eur. J. Prev. Cardiol.* **2016**, *23*, 1715–1733. [CrossRef] [PubMed]
21. Tian, D.Y.; Meng, J.Q. Exercise for Prevention and Relief of Cardiovascular Disease: Prognoses, Mechanisms, and Approaches. *Oxidative Med. Cell. Longev.* **2019**, *2019*, 3756750. [CrossRef]
22. Bull, F.C.; Al-Ansari, S.S.; Biddle, S.; Borodulin, K.; Buman, M.P.; Cardon, G.; Carty, C.; Chaput, J.P.; Chastin, S.; Chou, R.G.; et al. World Health Organization 2020 guidelines on physical activity and sedentary behaviour. *Br. J. Sports Med.* **2020**, *54*, 1451–1462. [CrossRef]
23. Mann, T.; Lamberts, R.P.; Lambert, M.I. Methods of Prescribing Relative Exercise Intensity: Physiological and Practical Considerations. *Sports Med.* **2013**, *43*, 613–625. [CrossRef]
24. Wita, K.; Kulach, A.; Wita, M.; Wybraniec, M.T.; Wilkosz, K.; Polak, M.; Matla, M.; Maciejewski, L.; Fluder, J.; Kalanska-Lukasik, B.; et al. Managed Care after Acute Myocardial Infarction (KOS-zawal) reduces major adverse cardiovascular events by 45% in 3-month follow-up—Single-center results of Poland's National Health Fund program of comprehensive post-myocardial infarction care. *Arch. Med. Sci.* **2020**, *16*, 551–558. [CrossRef]
25. Pilarska, A.; Zimmermann, A.; Zdun-Ryzewska, A. Access to Health Information in the Polish Healthcare System-Survey Research. *Int. J. Environ. Res. Public Health* **2022**, *19*, 7320. [CrossRef] [PubMed]
26. Sowada, C.; Sagan, A.; Kowalska-Bobko, I. Poland Health system review preface. In *Poland: Health System Review*; World Health Organization: Geneva, Switzerland, 2019; Volume 21.
27. Masters, R.; Anwar, E.; Collins, B.; Cookson, R.; Capewell, S. Return on investment of public health interventions: A systematic review. *J. Epidemiol. Community Health* **2017**, *71*, 827–834. [CrossRef] [PubMed]
28. Boet, S.; Sharma, S.; Goldman, J.; Reeves, S. Review article: Medical education research: An overview of methods. *Can. J. Anesth.* **2012**, *59*, 159–170. [CrossRef]
29. Mansouri, M.; Lockyer, J. A meta-analysis of Continuing Medical Education effectiveness. *J. Contin. Educ. Health Prof.* **2007**, *27*, 6–15. [CrossRef] [PubMed]
30. Ju, I.; Banks, E.; Calabria, B.; Ju, A.; Agostino, J.; Korda, R.J.; Usherwood, T.; Manera, K.; Hanson, C.S.; Craig, J.C.; et al. General practitioners' perspectives on the prevention of cardiovascular disease: Systematic review and thematic synthesis of qualitative studies. *BMJ Open* **2018**, *8*, e021137. [CrossRef] [PubMed]
31. Smeets, M.; Zervas, S.; Leben, H.; Vermandere, M.; Janssens, S.; Mullens, W.; Aertgeerts, B.; Vaes, B. General practitioners' perceptions about their role in current and future heart failure care: An exploratory qualitative study. *BMC Health Serv. Res.* **2019**, *19*, 432. [CrossRef]
32. Price, E.; Baker, R.; Krause, J.; Keen, C. Organisation of services for people with cardiovascular disorders in primary care: Transfer to primary care or to specialist-generalist multidisciplinary teams? *BMC Fam. Pract.* **2014**, *15*, 158. [CrossRef] [PubMed]
33. Guadagnoli, E.; Normand, S.L.T.; DiSalvo, T.G.; Palmer, R.H.; McNeil, B.J. Effects of treatment recommendations and specialist intervention on care provided by primary care physicians to patients with myocardial infarction or heart failure. *Am. J. Med.* **2004**, *117*, 371–379. [CrossRef] [PubMed]
34. Dubas-Jakobczyk, K.; Domagala, A.; Mikos, M. Impact of the doctor deficit on hospital management in Poland: A mixed-method study. *Int. J. Health Plan. Manag.* **2019**, *34*, 187–195. [CrossRef] [PubMed]
35. Astin, J.A. Why patients use alternative medicine—Results of a national study. *JAMA* **1998**, *279*, 1548–1553. [CrossRef] [PubMed]
36. The World Health Organization Quality of Life-100 Questionnaire. Available online: https://www.who.int/tools/whoqol/whoqol-100 (accessed on 18 August 2022).
37. The World Health Organization Quality of Life Questionnaire-BREF. Available online: https://www.who.int/tools/whoqol/whoqol-bref (accessed on 18 August 2022).
38. HCAHPS: Patients' Perspectives of Care Survey. Available online: https://www.cms.gov/Medicare/Quality-Initiatives-Patient-Assessment-Instruments/HospitalQualityInits/HospitalHCAHPS (accessed on 18 August 2022).
39. Hermans, A.N.L.; Gawalko, M.; Hillmann, H.A.K.; Sohaib, A.; van der Velden, R.M.J.; Betz, K.; Verhaert, D.; Scherr, D.; Meier, J.; Sultan, A.; et al. Self-Reported Mobile Health-Based Risk Factor and CHA(2)DS(2)-VASc-Score Assessment in Patients with Atrial Fibrillation: TeleCheck-AF Results. *Front. Cardiovasc. Med.* **2022**, *8*, 757587. [CrossRef]

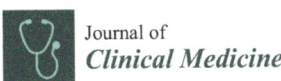

Article

Prevalence of Cigarette Smoking among Professionally Active Adult Population in Poland and Its Strong Relationship with Cardiovascular Co-Morbidities-POL-O-CARIA 2021 Study

Anna Rulkiewicz [1], Iwona Pilchowska [1,2], Wojciech Lisik [3], Piotr Pruszczyk [4] and Justyna Domienik-Karłowicz [1,4,*]

1. LUX MED, Postępu 21C, 02-676 Warsaw, Poland; anna.rulkiewicz@luxmed.pl (A.R.); iwona.pilchowska@luxmed.pl (I.P.)
2. Department of Psychology, SWPS University of Social Sciences and Humanities, 03-815 Warsaw, Poland
3. Department of General and Transplantation Surgery, Medical University of Warsaw, 02-014 Warsaw, Poland; wojciech.lisik@wum.edu.pl
4. Department of Internal Medicine and Cardiology, Medical University of Warsaw, 02-005 Warsaw, Poland; piotr.pruszczyk@wum.edu.pl
* Correspondence: jdomienik@tlen.pl or justyna.domienik@luxmed.pl; Tel.: +48-22-502-11-44

Abstract: Smoking is a leading cause of preventable mortality. It affects both the health and economic situation within societies. The aim of the study is to perform an epidemiological analysis of smoking among professionally active adults in Poland in the years 2016–2020 and its Strong Relationship with Cardiovascular Co-morbidities. The article retrospectively analyzed the records of 1,450,455 who underwent occupational medicine examinations between 2016 and 2020. Statistical analyses performed using IBM SPSS Statistics 25 software were performed. In general, irrespective of the year of measurement, 11.6% of women and 17.1% of men declared smoking. After sorting by year of measurement, we found that the percentage of female smokers was decreasing, while that of males remained relatively consistent. In the case of BMI, it was found that among tobacco smokers the percentage of people with normal body weight decreases with successive years of measurement, while the percentage of overweight and level I obesity increases. Moreover, we analyzed in detail the occurrence of particular comorbidities in the group of people who declared smoking. The most common diseases in this group were: arterial hypertension (39%), lipid disorders (26.7%), and hypertension and lipid disorders (16.5%). Active preventive measures are necessary to reduce the number of smokers and the negative impact of smoking on the occurrence of comorbid diseases.

Keywords: cardiovascular diseases; cigarette smoking; professionally active adult population

1. Introduction

The proportion of cigarette smokers in Europe remains high, with around 21% of adults reporting that they are active smokers [1]. However, cohort studies performed in Europe present the percentage of smokers in the group of 16–20-year-olds as being in decline. This phenomenon is observed in all parts of Europe (Northern, Eastern, and Western Europe) except Southern Europe, where smoking has remained at levels since 1990. The initiation rate in early adolescence (11–15 years) has increased since 1990, especially in Western Europe. The lowest rates of tobacco initiation are observed in Western Europe [2].

In recent years, there has been a decline in the percentage of people who declare themselves smokers. This is attributed to restrictions introduced by individual European countries [3,4]. The Framework Convention on Tobacco Control is a further impetus in the global fight against smoking [5]. However, studies on the age of initiation of smoking are still missing–according to the 2015 Eurobarometer, 19% of Europeans started smoking before the age of 15 [6].

Since 2015, active smoking has been linked to more than five million deaths per year coming from an estimated one billion smokers, while around 600,000 deaths are explained by exposure to passive smoking [7].

Smoking is a leading cause of preventable mortality. It is one of the factors that increase the risk of respiratory diseases, allergies, cardiovascular diseases, and cancer [8]. Young people whose organs are still developing are particularly vulnerable to these diseases. There are many studies that show that exposure to the effects of smoking during the growth period can have a significant impact on health between generations [9–11]. In addition, smoking cessation significantly reduces the risk of cancer and heart disease after 12 months of not smoking [12]. Ultimately, people who smoke tobacco products for many years have a lower willingness to quit smoking [13], which results from addiction and low motivation to change their habits [13,14].

Smoking tobacco affects both the health and economic situation within a society. Research by Baker [15] confirmed that tobacco smoking increases absenteeism and decreases professional activity at work among employees from the USA, Europe, and China. These trends improved significantly after cessation of smoking–workers who quit smoking up to four years prior experienced both significant increases in work productivity and fewer days of absence from work. Other studies have shown that US workers who smoke cigarettes lose an average of 2–3 working days per year due to health consequences when compared to workers who have never smoked [16–18]. Studies conducted in the Netherlands, Germany, and China gave similar results [19–21].

Apart from individual health disorders and occupational troubles, smoking entails very high collateral monetary costs. These are mainly felt as the added costs of providing health care to workers for treatment of diseases resulting from long-term smoking. Still, farther-reaching costs arise from aggregate losses to countries as a result of early smoking mortality [22].

Proper communication between the doctors and patients disclosing their smoking is a very significant factor. Doctors rarely recommend quitting smoking among older adults [23], mainly because the patient is highly addicted or lacks tangible health benefits. However, it is worth noting that quitting smoking in old age may still bring significant health benefits, extend life expectancy and quality [24], and reduce the risk of disability [25]. In addition, quitting smoking can significantly increase the potential benefits for employers, employees, and society as a whole [26].

One of the primary difficulties in developing programs to change the habits of smokers is understanding the more fundamental causes of tobacco addiction; analysis of the ages at which smoking initiation takes place also seems to be important–it should be noted, however, that most publications focus only on the sheer prevalence of smoking in societies. Understanding the reasons underlying tobacco use would almost certainly allow for the development of more effective prevention strategies. Current research indicates that undertaken actions are most effective in lower socioeconomic groups [27].

There have been multiple approaches taken to broadly curb tobacco use. One preventive approach was increasing the price of a pack of cigarettes. Analyses show that this mainly affected young people whose budgets tend to be more sensitive to price increases [28]. Another approach–limiting exposure to tobacco product advertising–was also introduced [29]. The most direct measure–introducing bans on smoking in public places–failed to yield any clear conclusions supporting its efficacy in reducing the percentage of people using tobacco products. European studies conducted in 2019 [30] show that raising prices for tobacco products and limiting places where it is permissible to smoke reduces the number of active smokers mainly in adults up to 65 years of age; the reverse relationship is visible in people over 65 years of age.

Post-quitting productivity gains have prompted many employers to support workers in quitting smoking by investing in tobacco cessation programs and behavioral interventions [31]. Employers incurring the costs of implementing smoking cessation programs also see measurable benefits–the average duration of professional activity of non-smokers is longer than that of active smokers [32].

The aim of the study is to perform a cross-sectional study of smoking among professionally active adults in Poland in the years 2016–2020 and its Strong Relationship with Cardiovascular Co-morbidities.

2. Materials and Methods

The article retrospectively analyzed the subsequent records of professionally active adults who underwent occupational medicine examinations between January 2016 and April 2020. In total, the results of 1,450,455 initial, control, and periodic visits as components of occupational medicine certifications were analyzed. During the study, sex, age, height, weight, voivodship of residence, period of validity of medical certification, and data from medical history (subjective assessment of health, smoking) were controlled. We did not exclude any patients. We present data of all subsequent patients. Detailed characteristics of the studied patients are presented in Appendix A.

Statistical Analysis

Statistical analyses performed using IBM SPSS Statistics 25 software for Windows, Version 27.0. Armonk, NY:IBM Corp were performed [26]. The percentages (with 95% CI) and numbers of observations were used to analyze qualitative data; to characterize the quantitative data: mean (M), standard deviation (SD), median (Me), skewness, kurtosis, and the minimum and maximum statistics were used. Significant statistical results were considered where the probability of making a type I error was less than 5% ($p < 0.05$). For statistical calculations we used: chi-square analysis (Bonferroni's correction was used to test column proportions) and U Mann–Whitney test.

3. Results

The chi-square analysis in the cross tables showed that the percentage of declared smokers slightly decreased with each passing year. It is worth noting, however, that the largest decrease in the percentage of declared smokers occurred between 2016 and other years, taken individually (see Table 1).

Table 1. Relationship between smoking and measurement time-data as percentage for the year of measurement (with 95% CI) [1].

	2016	2017	2018	2019	2020	Total
No	85.2% a (±0.2%)	85.5% b (±0.1%)	85.8% c (±0.2%)	85.7% b,c (±0.2%)	85.8% b,c (±0.3%)	85.6% (±0.2%)
Yes	14.8% a (±0.2%)	14.5% b (±0.1%)	14.2% c (±0.2%)	14.3% b,c (±0.2%)	14.2% b,c (±0.3%)	14.4% (±0.2%)
Total	100.00%	100.00%	100.00%	100.00%	100.00%	100.00%

[1] Each letter in subscript represents a subset of the year category whose column proportions do not differ significantly at the level of 5%.

3.1. Characteristics of Declared Smokers

In general, irrespective of the year of measurement, 11.6% of women and 17.1% of men declared smoking. After sorting by year of measurement, we found that the percentage of female smokers was decreasing, while that of males remained relatively consistent (see Figure 1).

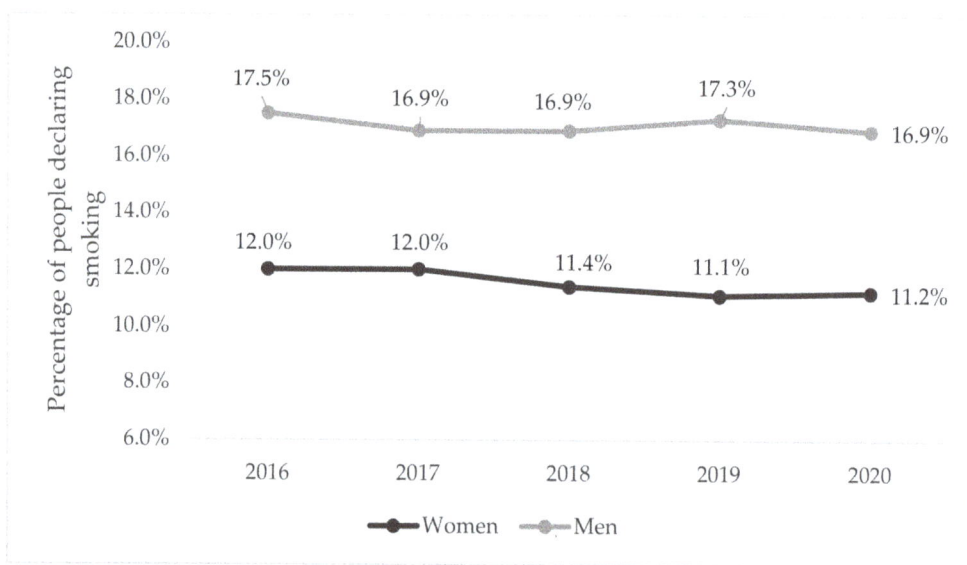

Figure 1. Percentage of declared smokers by sex and year of measurement (95% CI: women group: ±0.3%, men group: ±0.5%).

The age of people declaring smoking ranged from 15 to 88 years (M = 37.52; SD = 12.37). There were no considerable changes in declared tobacco smoking in individual age groups in the analyzed years–only in 2020 was there a slight increase in the percentage of smokers in the 35–54 and 55–69 age groups, along with a slight increase in the 18–35 age group (see Table 2).

Table 2. Relationship between age and measurement time–percentages (with 95% CI) by year of measurement (analysis only for people declaring smoking) [1].

	2016	2017	2018	2019	2020	Total
<18	0.1% a (±0.1%)	0.1% a (±0.1%)	0.1% a (±0.1%)	0.0% a (±0.1%)	n/a	0.1% (±0.1%)
18–35	51.1% a (±0.4%)	50.9% a (±0.3%)	51.2% a (±0.3%)	50.8% a (±0.3%)	45.9% b (±0.2%)	50.7% (±0.3%)
35–54	35.9% a (±0.3%)	36.1% a (±0.2%)	35.8% a (±0.3%)	36.3% a (±0.2%)	39.5% b (±0.3%)	36.2% (±0.3%)
55–69	12.8% a (±0.2%)	12.8% a (±0.2%)	12.7% a (±0.2%)	12.6% a (±0.2%)	14.4% b (±0.2%)	12.8% (±0.2%)
>69	0.1% a (±0.1%)	0.1% a (±0.1%)	0.2% b (±0.1%)	0.2% b (±0.1%)	0.2% b (±0.1%)	0.2% (±0.1%)
Total	100.0%	100.0%	100.0%	100.0%	100.0%	100.0%

[1] Each letter in subscript represents a subset of the year category whose column proportions do not differ significantly at the level of 5%.

In the case of BMI, it was found that among tobacco smokers the percentage of people with normal body weight decreases with successive years of measurement, while the percentage of overweight and level I obesity increases (see Table 3).

Table 3. Relationship between BMI and measurement time–percentages (with 95% CI) by the year of measurement (analysis only for people declaring smoking) [1].

	2016	2017	2018	2019	2020	Total
Underweight	2.8% a (±0.2%)	2.8% a (±0.2%)	2.7% a,b (±0.3%)	2.8% a (±0.3%)	2.4% b (±0.2%)	2.8% (±0.2%)
Normal body mass	47.0% a (±0.5%)	46.3% b (±0.4%)	45.5% c (±0.4%)	44.8% d (±0.4%)	43.1% e (±0.4%)	45.7% (±0.4%)
overweight	34.2% a (±0.7%)	34.2% a (±0.6%)	34.8% a,b (±0.6%)	34.5% a,b (±0.7%)	35.4% b (±0.7%)	34.5% (±0.6%)
Obesity type I	12.2% a (±0.2%)	12.8% b (±0.3%)	13.1% b,c (±0.3%)	13.4% c (±0.2%)	14.6% d (±0.2%)	13.0% (±0.2%)
Obesity type II	2.9% a (±0.2%)	3.0% a (±0.1%)	3.1% a (±0.2%)	3.4% b (±0.2%)	3.5% b (±0.2%)	3.1% (±0.2%)
Obesity type III	0.8% a (±0.1%)	0.8% a (±0.1%)	0.8% a (±0.1%)	1.0% b (±0.1%)	0.9% a,b (±0.1%)	0.8% (±0.1%)
Total	100.00%	100.00%	100.00%	100.00%	100.00%	100.00%

[1] Each letter in subscript represents a subset of the year category whose column proportions do not differ significantly at the level of 5%.

The average number of months for the occupational medicine certificates was approximately 29 months (M = 29.09; SD = 13.47).

3.2. Smoking and Diagnosis According to ICD-10

Table 4 shows the relationship between those who declared cigarette smoking and the occurrence of individual ICD-10 categories ($p < 0.001$). It turned out that in the case of selected categories (such as factors influencing health status and contact with health care and cardiovascular diseases) a higher percentage of diagnoses was associated with people who declared smoking.

Table 4. The relationship between cigarette smoking and the occurrence of individual ICD-10 categories—percentages (with 95% CI) of the smoking category [1].

	Smoking		Total
	No	Yes	
Selected infectious and parasitic diseases	0.6% a (±0.05%)	0.5% b (±0.04%)	0.6% (±0.05%)
Cancers	0.6% a (±0.06%)	0.4% b (±0.05%)	0.5% (±0.05%)
Diseases of blood and hematopoietic organs and selected diseases involving immunological mechanisms	0.1% a (±0.01%)	0.1% b (±0.01%)	0.1% (±0.01%)
Disorders of endocrine secretion, nutritional status, and metabolic changes	10.3% a (±0.5%)	8.8% b (±0.4%)	10.0% (±0.4%)
Mental and behavioral disorders	0.3% a (±0.04%)	0.4% b (±0.04%)	0.3% (±0.04%)
Nervous system diseases	0.5% a (±0.07%)	0.5% a (±0.06%)	0.5% (±0.06%)
Diseases of the eye and eye appendages	8.9% a (±0.10%)	9.4% b (±0.09%)	9.0% (±0.10%)
Diseases of the ear and mastoid process	0.9% a (±0.03%)	1.0% b (±0.04%)	0.9% (±0.3%)
Cardiovascular disease	9.0% a (±0.10%)	9.5% b (±0.08%)	9.0% (±0.10%)
Respiratory system diseases	5.4% a (±0.12%)	4.7% b (±0.14%)	5.3% (±0.12%)
Digestive system diseases	2.4% a (±0.15%)	2.1% b (±0.09%)	2.4% (±0.11%)

Table 4. *Cont.*

	Smoking		Total
	No	Yes	
Diseases of the skin and subcutaneous tissue	2.3% a (±0.22%)	1.7% b (±0.16%)	2.2% (±0.17%)
Diseases of the musculoskeletal system and connective tissue	3.9% a (±0.12%)	3.6% b (±0.17%)	3.9% (±0.13%)
Diseases of the genitourinary system	2.4% a (±0.14%)	1.6% b (±0.14%)	2.3% (±0.14%)
Pregnancy, childbirth and the postpartum period	0.4% a (±0.08%)	0.2% b (±0.06%)	0.4% (±0.06%)
Selected conditions starting in the perinatal period	0.0% a (±0.01%)	0.0% a (±0.02%)	0.0% (±0.01%)
Congenital malformations, distortions, and chromosomal aberrations	0.0% a (±0.01%)	0.0% b (±0.01%)	0.0% (±0.01%)
Symptoms, signs, and abnormal results of clinical and laboratory tests; not elsewhere classified	3.4% a (±0.18%)	2.9% b (±0.16%)	3.4% (±0.16%)
Injury, poisoning, and other specific effects of external factors	2.2% a (±0.03%)	2.1% b (±0.02%)	2.2% (±0.03%)
External causes of illness and death	0.2% a (±0.01%)	0.1% b (±0.02%)	0.2% (±0.01%)
Factors influencing health condition and contact with health services	46.2% a (±0.45%)	50.5% b (±0.41%)	46.8% (±0.42%)
Total	100.0%	100.0%	100.0%

[1] Each letter in subscript represents a subset of the year category whose column proportions do not differ significantly at the level of 5%.

Additionally, after dividing cardiovascular diseases into groups, we observed that in the case of ischemic heart disease a higher percentage of cases was found in people who declared smoking; however, for arterial hypertension, the opposite relationship was obtained. The exact results are shown in the Table 5 below.

Table 5. Relationship between cigarette smoking and the incidence of individual ICD-10 groups (cardiovascular diseases)–percentages (with 95% CI) for the smoking category [1].

	Smoking		Total
	No	Yes	
Acute rheumatic disease	0.0% a (±0.1%)	n/a	0.0% (±0.1%)
Chronic rheumatic heart disease	0.0% a (±0.1%)	0.0% a (±0.1%)	0.0% (±0.1%)
Hypertension	87.0% a (±0.3%)	86.3% b (±0.3%)	86.9% (±0.3%)
Ischemic heart disease	7.1% a (±0.2%)	8.8% b (±0.1%)	7.4% (±0.2%)
Cardiopulmonary syndrome and pulmonary circulation diseases	0.0% a (±0.1%)	0.0% a (±0.1%)	0.0% (±0.1%)
Other heart conditions	1.8% a (±0.1%)	1.8% a (±0.1%)	1.8% (±0.1%)
Cerebral vessel diseases	0.2% a (±0.1%)	0.3% a (±0.1%)	0.2% (±0.1%)
Diseases of arteries, arterioles, and capillaries	0.4% a (±0.1%)	0.4% a (±0.1%)	0.4% (±0.1%)
Diseases of the veins, lymph vessels, and lymph nodes, not elsewhere classified	3.3% a (±0.3%)	2.3% b (±0.2%)	3.1% (±0.2%)
Other and unspecified disorders of the circulatory system	0.1% a (±0.1%)	0.1% a (±0.1%)	0.1% (±0.1%)
Total		100.0%	100.0%	100.0%

[1] Each letter in subscript represents a subset of the year category whose column proportions do not differ significantly at the level of 5%.

Analyzing the relationship between selected diseases and declared smoking, it turned out that in the group of smokers a higher percentage of people with hypertension and type 2 diabetes was observed; in the case of lipid disorders, the opposite correlation was obtained (see Table 6).

Table 6. Relationship between cigarette smoking and the occurrence of selected diseases–percentages (with 95% CI) of the smoking category [1].

	Smoking		Total
	No	Yes	
Hypertension	44.5% a (±0.1%)	48.7% b (±0.1%)	45.1% (±0.1%)
Type 2 diabetes	8.2% a (±0.2%)	8.9% b (±0.2%)	8.3% (±0.2%)
Lipid disorders	43.6% a (±0.4%)	37.5% b (±0.3%)	42.8% (±0.3%)
Coronary artery disease	3.6% a (±0.1%)	5.0% b (±0.1%)	3.8% (±0.1%)
Total	100.0%	100.0%	100.0%

[1] Each letter in subscript represents a subset of the year category whose column proportions do not differ significantly at the level of 5%.

3.3. Cigarette Smoking and Comorbidities

The figure below shows the occurrence of particular comorbidities in the group of people who declared smoking. The most common diseases in this group were: arterial hypertension (39%), lipid disorders (26.7%), and hypertension and lipid disorders (16.5%). The remaining diseases occurred in less than 5% of the patients (see Figure 2).

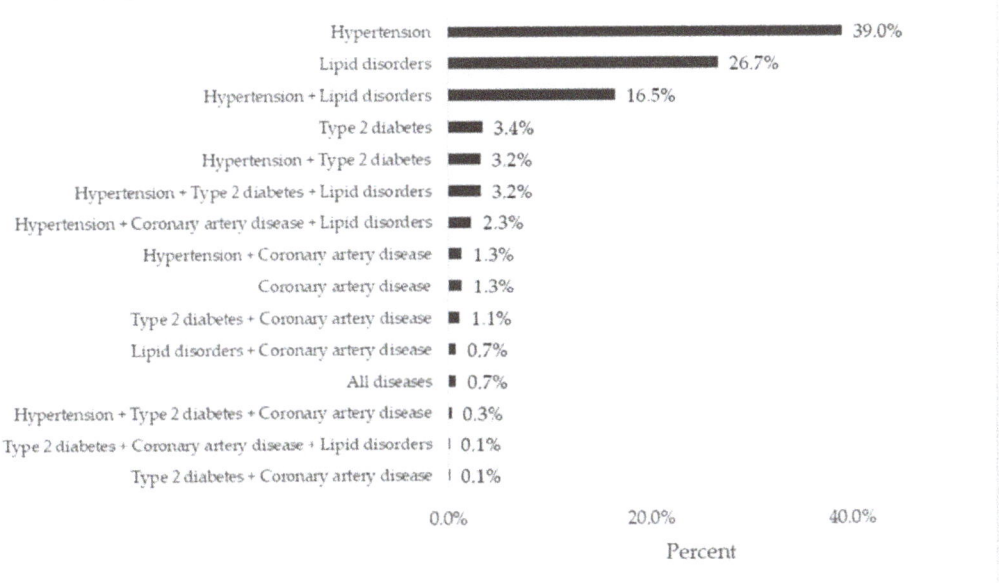

Figure 2. Occurrence of comorbidities in the group of people who declared smoking (95% CI: hypertension: ±0.1%, lipid disorders: ±0.3%; others: ±0.1%).

Moreover, we confirmed that people who declared smoking cigarettes have significantly more diagnosed diseases as compared to people who do not smoke ($p < 0.001$). The obtained results are presented graphically in the Figure 3 below.

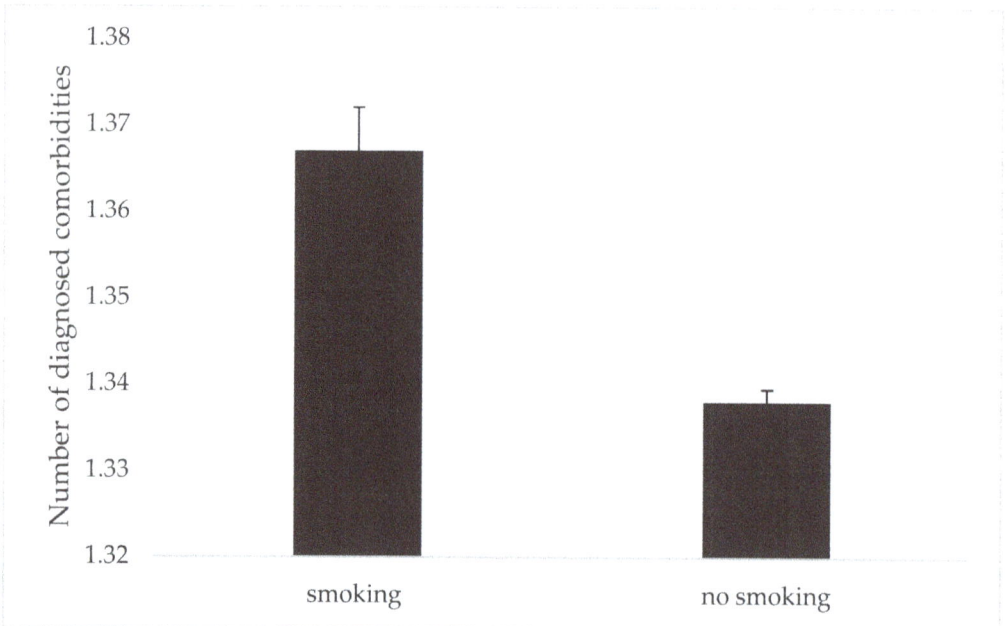

Figure 3. Number of diagnosed comorbidities in the group of people declaring or not smoking (with SD).

4. Discussion

In this study, we examined in detail the rates of smoking in Poland using data from 2016–2020. In general, irrespective of the year of measurement, 11.6% of women and 17.1% of men declared smoking. After sorting by year of measurement, we found that the percentage of female smokers was decreasing, while that of males remained relatively consistent. Clearly, the proportion of cigarette smokers in Poland remains high, it is lower than in other European countries [1,2]. In addition, we are very pleased with the delicate downward trend, which, in our opinion, requires intensive legislative changes to strengthen it, i.e., significantly lowering the percentage of active smokers in the group of professionally active Poles [33].

The relationship between smoking and obesity is not clear and published studies have produced conflicting results. Some studies showed no relationship between smoking and obesity, and some give quite different data based on the metabolic effects of nicotine (restricted absorption, reduced calorific intake, increased metabolic rate, and thermogenesis). The Mendelian randomization analysis of UK Biobank data indicated that each standard deviation increment in body mass index (4.6) increased the risk of being a smoker (odds ratio 1.18 (95% confidence interval 1.13 to 1.23), $p < 0.001$) [34–36].

In our study, it was clearly found that among tobacco smokers the percentage of people with normal body weight decreases with successive years of measurement, while the percentage of overweight and level I obesity increases. In our opinion, along with the increase in the number of obese patients, it is another factor contributing to the development of comorbidities in this group of patients [34,35].

The relationship between cigarette smoking and the occurrence of individual ICD-10 categories is obviously marked in the group of patients with cardiovascular diseases [37–40]. It is due to mechanisms, which we present in Figure 4.

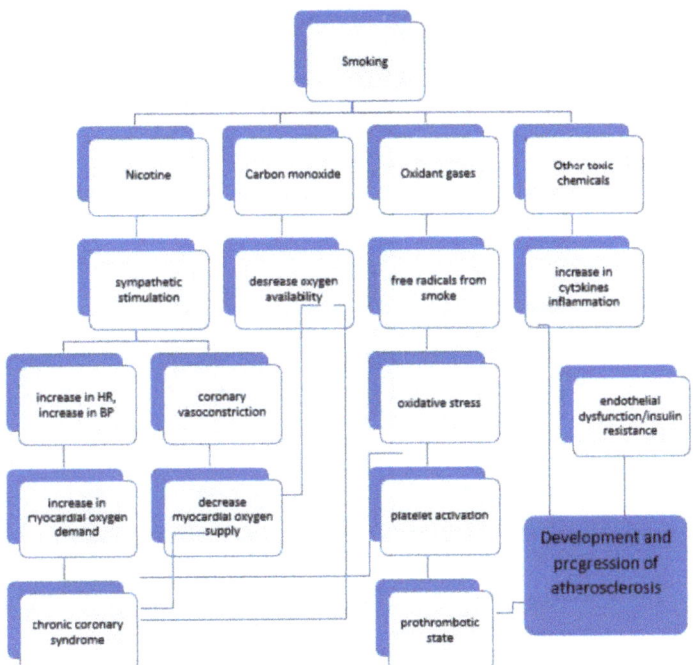

Figure 4. Pathophysiologic mechanisms of tobacco smoke in cardiovascular disease.

Moreover, it turned out that in the group of smokers a higher percentage of people with hypertension, ischemic heart disease, and type 2 diabetes was observed. therefore, in the largest Polish epidemiological study in the field of cigarette smoking, we are consistent with the results of international studies on cardiovascular risk [37–40]. Moreover, we confirmed that people who declared smoking cigarettes have significantly more diagnosed diseases as compared to people who do not smoke ($p < 0.001$)

5. Conclusions

Active preventive actions are necessary to reduce the number of smokers and the negative impact of smoking on the occurrence of comorbid diseases.

Author Contributions: Conceptualization, A.R., P.P. and J.D.-K.; Data curation, A.R. and I.P.; Formal analysis, I.P.; Investigation, A.R.; Methodology, I.P. and J.D.-K.; Project administration, I.P.; Supervision, J.D.-K.; Writing—original draft, I.P., W.L. and J.D.-K.; Writing—review & editing, J.D.-K. All authors have read and agreed to the published version of the manuscript.

Funding: This research received no external funding.

Data Availability Statement: Not applicable.

Conflicts of Interest: There is no conflict of interest (all Cases) Anna Rulkiewicz, Iwona Pilchowska and Justyna Domienik-Karłowicz are Lux med employees.

Appendix A. Additional Analyzes

The study included 1,450,455 visits to occupational medicine (collected from 931,985 unique Patients) from 2016–2020. The exact number of collected results depending on the year of measurement is presented below.

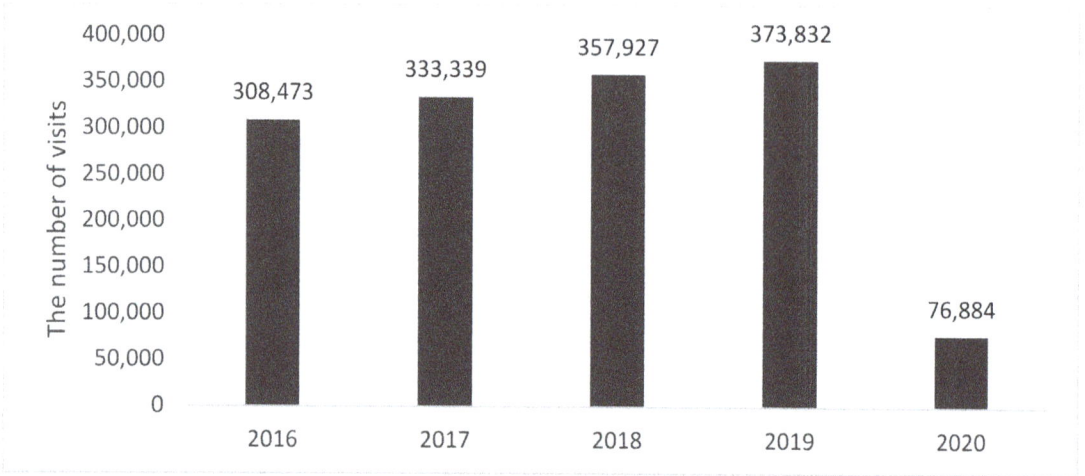

Figure A1. The number of visits analyzed versus the year of measurement.

In terms of sex, the results of men accounted for a slightly higher percentage (51.6%). Along with the successive stages of the study, the percentage of surveyed men slightly increased (see Figure A2).

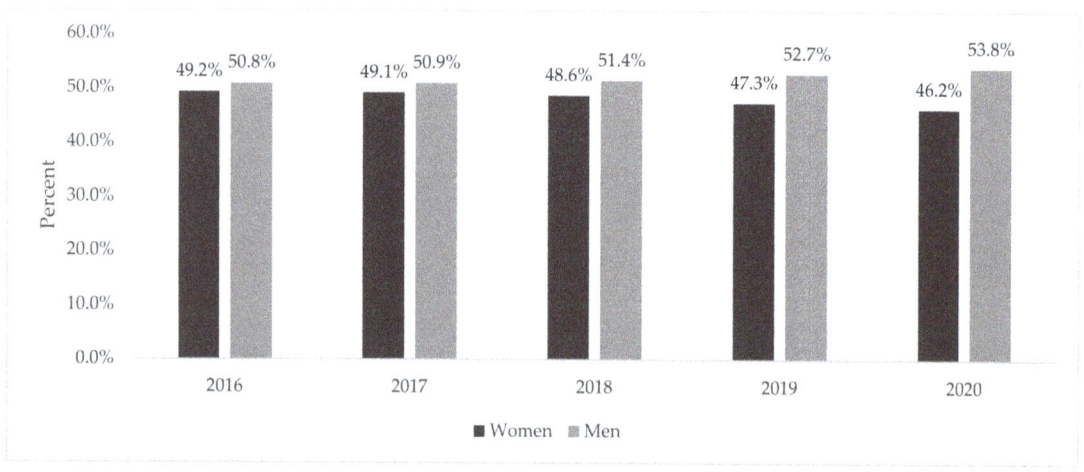

Figure A2. Sex distribution depending on the year of measurement (95% CI: ±0.2%).

The age of the respondents ranged between 14 and 90 years (M = 36.59; SD = 11.56). A slight trend was observed indicating the mean age of the examined patients slightly increased with each year of measurement (see Figure A3). Clarification: patients can change age categories if their change in age necessitates this; this is not to be misinterpreted as a tautological restatement of the patients aging with time.

The exact distribution of age groups depending on the year of measurement is presented in the table below. It was found that with successive years of measurement, a decreased percentage of people aged 18–35 and an increased percentage in the age group 35–54 were observed; in the case of the remaining age groups, the trends were not as clear as in the case of these two age categories.

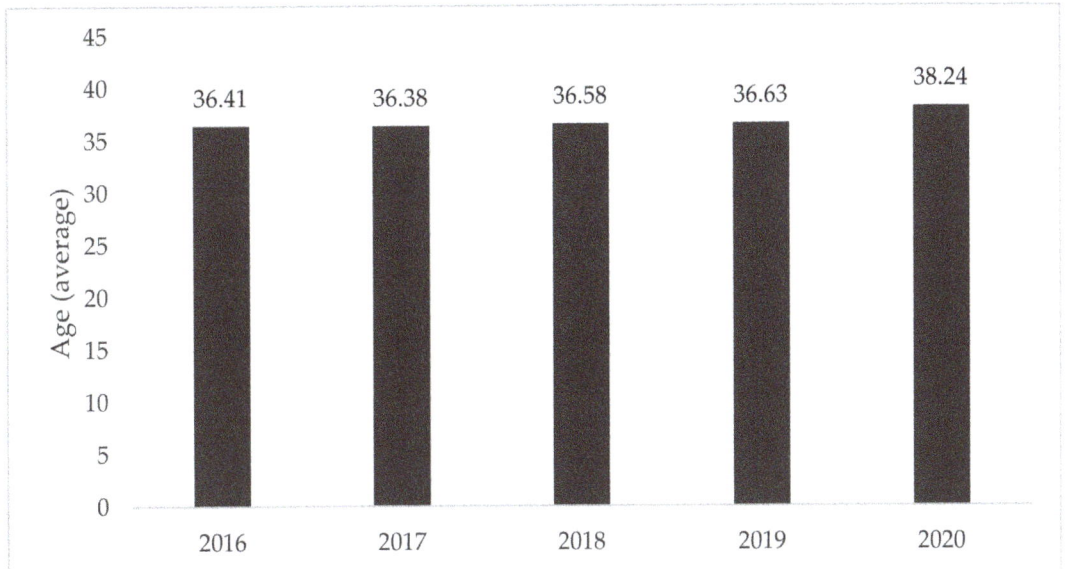

Figure A3. Patient age distribution versus the year of measurement.

Table A1. Distribution of age groups versus the year of measurement (with 95% CI).

	2016	2017	2018	2019	2020	Total
<18	0.0% (±0.1%)	0.0% (±0.1%)	0.1% (±0.1%)	0.1% (±0.1%)	0.0% (±0.2%)	0.1% (±0.2%)
18–35	54.5% (±0.2%)	54.3% (±0.3%)	53.3% (±0.2%)	52.5% (±0.2%)	46.8% (±0.2%)	53.2% (±0.2%)
35–54	35.7% (±0.2%)	35.8% (±0.2%)	36.7% (±0.2%)	37.6% (±0.2%)	41.9% (±0.3%)	36.8% (±0.2%)
55–69	9.6% (±0.1%)	9.7% (±0.1%)	9.8% (±0.1%)	9.7% (±0.1%)	11.1% (±0.1%)	9.8% (±0.1%)
>69	0.1% (±0.1%)	0.1% (±0.1%)	0.2% (±0.1%)	0.2% (±0.1%)	0.3% (±0.1%)	0.2% (±0.1%)
Total	100.0%	100.0%	100.0%	100.0%	100.0%	100.0%

There were also no significant differences in terms of the distribution of the respondents by year of measurement and the voivodeship of residence (see Table A2).

Table A2. Distribution of voivodships depending on the year of measurement (with 95% CI).

	2016	2017	2018	2019	2020	Total
Lower Silesia	12.6% (±0.2%)	13.1% (±0.2%)	12.7% (±0.1%)	13.0% (±0.1%)	13.6% (±0.2%)	12.9% (±0.2%)
Kuyavian-Pomeranian	3.9% (±0.1%)	4.1% (±0.1%)	4.1% (±0.1%)	3.8% (±0.1%)	3.7% (±0.1%)	4.0% (±0.1%)
Lublin	0.9% (±0.1%)	0.9% (±0.1%)	0.9% (±0.1%)	0.8% (±0.1%)	0.7% (±0.1%)	0.8% (±0.1%)
Lubusz	1.4% (±0.1%)	1.4% (±0.1%)	1.5% (±0.1%)	1.6% (±0.1%)	1.9% (±0.1%)	1.5% (±0.1%)
Lodz	7.2% (±0.1%)	7.1% (±0.1%)	6.6% (±0.1%)	6.7% (±0.2%)	6.3% (±0.1%)	6.9% (±0.1%)

Table A2. *Cont.*

	2016	2017	2018	2019	2020	Total
Lesser	10.9% (±0.1%)	11.2% (±0.2%)	11.8% (±0.2%)	11.3% (±0.2%)	11.6% (±0.2%)	11.3% (±0.2%)
Mazowieckie	33.6% (±0.2%)	32.0% (±0.3%)	30.8% (±0.3%)	28.6% (±0.2%)	29.0% (±0.2%)	31.0% (±0.2%)
Opole	1.1% (±0.1%)	1.1% (±0.1%)	1.1% (±0.1%)	1.2% (±0.1%)	1.2% (±0.1%)	1.1% (±0.1%)
Subcarpathian	2.0% (±0.1%)	2.4% (±0.1%)	3.4% (±0.1%)	3.1% (±0.1%)	2.8% (±0.1%)	2.8% (±0.1%)
Podlasie	1.8% (±0.1%)	1.9% (±0.1%)	1.7% (±0.1%)	1.6% (±0.1%)	1.5% (±0.1%)	1.7% (±0.1%)
Pomeranian	6.2% (±0.1%)	6.3% (±0.1%)	6.8% (±0.2%)	7.3% (±0.1%)	6.5% (±0.1%)	6.7% (±0.1%)
Silesian	6.1% (±0.1%)	6.2% (±0.1%)	6.2% (±0.1%)	8.2% (±0.1%)	8.3% (±0.1%)	6.8% (±0.1%)
Świetokrzyskie	0.7% (±0.1%)	0.7% (±0.1%)	0.7% (±0.1%)	0.7% (±0.1%)	0.7% (±0.1%)	0.7% (±0.1%)
Warmia-Masurian	2.1% (±0.1%)	1.9% (±0.1%)	2.0% (±0.1%)	2.1% (±0.1%)	2.1% (±0.1%)	2.0% (±0.1%)
Greater	7.0% (±0.2%)	6.8% (±0.2%)	6.7% (±0.3%)	6.4% (±0.2%)	6.7% (±0.2%)	6.7% (±0.2%)
West Pomeranian	2.6% (±0.1%)	3.0% (±0.1%)	3.0% (±0.1%)	3.5% (±0.1%)	3.5% (±0.1%)	3.1% (±0.1%)
Total	100.0%	100.0%	100.0%	100.0%	100.0%	100.0%

References

1. World Health Organization. Tobacco Control Country Profiles. 2014. Available online: http://www.who.int/tobacco/surveillance/policy/country_profile/en/ (accessed on 1 February 2022).
2. Marcon, A.; Pesce, G.; Calciano, L.; Bellisario, V.; Dharmage, S.C.; Garcia-Aymerich, J.; Gislasson, T.; Heinrich, J.; Holm, M.; Janson, C.; et al. Trends in smoking initiation in Europe over 40 years: A retrospective cohort study. *PLoS ONE* **2018**, *13*, e0201881. [CrossRef] [PubMed]
3. GBD 2015 SDG Collaborators. Measuring the health-related Sustainable Development Goals in 188 countries: A baseline analysis from the Global Burden of Disease Study 2015. *Lancet* **2016**, *388*, 1813–1850. [CrossRef]
4. Hoffman, S.J.; Tan, C. Overview of systematic reviews on the health-related effects of government tobacco control policies. *BMC Public Health* **2015**, *15*, 744. [CrossRef] [PubMed]
5. World Health Organization (WHO). *WHO Report on the Global Tobacco Epidemic, 2017: Monitoring Tobacco Use and Prevention Policies*; World Health Organization: Geneva, Switzerland, 2017.
6. *Eurobarometer, Special Report 429 (EB82.4): Attitudes of Europeans towards Tobacco and Electronic Cigarettes*; European Comission: Brussels, Belgium, 2021. Available online: https://europa.eu/eurobarometer/surveys/detail/2240 (accessed on 1 February 2022).
7. World Health Organization. Tobacco. 2015. Available online: http://www.who.int/me-diacentre/factsheets/fs339/en/ (accessed on 22 July 2020).
8. Mlinaric, A.; Popovic Grle, S.; Nadalin, S.; Skurla, B.; Munivrana, H.; Milosevic, M. Passive smoking and respiratory allergies in adolescents. *Eur. Rev. Med. Pharmacol. Sci.* **2011**, *15*, 973–977. [PubMed]
9. Svanes, C.; Koplin, J.; Skulstad, S.M.; Johannessen, A.; Bertelsen, R.J.; Benediktsdottir, B.; Bråbäck, L.; Elie Carsin, A.; Dharmage, S.; Dratva, J.; et al. Father's environment before conception and asthma risk in his children: A multi-generation analysis of the Respiratory Health In Northern Europe study. *Int. J. Epidemiol.* **2017**, *46*, 235–245. [CrossRef]
10. Northstone, K.; Golding, J.; Davey Smith, G.; Miller, L.L.; Pembrey, M. Prepubertal start of father's smoking and increased body fat in his sons: Further characterisation of paternal transgenerational responses. *Eur. J. Hum. Genet.* **2014**, *22*, 1382–1386. [CrossRef]
11. Accordini, S.; Calciano, L.; Johannessen, A.; Portas, L.; Benediktsdóttir, B.; Bertelsen, R.J.; Bråbäck, L.; Carsin, A.E.; Dharmage, S.C.; Dratva, J.; et al. A three-generation study on the association of tobacco smoking with asthma. *Int. J. Epidemiol.* **2018**, *47*, 1106–1117. [CrossRef]

12. Centers for Disease Control and Prevention (US); National Center for Chronic Disease Prevention and Health Promotion (US); Office on Smoking and Health (US). *How Tobacco Smoke Causes Disease: The Biology and Behavioral Basis for Smoking-Attributable Disease: A Report of the Surgeon Gen-Eral*; Publications and Reports of the Surgeon General; Centers for Disease Control and Prevention (US): Atlanta, GA, USA, 2010.
13. Warner, K.E.; Burns, D.M. Hardening and the hard-coresmoker: Concepts, evidence, and implications. *Nicotine Tob. Res.* **2003**, *5*, 37–48. [CrossRef]
14. Hughes, J.R. The hardening hypothesis: Is the ability to quitdecreasing due to increasing nicotine dependence? A reviewand commentary. *Drug Alcohol Depend.* **2011**, *117*, 111–117. [CrossRef]
15. Baker, C.L.; Flores, N.M.; Zou, K.H.; Bruno, M.; Harrison, V.J. Benefits of quitting smoking on work productivity and activity impairment in the United States, the European Union and China. *Int. J. Clin. Pract.* **2017**, *71*, e12900. [CrossRef]
16. Halpern, M.T.; Shikiar, R.; Rentz, A.M.; Khan, Z.M. Impact of smoking sta-tus on workplace absenteeism and productivity. *Tob. Control* **2001**, *10*, 233–238. [CrossRef] [PubMed]
17. Berman, M.; Crane, R.; Seiber, E.; Munur, M. Estimating the cost of a smoking employee. *Tob. Control* **2014**, *23*, 428–433. [CrossRef]
18. Bunn, W.B., 3rd; Stave, G.M.; Downs, K.E.; Alvir, J.M.; Dirani, R. Effect of smoking status on productivity loss. *J. Occup. Environ. Med.* **2006**, *48*, 1099–1108. [CrossRef] [PubMed]
19. Robroek, S.J.; van den Berg, T.I.; Plat, J.F.; Burdorf, A. The role of obesity and lifestyle behaviours in a productive workforce. *Occup. Environ. Med.* **2011**, *68*, 134–139. [CrossRef] [PubMed]
20. Wegner, C.; Gutsch, A.; Hessel, F.; Wasem, J. Smoking-attributable productivity loss in Germany–A partial sickness cost study based on the human capital potential method. *Gesundheitswesen* **2004**, *66*, 423–432. [CrossRef]
21. Yu, J.; Wang, S.; Yu, X. Health risk factors associated with presenteeism in a Chinese enterprise. *Occup. Med.* **2015**, *65*, 732–738. [CrossRef]
22. US Department of Health and Human Services (USDHHS). The health consequences of smoking—50 years of progress. In *A Report of the Sur-Geon General*; US Department of Health and Human Services, Centers for Disease Control and Prevention, National Center for Chronic Disease Prevention and Health Promotion, Office on Smoking and Health: Atlanta, GA, USA, 2014. Available online: http://www.surgeongeneral.gov/library/reports/50-years-of-progress/ (accessed on 1 February 2022).
23. Connolly, M.J. Smoking cessation in old age: Closing the stabledoor? *Age Ageing* **2000**, *29*, 193–195. [CrossRef]
24. La Croix, A.Z.; Lang, J.; Scherr, P.; Wallace, R.B.; Cornoni-Huntley, J.; Berkman, L.; Curb, J.D.; Evans, D.; Hennekens, C.H. Smoking and mortality amongolder men and women in three communities. *N. Engl. J. Med.* **1991**, *324*, 1619–1625. [CrossRef]
25. Friedman, R.J.; Sengupta, N.; Lees, M. Economic impact of venous thromboembolism after hip and knee arthroplasty: Potential impact of rivaroxaban. *Expert Rev. Pharmacoecon. Outcomes Res.* **2011**, *11*, 299–306. [CrossRef]
26. Rasmussen, S.R.; Prescott, E.; Sorensen, T.I.; Sogaard, J. The total life-time health cost savings of smoking cessation to society. *Eur. J. Public Health* **2005**, *15*, 601–606. [CrossRef]
27. Hill, S.; Amos, A.; Clifford, D.; Platt, S. Impact of tobacco control interventions on socioeconomic inequalities in smoking: Review of the evidence. *Tob. Control* **2014**, *23*, e89–e97. [CrossRef] [PubMed]
28. Kostova, D.; Ross, H.; Blecher, E.; Markowitz, S. Is youth smoking responsive to cigarette prices? Evidence from low-and middle-income countries. *Tob. Control* **2011**, *20*, 419–424. [CrossRef] [PubMed]
29. Hanewinkel, R.; Isensee, B.; Sargent, J.D.; Morgenstern, M. Cigarette advertising and teen smoking initiation. *Pediatrics* **2011**, *127*, e271-8. [CrossRef] [PubMed]
30. Serrano-Alarcón, M.; Kunst, A.E.; Bosdriesz, J.R.; Perelman, J. Tobacco control policies and smoking among older adults: A longitudinal analysis of 10 European countries. *Addiction* **2019**, *114*, 1076–1085. [CrossRef]
31. Fitch, K.; Iwasaki, K.; Pyenson, B. Covering Smoking Cessation as a Health Benefit: A Case for Employers. 2006. Available online: http://www.dfwbgh.org/events07/9-27-2007.pdf (accessed on 1 February 2022).
32. Jackson, K.C., 2nd; Nahoopii, R.; Said, Q.; Dirani, R.; Brixner, D. An employer-based cost-benefit analysis of a novel pharmaco-therapy agent for smoking cessation. *J. Occup. Environ. Med.* **2007**, *49*, 453–460. [CrossRef] [PubMed]
33. Bala, M.M.; Strzeszynski, L.; Topor-Madry, R. Mass media interventions for smoking cessation in adults. *Cochrane Database Syst. Rev.* **2017**, *11*, CD004704. [CrossRef]
34. Carreras-Torres, R.; Johansson, M.; Haycock, P.C.; Relton, C.L.; Davey Smith, G.; Brennan, P.; Martin, R.M. Role of obesity in smoking behaviour: Mendelian randomisation study in UK Biobank. *BMJ* **2018**, *361*, k1767. [CrossRef] [PubMed]
35. Dare, S.; Mackay, D.F.; Pell, J.P. Relationship between smoking and obesity: A cross-sectional study of 499,504 middle-aged adults in the UK general population. *PLoS ONE* **2015**, *10*, e0123579. [CrossRef]
36. Chiolero, A.; Faeh, D.; Paccaud, F.; Cornuz, J. Consequences of smoking for body weight, body fat distribution, and insulin resistance. *Am. J. Clin. Nutr. United States* **2008**, *87*, 801–809. [CrossRef]
37. GBD 2016 Mortality and Causes of Death Collaborators. Global, regional, and national age-sex specific mortality for 264 causes of death, 1980–2016: A systematic analysis for the Global Burden of Disease Study 2016. *Lancet* **2017**, *390*, 1151–1210. [CrossRef]
38. GBD 2016 Risk Factors Collaborators. Global, regional, and national comparative risk assessment of 84 behavioural, environmental and occupational, and metabolic risks or clusters of risks, 1990–2016: A systematic analysis for the Global Burden of Disease Study 2016. *Lancet* **2017**, *390*, 1345–1422. [CrossRef]

39. Doll, R.; Peto, R.; Boreham, J.; Sutherland, I. Mortality in relation to smoking: 50 years' observations on male British doctors. *BMJ* **2004**, *328*, 1519. [CrossRef] [PubMed]
40. Thun, M.J.; Carter, B.D.; Feskanich, D.; Freedman, N.D.; Prentice, R.; Lopez, A.D.; Hartge, P.; Gapstur, S.M. 50-year trends in smoking-related mortality in the United States. *N. Engl. J. Med.* **2013**, *368*, 351–364. [CrossRef] [PubMed]

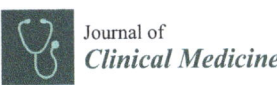

Article

Prevalence of Obesity and Severe Obesity among Professionally Active Adult Population in Poland and Its Strong Relationship with Cardiovascular Co-Morbidities-POL-O-CARIA 2016–2020 Study

Anna Rulkiewicz [1], Iwona Pilchowska [1,2], Wojciech Lisik [3], Piotr Pruszczyk [4], Michał Ciurzyński [4] and Justyna Domienik-Karłowicz [1,4,*]

1. LUX MED, Postępu 21C, 02-676 Warsaw, Poland; anna.rulkiewicz@luxmed.pl (A.R.); iwona.pilchowska@luxmed.pl (I.P.)
2. Department of Psychology, SWPS University of Social Sciences and Humanities, 03-815 Warsaw, Poland
3. Department of General and Transplantation Surgery, Medical University of Warsaw, 02-014 Warsaw, Poland; wojciech.lisik@wum.edu.pl
4. Department of Internal Medicine and Cardiology, Medical University of Warsaw, 02-005 Warsaw, Poland; piotr.pruszczyk@wum.edu.pl (P.P.); michal.ciurzynski@wum.edu.pl (M.C.)
* Correspondence: jdomienik@tlen.pl or justyna.domienik@wum.edu.pl; Tel.: +48-(22)-502-11-44

Abstract: For several decades, a steady increase in the percentage of overweight and obese people has been observed all over the world. There are many studies available in the literature emphasizing the relationship of overweight and obesity with the occurrence of other diseases. The aim of this study is to characterize the prevalence of obesity and severe obesity, as well as their changes over time, among professionally active adults who underwent occupational medicine examinations in Poland in 2016–2020, for the POL-O-CARIA 2016–2020 study. In total, the results of 1,450,455 initial, control and periodic visits as part of the occupational medicine certificate were analyzed. Statistical calculations were performed with the use of IBM SPSS Statistics 25. In both groups (men/women), a significant decrease was observed every year for people who had normal body weight. In addition, the tendency to increase in people with I and III degrees of obesity was more strongly observed in the male group. A significant relationship was also observed between BMI categories and the occurrence of all analyzed comorbidities: hypertension, type 2 diabetes, lipid disorders and coronary artery disease (chi^2 (70) = 12,228.11; $p < 0.001$). Detailed results showed that in the group of patients diagnosed with hypertension or lipid disorders, significant differences were observed between all groups; it turned out that as the BMI level increased (I, I, III), there was an increase in the percentage of occurrence of hypertension (38.1%, 41% and 45.3%, respectively) and type 2 diabetes (3.2%, 4.6% and 5.8%, respectively) ($p < 0.001$). Our analysis indicates that the prevalence of adult obesity and severe obesity will continue to increase nationwide, with an accompanying large increase in comorbidities.

Keywords: BMI index; professionally active adult population; cardiovascular diseases; obesity

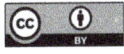

1. Introduction

For several decades, a steady increase in the percentage of overweight and obese people has been observed all over the world. More and more countries declare problems with controlling this epidemic. This disease affects children as well as adults [1]. According to the WHO definition, obesity is abnormal or excessive accumulation of fat that negatively affects health. Obesity is diagnosed when the BMI level exceeds or is equal to 30 kg/m^2 [2]. According to data published by WHO in 2014, the percentage of people with obesity in Poland is 25.1% [3]. The main cause of obesity is a long-term imbalance between the amount of calories consumed and the body's demands [4]. Diet, lifestyle and genetics have a significant influence on the occurrence of obesity [5].

1.1. Obesity and Comorbidities

There are many studies available in the literature emphasizing the relationship of overweight and obesity with the occurrence of other diseases. A meta-analysis carried out in 2015 showed that each increase in weight by 5 kg significantly increases the risk of developing post-menopausal breast (11%), endometrial (39%), ovarian cancer (13%) and male colon cancer (9%) [6]. Cohort studies conducted in Europe (Austria, Norway, Sweden) under the Me-Can 2.0 program showed that overweight people up to 40 years of age significantly increase their chance of developing endometrial, male renal cell and male colon cancer [7]. Obesity is a chronic and metabolic disease; therefore, it affects the occurrence of cardiovascular diseases [8]. It affects the structural and functional changes in the cardiovascular system, e.g., causing decreased cardiac output, increased left ventricular mass and wall thickness [9]. The association of obesity with hypertension, coronary artery disease and diabetes is also scientifically confirmed [10,11].

1.2. The Global Obesity Epidemic

For several decades, a steady increase in the percentage of overweight and obese people has been observed. Most countries in the world are affected. Current reports show that more people worldwide die from overweight and obesity than from underweight [12]. Obesity is the main reason for the development of NCDs (non-communicable diseases), which since 2010 have been responsible for 86% of deaths and 77% of other diseases in Europe. Over the past 40 years, there has been a sharp increase in the percentage of people with obesity; since 1975, the percentage of people with obesity has increased from 1% to 6–8%. Women saw an increase from 6% to 15%, while men increased from 3% to 11% [13]. There are four levels of obesity, distinguished on the basis of an analysis of the 30 most populous countries in the world [14]:

- Level 1—characterized by a higher prevalence of obesity in women than men (more often in adults than children) and in people with a higher socioeconomic status. This level is most commonly observed in South Asia and Sub-Saharan Africa.
- Level 2—at this stage there is a significant increase in obesity in the adult group and a decrease in children. The importance of gender and socioeconomic status is not as clear as in level 1. This stage is most often observed in Latin America and the Middle East.
- Level 3—the most characteristic for the inhabitants of Europe. A higher obesity rate is observed more often in the group of people with a low socioeconomic status, but it is worth noting the increase in the percentage of obese people in the group of women with high economic status and in the group of children.
- Level 4—there are few countries classified to this stage. It is characterized by a decrease in the prevalence of obesity. The research results do not allow for an unequivocal determination of the relationship between the prevalence of obesity and gender and socioeconomic status.

The two regions with a dynamic increase in obesity are North America and Europe [14].

1.3. Actions to Reduce the Obesity Epidemic

Obesity is a multidimensional disease that affects many spheres of life. Hence, it is advisable to provide long-term support for patients suffering from this disease. Current activities aimed at controlling and reducing obesity in society focus on the analysis of the occurrence of civilization diseases, followed by body weight. It seems important to focus on the many dimensions of the fight against obesity (diet, physical activity, changes in behavior), which will translate into an improvement in the quality of life. Attention is also paid to the growing interest in surgical methods of obesity treatment [15]. In Europe, the prevalence of overweight increased from 48% in 1980 to 59.6% in 2015; in the case of obesity, the incidence increased fromd 15.5% in 1980 to 22.9% in 2015. Moreover, a lower probability of obesity was reported among women (in the group of people aged 20 to 44); an inverse relationship was observed in the group of people over 45 years of age.

1.4. Obesity and Professional Activity

Work is recognized as a source that may influence overweight and obesity [16]. Employers take measures to promote healthy eating habits and increase physical activity among employees [17]. Employers increasingly organize free fruits and vegetables in their offices for their employees [18]. The factors that may increase the chance of overweight and obesity in the workplace are sedentary work, stress and sleep problems [19]. Office work and sedentary work increase the likelihood of obesity among employees [20]. The research by Shields and Tremlay (2008) confirmed the existence of a positive relationship between obesity and spending free time sitting (e.g., while using a computer) [21]. There are also several studies that do not confirm the relationship between sedentary work or leisure activities and the prevalence of overweight and obesity [22]. An important factor associated with overweight and obesity is also stress experienced in the workplace [23].

1.5. Aim of the Study

The aim of the study is to characterize professionally active adults who underwent occupational medicine examinations in Poland in 2016–2020. Due to the exploratory nature of the research, the article did not put forward research hypotheses. Instead, research questions were asked that define the main subject of the analysis: how the intensity of obesity changes over time and how it coexists with other diseases [24].

2. Materials and Methods

The article analyzes the results of the POL-O-CARIA 2016–2020 study, concerning adults who are professionally active and visited in the years January 2016–April 2020 as part of occupational medicine. The data for analysis was provided by the LUX MED Group. In total, the results of 1,450,455 initial, control and periodic visits as part of the occupational medicine certificate were analyzed. During the study, sex, age, province of residence, information on the period of the issued medical certificate and data contained in the medical history (subjective assessment of health, smoking) were controlled. Detailed characteristics of the studied patients are presented in Appendix A.

For several decades, a steady increase in the percentage of overweight and obese people has been observed. For this reason, it seems extremely important to monitor the prevalence of obesity in individual social groups. The study of professionally active adults is important for several reasons. It is important to monitor the health condition and forecast the occurrence of specific civilization diseases in a given society. The occurrence of certain diseases (e.g., obesity, hypertension, diabetes) translates into shorter medical certificates enabling employment.

Statistical Analysis

Statistical calculations were performed with the use of IBM SPSS Statistics 25 [25]. Percentage and number of occurrences were used to analyze qualitative data, while the following were used to characterize qualitative data: mean (M), standard deviation (SD), median, skewness, kurtosis, and the minimum and maximum values. Significant statistical results were considered to be those where the probability of making a type I error was lower than 5% ($p < 0.05$). The following were used for statistical calculations: chi-square analysis in cross tables (Bonferroni correction was used to test column proportions) and one-way analysis of variance (Scheffe's post hoc test was used for mean comparisons). The charts were made in the R program [26].

3. Results

3.1. Information on BMI

It was observed that, with successive years of measurement, the percentage of overweight and obesity (regardless of degree) increased, while the percentage of people with normal body weight significantly decreased. Detailed results are presented in Table 1.

Table 1. Body mass index (BMI) distribution depending on the year of measurement.

	2016	2017	2018	2019	2020	Total
underweight	3.40% a	3.40% a	3.40% a	3.20% a	2.90% a	3.30%
normal body weight	51.60% a	51.10% a	50.20% b	49.30% b	46.90% c	50.30%
overweight without obesity	31.40% a	31.50% a	32.00% a	32.20% a	33.50% a	31.90%
I degree of obesity	10.40% a	10.70% a,b	11.00% b,c	11.50% c	12.50% d	11.00%
II degree of obesity	2.50% a	2.60% a	2.70% a,b	2.90% b	3.30% b	2.70%
III degree of obesity	0.70% a	0.70% a	0.80% a,b	0.80% a,b	0.90% b	0.80%
Total	100.0%	100.0%	100.0%	100.0%	100.0%	100.0%

Each letter in subscript represents a subset of the year category whose column proportions do not differ significantly at the level of 5%.

In the case of BMI, it was shown that the longest medical certificates for professionally active Poles were received by people with normal body weight, which equaled about 34 months. In the group of people with overweight and obesity, it was observed that, along with the degree of obesity, the average number of months in which the decision was issued decreased significantly (see Table 2). According to doctor decision, patients with overweight received medical certificates for work for an average of about 30 months. The ability to work was significantly worse in patients with obesity of the I degree (about 28 months), obesity of the II degree (about 27 months) and obesity of the III degree (almost 26 months); the details are presented in Table 2.

Table 2. Descriptive statistics on the average number of months of the issued medical certificate depending on BMI.

	Underweight	Normal Body Weight	Overweight without Obesity	I Degree of Obesity	II Degree of Obesity	III Degree of Obesity
M	35.46	34.01	30.63	28.24	27.10	25.99
Me	36.00	36.00	36.00	24.00	24.00	24.00
SD	12.28	12.63	13.06	13.07	12.90	12.72
Skewness	−0.71	−0.57	−0.25	−0.05	0.05	0.14
Kurtosis	−0.02	−0.50	−0.80	−0.91	−0.66	−0.83
Min	0.00	0.00	0.00	0.00	0.00	0.00
Max	156.00	156.00	178.00	155.00	156.00	60.00

M—mean; Me—median; SD—standard deviation.

3.2. Patient Characteristics Depending on the BMI Level

Chi-square analysis showed that, for both women and men, similar trends were observed regarding the dynamics of occurrence of individual BMI categories. In both groups, a significant decrease was observed every year for people who had normal body weight. In addition, the tendency to increase in people with I and III degrees of obesity was more strongly observed in the male group (see Table 3).

Table 3. Relationship between BMI and measurement time, as well as patients' sex; data presented as percentage of the year of measurement [1].

		2016	2017	2018	2019	2020	Total
Women	underweight	6.1% a	6.2% a	6.0% a	5.8% b	5.4% c	6.00%
	normal body weight	64.4% a	63.7% b	62.7% c	62.0% d	60.3% e	63.00%
	overweight without obesity	19.6% a	19.9% a	20.7% b	20.9% b	22.0% c	20.40%
	I degree of obesity	7.1% a	7.3% a	7.5% b	8.0% c	8.6% d	7.50%
	II degree of obesity	2.1% a	2.2% b	2.2% b	2.4% c	2.8% d	2.30%
	III degree of obesity	0.7% a	0.8% b	0.8% b,c	0.8% c,d	0.9% d	0.80%
	Total	100.00%	100.00%	100.00%	100.00%	100.00%	100.00%

Table 3. Cont.

		2016	2017	2018	2019	2020	Total
Men	underweight	0.8% a	0.8% a,b	0.9% b,c	0.9% c	0.8% a,b	0.80%
	normal body weight	39.3% a	38.9% b	38.3% c	37.9% d	35.5% e	38.40%
	overweight without obesity	42.7% a,b,c,d	42.8% c,d	42.7% b,d	42.4% b	43.2% a,c	42.70%
	I degree of obesity	13.6% a	14.0% b	14.3% c	14.7% d	15.9% e	14.30%
	II degree of obesity	2.9% a	2.9% a	3.2% b	3.3% b	3.7% c	3.10%
	III degree of obesity	0.6% a	0.7% a	0.8% b	0.8% c	0.9% c	0.70%
	Total	100.00%	100.00%	100.00%	100.00%	100.00%	100.00%

[1] Each letter in subscript represents a subset of the year category whose column proportions do not differ significantly at the level of 5%.

Significant differences, regardless of the year of measurement, were observed using a one-way analysis of variance for the age and time for which the measurement was issued (in both cases, the significance of differences between the groups was $p < 0.001$). The exact results are discussed below.

In the case of patients' age, post hoc analysis with Scheffe's correction showed that only between people with II and III degrees of obesity were there no differences for the average age; in other cases, the significance of differences between individual groups was $p < 0.001$. The highest average age was observed for people with obesity, while the lowest was observed for people with underweight or normal weight (see Figure 1).

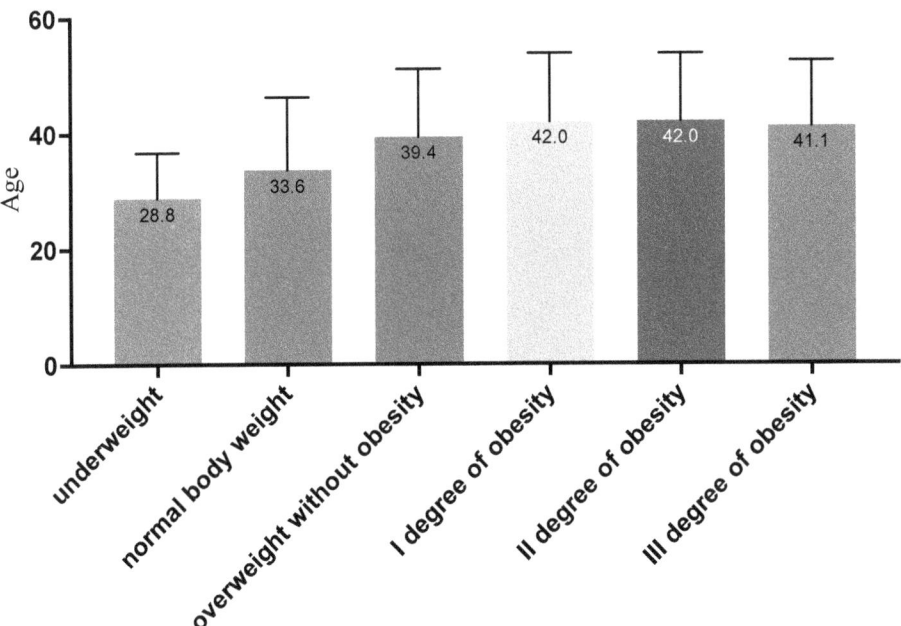

Figure 1. Average age depending on the BMI category (in the figure, all groups are statistically significantly different, at least at the $p < 0.001$ level; due to the number of groups compared, results for differences are not shown in the figure).

Patients with normal body weight most often occurred in the group under 35 years of age, while the percentage of people with obesity (especially I degree) increased significantly in each age category (see Table 4).

Table 4. Relationship between BMI and patients' age; data presented as percentage of age group [1].

	<18	18–35	35–54	55–69	>69	Total
underweight	14.3% a	5.1% b	1.4% c	0.5% d	0.6% d	3.30%
normal body weight	61.7% a	60.1% a	41.7% b	27.5% c	26.9% c	50.20%
overweight without obesity	17.5% a	25.6% b	37.8% c	44.8% d	49.9% e	32.00%
I degree of obesity	4.0% a	7.0% b	14.4% c	20.9% d	18.2% d	11.10%
II degree of obesity	1.9% a	1.7% a	3.7% b	5.0% c	4.0% b	2.70%
III degree of obesity	0.5% a,b,c,d	0.5% d	1.1% c	1.2% b	0.4% a,d	0.80%
Total	100.00%	100.00%	100.00%	100.00%	100.00%	100.00%

[1] Each letter in subscript represents a subset of the year category whose column proportions do not differ significantly at the level of 5%.

Table 5 presents the same data by changing the percentage to the BMI category. The obtained results showed that, together with the higher BMI level, the percentage of people under 35 years of age decreased in each group. In the case of people aged 35–69, it was obtained that they were more often classified into the group with obesity or overweight, compared to groups with normal body weight.

Table 5. Relationship between BMI and age of patients; data presented as percentage of the BMI category [1].

	Underweight	Normal Body Weight	Overweight Without Obesity	I Degree of Obesity	II Degree of Obesity	III Degree of Obesity	Total
<18	0.2% a	0.1% b	0.0% c	0.0% d	0.0% c	0.0% b,c,d	0.10%
18–35	83.2% a	64.1% b	42.9% c	33.7% d	32.8% e	34.7% f	53.50%
35–54	15.0% a	30.5% b	43.3% c	47.8% d	49.3% e	50.5% f	36.70%
55–69	1.5% a	5.3% b	13.5% c	18.2% d	17.6% e	14.7% f	9.60%
>69	0.0% a	0.1% b	0.3% c	0.3% c	0.2% c	0.1% b	0.20%
Total	100.0%	100.0%	100.0%	100.0%	100.0%	100.0%	100.0%

[1] Each letter in subscript represents a subset of the year category whose column proportions do not differ significantly at the level of 5%.

When analyzing the time periods for issuing a medical certificate, significant differences between the groups were also observed. A linear trend was obtained showing that, along with the BMI level, the average number of months of the issued decision decreased. In addition, post hoc analysis with Scheffe's correction showed that significant differences were observed between all BMI categories. Detailed results are presented below (see Figure 2).

Patients with normal weight or underweight were less likely to smoke than overweight or obese patients. This relationship was observed regardless of the year of measurement (see Figure 3).

The relationship between BMI categories and subjective health assessment was also examined. It was found that people who subjectively assessed their own health as good, less often than people who assessed their health as very good, were classified into the group of people with normal body weight. An inverse relationship was obtained for overweight and obese people. Detailed results are presented below Table 6.

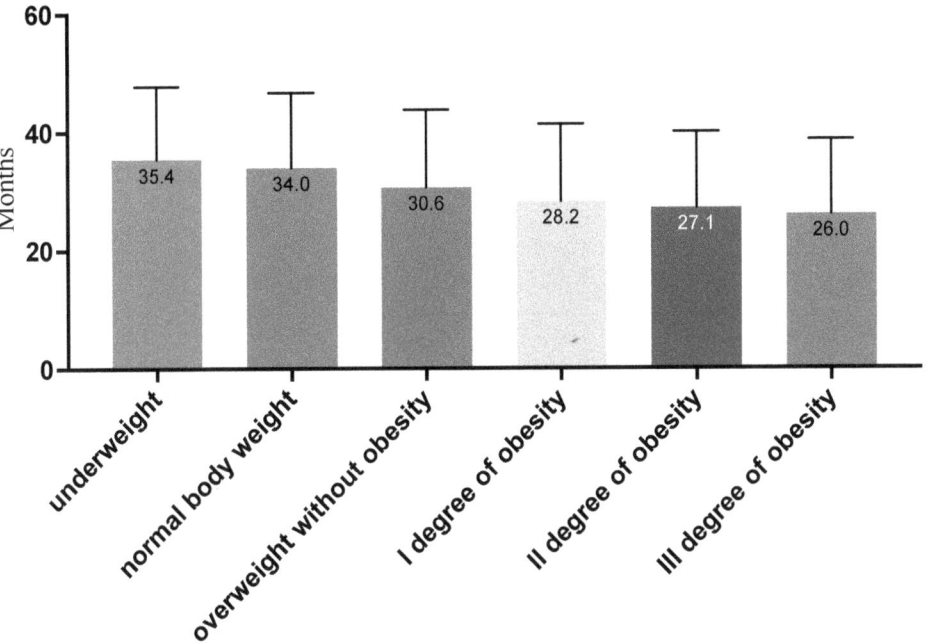

Figure 2. Average number of months for the issued medical certificate depending on the BMI category (in the figure, all groups are statistically significantly different, at least at the $p < 0.05$ level; due to the number of groups compared, results for differences are not shown in the figure).

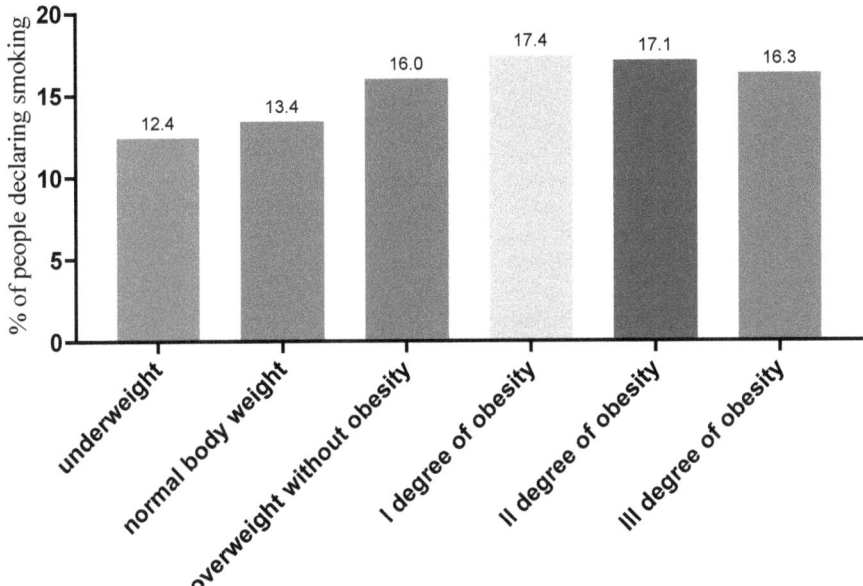

Figure 3. Percentage of people declaring smoking depending on the BMI category (due to the number of groups compared, results for differences are not shown in the figure).

Table 6. Relationship between BMI and subjective assessment of health; data presented as percentage of the health assessment.

	Subjective Health Assessment		Total
	Good	Very Good	
underweight	3.00%	3.80%	3.40%
normal body weight	47.00%	55.20%	50.70%
overweight without obesity	33.10%	30.20%	31.80%
I degree of obesity	12.60%	8.60%	10.80%
II degree of obesity	3.30%	1.80%	2.60%
III degree of obesity	1.00%	0.40%	0.70%
Total	100.00%	100.00%	100.00%

Table 7 shows the relationship between selected diseases and BMI categories. A significant relationship between variables was obtained ($p < 0.001$). The most pronounced differences were observed for hypertension (with increasing BMI level, the percentage of people with this disease increased), and for lipid disorders and type 2 diabetes.

Table 7. Relationship between BMI and the incidence of selected diseases; data presented as percentage of the BMI category [1].

	Underweight	Normal Body Weight	Overweight without Obesity	I Degree of Obesity	II Degree of Obesity	III Degree of Obesity	Total
Hypertension	29.6% a	38.4% b	45.3% c	50.5% d	52.3% e	55.4% f	44.9%
Type 2 diabetes	8.6% a	5.8% b	6.9% c	10.6% d	15.6% e	18.3% f	8.1%
Lipid disorders	58.9% a	52.3% b	43.9% c	35.1% d	28.9% e	23.8% f	43.4%
Coronary disease	2.9% a,b,c,d	3.4% d	4.0% c	3.8% c	3.2% b,d	2.5% a	3.7%
Total	100.0%	100.0%	100.0%	100.0%	100.0%	100.0%	100.0%

[1] Each letter in subscript represents a subset of the year category whose column proportions do not differ significantly at the level of 5%.

3.3. BMI and Observed Comorbidities

A significant relationship was also observed between BMI categories and the occurrence of comorbidities (chi^2 (70) = 12,228.11; $p < 0.001$). Detailed results showed that in the group of patients diagnosed with hypertension or lipid disorders, significant differences were observed between all groups; it turned out that, as the BMI level increased, the percentage of occurrence of a given disease increases. A comparison of all comorbidities depending on BMI level is shown in the Table 8 below.

Table 8. Relationship between BMI and comorbidities; data presented as percentage of BMI [1].

	Underweight	Normal Body Weight	Overweight without Obesity	I Degree of Obesity	II Degree of Obesity	III Degree of Obesity	Total
Hypertension	26.1% a	30.5% b	33.7% c	38.8% d	41.0% e	45.3% f	34.1%
Type 2 diabetes	7.8% a	4.1% b	2.8% c	3.2% d	4.6% b	5.8% e	3.5%
Lipid disorders	57.7% a	47.3% b	33.0% c	19.7% d	11.6% e	7.5% f	33.8%
Coronary disease	2.0% a	1.2% b	1.0% c	0.6% d	0.4% d,e	0.2% e	0.9%
Hypertension + Type 2 diabetes	0.6% a	0.9% a	2.0% b	4.3% c	7.7% d	10.7% e	2.5%
Hypertension + Lipid disorders	4.2% a	11.6% b	19.5% c	21.9% d	20.1% c	17.0% e	17.3%
Hypertension + Coronary disease	0.3% a	0.6% a	0.9% b	1.0% b	0.9% b	1.1% b	0.8%
Type 2 diabetes + Lipid disorders	0.4% a	0.7% a	1.1% b	1.5% c	1.8% d	1.4% b,c,d	1.1%
Type 2 diabetes + Coronary disease	0.1% a,b,c	0.0% c	0.1% b	0.1% a	0.2% a	0.1% a,b,c	0.1%
Lipid disorders + Coronary disease	0.4% a,b,c	0.7% c	0.7% c	0.4% b	0.3% a,b	0.1% a	0.6%
Hypertension + Type 2 diabetes + Lipid disorders	0.2% a	0.9% b	2.7% c	5.0% d	8.1% e	8.5% e	2.9%
Hypertension + Type 2 diabetes + Coronary disease	0.1% a,b,c	0.1% c	0.2% b	0.4% a	0.4% a	0.4% a	0.2%

Table 8. Cont.

	Underweight	Normal Body Weight	Overweight without Obesity	I Degree of Obesity	II Degree of Obesity	III Degree of Obesity	Total
Hypertension + Lipid disorders + Coronary disease	0.3% a	1.2% b,c	2.0% d	2.0% d	1.5% c	0.8% a,b	1.7%
Type 2 diabetes + Lipid disorders + Coronary disease	0.1% a,b,c,d	0.0% c,d	0.0% b,d	0.1% a	0.1% a,b,c,d	0.1% a,b,c,d	0.1%
All		0.2% a	0.6% b	1.0% c	1.3% d	1.1% c,d	0.6%
Total	100.0%	100.0%	100.0%	100.0%	100.0%	100.0%	100.0%

[1] Each letter in subscript represents a subset of the year category whose column proportions do not differ significantly at the level of 5%.

The cross-tabulation chi-square analysis performed confirmed that there was an association between age and comorbidities (chi^2(56) = 16,758.06; $p < 0.001$). In the case of hypertension, it was obtained that the prevalence of hypertension was more common in those aged 18–54 compared to other age groups. In addition, the prevalence of lipid disorders was significantly different in each of the age groups; a trend was observed showing that the diagnosis of this disease decreased with age. A detailed comparison of the age groups for the other diseases is shown below Table 9.

Table 9. Relationship between age and comorbidities; data presented as percentage of age group [1].

	Age					Total
	<18	18–35	35–54	55–69	>69	
Hypertension	66.7% a,b,c	37.7% c	34.3% b	31.6% a	30.2% a	34.3%
Type 2 diabetes	33.3% a	6.7% a	2.8% b	2.6% c	2.5% b,c	3.5%
Lipid disorders		44.3% d	35.8% c	18.6% b	7.1% a	33.2%
Coronary disease		0.5% c	0.8% b	1.8% a	2.0% a	1.0%
Hypertension + Type 2 diabetes		0.9% d	2.1% c	4.8% b	6.6% a	2.6%
Hypertension + Lipid disorders		8.7% d	18.3% c	22.1% b	19.0% a,c	17.3%
Hypertension + Coronary disease		0.1% d	0.5% c	2.1% b	4.5% a	0.8%
Type 2 diabetes + Lipid disorders		0.6% c	1.1% b	1.5% a	1.4% a,b	1.1%
Type 2 diabetes + Coronary disease		0.0% d	0.0% c	0.2% b	0.6% a	0.1%
Lipid disorders + Coronary disease		0.1% c	0.5% b	1.3% a	1.9% a	0.6%
Hypertension + Type 2 diabetes + Lipid disorders		0.4% c	2.2% b	6.5% a	8.1% a	3.0%
Hypertension + Type 2 diabetes + Coronary disease		0.0% d	0.1% c	0.6% b	1.9% a	0.2%
Hypertension + Lipid disorders + Coronary disease		0.1% d	1.1% c	4.3% b	9.0% a	1.7%
Type 2 diabetes + Lipid disorders + Coronary disease		0.0% b	0.0% b	0.2% a	0.4% a	0.1%
All		0.0% d	0.2% c	1.8% b	4.7% a	0.6%
Total	100.0%	100.0%	100.0%	100.0%	100.0%	100.0%

[1] Each letter in subscript represents a subset of the age category whose column proportions do not differ significantly at the level of 5%.

4. Discussion

In this study, we used data from 931,985 unique adult patients and applied an analytical approach that provided estimates of BMI trends. Analyses on the prevalence of obesity in Poland were present in previous years; however, none of them were concerning the current years, and they were not based on such a large group of patients.

Unique in our analysis is also the correlation with the average number of months for the issued medical certificate, and the correlation with the coexistence of other serious diseases, mainly of the cardiovascular system. It is very worrying that, with the increase in BMI, the ability to work is limited, and we did not include patients who, due to obesity and comorbidities, do not try to work at all.

We would like to point out that, in this very large group of patients, we have confirmed the coexistence of diseases that significantly reduce the quality of life of patients, and their coexistence clearly depends on the degree of obesity.

Our data showed that one third of the professionally active women and almost two thirds of the professionally active men are overweight or obese. This result is extremely disturbing. Moreover, we demonstrated a trend showing an increase in the phenomenon over time, which raises concerns in terms of access to medical care and the cost of medical care. The data clearly indicate that the phenomenon is not uniform in all regions of the country. In additional materials, we present unique data indicating the diversification of obesity depending on the region of the country. Although grade II and grade III obesity were once a rare condition, our findings may suggest that they will soon be the most common BMI category in the patient populations. Given that physicians are not well equipped to treat obese patients, the continuing trend will be a major challenge for healthcare as a whole.

5. Conclusions

Further annual assessment of the prevalence of obesity and comorbidities seems necessary to prepare the health care system for treating growing number of obese, professionally active Poles, and to take the most effective measures to inhibit the trend.

Author Contributions: Conceptualization, A.R., W.L., P.P., M.C. and J.D.-K.; Data curation, A.R., I.P. and J.D.-K.; Formal analysis, I.P. and J.D.-K.; Investigation, I.P.; Methodology, A.R. and J.D.-K.; Project administration, A.R., I.P. and J.D.-K.; Supervision, J.D.-K.; Visualization, I.P.; Writing—original draft, I.P. and J.D.-K.; Writing—review & editing, W.L., P.P., M.C. and J.D.-K. All authors have read and agreed to the published version of the manuscript.

Funding: This research received no external funding.

Institutional Review Board Statement: Ethical review and approval were waived for this study due to REASON: retrospective anonymized analysis.

Informed Consent Statement: Not applicable.

Conflicts of Interest: There is no conflict of interest (all cases). Anna Rulkiewicz, Iwona Pilchowska and Justyna Domienik-Karłowicz are LUX MED employees.

Appendix A. Additional Analyzes

The study included 1,450,455 visits to occupational medicine (collected from 931,985 unique patients) from 2016–2020. The exact number of collected results depending on the year of measurement is presented below.

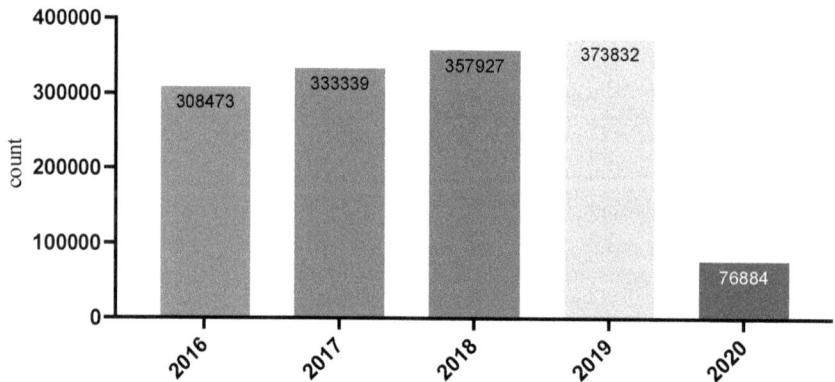

Figure A1. The number of visits analyzed versus the year of measurement.

In terms of sex, the results of the men accounted for a slightly higher percentage (51.6%). Along with the successive stages of the study, the percentage of surveyed men slightly increased (see Figure A2).

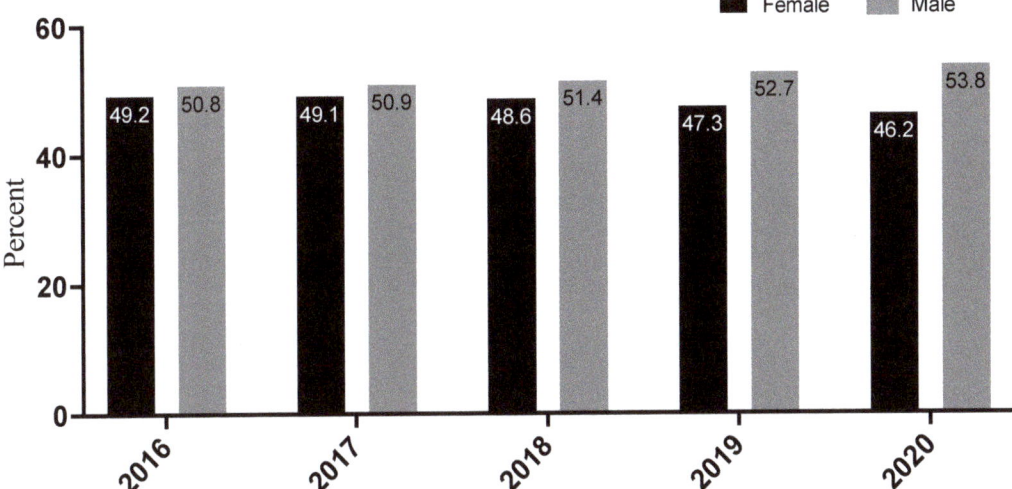

Figure A2. Sex distribution depending on the year of measurement.

The age of the respondents ranged between 14 and 90 years (M = 36.59; SD = 11.56). A slight trend was observed indicating the mean age of the examined patients slightly increased with each year of measurement (see Figure A3). Clarification: patients can change age categories if their change in age necessitates this; this is not to be misinterpreted for a tautological restatement of the patients aging with time.

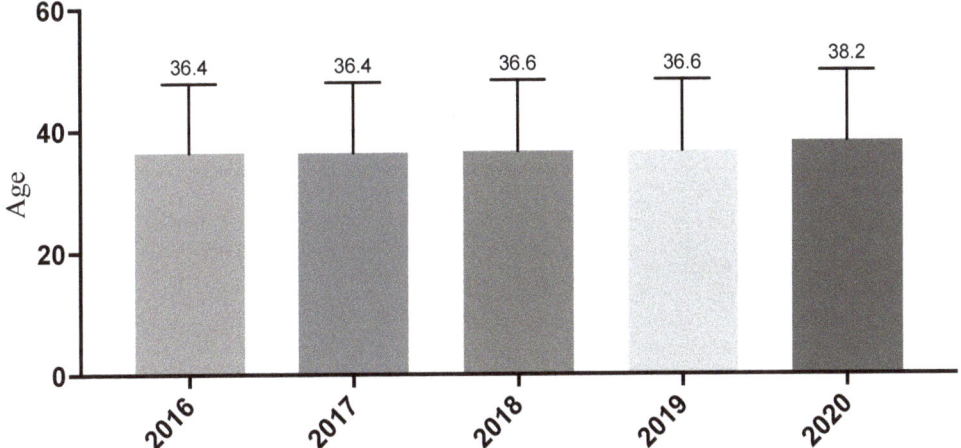

Figure A3. Patient age distribution versus the year of measurement.

The exact distribution of age groups depending on the year of measurement is presented in the table below. It was found that, with successive years of measurement, a decreased percentage of people aged 18–35 and an increased percentage in the age group 35–54 were observed. In the case of the remaining age groups, the trends were not as clear as in the case of these two age categories.

Table A1. Distribution of age groups versus the year of measurement.

	2016	2017	2018	2019	2020	Total
<18	0.00%	0.00%	0.10%	0.10%	0.00%	0.10%
18–35	54.50%	54.30%	53.30%	52.50%	46.80%	53.20%
35–54	35.70%	35.80%	36.70%	37.60%	41.90%	36.80%
55–69	9.60%	9.70%	9.80%	9.70%	11.10%	9.80%
>69	0.10%	0.10%	0.20%	0.20%	0.30%	0.20%
Total	100.00%	100.00%	100.00%	100.00%	100.00%	100.00%

There were also no significant differences in terms of the distribution of the respondents by year of measurement and the voivodeship of residence (see Table A2).

Table A2. Distribution of voivodeships depending on the year of measurement.

	2016	2017	2018	2019	2020	Total
Lower Silesia	12.60%	13.10%	12.70%	13.00%	13.60%	12.90%
Kuyavian-Pomeranian	3.90%	4.10%	4.10%	3.80%	3.70%	4.00%
Lublin	0.90%	0.90%	0.90%	0.80%	0.70%	0.80%
Lubusz	1.40%	1.40%	1.50%	1.60%	1.90%	1.50%
Lodz	7.20%	7.10%	6.60%	6.70%	6.30%	690%
Lesser	10.90%	11.20%	11.80%	11.30%	11.60%	11.30%
Mazowieckie	33.60%	32.00%	30.80%	28.60%	29.00%	31.00%
Opole	1.10%	1.10%	1.10%	1.20%	1.20%	1.10%
Subcarpathian	2.00%	2.40%	3.40%	3.10%	2.80%	2.80%
Podlasie	1.80%	1.90%	1.70%	1.60%	1.50%	1.70%
Pomeranian	6.20%	6.30%	6.80%	7.30%	6.50%	6.70%
Silesian	6.10%	6.20%	6.20%	8.20%	8.30%	6.80%
Świetokrzyskie	0.70%	0.70%	0.70%	0.70%	0.70%	0.70%
Warmia-Masurian	2.10%	1.90%	2.00%	2.10%	2.10%	2.00%
Greater	7.00%	6.80%	6.70%	6.40%	6.70%	6.70%
West Pomeranian	2.60%	3.00%	3.00%	3.50%	3.50%	3.10%
Total	100.00%	100.00%	100.00%	100.00%	100.00%	100.00%

References

1. Ng, M.; Fleming, T.; Robinson, M.; Thomson, B.; Graetz, N.; Margono, C.; Gakidou, E. Global, regional, and national prevalence of overweight and obesity in children and adults during 1980–2013: A systematic analysis for the Global Burden of Disease Study 2013. *Lancet* **2014**, *384*, 766–781. [CrossRef]
2. Prospective Studies Collaboration. Body- mass index and cause- specific mortality in 900,000 adults: Collaborative analyses of 57 prospective studies. *Lancet* **2009**, *373*, 1083–1096. [CrossRef]
3. Blundell, J.E.; Baker, J.L.; Boyland, E.; Blaak, E.; Charzewska, J.; De Henauw, S.; Frühbeck, G.; Gonzalez-Gross, M.; Hebebrand, J.; Holm, L.; et al. Variations in the Prevalence of Obesity Among European Countries, and a Consideration of Possible Causes. *Obes. Facts* **2017**, *10*, 25–37. [CrossRef] [PubMed]
4. Blüher, M. Obesity: Global epidemiology and pathogenesis. *Nat. Rev. Endocrinol.* **2019**, *15*, 288–298. [CrossRef]
5. Yarborough, C.M., III; Brethauer, S.; Burton, W.N.; Fabius, R.J.; Hymel, P.; Kothari, S.; Roslin, M.S. ACOEM Guidance Statement: Obesity in the Workplace: Impact, Outcomes, and Recommendations. *J. Occup. Environ. Med.* **2018**, *60*, 97. [CrossRef]
6. Keum, N.; Greenwood, D.C.; Lee, D.H.; Kim, R.; Aune, D.; Ju, W.; Giovannucci, E.L. Adult weight gain and adiposity-related cancers: A dose-response meta-analysis of prospective observational studies. *J. Natl. Cancer Inst.* **2015**, *2015*, 107. [CrossRef]
7. Bjørge, T.; Häggström, C.; Ghaderi, S.; Nagel, G.; Manjer, J.; Tretli, S.; Ulmer, H.; Harlid, S.; Rosendahl, A.H.; Lang, A.H.; et al. BMI and weight changes and risk of obesity-related cancers: A pooled European cohort study. *Int. J. Epidemiol.* **2019**, *48*, 1872–1885. [CrossRef]
8. Poirier, P.; Eckel, R.H. Obesity and cardiovascular disease. *Curr. Atheroscler. Rep.* **2002**, *4*, 448–453. [CrossRef]
9. Bastien, M.; Poirier, P.; Lemieux, I.; Després, J.-P. Overview of Epidemiology and Contribution of Obesity to Cardiovascular Disease. *Prog. Cardiovasc. Dis.* **2013**, *56*, 369–381. [CrossRef]
10. Wilson, P.W.; D'Agostino, R.B.; Sullivan, L.; Parise, H.; Kannel, W.B. Overweight and obesity as determinants of cardiovascular risk: The Framingham experience. *Arch. Intern Med.* **2002**, *162*, 1867–1872. [CrossRef]
11. Bastard, J.-P.; Maachi, M.; Lagathu, C.; Kim, M.J.; Caron, M.; Vidal, H.; Capeau, J.; Feve, B. Recent advances in the relationship between obesity, inflammation, and insulin resistance. *Eur. Cytokine Netw.* **2006**, *17*, 4–12. [PubMed]

12. World Health Organization. Obesity and Overweight. 2016. Available online: https://www.who.int/mediacentre/factsheets/fs311/en/ (accessed on 1 July 2020).
13. Jaacks, L.M.; Vandevijvere, S.; Pan, A.; McGowan, C.; Wallace, C.; Imamura, F.; Mozaffarian, D.; Swinburn, B.; Ezzati, M. The obesity transition: Stages of the global epidemic. *Lancet Diabetes Endocrinol.* **2019**, *7*, 231–240. [CrossRef]
14. Chooi, Y.C.; Ding, C.; Magkos, F. The epidemiology of obesity. *Metabolism* **2019**, *92*, 6–10. [CrossRef] [PubMed]
15. Ryan, D.H.; Kahan, S. Guideline Recommendations for Obesity Management. *Med. Clin. N. Am.* **2018**, *102*, 49–63. [CrossRef] [PubMed]
16. Sorensen, G.; McLellan, D.L.; Sabbath, E.L.; Dennerlein, J.T.; Nagler, E.M.; Hurtado, D.A.; Pronk, N.P.; Wagner, G.R. Integrating worksite health protection and health promotion: A conceptual model for intervention and research. *Prev. Med.* **2016**, *91*, 188–196. [CrossRef] [PubMed]
17. Katz, D.; O'Connell, M.; Yeh, M.-C.; Nawaz, H.; Njike, V.; Anderson, L.M.; Cory, S.; Dietz, W. *Public Health Strategies for Preventing and Controlling Overweight and Obesity in School and Worksite Settings: A Report on Recommendations of the Task Force on Community Preventive Services*; Mortality and Morbidity Weekly Report; Department of Health and Human Services, Centers for Disease Control and Prevention: Atlanta, GA, USA, 2005. Available online: http://www.cdc.gov/mmwr/preview/mmwrhtml/rr5410a1.htm (accessed on 1 July 2020).
18. Beresford, S.A.; Thompson, B.; Feng, Z.; Christianson, A.; McLerran, D.; Patrick, D.L. Seattle 5 a Day Worksite Program to Increase Fruit and Vegetable Consumption. *Prev. Med.* **2001**, *32*, 230–238. [CrossRef]
19. Iii, C.M.Y.; Brethauer, S.; Burton, W.N.; Fabius, R.J.; Hymel, P.; Kothari, S.; Roslin, M.S. Obesity in the Workplace: Impact, Outcomes, and Recommendations. *J. Occup. Environ. Med.* **2018**, *60*, 97–107.
20. Lin, T.-C.; Courtney, T.; Lombardi, D.A.; Verma, S.K. Association between Sedentary Work and BMI in a U.S. National Longitudinal Survey. *Am. J. Prev. Med.* **2015**, *49*, e117–e123. [CrossRef]
21. Shields, M.; Tremblay, M.S. Sedentary behaviour and obesity. *Health Rep.* **2008**, *19*, 19.
22. Mitchell, J.A.; Bottai, M.; Park, Y.; Marshall, S.J.; Moore, S.C.; Matthews, C.E. A prospective study of sedentary behavior and changes in the body mass index distribution. *Med. Sci. Sports Exerc.* **2014**, *46*, 2244–2252. [CrossRef]
23. Kottwitz, M.U.; Grebner, S.I.; Semmer, N.K.; Tschan, F.; Elfering, A. Social Stress at Work and Change in Women's Body Weight. *Ind. Health* **2014**, *52*, 163–171. [CrossRef] [PubMed]
24. Bandalos, D.L.; Finney, S.J. *Exploratory and Confirmatory. The Reviewer's Guide to Quantitative Methods in the Social Sciences*; Routledge: New York, NY, USA, 2010; Volume 93.
25. Field, A. *Discovering Statistics Using IBM SPSS Statistics*; Sage Publications: Thousand Oaks, CA, USA, 2013.
26. Field, A.; Miles, J.; Field, Z. *Discovering Statistics Using R*; Sage Publications: Thousand Oaks, CA, USA, 2012.

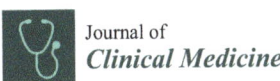 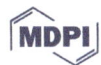

Article

Transversal Arch Clamping for Complete Resection of Aneurysms of the Distal Ascending Aorta without Open Anastomosis

Andreas Rukosujew [1,*,†], Arash Motekallemi [1,†], Konrad Wisniewski [1], Raluca Weber [1], Fernando De Torres-Alba [2], Abdulhakim Ibrahim [3], Raphael Weiss [4], Sven Martens [1] and Angelo Maria Dell'Aquila [1]

1 Department of Cardiothoracic Surgery, University Hospital Muenster, 48149 Münster, Germany; arash.motekallemi@ukmuenster.de (A.M.); konrad.wisniewski@ukmuenster.de (K.W.); raluca.weber@ukmuenster.de (R.W.); sven.martens@ukmuenster.de (S.M.); angelo.dellaquila@ukmuenster.de (A.M.D.)
2 Department of Cardiology, University Hospital Muenster, 48149 Münster, Germany; fernando.detorresalba@ukmuenster.de
3 Department of Vascular and Endovascular Surgery, University Hospital Münster, 48149 Münster, Germany; abdulhakim.ibrahim@ukmuenster.de
4 Department of Anesthesiology, Intensive Care Medicine and Pain Therapy, University Hospital Münster, 48149 Münster, Germany; raphael.weiss@ukmuenster.de
* Correspondence: andreas.rukosujew@ukmuenster.de; Tel.: +49-251-83-56111; Fax: +49-251-83-47469
† These authors contributed equally to this work.

Abstract: Background: The extent of aortic replacement for aneurysms of the distal ascending aorta remains controversial and opinions vary between standard cross-clamp resection and open hemiarch anastomosis in circulatory arrest and selective cerebral perfusion. As the deleterious effects of extended circulatory arrest are well-known, borderline indication for distal ascending aorta aneurysm repair must be outweighed against the potential risk of complications related to the open anastomosis. In the present study, we describe our own approach consisting of "transversal arch clamping" for exhaustive resection of aneurysms of the distal ascending aorta without open anastomosis and we present the postoperative outcomes. Methods: Between May 2017 and December 2019, 35 patients with aneurysm of the ascending aorta (20 male, 15 female) underwent replacement with repair of the lesser curvature without circulatory arrest. Pre-operative, intraoperative, and postoperative clinical outcomes were retrospectively withdrawn from our institutional database and analyzed. Results: Maximal diameter of distal ascending aorta was 47.5 mm. Patient median age was 66 years (IQR 14) (range 42–86). Preoperative logistic median EuroSCORE II was 17% (IQR 11.3). Median duration of cardiopulmonary bypass and cardiac arrest were 137 (IQR 64) and 93 (IQR 59) min, respectively. In-hospital and 30-day mortality were 0%. There were no cases with acute low output syndrome, surgical re-exploration for bleeding, kidney injury requiring dialysis, or wound infection. Disabling stroke was observed in one patient (2.9%). There was one case of major ventricular arrhythmia (2.9%). Conclusions: Our institutional experience suggests that this novel technique is safe and feasible. It facilitates complete resection of the aortic ascending aneurysm avoiding circulatory arrest, antegrade cerebral perfusion, additional peripheral cannulation, and all related complications.

Keywords: ascending aorta aneurysm; aortic replacement; technique of distal anastomosis

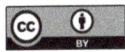

1. Introduction

Regarding current evidence, the extent of aortic replacement in borderline aneurysms of the distal ascending aorta remains controversial and opinions vary between standard cross-clamp aortic resection and open hemiarch anastomosis in hypothermic circulatory arrest [1–3]. During the so-called "conventional" ascending aorta replacement, approximately 2 cm of the distal aorta ascendens may remain unresected without open anastomosis technique. This could lead to a certain degree of diameter mismatch between graft and proximal arch. As a consequence, the remaining aneurysmatic tissue may predispose patients to a further arch dilatation with aneurysm formation on the long run. On the other hand, "open" distal anastomosis and hemiarch reconstruction in hypothermic circulatory arrest (HCA) allows a more complete resection of aneurysmatic tissue [3–5]. However, the use of HCA results in prolonged extracorporeal circulation with potential end organ ischemia. In addition, this procedure requires a peripheral arterial cannulation that can potentially cause further related complications.

There are several surgical techniques concerning distal anastomosis for the resection of the ascending aorta aneurysms with or without HCA [1,6,7]. At our institution, we developed a new approach of transversal arch clamping with closed distal anastomosis for avoiding circulatory arrest, antegrade cerebral perfusion, and additional peripheral cannulation while allowing a more complete resection of aneurysmatic tissue.

In this study, we present our technique and discuss our institutional experience and outcomes in patients with borderline indication for aneurysms of the distal ascending aorta. Moreover, we retrospectively analyzed aortic diameter size of the resected aneurysmatic aorta in order to identify a potential reference value for the application of our institutional method.

2. Patients and Methods

Local ethics committee approval was granted for the collection of patient data as well as follow up (approval number 2020-076-f-S). The present study includes 35 patients between May 2017 and December 2019 who underwent an elective replacement of an ascending aorta aneurysm with our institutional method of transversal arch clamping. The preoperative workup included either computed tomography angiography (CTA), echocardiography, or coronary angiography (in patients older than 50 years). The indication for surgical aortic replacement was according to the 2014 ESC Guidelines [8]. The decision whether patients were suitable for "transversal arch clamping" was made intraoperatively, based on surgical assessment and the extent of aneurysm reaching into the aortic arch. All baseline data of patients, including ascending aorta diameter, aortic valve characteristics, and major comorbidities are presented in Table 1.

Table 1. Demographic patient data.

Preoperative Variables	Median/N	IQR/%
Age (years)	66	14
Sex (female)	15	43%
BMI	29	5
History of stroke	14	40%
Diabetes mellitus	3	8.6%
Dyslipidemia	13	37.1%
Arterial hypertension	28	80%
Peripheral vascular disease	1	2.9%
Cerebrovascular disease	2	5.7%
Abdominal aortic aneurysm	1	2.9%
COPD	7	20%
Preoperative history of stroke	3	8.6%
NYHA	1.8	1
Creatinine peak (mg/dL)	1.0	0.3
Hemoglobin (g/dL)	13.9	2.6
Atrial fibrillation	7	20%
Aortic diameter (mm)	57	7
Bicuspid aortic valve	18	51%
Redo	2	5.7%
EuroSCORE II	8.7	2.5

IBM SPSS Statistics for Windows, Version 22 (IBM Corp, Armonk, NY, USA) was used for statistical analysis. A Kolmogorow–Smirnow test with Lilliefors correction was applied across the data and revealed a normal distribution of data regarding aortic diameter (K = 0.19635, p = 0.05217). Median was used presenting the variables.

2.1. Surgical Technique

NIRS control with left radial and femoral pressure monitoring was applied during all procedures. Cardiopulmonary bypass was established using arterial cannulation of the distal aortic arch directly below the left subclavian artery and venous cannulation of the right atrium. In most cases, Seldinger technique with echocardiographic control of the wire position in the aorta descendens was used for arterial cannulation. In our opinion based on our institutional experience, in this way, the cannula can be safely introduced at an acute angle in the descending aorta facilitating cannulation. Without Seldinger technique there is the risk of potential aortic dissection due to tangential introduction of the cannula. Myocardial protection is achieved either by retrograde cold blood cardioplegia in case of full median sternotomy or, in case of L-shaped partial upper sternotomy, initially anterograde through the aortic wall followed by selective cannulation of coronary ostia. Figure 1 demonstrates our institutional approach step by step.

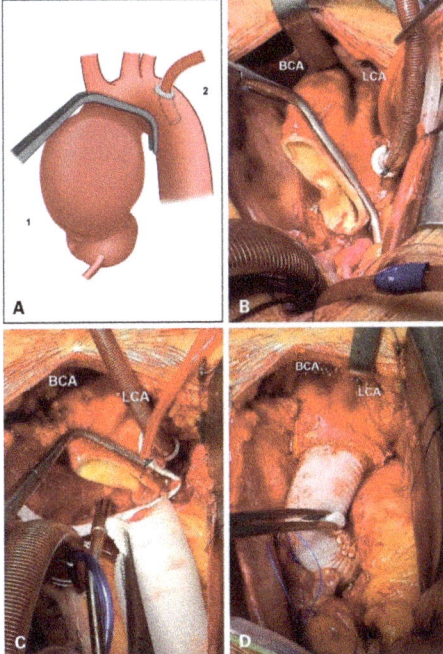

Figure 1. Stepwise approach of our institutional method of transversal arch clamping. (**A**) A schematic picture of the Satinsky clamp placement in relation to ascending aneurysm (1) and the position of the aortic cannula (2). (**B**) Intraoperative view showing complete resection of ascending aortic aneurysm. (**C**) Display of the Satinsky clamp for the "transversal arch clamping". (**D**) A picture after the completion of ascending aorta replacement and repair of the lesser curvature of the aortic arch. BCA: brachiocephalic artery; LCA: left carotid artery.

First, a conventional clamping is performed proximal to the brachiocephalic artery (BCA) (Figure 1A). Second, in cardiac arrest, aneurysmatic tissue is resected right below the clamp (at the level of the BCA) and at the sinotubular junction (STJ). Once the ascending aorta has been trimmed, the aortic arch should be mobilized dorsally by separating the aorta from the periaortic tissue. In this regard, it is of utmost importance to extend the distal preparation exposing zone 3 of the aorta. At this point, the Satinsky clamp can be safely placed in order to expose the lesser curvature for removal. This maneuver enables complete mobilization of the aortic arch under visual control. Third, a Satinsky clamp is then (under low-flow cardiopulmonary bypass) placed distal to the first clamp at the outflow of the brachiocephalic artery and transversal to the aortic arch allowing maximal removal of the lesser curvature (Figure 1B,C). Prosthesis size is determined according to the diameter of the sinotubular junction in case of a supracoronary replacement or to conduit size when aortic root is replaced. The selected prosthesis is trimmed and tailored for distal anastomosis leaving a prosthesis bevel for accommodation to the lesser curvature. After proximal arch resection the distal anastomosis is carried out by means of continuous 4-0 polypropylene suture using a periaortic Teflon felt strip. The proximal anastomosis was then tailored according to the necessity of concomitant procedures (i.e., composite graft implantation, aortic root reconstruction). BioGlue® (CryoLife, Inc., Kennesaw, GA, USA) was applied for sealing of the suture line (Figure 1D).

2.2. Retrospective Biplanar Measurement

In order to identify a potential reference value for the application of our institutional method regarding suitable aneurysmatic diameter at the different levels of the ascending aorta we retrospectively performed biplanar measurement. CT angiography scans were reconstructed automatically using Aquarius iNtuition (TeraRecon Inc., Foster City, CA, USA).

Based on ECG-gated computed tomography angiograms (CTAs) biplanar measurements at the level of the sinotubular junction (STJ) and immediately proximal to the origin of the brachiocephalic artery (BCA), the supposed position of the clamp, have been performed. Exemplary biplanar measurement with automated 3D reconstruction is displayed in Figure 2. According to the data, a suggested reference value for suitable diameter size of the respected levels of aneurysmatic aorta for the application of our institutional method of transversal arch clamping was evaluated.

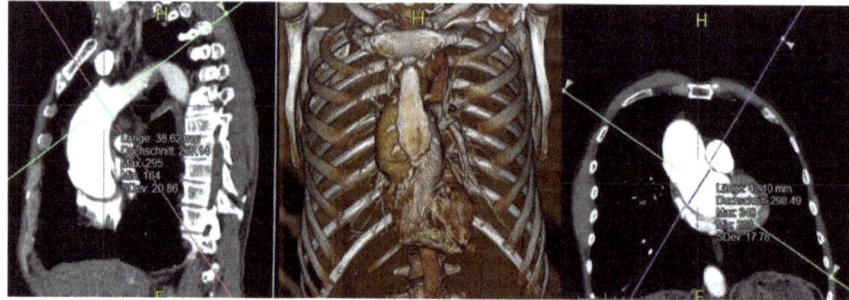

Figure 2. Exemplary biplanar measurement with automated 3D reconstruction using Aquarius iNtuition.

3. Results

Patient median age was 66 years (IQR 14) (range 42–86). Patient demographics and concomitant procedures are summarized in Table 1. The median diameter of the ascending aorta was 57 mm (IQR 7) (range 50–72 mm). Half of the patients (51%) had a bicuspid aortic valve. Preoperative EuroSCORE II was 8.7 (IQR 2.5).

The median duration of surgery, CPB time and cross clamp time were 232, 137, and 93 min, respectively. Mild hypothermia was applied in all cases with average nadir temperature about 32 °C. Concomitant CABG procedure took place in 10 (28.6%) patients. Additional Bentall operation, partial Yacoub procedure, and Wheat procedure were performed in 14 (40.0%), 5 (14.3%), and 3 (8.6%) patients of the study group, respectively. Minimally invasive approach through L-shaped partial upper sternotomy was performed in 8 (22.9%) patients. Intraoperative data and concomitant procedures are summarized in Table 2.

Table 2. Intraoperative data and concomitant procedures.

Operative Variables	Median/N	IQR/%
Duration of surgery (min.)	232	99
CPB time (min.)	137	64
Cross clamp time (min.)	93	59
Nadir temperature (min.)	32	1
Concomitant CABG	10	28.6%
Bentall operation	14	40.0%
Partial Yacoub procedure	5	14.3%
Wheat procedure	2	5.7%
Partial upper sternotomy	8	22.9%

The postoperative results are shown in Table 3. There were neither in-hospital nor 30-day mortality cases. The length of ICU and IMC stay was 2.8 (IQR 2.5) days, the median mechanical ventilation time lasted 9.4 (IQR 3) h. The mean amount of blood loss was 724 (IQR 320) mL and none of the patients required a re-exploration for revision. One patient (2.9%) had a postoperative stroke with residual hemiparesis at discharge. Delirium requiring drug treatment was reported in nine patients (27.7%) There was no postoperative kidney injury requiring dialysis. In one patient with postoperative creatinine value of 2.6 mg/dL the renal function was restored due to medical treatment and volume management. Deep wound infections were not observed. In 19 out of 35 patients, CTA based, biplanar measurements of the sinotubular junction (STJ) and the base of the brachiocephalic artery (the designated clamping site) were analyzed retrospectively in order to objectify the surgeon's "instinct" and identify a potential reference size (regarding suitable diameter) for the application of this technique.

Table 3. Postoperative outcomes.

Postoperative Variables	Median/N	IQR/%
Hospital stay (d)	10	2.5
In-hospital mortality	0	0%
30-day mortality	0	0%
Length of ICU/IMC stay (d)	2.8	2.5
Duration of mechanical ventilation (h)	9.4	3
Tracheostomy	0	0%
Low output syndrome	0	0%
Surgical re-exploration for bleeding	0	0%
Drainage loss (mL)	724	320
CPR	1	2.9%
Disabling stroke	1	2.9%
Delirium	9	27.7%
Dialysis	0	0%
Creatinine peak mg/dL	0.9	0.4
Wound/sternal infection	0	0%
NYHA	1.6	1

The missing CTAs are due to the following reasons: In ten patients with bicuspid valve and dilatated aorta echocardiography was used for indication. In two patients, indication was based on aortography due to concomitant CABG procedure. In four patients the decision was made intraoperatively without additional preoperative imaging. Using Aquarius iNtuition® for biplanar measurement the median diameter of the STJ and BCA origin (designated clamping site) were 45.7 mm (range: 24.5–57 mm) and 40.9 mm (range: 35.7–47.5 mm), respectively.

4. Discussion

To date, there is no consensus regarding the optimal surgical approach for borderline aneurysms of the distal ascending aorta. Although open hemiarch anastomosis requiring initial peripheral cannulation and HCA is necessary for the treatment of type A aortic dissection, the same approach seems exaggerated for the purpose of extensive repair of borderline aneurysms of the distal ascending aorta, even if parts of the aortic arch are involved. However, several retrospective studies [9,10] have shown that the open hemiarch approach is a similarly safe method and does not increase the risk for cardiac, neurological, pulmonary, or hemorrhagic complications in the immediate postoperative period. On the other hand, no prospective studies are available. We know from our own experience that aortic surgery with HCA is not an "easy walk" and contains a potential risk of coagulation disorder with postoperative bleeding as well as potential cerebral injury as a result of air embolism, insufficient perfusion, or other potential complications like ischemia of the abdominal organs or extremities. Furthermore, the extrathoracic arterial cannulation itself via right axillary artery and/or femoral artery carries the risk for associated complications such as brachial plexus injury, ischemia, bleeding, and lymphatic fistula.

In our opinion, the above-mentioned potential risks for the treatment of borderline aneurysms of the distal ascending aorta do not justify a rigid application for aneurysms of the distal ascending aorta. Rather, a tailored approach seems to be indicated as it enables to maximize resection of aneurysmatic tissue—even in cases with aortic arch involvement.

Our institutional approach claims to achieve both, balancing exhaustive resection of aneurysmatic tissue while preventing additional damage. In our setting, despite the double clamping of the aorta (first, in a conventional manner and then transversally—see Figure 1), the surgeon can achieve a more exhaustive resection and thus reduce the associated risks of undissected aneurysmatic tissue. This is reached through the maneuver of clamp replacement under visual control through mobilization of the dorsal wall of the aortic arch. This allows the application of the Satinsky clamp without multiple attempts and thus avoids possible iatrogenic aortic wall injury.

In our institutional experience, this technique can be applied safely in the majority of patients with borderline aneurysms. However, one must consider that any multiple replacements of the clamp could lead to potential plaque loosing or rupture. It is self-explanatory that this should be avoided in patients with sclerotic distal ascending aortas or visible (via sonography) or manual palpation at the intended clamping site.

In our patient population, there was no bleeding at the distal anastomosis region as a result of the suture penetration due to aortic tension during clamping. The application of the transversal arch clamping generally did not result in a deviation from the initial surgical plan. In our opinion, this is due to the accurate preoperative planning. Moreover, our outcomes suggest that this method does not increase the risk for additional neurological deficits, strokes, or an increase in cardiac or non-cardiac associated death.

We also believe that our technique with formation of a "prosthesis bevel" for repair of the lesser curvature of the aortic arch stabilizes the aortic arch and thus prevents the formation of new aneurysms, even if performed in an open manner.

Another benefit of this approach might be the prevention of hypothermic circulatory arrest enabling even the "lesser experienced" surgeon to reach maximized resection of all aneurysmatic tissue in even more complex cases of borderline aneurysms of the distal ascending aorta. This enables low volume centers to reach better outcomes. We have identified some limitations of our study, which are mainly expressed by the retrospective design and the lack of a control group. We aimed to reduce the subjective assessment of the surgeon by identifying a potential reference value for the application of our institutional method regarding suitable aneurysmatic diameter at the different levels of the ascending aorta through biplanar measurement.

Our data suggests that up to an aortic diameter of 47.5 mm at the BCA origin designated clamping site our method of transversal arch clamping can safely be applied.

Routinely implemented biplanar measurement might become a standardized approach for the assessment of aneurysmatic aneurysms to identify suitable candidates for this approach.

5. Conclusions

Transversal arch clamping of aneurysms of the distal ascending aorta (reaching into the aortic arch) seems to be a safe and feasible method in order to achieve maximized resection of aneurysmatic tissue. Waiving the disadvantages of hypothermic circulatory arrest with antegrade cerebral perfusion and potential risks of peripheral cannulation may qualify this approach to become a standard approach in low volume centers and for less experienced surgeons.

Author Contributions: Conceptualization, A.R., A.M., S.M. and A.M.D.; methodology, A.R., A.M., K.W., A.I., S.M. and A.M.D.; software, A.M., K.W., F.D.T.-A. and A.I.; validation, A.R., A.M., S.M. and A.M.D.; formal analysis, A.R., A.M., K.W., A.I. and A.M.D.; investigation, A.R., A.M. and R.W. (Raphael Weiss); resources, A.R., A.M., R.W. (Raluca Weber), F.D.T.-A., A.I., R.W. (Raphael Weiss), S.M. and A.M.D.; data curation, A.R., A.M., K.W., R.W. (Raluca Weber), A.I. and R.W. (Raphael Weiss); writing—original draft preparation, A.R., A.M. and A.M.D.; writing—review and editing, A.R., A.M., K.W., S.M. and A.M.D.; visualization, A.R., A.M., K.W. and F.D.T.-A.; supervision, A.R., F.D.T.-A., S.M. and A.M.D.; project administration, A.R., A.M. and A.M.D.; funding acquisition, S.M. All authors have read and agreed to the published version of the manuscript.

Funding: This research received no external funding.

Institutional Review Board Statement: Local ethics committee (Ethik-Kommission der Ärztekammer Westfalen-Lippe und der Westfälischen Wilhelms-Universität) approval was granted for the collection of patient data as well as follow up (approval number 2020-076-f-S, approved on 17 May 2020).

Data Availability Statement: Raw data were generated at the Department of Cardiothoracic Surgery, University Hospital Muenster, Muenster, Germany. Derived data supporting the findings of this study are available from the corresponding author Andreas Rukosujew on request.

Conflicts of Interest: The authors declare no conflict of interest.

References

1. Amulraj, E.A.; Kent, W.D.T.; Malaisrie, S.C. Aortoplasty for management of the dilated distal ascending aorta during proximal aortic reconstruction. *Ann. Thorac. Surg.* **2013**, *96*, 1499–1501. [CrossRef] [PubMed]
2. Lentini, S.; Specchia, L.; Nicolardi, S.; Mangia, F.; Rasovic, O.; Di Eusanio, G.; Gregorini, R. Surgery of the Ascending Aorta with or without Combined Procedures through an Upper Ministernotomy: Outcomes of a Series of More Than 100 Patients. *Ann. Thorac. Cardiovasc. Surg.* **2016**, *22*, 44–48. [CrossRef] [PubMed]
3. Singh, R.; Yamanaka, K.; Reece, T.B. Hemiarch: The Real Operation for Ascending Aortic Aneurysm. *Semin. Cardiothorac. Vasc. Anesth.* **2016**, *20*, 303–306. [CrossRef] [PubMed]
4. Kaplan, M.; Temur, B.; Can, T.; Abay, G.; Olsun, A.; Aydogan, H. Open distal anastomosis technique for ascending aortic aneurysm repair without cerebral perfusion. *Heart Surg. Forum* **2015**, *18*, E124–E128. [CrossRef] [PubMed]
5. Sultan, I.; Bianco, V.; Yazji, I.; Kilic, A.; Dufendach, K.; Cardounel, A.; Althouse, A.D.; Masri, A.; Navid, F.; Gleason, T.G. Hemiarch Reconstruction Versus Clamped Aortic Anastomosis for Concomitant Ascending Aortic Aneurysm. *Ann. Thorac. Surg.* **2018**, *106*, 750–756. [CrossRef] [PubMed]
6. Higuchi, K.; Koseni, K.; Takamoto, S. Graft insertion technique for distal anastomosis in cases of ascending aortic aneurysm. *J. Cardiovasc. Surg.* **2005**, *46*, 537–538.
7. Kim, T.Y.; Kim, K.H. Dual inflow without circulatory arrest for hemiarch replacement. *J. Cardiothorac. Surg.* **2019**, *14*, 9. [CrossRef] [PubMed]
8. Erbel, R.; Aboyans, V.; Boileau, C.; Bossone, E.; di Bartolomeo, R.; Eggebrecht, H.; Evangelista, A.; Falk, V.; Frank, H.; Gaemperli, O.; et al. 2014 ESC Guidelines on the diagnosis and treatment of aortic diseases: Document covering acute and chronic aortic diseases of the thoracic and abdominal aorta of the adult. The Task Force for the Diagnosis and Treatment of Aortic Diseases of the European Society of Cardiology (ESC). *Eur. Heart J.* **2014**, *35*, 2873–2926. [PubMed]
9. Malaisrie, S.C.; Duncan, B.F.; Mehta, C.K.; Badiwala, M.V.; Rinewalt, D.; Kruse, J.; Li, Z.; Andrei, A.C.; McCarthy, P.M. The addition of hemiarch replacement to aortic root surgery does not affect safety. *J. Thorac. Cardiovasc. Surg.* **2015**, *150*, 118–124. [CrossRef] [PubMed]
10. Kozlov, B.N.; Panfilov, D.S.; Zherbakhanov, A.V.; Khodashinsky, I.A.; Sonduev, E.L. Early results of various surgical approaches in reconstruction of ascending aortic aneurysms. *Angiol. Sosud. Khir.* **2019**, *25*, 101–106. [CrossRef] [PubMed]

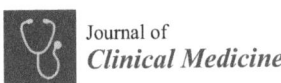

Article

Prognostic Impact of Hybrid Comprehensive Telerehabilitation Regarding Diastolic Dysfunction in Patients with Heart Failure with Reduced Ejection Fraction—Subanalysis of the TELEREH-HF Randomized Clinical Trial

Robert Irzmański [1,†], Renata Glowczynska [2,*,†], Maciej Banach [3], Dominika Szalewska [4], Ryszard Piotrowicz [5,6], Ilona Kowalik [5], Michael J. Pencina [7], Wojciech Zareba [8], Piotr Orzechowski [9], Slawomir Pluta [10], Zbigniew Kalarus [10], Grzegorz Opolski [2] and Ewa Piotrowicz [9]

Citation: Irzmański, R.; Glowczynska, R.; Banach, M.; Szalewska, D.; Piotrowicz, R.; Kowalik, I.; Pencina, M.J.; Zareba, W.; Orzechowski, P.; Pluta, S.; et al. Prognostic Impact of Hybrid Comprehensive Telerehabilitation Regarding Diastolic Dysfunction in Patients with Heart Failure with Reduced Ejection Fraction—Subanalysis of the TELEREH-HF Randomized Clinical Trial. J. Clin. Med. 2022, 11, 1844. https://doi.org/10.3390/jcm11071844

Academic Editors: Patrick De Boever and Renato Pietro Ricci

Received: 2 March 2022
Accepted: 22 March 2022
Published: 26 March 2022

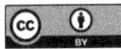

Copyright: © 2022 by the authors. Licensee MDPI, Basel, Switzerland. This article is an open access article distributed under the terms and conditions of the Creative Commons Attribution (CC BY) license (https://creativecommons.org/licenses/by/4.0/).

1. Department of Internal Medicine and Cardiac Rehabilitation, Medical University of Łódź, 90-647 Lodz, Poland; robert.irzmanski@umed.lodz.pl
2. 1st Chair and Department of Cardiology, Medical University of Warsaw, 02-097 Warsaw, Poland; grzegorz.opolski@wum.edu.pl
3. Department of Hypertension, Medical University of Łódź, 90-647 Lodz, Poland; maciej.banach@umed.lodz.pl
4. Clinic of Rehabilitation Medicine, Faculty of Health Sciences, Medical University of Gdańsk, 80-210 Gdańsk, Poland; dominika.szalewska@gumed.edu.pl
5. National Institute of Cardiology, 04-628 Warsaw, Poland; rpiotrowicz@ikard.pl (R.P.); ikowalik@ikard.pl (I.K.)
6. Warsaw Academy of Medical Rehabilitation, 01-234 Warsaw, Poland
7. The Department of Biostatistics and Bioinformatics, Duke University School of Medicine, Durham, NC 27710, USA; michal.pencina@duke.edu
8. Cardiology Unit of the Department of Medicine, University of Rochester Medical Center, Rochester, NY 14642, USA; wojciech_zareba@urmc.rochester.edu
9. Telecardiology Center, National Institute of Cardiology, 04-628 Warsaw, Poland; porzechowski@ikard.pl (P.O.); epiotrowicz@ikard.pl (E.P.)
10. Department of Cardiology, Congenital Heart Diseases and Electrotherapy, Silesian Center for Heart Diseases, Silesian Medical University, 41-800 Zabrze, Poland; spluta77@gmail.com (S.P.); zbigniewkalarus@kalmet.com.pl (Z.K.)

* Correspondence: renata.glowczynska@wum.edu.pl
† These authors contributed equally to this work.

Abstract: Aims: The objective of the study was to evaluate the effects of individually prescribed hybrid comprehensive telerehabilitation (HCTR) implemented at patients' homes on left ventricular (LV) diastolic function in heart failure (HF) patients. Methods and results: The Telerehabilitation in Heart Failure Patients trial (TELEREH-HF) is a multicenter, prospective, randomized (1:1), open-label, parallel-group, controlled trial involving HF patients assigned either to HCTR involving a remotely monitored home training program in conjunction with usual care (HCTR group) or usual care only (UC group). The patient in the HCTR group underwent a 9-week HCTR program consisting of two stages: an initial stage (1 week) conducted in hospital and the subsequent stage (eight weeks) of home-based HCTR five times weekly. Due to difficulties of proper assessment and differences in the evaluation of diastolic function in patients with atrial fibrillation, we included in our subanalysis only patients with sinus rhythm. Depending on the grade of diastolic dysfunction, patients were assigned to subgroups with mild diastolic (MDD) or severe diastolic dysfunction (SDD), both in HCTR (HCTR-MDD and HCTR-SDD) and UC groups (UC-MDD and UC-SDD). Changes from baseline to 9 weeks in echocardiographic parameters were seen only in A velocities in HCTR-MDD vs. UC-MDD; no significant shifts between groups of different diastolic dysfunction grades were observed after HCTR. All-cause mortality was higher in UC-SDD vs. UC-MDD with no difference between HCTR-SDD and HCTR-MDD. Higher probability of HF hospitalization was observed in HCTR-SDD than HCTR-MDD and in UC-SDD than UC-MDD. No differences in the probability of cardiovascular mortality and hospitalization were found. Conclusions: HCTR did not influence diastolic function in HF patients in a significant manner. The grade of diastolic dysfunction had an impact on mortality only in the UC group and HF hospitalization over a 12–24 month follow-up in HCTR and UC groups.

Keywords: hybrid telerehabilitation; heart failure with reduced ejection fraction; diastolic function

1. Introduction

Heart failure (HF) is a major challenge in modern healthcare and is increasing with the aging of the population. The pathophysiology in HF is determined by altered cardiac output, reduced cardiac contractility, myocardial stiffness, increased filling pressure of LV and diastolic dysfunction [1]. Diastolic HF has been found to occur in more than 50% of patients with systolic HF [2,3]. The diastolic phase becomes shorter, which exacerbates the pre-existing impairment of left ventricular (LV) filling. Thus, diastolic irregularities lead to elevated pressure in the pulmonary circulation, causing shortness of breath [4]. Diastolic dysfunction is usually accompanying systolic dysfunction. Echocardiography is a key imaging method for the evaluation of diastolic function. Echocardiographic estimation of LV filling pressure can be drawn from algorithms accounting for Doppler velocities at the mitral valve, tissue Doppler imaging techniques and data of left atrium size [5,6].

There is a need for echocardiographic evaluation in all patients with HF in the qualification process for cardiac rehabilitation.

The most typical clinical symptoms reported by the patients are dyspnea and low exercise tolerance (fatigue and weakness upon exertion). Exercise dyspnea is also the earliest clinical manifestation in patients with diastolic HF, as tachycardia upon exertion triggers the pathomechanism of dyspnea. Thus, it is interesting to determine if cardiac rehabilitation can influence diastolic dysfunction in HF patients. HF is associated with progressive exercise intolerance. According to the 2020 Sports Cardiology ESC guidelines, exercise-based cardiac rehabilitation is recommended in all stable individuals with HF [7] to improve exercise capacity, quality of life, and to reduce the risk of the rehospitalization [8]. Because of the high mortality associated with chronic heart failure [9], there is need for wider implementation of evidence-based management.

The Telerehabilitation in Heart Failure Patients trial (TELEREH-HF) study [10,11] is the largest prospective, multicenter, and randomized clinical trial to date that assessed a 9-week hybrid comprehensive telerehabilitation (HCTR) compared to usual care (UC) in HF patients, and had the data regarding diastolic dysfunction in HF with reduced ejection fraction.

The TELEREH-HF trial supported the statement that telemedicine may offer a novel model of organization and HCTR may facilitate the implementation of the comprehensive management of HF patients. TELEREH proved that telerehabilitation is well accepted, safe, and effective with high adherence in HF patients. Our trial confirmed that HCTR improved quality of life in HF patients.

There are scarce data regarding the prognostic impact of diastolic dysfunction in HF patients, participating or not in cardiac telerehabilitation. What is more, HCTR is an attractive option for HF treatment during the COVID-19 pandemic.

Research Objectives

The objective of the study was to evaluate the effects of individually prescribed HCTR on left ventricular diastolic function in HF patients. We focused on the impact of HCTR regarding the severity of diastolic dysfunction, mild versus severe. We assessed the survival probability depending on discrepancies in left ventricular diastolic function.

2. Methods

TELEREH-HF is a multicenter, prospective, randomized (1:1), open-label, parallel-group, controlled trial involving patients with HF assigned either to the HCTR program in conjunction with UC (HCTR group) or UC only (UC group). Patients were qualified for the TELEREH-HF study (ClinicalTrials.gov NCT 02523560) with New York Heart Association (NYHA) class I, II or III HF with LV ejection fraction (LVEF) 40% or less after hospitalization due to worsening of HF within 6 months prior to randomization. The aim of the study was to determine whether the potential improvement in functional outcomes and quality of life after a 9-week training period improves clinical outcomes during an extended follow-up of 12 to 24 months.

The study was performed in accordance with the Helsinki Declaration and Polish legal regulations. Each patient gave informed consent. The study was approved by the Bioethics Committee at the National Institute of Cardiology in Warsaw. Patient data were verified by an independent Data Security Monitoring Council. The task of the Clinical Endpoint Committee, without knowledge of randomization, was to review hospitalizations and deaths.

The inclusion and exclusion criteria are presented elsewhere in design documents [10,11]. In the presented subanalysis, only patients with sinus rhythm were qualified. A patient in the HCTR group underwent a 9-week HCTR program with two stages: the first stage (1 week) was conducted in the hospital and the next stage (8 weeks) of HCTR was conducted at home 5 times a week. The telerehabilitation program includes three training ranges: aerobic endurance training, Nordic walking, breathing muscles training, exercises with light resistance and strength exercises.

2.1. Echocardiography Assessment

Echocardiography exams were performed by experienced echocardiographists on different echo machines on each site (GE Vivid 6, GE Vivid 4, Philips Epiq 8, Acuson CV70). Diameters of heart chambers were measured on long axis view, while left atrium volume was assessed in four-chamber apical view. The LVEF was determined by biplane Simpson's method. Mitral inflow was evaluated by PW Doppler sample volume between mitral leaflet tips.

Mitral inflow was assessed by measurement of: early diastolic mitral inflow velocity (E wave), late diastolic mitral inflow velocity (A wave), deceleration time of E wave (DTE), and E/A ratio. On pulsed-wave tissue Doppler imaging, annular E' velocity was measured on medial wall (E' med.) and lateral wall of left ventricle (E' lat). E velocity divided by mitral annular E' velocity was calculated at medial wall (E/E' med) and lateral wall (E/E' lat), and then average value was calculated (E/E' avg). Jet velocity of tricuspid regurgitation (TR) was calculated on continues wave Doppler. Normal mitral inflow was determined as both E/A $\leq$ 0.8 and E $\leq$ 50 cm/s. When mitral inflow shows an E/A $\leq$ 0.8 but the peak E velocity is >50 cm/sec, or if the E/A ratio is >0.8 but <2, other signals are necessary for accurate evaluation. Due to the lack of measurement of left atrium volume, we used only 2 criteria: TR jet peak velocity by color Doppler and average E/E' ratio.

To determine diastolic dysfunction, we used algorithm for estimation of LV filling pressures and grading LV diastolic function in patients with HFrEF recommended by the American Society of Echocardiography and the European Association of Cardiovascular Imaging [5]. We excluded patients with AF because of differences of assessment of diastolic function in case of AF (altered pattern of mitral inflow, lack of A wave, variability in cycle length, common occurrence of LA enlargement regardless of filling pressures). I grade diastolic dysfunction with normal left atrium pressure was called as mild diastolic dysfunction (MDD). Severe diastolic dysfunction was defined as characterized by increased left atrium pressure, and so it consisted of both grade II and III dysfunction.

Thus, regarding grade of diastolic dysfunction, patients assigned to HCTR group were divided into HCTR-MDD and HCTR-SDD. Analogically, among patients from UC care, there were UC-MDD and UC-SDD subgroups.

Patients were followed during 14–26 months after for all-cause mortality, cardiovascular (CV) mortality, all-cause mortality, CV hospitalizations, HF hospitalizations, and composite points previously listed.

2.2. Statistical Analyses

Results are reported as numbers and percentages for categorical variables, or means ± SD (baseline characteristic) or means and 95% confidence intervals (difference between 9-week value and baseline) for continuous variables. Comparisons between groups on baseline characteristics were performed by the chi-square test of independence or the Fisher exact test (when the number of expected events was less than 5), the Cochran Mantel-Haenszel test, or Student's *t*-test (or Satterthwaite method), respectively. Differences in change over time between groups were compared using a correction of variance analysis for baseline measurement level and body surface area, hypertension, loop diuretics, and NYHA class. Interactions between groups and diastolic dysfunction were studied. The rate of events (all-cause mortality, all-cause hospitalization, cardiovascular mortality, and cardiovascular hospitalization) was estimated using Kaplan–Meier curves and made using the log-rank test with the Tukey–Kramer correction for multiple comparisons. Two-sided $p < 0.05$ was considered statistically significant. The analyses were made using SAS statistical software version 9.4 (SAS Institute, Inc., Cary, NC, USA).

3. Results

Between the beginning of June 2015 and the end of June 2017, we randomized 850 eligible patients in a 1:1 ratio to either a HCTR plus usual care group (HCTR group) or a usual care only (UC group).

Among enrolled patients, sinus rhythm necessary for proper assessment of diastolic function was present in 512 patients. Echocardiography was performed twice before and after intervention (HCTR group) or observation (UC group) in 472 patients. The study flow diagram is shown in Figure 1.

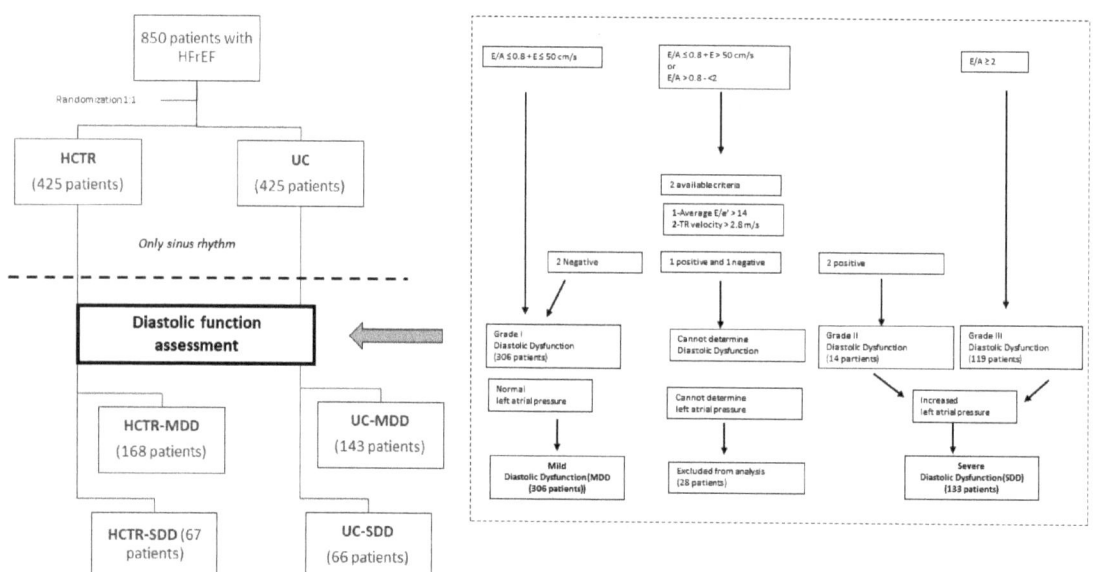

Figure 1. Study flow with algorithm for estimation of LV filling pressures and grading LV diastolic function in patients with HFrEF.

Normal mitral inflow was found in 329 patients. First grade and mild diastolic dysfunction was found in 306 patients. Second grade diastolic dysfunction was present in 14 patients, when the restrictive pattern of mitral inflow with $E/A \geq 2$ in 119 patients. Severe diastolic dysfunction was diagnosed in 119 patients. It was impossible to determine left atrial pressure and diastolic dysfunction in 28 patients.

Among patients assigned to the HCTR group with sinus rhythm, 168 patients had mild diastolic dysfunction (HCTR-MDD) and 67 patients had severe diastolic dysfunction (HCTR-SDD). Among patients assigned to the UC group with sinus rhythm, 143 patients had mild diastolic dysfunction (UC-MDD) and 66 patients had severe diastolic dysfunction (UC-SDD). On Figure 1, diastolic dysfunction criteria and groups are presented.

The study groups HCTR and UC did not significantly differ in terms of baseline clinical parameters, demographic data, and treatment, except for a higher prevalence of hypertension and more frequent use of loop diuretics in UC-SDD than in HCTR-SDD. Moreover, patients in the UC-MDD and HCTR-MDD groups differed in NYHA classes and body surface area. The baseline characteristics of the cohort at randomization are presented in Table 1. Echocardiographic parameters at randomization are listed in Table 2. There were only differences between HCTR-MDD and UC-MDD in DTE parameters at baseline.

Table 1. Baseline characteristics.

	MDD (n = 311)			SDD (n = 133)		
	HCTR-MDD n = 168	UC-MDD n = 143	$p1$	HCTR-SDD n = 67	UC-SDD n = 66	$p2$
Males. n (%)	151 (89.9)	131 (91.6)	0.602	59 (88.1)	57 (86.4)	0.770
Age (years). mean ± SD	60.9 ± 10.8	60.9 ± 10.3	0.977	62.3 ± 13.6	62.6 ± 10.2	0.911
Left Ventricular Ejection Fraction (%). mean ± SD	32.7 ± 6.2	32.2 ± 6.7	0.552	27.8 ± 6.3	27.7 ± 7.4	0.931
BSA (m^2)	2.01 ± 0.22	2.06 ± 0.21	0.038	1.93 ± 0.20	1.96 ± 0.20	0.419
Etiology of heart failure. n (%)						
Ischaemic	117 (69.6)	90 (62.9)	0.212	43 (64.2)	45 (68.2)	0.626
Non-ischeamic	51 (30.4)	53 (37.1)		24 (35.8)	21 (31.8)	
Previous medical history. n (%)						
Coronary artery disease	115 (65.4)	88 (61.5)	0.202	44 (65.7)	45 (68.2)	0.758
Myocardial infarction	104 (61.9)	81 (56.6)	0.346	44 (65.7)	39 (59.1)	0.433
Angioplasty	79 (47.0)	66 (46.1)	0.878	33 (49.2)	36 (54.5)	0.541
Coronary artery bypass grafting	25 (14.9)	21 (11.7)	0.961	11 (16.4)	8 (12.1)	0.480
Hypertension	101 (60.1)	97 (67.8)	0.159	34 (50.7)	45 (68.2)	0.041
Stroke	9 (5.4)	7 (4.9)	0.854	2 (3.0)	8 (12.1)	0.055
Chronic kidney disease	21 (12.5)	19 (13.3)	0.836	18 (26.9)	14 (21.2)	0.446
Hyperlipidemia	85 (50.6)	63 (44.1)	0.250	31 (46.3)	27 (40.9)	0.533
Diabetes	56 (33.3)	47 (32.9)	0.931	21 (31.3)	24 (36.4)	0.541
Functional status						
NYHA I. n (%)	19 (11.3)	32 (22.4)	0.007	8 (11.9)	3 (4.5)	0.254
NYHA II. n (%)	127 (75.6)	85 (59.4)		45 (67.2)	45 (68.2)	
NYHA III. n (%)	22 (13.1)	26 (18.2)		14 (20.9)	18 (27.3)	
Treatment						
Beta-blocker	161 (95.8)	137 (95.8)	0.990	63 (94.0)	66 (100)	0.119
ACEI/ARB	159 (94.6)	137 (95.8)	0.634	58 (86.6)	58 (87.9)	0.821
Digoxin	9 (5.4)	5 (3.5)	0.430	8 (11.9)	5 (7.6)	0.397
Loop diuretics	116 (69.0)	100 (69.9)	0.866	52 (77.6)	61 (92.4)	0.017
Spironolactone/eplerenone	138 (82.1)	118 (82.5)	0.931	54 (80.6)	53 (80.3)	0.966
Aspirin/clopidogrel	121 (72.0)	89 (62.2)	0.066	37 (55.2)	43 (65.1)	0.243
Anticoagulants	23 (13.7)	22 (15.4)	0.672	19 (28.4)	18 (27.3)	0.889

Table 1. Cont.

	MDD (n = 311)			SDD (n = 133)		
	HCTR-MDD n = 168	UC-MDD n = 143	p1	HCTR-SDD n = 67	UC-SDD n = 66	p2
Statins	146 (86.9)	120 (83.9)	0.455	50 (74.6)	52 (78.8)	0.570
CIEDs	122 (72.6)	117 (81.8)	0.055	58 (86.6)	54 (81.8)	0.453
Implantable cardioverter-defibrillator	75 (61.5)	78 (66.7)		39 (67.2)	33 (61.1)	
CRT-P	3 (2.5)	2 (1.7)	0.482	0	0	0.310
CRT-D	42 (34.4)	37 (31.6)		19 (32.8)	19 (35.2)	

Abbreviations: NYHA—New York Heart Association class; ACEI—angiotensin-converting enzyme inhibitors; ARB—angiotensin receptor blockers; CIEDs—cardiovascular implantable electronic devices; CRT-P—cardiac resynchronization therapy; CRT-D—cardiac resynchronization therapy and cardioverter-defibrillator; DM—diabetes mellitus; BSA—body surface area; HCTR-MD—patients in hybrid comprehensive telerehabilitation arm with mild diastolic dysfunction; HCTR-SDD—patients in hybrid comprehensive telerehabilitation arm with severe diastolic dysfunction; HFrEF—heart failure with reduced ejection fraction; UC-MDD—patients in usual care arm with mild diastolic dysfunction; UC-SDD—patients in usual care arm with severe diastolic dysfunction.

Table 2. Baseline parameters of echocardiographic parameters.

	MDD (n = 311)			SDD (n = 133)		
	HCTR-MDD n = 168	UC-MDD n = 143	p1	HCTR-SDD n = 67	UC-SDD n = 66	p2
E	0.53 ± 0.16	0.55 ± 0.17	0.421	0.93 ± 0.24	0.93 ± 0.24	0.962
A	0.70 ± 0.17	0.73 ± 0.17	0.219	0.39 ± 0.18	0.43 ± 0.18	0.224
E/A	0.79 ± 0.29	0.79 ± 0.33	0.983	2.63 ± 0.91	2.43 ± 0.97	0.267
DTE	230 ± 59	222 ± 64	0.241	164 ± 49	172 ± 54	0.432
E/E' lat	8.09 ± 3.07	8.03 ± 3.02	0.883	17.3 ± 8.6	15.4 ± 7.1	0.223
E/E' med	9.53 ± 3.2	9.50 ± 3.07	0.935	19.1 ± 10.0	22.5 ± 10.1	0.067
E/E' avg	8.81 ± 2.61	8.77 ± 2.46	0.904	18.2 ± 8.3	19.0 ± 7.6	0.586
LA	42.8 ± 6.0	43.2 ± 5.8	0.546	46.3 ± 7.0	47.6 ± 6.4	0.254
LAA	23.0 ± 4.8	24.0 ± 5.9	0.113	28.5 ± 6.2	28.2 ± 6.8	0.854
TR velocity	2.03 ± 0.46	2.04 ± 0.49	0.894	2.8 ± 0.7	2.9 ± 0.7	0.557
EF	32.8 ± 6.1	32.1 ± 6.7	0.330	27.9 ± 6.4	28.0 ± 7.4	0.937
E/A ≤ 0.8 (n, %)	112 (66.7)	98 (68.5)		1 (1.5)	1 (1.5)	
E/A 0.8–2 (n, %)	56 (33.3)	45 (31.5)	0.727	3 (4.5)	9 (13.6)	0.185
E/A > 2 (n, %)	0	0		63 (94.0)	56 (84.8)	
DTE ≤ 160 (n, %)	15 (9.0)	18 (12.6)		37 (56.1)	34 (53.1)	
DTE 160–200 (n, %)	26 (15.7)	10 (29.4)	0.004	17 (25.8)	16 (25.0)	0.870
DTE ≥ 200 (n, %)	125 (75.3)	83 (58.0)		12 (18.2)	25 (21.9)	
E/E' avg > 14 (n, %)	1 (0.6)	2 (1.4)	0.595	44 (65.7)	49 (75.4)	0.221
TR velocity > 2.8 (n, %)	1 (0.6) (n = 141)	0 (0) (n = 119)	1.00	23 (43.4) (n = 52)	27 (51.9) (n = 53)	0.382

Abbreviations: HCTR-MDD—patients in hybrid comprehensive telerehabilitation arm with mild diastolic dysfunction; HCTR-SDD– patients in hybrid comprehensive telerehabilitation arm with severe diastolic dysfunction; HFrEF—heart failure with reduced ejection fraction; UC-MDD—patients in usual care arm with mild diastolic dysfunction; UC-SDD—patients in usual care arm with severe diastolic dysfunction; LVEF—Left Ventricular Ejection Fraction; E—early diastolic mitral inflow velocity; A—late diastolic mitral inflow velocity; DTE—deceleration time of E wave; E' med—E' velocity at medial wall; E' lat—E' velocity at lateral wall; E/E' avg—average value of E/E' at medial and lateral wall of the left ventricle; TR velocity—tricuspid regurgitation (TR) jet velocity; LA—left atrium diameter; LAA—left atrium area.

Changes from baseline to 9 weeks in echocardiographic parameters were seen only in A velocities (delta from baseline to 9 weeks 0.06 (0.01;0.11) in HCTR-MDD vs. −0.03 (−0.11;0.04) in UC-MDD; p interaction = 0.008) and tricuspid regurgitation velocity (−0.10 (−0.28;0.08) in HCTR-SDD vs. 0.23 (−0.03;0.49) in UC-SDD; p interaction = 0.007). No significant shifts between groups of different diastolic dysfunction grade were observed after HCTR (Table 3).

Table 3. Changes from baseline to 9 weeks in echocardiographic parameters (adjusted for baseline measure, body Surface area, hypertension, loop diuretics, NYHA class).

	MDD (n = 311)				SDD (n = 133)				p Interaction
	HCTR-MDD n = 168	UC-MDD n = 143	Difference [95% CI] *	p *	HCTR-SDD n = 67	UC-SDD n = 66	Difference [95% CI] *	p *	
	Δ 9 week—baseline [95% CI] *				Δ 9 week—baseline [95% CI] *				
E [m/s]	0.01 (−0.03;0.08)	−0.02 (−0.05;0.01)	0.03 (−0.02;0.08)	0.526	0.01 (−0.05;0.05)	0.03 (−0.02;0.08)	−0.02 (−0.10;−0.05)	0.864	0.163
A	0.03 (−0.01;0.06)	−0.03 (−0.06;−0.01)	0.06 (0.01;0.11)	<0.010	−0.01 (−0.06;0.04)	0.02 (−0.02;0.07)	−0.03 (−0.11;0.04)	0.648	0.008
E/A	−0.03 (−0.14;0.09)	−0.02 (−0.13;0.10)	−0.01 (−0.19;0.17)	0.992	−0.03 (−0.24;0.19)	0.00 (−0.20;0.21)	−0.03 (−0.32;0.25)	0.989	0.844
DTE	7.7 (−3.9;19.4)	4.5 (−6.7;15.8)	3.2 (−16.0;22.4)	0.973	−23.9 (−41.6;−6.1)	−22.6 (−39.9;−5.3)	−1.3 (−31.1;28.6)	0.999	0.744
E/E' lat	−0.08 (−1.05;0.90)	−0.27 (−1.21;0.67)	0.19 (−1.37;1.76)	0.989	2.07 (0.53;3.61)	1.42 (−0.02;2.86)	0.65 (−1.78;3.61)	0.901	0.684
E/E' med	−0.78 (−1.92;0.35)	−0.97 (−2.07;0.13)	0.19 (−1.63;2.01)	0.993	1.86 (0.14;3.58)	2.38 (0.56;4.20)	−0.52 (−3.36;2.32)	0.965	0.587
E/E' avg	−0.32 (−1.25;0.61)	−0.51 (−1.41;0.40)	0.19 (−1.29;1.66)	0.988	1.79 (0.34;3.24)	1.55 (0.09;3.01)	0.24 (−2.04;2.52)	0.993	0.958
LA LAX	0.03 (−0.83;0.89)	−0.66 (−1.49;0.17)	0.69 (−0.73;2.11)	0.597	0.72 (−0.55;1.98)	−0.24 (−1.50;1.02)	0.96 (−1.22;3.13)	0.670	0.789
LAA 4CH	−0.24 (−0.98;0.49)	−0.69 (−1.40;0.01)	0.45 (−0.75;1.66)	0.764	1.70 (0.55;2.85)	1.14 (0.05;2.23)	0.56 (−1.35;2.46)	0.875	0.904
TR velocity	−0.17 (−0.28;−0.06)	−0.07 (−0.18;0.04)	−0.10 (−0.28;0.08)	0.462	0.18 (0.02;0.34)	−0.05 (−0.21;0.10)	0.23 (−0.03;0.49)	0.106	0.007
EF	2.17 (1.45;2.88)	1.14 (0.45;1.82)	1.03 (−0.15;2.21)	0.111	1.06 (0.01;2.11)	1.27 (0.23;2.31)	−0.21 (−2.03;1.60)	0.990	0.138

Abbreviations: HCTR-MDD—patients in hybrid comprehensive telerehabilitation arm with mild diastolic dysfunction; HCTR-SDD–patients in hybrid comprehensive telerehabilitation arm with severe diastolic dysfunction; HFrEF—heart failure with reduced ejection fraction; UC-MDD—patients in usual care arm with mild diastolic dysfunction; UC-SDD—patients in usual care arm with severe diastolic dysfunction; LVEF—left ventricular ejection fraction; E—early diastolic mitral inflow velocity; A—late diastolic mitral inflow velocity; DTE—deceleration time of E wave; E' med—E' velocity at medial wall; E' lat—E' velocity at lateral wall; E/E' avg—average value of E/E' at medial and lateral wall of the left ventricle; TR velocity—tricuspid regurgitation (TR) jet velocity; LA—left atrium diameter; LAA—left atrium area. * regarding Difference [95% CI].

Understanding the impact of volume overload in HF patients, we were checking the weight gain before every session of cardiac rehabilitation. We did not notice any BMI changes of statistical importance between analyzed subgroups regarding diastolic dysfunction.

All-cause mortality was higher in UC-SDD vs. UC-MDD (24 (36.4%) vs. 42 (29.4%), $p < 0.001$, with no difference between HCTR-SDD and HCTR-MDD (24 (35.8%) vs. 49 (29.2%), $p = 0.064$) (Figure 2). No difference in the probability of CV mortality and hospitalization were found in HCTR and UC groups (Figures 3 and 4). The probability of CV hospitalization was not associated with diastolic dysfunction. A higher probability of HF hospitalization (Figure 5) was seen in HCTR-SDD compared to HCTR-MDD (46 (68.6%) vs. 65 (38.7%), $p < 0.001$, retrospectively) and in UC-SDD compared to UC-MDD (40 (60.6%) vs. 55 (38.5%), $p < 0.001$, retrospectively).

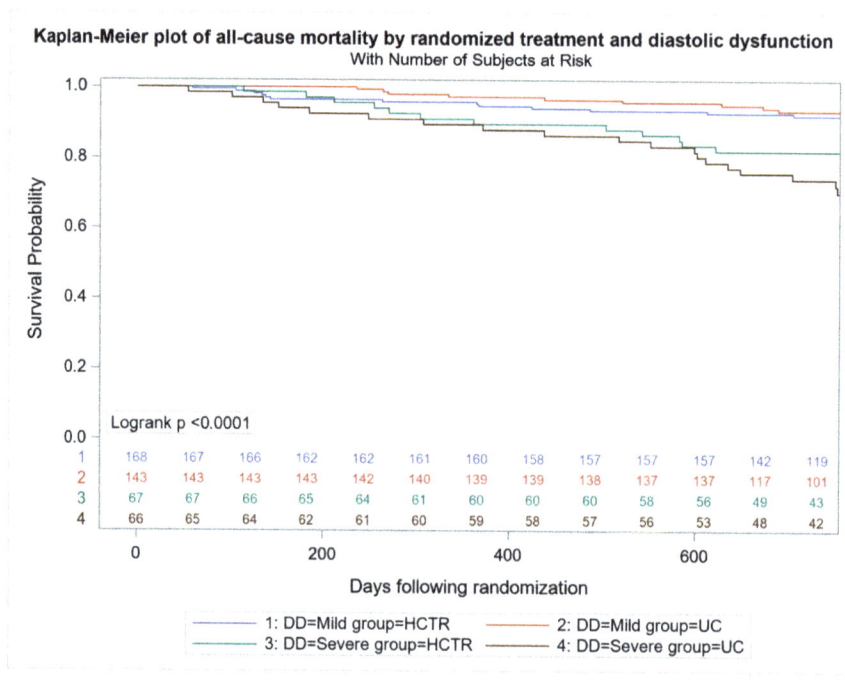

Figure 2. Kaplan–Meier Plot of all-cause mortality-free survivals in subgroups regarding diastolic function and rehabilitation.

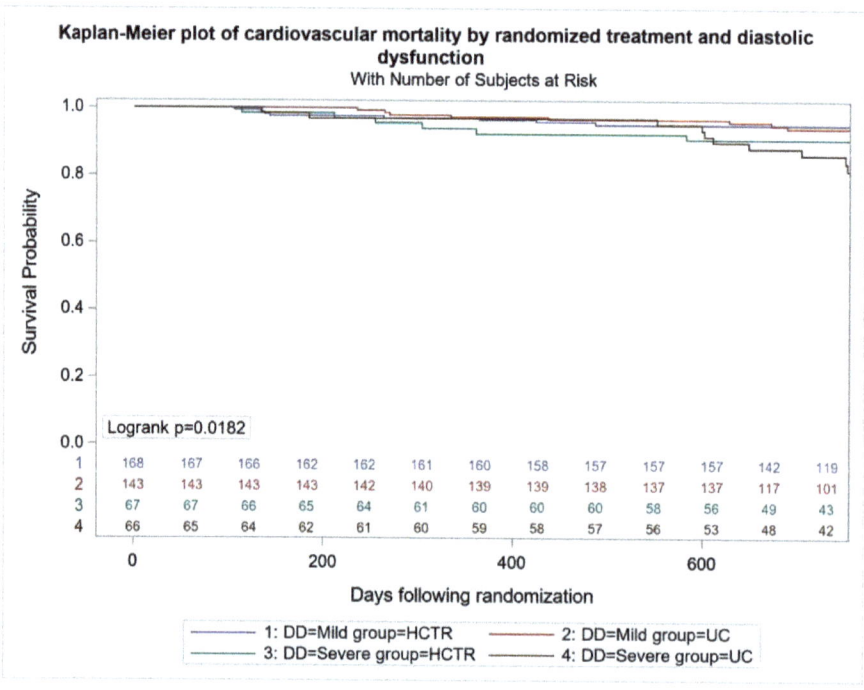

Figure 3. Kaplan–Meier plot of cardiovascular mortality-free survival in subgroups regarding diastolic function and rehabilitation.

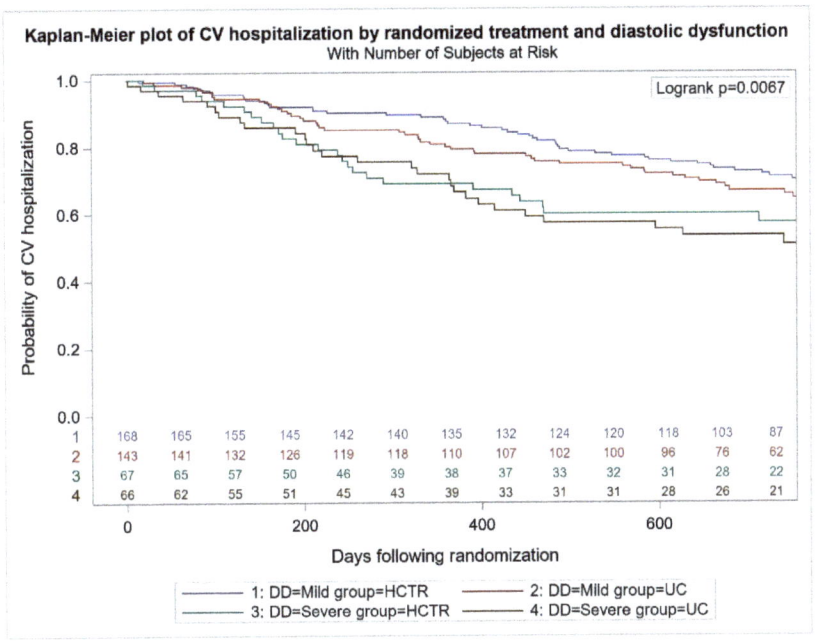

Figure 4. Kaplan–Meier plot of cardiovascular hospitalization in subgroups regarding diastolic function and rehabilitation.

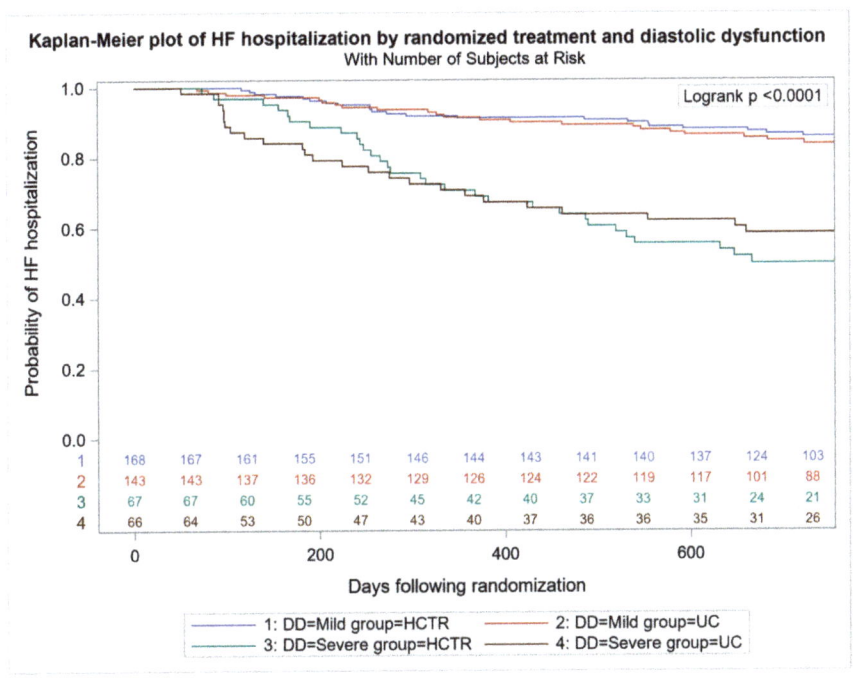

Figure 5. Kaplan–Meier plot of heart failure hospitalization in subgroups regarding diastolic function and rehabilitation.

4. Discussion

Currently, many research centers conduct projects aimed at optimizing non-invasive therapy in order to prevent HF progression [12]. Telemedicine is one of the solutions dedicated to this group of patients, also with HF [13]. Until now, there have been no large available data on the diastolic dysfunction in patients with HFrEF who were randomized to HCTR or UC. Our study, for the first time, describes the impact of diastolic dysfunction severity on prognosis in HF patients, in the context of a telerehabilitation program.

Imaging tests provide many important information necessary in the diagnosis and prognosis of patients with HF. In a group of 31 patients after an acute cardiovascular event, we assessed the effect of rehabilitation on the functional remodeling of the LV. It has been observed that rehabilitation leads to a reverse functional remodeling of the LV and an improvement in functional reserve [14]. Cardoso et al. also investigated the mechanisms associated with myocardial reverse remodeling in patients with HF with reduced and preserved LVEF, but still detailed data regarding the impact of cardiac rehabilitation on parameters of cardiac magnetic resonance imaging, vasomotor endothelial function, cardiac sympathetic activity imaging and serum biomarker are not available [15].

An important reason for examining diastolic function in patients with decreased LVEF is the assessment of LV filling pressure. Diastolic dysfunction with increased LV filling pressure determines the prognosis [16].

Diastolic dysfunction of the LV results in decreased exercise tolerance, and is associated with poor prognosis in patients, particularly the elderly [17]. Physical activity may improve clinical outcomes in patients with HF, including patients with end-stage HF treated with implantable devices to assist the LV [18]. However, the influence of exercise training on the diastolic function of the LV in patients with cardiovascular diseases remains controversial [19].

There are only a few papers regarding the influence of cardiac rehabilitation on diastolic function, mostly in patients with chronic coronary syndromes or after myocardial infarction.

Wuthiwaropas et al. analyzed the influence of a 3-month-old rehabilitation on the hemodynamic parameters of the myocardium in patients with coronary artery disease. Out of 24 (96%) patients: 12 (50%) had an improvement in diastolic function, 2 (8%) had a normal diastolic function all the time, 9 (38%) remained at the same level, and one (4%) had a deterioration in diastolic function [20]. At this point, it is worth emphasizing that the second largest group of patients studied did not benefit—the diastolic function, despite rehabilitation, did not change. Those results correspond to ours, but in the HF population.

Lee et al. determined the impact of cardiac rehabilitation on diastolic function and prognosis in patients after a history of acute myocardial infarction. The parameters E/E' >14, velocity e' of the septum <7 cm/s, left atrial volume index (LAVI) > 34 mL/m^2 and maximum TR velocity > 2.8 m/s were compared. In the group undergoing cardiac rehabilitation, an improvement in the examined parameters was observed. The authors proved that cardiac rehabilitation was significantly associated with favorable diastolic function after myocardial infarction. Those results are in contrast to our study in the HF population, but in that study authors compared patients participating in cardiac rehabilitation sufficiently with those not participating sufficiently [21].

In the next study, 98 patients with moderate-to-severe, mild, and preserved LVEF were randomly assigned to exercise training plus UC or UC alone in a randomization ratio of 2:1. Cardiac rehabilitation increased the mean ratio of early-to-late mitral inflow velocities (E/A ratio) and decreased deceleration time (DT) of early filling in patients with mild and preserved LVEF. In patients with advanced diastolic dysfunction (DT < 160 ms), rehabilitation decreased E/A ratio and increased DT, both of which were unchanged after UC alone. Importantly, cardiac rehabilitation decreased left ventricular dimensions in patients with mild and moderate-to-severe reductions in LVEF but not in patients with preserved LVEF [22].

Pearson et al. evaluated the effect of exercise training on diastolic function in patients with HF. Data from five studies in HF with preserved ejection fraction (HFpEF) patients, with a total of 204 participants, also demonstrated a significant improvement in E/E' in exercise group [23].

In the recent study on patients with acute coronary syndromes, the adopted criteria and detailed analysis of the tested diastolic dysfunction parameters did not show a significant effect of cardiac rehabilitation on diastolic function in the studied group. At this point, it is worth emphasizing that most of the patients enrolled in the study underwent STEMI. Moreover, the majority of respondents had a history of several years of high blood pressure. The matrix and the collagen fibers in the heart determine the effectiveness of the mechanical systole and diastole. Cardiac perfusion disorders activate macrophages and increase the concentration of transforming factors, e.g., TGF-beta1 (transforming growth factor beta 1). As a result, there is proliferation of fibroblasts and an increase in collagen content in the cell stroma and around the vessels [24]. STEMI is dominated by the process of structural degradation of collagen fibers under the influence of activated proteolytic enzymes. This starts stromal fibrosis with a disturbed ratio of collagen fibers, which increases muscle stiffness and generates disorders of its relaxation, and finally compliance. According to Soholm et al. Diastolic dysfunction in the early phase after STEMI determines the extent of myocardial damage and significantly reduces the effect of myocardial salvage treatment after three months. Thus, the presence of post-STEMI diastolic dysfunction is indicative of a poorer prognosis [25]. It is possible that the changes described in the study groups overlap with early changes generated by long-term hypertension, myocardial fibrosis and existing LV filling abnormalities. Therefore, they could observe permanent diastolic disorders, which, due to the irreversible nature of changes in the stroma, we are unable to reverse. Moreover, it is highly prevalent in hypertensive patients and is associated with increased cardiovascular morbidity and mortality [26]. Those results are not consistent with our results, because our population was HF patients.

The analysis carried out by Acar RD et al. was aimed at assessing the influence of cardiac rehabilitation on the LV diastolic function. The study was performed in a group of 82 patients after acute myocardial infarction. A significant improvement in the E/A wave ratio was observed; however, DTE and isovolumic relaxation time (IVRT) did not change significantly [27].

On the other hand, in another study, after an eight-week rehabilitation program in the group of patients after myocardial infarction, the authors also did not find a significant improvement in the examined echocardiographic parameters [28]. Similarly, after an 8-week endurance exercise program, despite the improvement in exercise capacity parameters, they did not notice a significant improvement in diastolic or systolic function [29]. The similarity to our work is the typical duration of cardiac rehabilitation.

Our study is the first randomized trial investigating the effect of comprehensive cardiac rehabilitation in HF patients with reduced ejection fraction on diastolic function. Some observed changes in echocardiographic parameters of diastolic function were not pronounced enough after 8-week HCTR. With the intention to see more clear beneficial effects of hybrid comprehensive telerehabilitation versus usual care rehabilitation on the diastolic function, the duration and volume of HCTR might be greater. We noticed an interesting observation regarding the prognostic impact of diastolic dysfunction severity on all-cause mortality in UC patients. Moreover, we observed a higher probability of HF hospitalization in case of SDD in both HCTR and UC arms.

5. Conclusions

Hybrid comprehensive telerehabilitation did not influence diastolic function in HF patients in a significant manner. The grade of diastolic dysfunction had an impact on mortality only in the UC group and HF hospitalization over a 12–24-month follow-up in HCTR and UC groups. Nevertheless, it is well known that cardiac rehabilitation in patients with HF may reduce the risk of rehospitalization and may reduce HF-related hospital admissions. The use of modern technologies for HCTR is helpful to overcome accessibility barriers to cardiac rehabilitation. HCTR should be considered a tool of great importance in HF patients.

Limitations

Our conclusions are drawn up only in patients with sinus rhythm, when atrial fibrillation is not uncommon in HF patients. In our study, the lack of influence of HCTR on diastolic function can be explained by its duration of 8 weeks. To see a better effect, longer probably and a more intensive program are needed. We could not determine the grade of diastolic dysfunction in some patients because of the lack of biplane measurement of left atrium volume. According to the recent echocardiographic guidelines, we used two criteria during the second step of diastolic function assessment after the characterization of mitral inflow.

Author Contributions: Conceptualization, R.G., M.B., R.P., M.J.P., W.Z., Z.K., G.O. and E.P.; Data curation, I.K.; Formal analysis, I.K. and M.J.P.; Funding acquisition, E.P.; Investigation, R.I., R.G., D.S., P.O., S.P. and E.P.; Methodology, R.G., D.S., P.O. and E.P.; Supervision, R.P., W.Z., Z.K., G.O. and E.P.; Validation, M.J.P.; Visualization, R.G.; Writing—original draft, R.I. and R.G.; Writing—review & editing, M.B., D.S., R.P., W.Z., P.O., S.P. and G.O. All authors have read and agreed to the published version of the manuscript.

Funding: The study was financed by the National Centre for Research and Development, Warsaw, Poland (grant number STRATEGMED1/233547/13/NCBR/2015). The authors are solely responsible for the design and implementation of this study, all analyses, the drafting and editing of the paper, and its final content.

Institutional Review Board Statement: The study was conducted in accordance with the Declaration of Helsinki, and approved by the Ethics Committee of Institute of Cardiology in Warsaw (protocol code IK-NP-0021-85/1402/13).

Informed Consent Statement: Informed consent was obtained from all subjects involved in the study.

Data Availability Statement: The data used to support the findings of this study are included within the article.

Conflicts of Interest: The authors received support from the National Centre for Research and Development, Warsaw, Poland.

References

1. Katz, S.D. Pathophysiology of Chronic Systolic Heart Failure. A View from the Periphery. *Ann. Am. Thorac. Soc.* **2018**, *15* (Suppl. 1), S38–S41. [CrossRef] [PubMed]
2. Naing, P.; Forrester, D.; Kangaharan, N.; Muthumala, A.; Myint, S.M.; Playford, D. Heart failure with preserved ejection fraction: A growing global epidemic. *AJGP* **2019**, *48*, 465–471. [CrossRef] [PubMed]
3. Jørgensen, M.E.; Andersson, C.; Vasan, R.S.; Køber, L.; Abdulla, J. Characteristics and prognosis of heart failure with improved compared with persistently reduced ejection fraction: A systematic review and meta-analyses. *Eur. J. Prev. Cardiol.* **2018**, *25*, 366–376. [CrossRef] [PubMed]
4. Sharifov, O.F.; Gupta, H. What Is the Evidence That the Tissue Doppler Index E/e' Reflects Left Ventricular Filling Pressure Changes After Exercise or Pharmacological Intervention for Evaluating Diastolic Function? A Systematic Review. *J. Am. Heart Assoc.* **2017**, *6*, e004766. [CrossRef] [PubMed]
5. Nagueh, S.F.; Smiseth, O.A.; Appleton, C.P.; Byrd, B.F.; Dokainish, H.; Edvardsen, T.; Flachskampf, F.A.; Gillebert, T.C.; Klein, A.L.; Lancellotti, P.; et al. Recommendations for the Evaluation of Left Ventricular Diastolic Function by Echocardiography: An Update from the American Society of Echocardiography and the European Association of Cardiovascular Imaging. *J. Am. Soc. Echocardiogr.* **2016**, *29*, 277–314. [CrossRef]
6. Silbiger, J.J. Pathophysiology and Echocardiographic Diagnosis of Left Ventricular Diastolic Dysfunction. *J. Am. Soc. Echocardiogr.* **2019**, *32*, 216–232.e2. [CrossRef] [PubMed]
7. Pelliccia, A.; Sharma, S.; Gati, S.; Bäck, M.; Börjesson, M.; Caselli, S.; Collet, J.-P.; Corrado, D.; Drezner, J.A.; Halle, M.; et al. 2020 ESC Guidelines on sports cardiology and exercise in patients with cardiovascular disease The Task Force on sports cardiology and exercise in patients with cardiovascular disease of the European Society of Cardiology (ESC). *Eur. Heart J.* **2021**, *42*, 17–96. [CrossRef] [PubMed]

8. Long, L.; Mordi, I.R.; Bridges, C.; Sagar, V.A.; Davies, E.J.; Coats, A.J.; Dalal, H.; Rees, K.; Singh, S.J.; Taylor, R.S. Exercise-based cardiac rehabilitation for adults with heart failure. *Cochrane Database Syst. Rev.* **2019**, *1*, CD003331. [CrossRef] [PubMed]
9. Jones, N.R.; Roalfe, A.K.; Adoki, I.; Hobbs, F.D.R.; Taylor, C.J. Survival of patients with chronic heart failure in the community: A systematic review and meta-analysis. *Eur. J. Heart Fail.* **2019**, *21*, 1306–1325. [CrossRef] [PubMed]
10. Piotrowicz, E.; Pencina, M.J.; Opolski, G.; Zareba, W.; Banach, M.; Kowalik, I.; Orzechowski, P.; Szalewska, D.; Pluta, S.; Glówczynska, R.; et al. Effects of a 9-Week Hybrid Comprehensive Telerehabilitation Program on Long-term Outcomes in Patients With Heart Failure: The Telerehabilitation in Heart Failure Patients (TELEREH-HF) Randomized Clinical Trial. *JAMA Cardiol.* **2020**, *5*, 300–308. [CrossRef]
11. Piotrowicz, E.; Piotrowicz, R.; Opolski, G.; Pencina, M.; Banach, M.; Zaręba, W. Hybrid comprehensive telerehabilitation in heart failure patients (TELEREH-HF): A randomized, multicenter, prospective, open-label, parallel group controlled trial-Study design and description of the intervention. *Am. Heart J.* **2019**, *217*, 148–158. [CrossRef]
12. Patti, A.; Merlo, L.; Ambrosetti, M.; Sarto, P. Exercise-Based Cardiac Rehabilitation Programs in Heart Failure Patients. *Heart Fail. Clin.* **2021**, *17*, 263–271. [CrossRef] [PubMed]
13. Tousignant, M.; Mampuya, W.M. Telerehabilitation for patients with heart failure. *Cardiovasc. Diagn. Ther.* **2015**, *5*, 74–78. [PubMed]
14. McGregor, G.; Stöhr, E.J.; Oxborough, D.; Kimani, P.; Shave, R. Effect of exercise training on left ventricular mechanics after acute myocardial infarction–an exploratory study. *Ann. Phys. Rehabil. Med.* **2018**, *61*, 119–124. [CrossRef] [PubMed]
15. Bianchini Cardoso, F.; Antunes-Correa, L.M.; Quinaglia, T.; Silva, A.C. Noninvasive imaging assessment of rehabilitation therapy in heart failure with preserved and reduced left ventricular ejection fraction (IMAGING-REHAB-HF): Design and rationale. *Ther. Adv. Chronic. Dis.* **2019**, *10*, 1–15. [CrossRef]
16. Nagueh, S.F. Left Ventricular Diastolic Function: Understanding Pathophysiology, Diagnosis, and Prognosis With Echocardiography. *JACC Cardiovasc. Imaging* **2020**, *13*, 228–244. [CrossRef] [PubMed]
17. Pavasini, R.; Cardelli, L.S.; Piredda, A.; Tonet, E.; Campana, R.; Vitali, F.; Cimaglia, P.; Maietti, E.; Caglioni, S.; Morelli, C.; et al. Diastolic dysfunction, frailty and prognosis in elderly patients with acute coronary syndromes. *Int. J. Cardiol.* **2021**, *327*, 31–35. [CrossRef]
18. Di Nora, C.; Guidetti, F.; Livi, U.; Antonini-Canterin, F. Role of Cardiac Rehabilitation after Ventricular Assist Device Implantation. *Heart Fail. Clin.* **2021**, *17*, 273–278. [CrossRef] [PubMed]
19. Smart, N.; Haluska, B.; Jeffriess, L.; Marwick, T.H. Exercise training in systolic and diastolic dysfunction: Effects on cardiac function, functional capacity, and quality of life. *Am. Heart J.* **2007**, *153*, 530–536. [CrossRef] [PubMed]
20. Wuthiwaropas, P.; Bellavia, D.; Omer, M.; Squires, R.W.; Scott, C.G.; Pellikka, P.A. Impact of cardiac rehabilitation exercise program on left ventricular diastolic function in coronary artery disease: A pilot study. *Int. J. Cardiovasc. Imaging* **2013**, *29*, 777–785. [CrossRef]
21. Lee, J.; Kim, J.; Sun, B.J.; Jee, S.J.; Park, J. Effect of Cardiac Rehabilitation on Left Ventricular Diastolic Function in Patients with Acute Myocardial Infarction. *J. Clin. Med.* **2021**, *10*, 2088. [CrossRef] [PubMed]
22. Alves, A.J.; Ribeiro, F.; Goldhammer, E.; Rivlin, Y.; Rosenschein, U.; Viana, J.L.; Duarte, J.A.; Sagiv, M.; Oliveira, J. Exercise Training Improves Diastolic Function in Heart Failure Patients. *Med. Sci. Sports Exerc.* **2012**, *44*, 776–785. [CrossRef] [PubMed]
23. Pearson, M.J.; Mungovan, S.F.; Smart, N.A. Effect of exercise on diastolic function in heart failure patients: A systematic review and meta-analysis. *Heart Fail. Rev.* **2017**, *22*, 229–242. [CrossRef] [PubMed]
24. Hanna, A.; Frangogiannis, N. The Role of the TGF-β Superfamily in Myocardial Infarction. *Front. Cardiovasc. Med.* **2019**, *6*, 140. [CrossRef] [PubMed]
25. Søholm, H.; Lønborg, J.; Andersen, M.J.; Vejlstrup, N.; Engstrøm, T.; Hassager, C.; Møller, J.E. Association diastolic function by echo and infarct size by magnetic resonance imaging after STEMI. *Scand. Cardiovasc. J.* **2016**, *50*, 172–179. [CrossRef] [PubMed]
26. Leao, N.; da Silva, M. Diastolic dysfunction in hypertension. *Hipertens. Riesgo Vasc Jul.* **2017**, *34*, 128–139. [CrossRef] [PubMed]
27. Acar, R.D.; Bulut, M.; Ergün, S.; Yesin, M.; Eren, H.; Akçakoyun, M. Does cardiac rehabilitation improve left ventricular diastolic function of patients with acute myocardial infarction? *Turk Kardiyol Dern Ars* **2014**, *42*, 710–716. [CrossRef] [PubMed]
28. Golabchi, A.; Basati, F.; Kargarfard, M.; Sadeghi, M. Can cardiac rehabilitation programs improve functional capacity and left ventricular diastolic function in patients with mechanical reperfusion after ST elevation myocardial infarction? A double-blind clinical trial. *ARYA Atheroscler.* **2012**, *8*, 125–129. [PubMed]
29. Fontes-Carvalho, R.; Azevedo, A.I.; Sampaio, F.; Teixeira, M.; Bettencourt, N.; Campos, L.; Gonçalves, F.R.; Ribeiro, V.G.; Azevedo, A.; Leite-Moreira, A. The Effect of Exercise Training on Diastolic and Systolic Function After Acute Myocardial Infarction A Randomized Study. *Medicine* **2015**, *94*, e1450. [CrossRef]

Article

Assessment of Selected Baseline and Post-PCI Electrocardiographic Parameters as Predictors of Left Ventricular Systolic Dysfunction after a First ST-Segment Elevation Myocardial Infarction

Tomasz Fabiszak [1,*], Michał Kasprzak [1], Marek Koziński [2] and Jacek Kubica [1]

1. Department of Cardiology and Internal Medicine, Collegium Medicum, Nicolaus Copernicus University, ul. Skłodowskiej-Curie 9, 85-094 Bydgoszcz, Poland; medkas@o2.pl (M.K.); jwkubica@gmail.com (J.K.)
2. Department of Cardiology and Internal Medicine, Medical University of Gdańsk, ul. Powstania Styczniowego 9B, 81-519 Gdynia, Poland; marek.kozinski@gumed.edu.pl
* Correspondence: tfabiszak@wp.pl; Tel.: +48-52-585-40-23; Fax: +48-52-585-40-24

Abstract: Objective: To assess the performance of ten electrocardiographic (ECG) parameters regarding the prediction of left ventricular systolic dysfunction (LVSD) after a first ST-segment-elevation myocardial infarction (STEMI). Methods: We analyzed 249 patients (74.7% males) treated with primary percutaneous coronary intervention (PCI) included into a single-center cohort study. We sought associations between baseline and post-PCI ECG parameters and the presence of LVSD (defined as left ventricular ejection fraction [LVEF] $\leq$ 40% on echocardiography) 6 months after STEMI. Results: Patients presenting with LVSD (n = 52) had significantly higher values of heart rate, number of leads with ST-segment elevation and pathological Q-waves, as well as total and maximal ST-segment elevation at baseline and directly after PCI compared with patients without LVSD. They also showed a significantly higher prevalence of anterior STEMI and considerably wider QRS complex after PCI, while QRS duration measurement at baseline showed no significant difference. Additionally, patients presenting with LVSD after 6 months showed markedly more severe ischemia on admission, as assessed with the Sclarovsky-Birnbaum ischemia score, smaller reciprocal ST-segment depression at baseline and less profound ST-segment resolution post PCI. In multivariate regression analysis adjusted for demographic, clinical, biochemical and angiographic variables, anterior location of STEMI (OR 17.78; 95% CI 6.45–48.96; p < 0.001), post-PCI QRS duration (OR 1.56; 95% CI 1.22–2.00; p < 0.001) expressed per increments of 10 ms and impaired post-PCI flow in the infarct-related artery (IRA; TIMI 3 vs. <3; OR 0.14; 95% CI 0.04–0.46; p = 0.001) were identified as independent predictors of LVSD (Nagelkerke's pseudo R^2 for the logistic regression model = 0.462). Similarly, in multiple regression analysis, anterior location of STEMI, wider post-PCI QRS, higher baseline number of pathological Q-waves and a higher baseline Sclarovsky-Birnbaum ischemia score, together with impaired post-PCI flow in the IRA, higher values of body mass index and glucose concentration on admission were independently associated with lower values of LVEF at 6 months (corrected R^2 = 0.448; p < 0.00001). Conclusions: According to our study, baseline and post-PCI ECG parameters are of modest value for the prediction of LVSD occurrence 6 months after a first STEMI.

Keywords: myocardial infarction; ECG; risk stratification; left ventricular systolic dysfunction; primary PCI

1. Introduction

Electrocardiography (ECG), invented by Willem Einthoven nearly 120 years ago, remains one of the essential diagnostic modalities in cardiology [1], shaping the elementary division of acute coronary syndromes into those with and without persistent ST-segment depression, affecting the timing and mode of management and adding to short- and long-term risk stratification [2–4].

It is estimated that left ventricular systolic dysfunction (LVSD), recognized as a long-term consequence of myocardial infarction (MI), may affect up to 60% of post-MI patients [5]. Its occurrence mainly depends on the presence of frozen myocardium, size of post-MI necrosis, and occurrence of left ventricular remodeling [6,7].

Left ventricular ejection fraction (LVEF), measured with echocardiography, is by far the most popular method for diagnosing LVSD in the clinical setting [8].

LVSD is a well-recognized marker of unfavorable prognosis in post-MI patients [8], translating into a 3–4-fold increase in mortality and higher rates of cardiovascular adverse outcomes, such as cardiac rupture, sudden cardiac arrest, recurrent myocardial infarction, ventricular arrhythmias, stroke, prolonged hospitalization and rehospitalization [7,9–11]. The mortality rate among post-MI patients with asymptomatic LVSD after 12 months of MI is as high as 12% and amounts to 36% in symptomatic patients [12]. LVSD independently predicts short-, mid- and long-term mortality after MI [12–15].

There are many reports regarding the predictive value of ECG with respect to the development of LVSD after STEMI [4,16,17]. A vast part of these reports however, comes from the era of thrombolytic treatment of STEMI and was derived from non-uniform cohorts of patients regarding forms of MI, reperfusion treatment and pharmacotherapy. Nowadays, in consequence of current standards of STEMI management, incorporating percutaneous coronary intervention (PCI) as a means of effective and safe reperfusion, together with dual antiplatelet treatment, we have witnessed a spectacular reduction in the rates of death, reinfarction, heart failure and strokes.

Our investigation aims to assess the relationship between selected baseline and post-PCI ECG variables and the presence of LVSD 6 months after a first STEMI.

2. Methods

2.1. Study Design

The investigation was a prospective cohort trial including patients receiving primary PCI with stent implantation for a first STEMI. Study design, including the inclusion and exclusion criteria, was described in detail in our previous publication exploring associations of ECG with post-MI left ventricular remodeling (LVR) [18]. Here, we provide only a brief overview of the study design. Major exclusion criteria were as follows: any previous myocardial infarction or coronary revascularization, presence of advanced acute or chronic heart failure (defined as class IV according to the Killip classification or class ≥III according to the New York Heart Association), presence of ECG abnormalities that might become study confounders (i.e., left bundle branch block, isolated posterior myocardial infarction, isolated right ventricular myocardial infarction, permanent atrial fibrillation), severe valvular heart disease, any cardiomyopathy, poorly controlled arterial hypertension (defined as blood pressure ≥180/110 mmHg on hospital admission) and significant kidney dysfunction on hospital admission (defined as creatinine concentration exceeding 2 mg/dL).

The analyzed ECG parameters included:
1. heart rate,
2. location of STEMI,
3. number of leads with ST-segment elevation,
4. sum of ST-segment elevation in all leads,
5. maximal ST-segment elevation in a single lead,
6. ST-segment resolution,
7. presence of reciprocal ST-segment depression ≥0.1 mV on admission to hospital,
8. number of leads with pathological Q-waves [19],
9. Sclarovsky-Birnbaum ischemia score [2],
10. QRS complex duration.

The primary study endpoint was the occurrence of LVSD 6 months after STEMI. LVSD was defined as LVEF ≤40% on transthoracic echocardiography. This cut-off value was previously shown to be associated with unfavorable prognosis [10,20–24]. Additionally, LVEF ≤40% is used by the European Society of Cardiology guidelines for defining heart failure with reduced ejection fraction [25] and post-infarct patients who benefit from therapy with a beta-blocker, angiotensin-converting enzyme inhibitor or mineralocorticoid receptor antagonist [26].

First, we planned to compare the clinical, biochemical, angiographic and echocardiographic characteristics. We also assessed differences in ECG parameters between patients with and without LVSD 6 months after STEMI. Second, we prespecified uni- and multivariate analyses aimed at identifying predictors of post-infarct LVSD. A particular focus was placed on the investigated ECG parameters.

As a final step, we planned to check whether the variables predictive of the primary study endpoint were associated with lower values of LVEF (expressed as a continuous parameter) 6 months after STEMI.

Details of coronary angiography, PCI technique and ECG evaluation were also published in our previous publication [18]. Importantly, we aimed to restore normal blood flow in the infarct-related artery (IRA) during the primary PCI. Other non-culprit lesions of $\geq 90\%$ in major coronary vessels were treated during the index hospitalization, while PCIs of the remaining significant stenoses (70–90%) were done electively (within 1 month of STEMI occurrence).

Informed consent for participation in the study was obtained from each participant. The study received approval from the local Bioethics Committee of Collegium Medicum, Nicolaus Copernicus University in Toruń (protocol code KB 440/2004). Throughout the entire course of the study, the Declaration of Helsinki and the principles of good clinical practice were applied.

2.2. Echocardiographic Assessment

Two-dimensional transthoracic echocardiography was performed in order to evaluate left ventricular systolic function using a Philips Sonos 7500 device (Philips, Andover, MA, USA) at two time points: before hospital discharge and after 6 months. Image acquisitions and measurements were performed according to the recommendations of the European Association of Echocardiography and the American Society of Echocardiography [27,28]. The biplane method of discs (modified Simpson's rule) based on apical 4-chamber and 2-chamber view was utilized for LVEF estimation. The echocardiographer was blinded to the ECG analysis. The intra-observer coefficient of variation for LVEF estimation for the first 50 patients was 2.5%.

2.3. Data Collection and Statistical Analysis

Relevant data were collected and initially analyzed using Microsoft Excel spreadsheet software (Microsoft Corporation, Redmond, WA, USA). No missing data were present.

Descriptive analysis was used to summarize participant characteristics. Categorical data are presented as frequencies and percentages. Continuous variables are reported as medians and interquartile ranges. Correspondence with normal distribution was verified with the Shapiro-Wilk test. Between-group differences were tested using the Mann-Whitney U test for continuous variables and the Pearson Chi-square and Mantel-Haensztel tests for categorical variables. In order to identify predictors of LVSD at 6 months, logistic regression was used. The results are presented as odds ratios (OR) with 95% confidence intervals. Only variables with univariate p-values of <0.1 were included in the multivariate models. Stepwise backward selection was employed to select variables included in the best-fitting models. To identify predictors of LVEF at 6 months, we used multiple linear regression. Variables showing univariate p-values of <0.1 were considered eligible for multivariate analyses. The variables were then removed via stepwise backward selection. p-values of <0.05 were considered significant. Data analysis was conducted using Statistica version 13 (TIBCO Software Inc., Palo Alto, CA, USA) and SPSS version 23 (IBM, Armonk, NY, USA).

3. Results

3.1. The Course of the Study

The final analysis included 249 patients. A detailed description of the course of the study can be found in our previous publication [18].

3.2. Clinical, Demographic, Angiographic and Biochemical Parameters

The study cohort was primarily composed of middle-aged men. At baseline, patients who presented with LVSD after 6 months of follow-up showed a higher prevalence of diabetes mellitus, left anterior descending artery (LAD) as the IRA and TIMI 0 flow before PCI, but less frequent TIMI 3 flow post PCI. Slightly worse kidney function (assessed based on glomerular filtration rate), higher plasma glucose concentration on admission to hospital, larger enzymatic infarct size (as assessed with maximal concentration of troponin I and maximal activity of isoenzyme MB of creatinine kinase [CK-MB]), higher concentration of B-type natriuretic peptide (BNP) and more common usage of GPIIb/IIIa inhibitors during PCI could also be found in this group. Detailed characteristics of the study population are presented in Table 1.

Table 1. Clinical characteristics of the study population in relation to the occurrence of LVSD. Data are presented as median (lower quartile-upper quartile) or number (percent) when appropriate.

Variable	Overall Study Population (n = 249)	Patients with LVSD at 6 Months (n = 52)	Patients without LVSD at 6 Months (n = 197)	p *
Age [years]	57.0 (51.0–64.0)	61.0 (52.0–67.0)	56.0 (51.0–64.0)	0.090
Gender [male/female]	186 (74.7%)/63 (25.3%)	42 (80.8%)/10 (19.3%)	144 (73.1%)/53 (26.9%)	0.258
Time from symptom onset to PCI [min]	220.0 (150.0–331.5)	223.5 (148.5–346.0)	220.0 (150.0–321.5)	0.727
Risk factors for coronary artery disease				
BMI [kg/m^2]	26.8 (24.2–29.4)	27.4 (25.0–30.2)	26.5 (24.1–29.1)	0.058
Hypertension	103 (41.4%)	24 (46.2%)	79 (40.1%)	0.431
Diabetes mellitus	50 (20.1%)	16 (30.8%)	34 (17.3%)	0.031
Current or ex-smoker	164 (65.9%)	29 (55.8%)	135 (68.5%)	0.084
Positive family history of IHD	61 (24.5%)	10 (19.2%)	51 (25.9%)	0.321
Angiographic characteristics				
IRA: LAD/other	121 (48.6%)/128 (52.4)	47 (90.4%)/5 (9.6%)	74 (37.6%)/123 (62.4%)	<0.001
IRA TIMI 0 flow prior to PCI	144 (57.8%)	39 (75.0%)	105 (53.3%)	0.005
IRA TIMI 3 flow post PCI	229 (92.0%)	41 (78.8%)	188 (95.4%)	0.001
Multivessel coronary artery disease	143 (57,4%)	34 (65.4%)	109 (55.3%)	0.192
Stent implantation	245 (98.4%)	51 (98.1%)	194 (98.5%)	0.678
GP IIb/IIIa inhibitor usage	66 (26.5%)	25 (48.1%)	41 (21.0%)	<0.001
Biochemical characteristics				
eGFR (CKD-EPI equation) [mL/min/1.73 m^2]	84.4 (74.1–94.5)	80.3 (72.8–88.1)	86.5 (75.0–96.6)	0.036
Glucose on admission [mg/dL]	138.5 (122.0–169.0)	157.0 (133.0–193.0)	135 (118.0–168.0)	0.001
cTnI$_{max}$ [ng/mL]	41.2 (11.8–50.0)	50.0 (50.0–50.0)	29.1 (9.7–50.0)	<0.001
CK-MB$_{max}$ [U/L]	242.0 (116.5–414.0)	489.0 (361.5–747.0)	178.5 (95.0–347.5)	<0.001
Total cholesterol [mg/dL]	223.0 (195.0–251.0)	223.0 (195.0–252.0)	223.0 (195.0–251.0)	0.688
LDL-C [mg/dL]	145.0 (125.0–173.0)	145.0 (131.5–170.0)	146.0 (124.0–174.0)	0.712
HDL-C [mg/dL]	52.0 (46.0–59.0)	51.0 (43.0–56.0)	52.0(46.0–59.0)	0.128
Triglycerides [mg/dL]	82.0 (59.0–128.0)	89.5 (62.5–130.5)	78.0(58.0–125.0)	0.103
BNP on admission [pg/mL]	53.9 (27.9–106.5)	74.8 (31.8–155.7)	50.6(27.3–101.9)	0.045
BNP at discharge [pg/mL]	139.8 (74.7–284.2)	436.7 (223.6–735.5)	111.9 (65.3–198.3)	<0.001

BMI, body mass index; BNP, B-type natriuretic peptide; CKD-EPI, Chronic Kidney Disease Epidemiology Collaboration; CK-MB$_{max}$, maximal activity of isoenzyme MB of creatinine kinase; cTnI$_{max}$, maximal activity of troponin I; eGFR, estimated glomerular filtration rate; HDL-C, high-density-lipoprotein cholesterol; IHD, ischemic heart disease; IRA, infarct-related artery; LAD, left anterior descending artery; LDL-C, low-density-lipoprotein cholesterol; LVSD, left ventricular systolic dysfunction; PCI, percutaneous coronary intervention; TIMI, thrombolysis in myocardial infarction score. * for comparison between groups with and without LVSD at 6 months.

3.3. Echocardiographic Characteristics

Table 2 presents major echocardiographic parameters at the time of discharge from hospital and after 6 months in the overall study population and in the subgroups with and without LVSD. Within 6 months of STEMI, a significant increase in median values of LVEF from 44% to 46% could be noted, leading to a decline in the percentage of patients with LVEF ≤40% from a baseline value of 33.7% to 20.9% after 6 months ($p < 0.001$; Table 3).

Table 2. Echocardiographic characteristics of the study population in relation to LVSD occurrence. Data are presented as median (lower quartile-upper quartile).

Variable	Overall Study Population (n = 249)	Patients with LVSD at 6 Months (n = 52)	Patients without LVSD at 6 Months (n = 197)	p *
		At discharge		
LA [mm]	40.0 (37.0–43.0)	41.0 (38.0–45.0)	39.0 (37.0–42.0)	0.007
LVEDd [mm]	49.0 (45.0–53.0)	53.0 (49.0–56.0)	47.0 (45.0–52.0)	<0.001
LVESd [mm]	34.0 (30.0–37.0)	38.0 (35.0–40.5)	33.0 (30.0–36.0)	<0.001
LVEDV [mL]	99.4 (84.0–121.0)	121.5 (102.5–132.5)	93.0 (81.0–111.0)	<0.001
LVESV [mL]	55.0 (45.0–69.0)	75.0 (66.0–84.5)	51.0 (42.5–62.0)	<0.001
LVEF [%]	44.0 (39.0–48.4)	36.0 (33.5–38.5)	45.9 (42.0–50.0)	<0.001
LVSD (LVEF ≤ 40%)	84.0 (33.7%)	45 (86.5%)	39 (19.8%)	<0.001
WMSI [points]	1.56 (1.38–1.75)	1.88 (1.78–1.94)	1.44 (1.38–1.69)	<0.001
		6 months after discharge		
LA [mm]	40.0 (38.0–44.0)	44.0 (40.0–46.0)	40.0 (37.0–42.0)	<0.001
LVEDd [mm]	50.0 (46.0–54.0)	55.0 (52.0–57.0)	48.0 (45.0–53.0)	<0.001
LVESd [mm]	34.0 (31.0–37.0)	40.0 (36.0–44.0)	33.0 (31.0–36.0)	<0.001
LVEDV [mL]	110.0 (94.0–134.0)	145.0 (129.5–163.0)	105.0 (91.0–125.0)	<0.001
LVESV [mL]	57.0 (48.0–76.0)	92.0 (79.0–103.0)	53.0 (45.0–65.0)	<0.001
LVEF [%]	46.0 (42.0–51.5)	36.0 (33.7–38.5)	48.0 (44.8–52.5)	<0.001
WMSI [points]	1.44 (1.31–1.69)	1.88 (1.75–1.94)	1.38 (1.31–1.50)	<0.001

LA, left atrium end-systolic diameter; LVEDd, left ventricular end-diastolic diameter; LVEDV, left ventricular end-diastolic volume; LVEF, left ventricular ejection fraction; LVESd, left ventricular end-systolic diameter; LVESV, left ventricular end-systolic volume; LVSD, left ventricular systolic dysfunction; WMSI, wall motion score index. * for comparison between groups with and without LVSD at 6 months.

Table 3. Occurrence of LVEF ≤ 40 % on transthoracic echocardiography at hospital discharge and at 6 months.

		LVEF ≤ 40 % (LVSD) at 6 Months	
		Absent (n = 197)	Present (n = 52)
LVEF ≤40 % at hospital discharge	Absent (n = 165)	158 (63.5%)	7 (2.8%)
	Present (n = 84)	39 (15.7%)	45 (18.1%)

LVEF, left ventricular ejection fraction; LVSD, left ventricular systolic dysfunction.

Interestingly, patients with LVEF ≤40% at the time of discharge from hospital, but not 6 months after STEMI (n = 39), when compared with those presenting with LVEF ≤ 40% both at hospital discharge and LVSD 6 months after STEMI (n = 45), had a lower proportion of the LAD as the IRA (31 [79.5%] vs. 42 [93.3%]; $p = 0.058$), more frequent TIMI 3 flow in the IRA following PCI (38 [97.4%] vs. 34 [75.6%]; $p = 0.002$) and lower values of cardiac biomarkers, including maximal concentration of cardiac troponin I (50.0 [27.7–50.0] vs. 50.0 [50.0–50.0] ng/mL; $p = 0.039$), maximal activity of CK-MB (354 [159–404] vs. 555 [378–761] U/L; $p < 0.001$) and BNP concentration on hospital discharge (177.3 [113.5–282.0] vs. 439.3 [233.0–751.5] pg/mL; $p < 0.001$).

3.4. Electrocardiographic Characteristics

Detailed baseline and post-PCI electrocardiographic data are reported in Table 4.

Table 4. Electrocardiographic characteristics of the study population in relation to LVSD occurrence. Data are presented as median (lower quartile-upper quartile) or number (percent) when appropriate.

Variable	Overall Study Population (n = 249)	Patients with LVSD at 6 Months (n = 52)	Patients without LVSD at 6 Months (n = 197)	p *
		Baseline		
Heart rate [BPM]	75.0 (62.0–88.0)	81.0 (68.5–97.0)	74.0 (60.0–85.0)	<0.001
Anterior location of STEMI	116 (47.0%)	47 (90.4%)	69 (35.0%)	<0.001
Number of leads with ST-segment elevation [n]	4.0 (3.0–6.0)	6.0 (5.0–7.0)	3.0 (3.0–5.0)	<0.001
Sum of ST-segment elevation [mm]	8.5 (4.0–14.0)	13.8 (9.8–18.0)	7.0 (4.0–12.0)	<0.001
Maximal ST-segment elevation [mm]	3.0 (2.0–4.0)	3.5 (3.0–5.0)	2.5 (1.5–4.0)	<0.001
Number of leads with pathologic Q waves [n]	2.0 (1.0–4.0)	4.0 (3.0–5.0)	2.0 (1.0–3.0)	<0.001
Presence of reciprocal ST-segment depression ≥ 1mm	193 (77.5%)	34 (65.4%)	159 (80.7%)	0.019
QRS duration [ms]	95.0 (85.0–100.0)	95.0 (86.0–110.0)	95.0 (85.0–100.0)	0.399
Sclarovsky-Birnbaum ischemia score	grade 2: 198 (79.5%); grade 3: 51 (20.5%)	grade 2: 35 (67.3%); grade 3: 17 (32.7%)	grade 2: 163 (82.7%); grade 3: 34 (17.3%)	0.014
		Post PCI		
Heart rate [BPM]	77.0 (66.0–89.0)	83.0 (72.0–94.0)	75.0 (64.0–88.0)	0.003
ST-segment resolution [%]	60.6 (30.0–88.9)	39.4 (0.0–69.3)	70.0 (40.0–100.0)	<0.001
ST-segment resolution (≥50%)	160 (64.3%)	22 (42.3%)	138 (70.1%)	<0.001
ST-segment resolution after PCI (trichotomised)	<30%–62 (24.9%) ≥30–69%–82 (32.9%) ≥70%–105 (42.2%)	<30%–22 (42.3%) ≥30–69%–24 (46.2%) ≥70%–6 (11.5%)	<30%–40 (20.3%) ≥30–69%–58 (29.4%) ≥70%–99 (50.3%)	<0.001
Number of leads with ST-segment elevation [n]	3.0 (1.0–5.0)	5.5 (4.0–7.0)	3.0 (0.0–4.0)	<0.001
Sum of ST-segment elevation [mm]	3.0 (1.0–7.0)	8.3 (5.0–13.0)	2.0 (0.0–4.5)	<0.001
Maximal ST-segment elevation [mm]	1.0 (0.5–2.0)	2.3 (1.5–4.0)	1.0 (0.5–1.5)	<0.001
Number of leads with pathologic Q waves [n]	3.0 (2.0–5.0)	5.0 (4.0–7.0)	3.0 (1.0–4.0)	<0.001
QRS duration [ms]	90.0 (84.0–100.0)	99.5 (87.5–111.0)	90.0 (83.0–100.0)	0.003

BPM, beats per minute; LVSD, left ventricular systolic dysfunction; PCI, percutaneous coronary intervention; STEMI, ST-segment elevation myocardial infarction. * for comparison between groups with and without LVSD at 6 months.

3.5. Characteristics Comparison of Patients with and without LVSD

As reported in Table 1, both groups showed no significant demographic nor clinical differences, except for a higher prevalence of diabetes in the LVSD (+) group. LVSD (+) patients also presented a less favorable angiographic profile, including more frequent involvement of LAD as the IRA, more widespread usage of GP IIb/IIIa inhibitor, a higher incidence of TIMI 0 and less frequent occurrence of TIMI 3 flow before and after PCI, respectively. Patients who presented with LVSD after 6 months were also characterized at baseline by worse renal function as assessed with glomerular filtration rate, higher blood glucose concentration on admission, more extensive release of myocardial necrosis markers and higher concentrations of B-type natriuretic peptide both on admission and at discharge. At discharge, both groups were receiving similar pharmacological treatment regarding aspirin, clopidogrel, statin, beta-blocker and ACEI/ARB (all used in ≥98.5% of patients); however, LVSD (+) patients were receiving aldosterone antagonist (28.8% vs. 5.1%; $p < 0.001$) and diuretic (28.8% vs. 4.6%; $p < 0.001$) more frequently than their LVSD (−) counterparts.

3.6. Electrocardiographic Characteristics of Patients with LVSD

The analyzed ECG parameters, both at baseline and post PCI, point to more severe ischemia and a more extensive MI in the LVSD (+) group. These include faster heart rate, more widespread ST-segment elevation and Q-wave development and higher total and maximal ST-segment elevation. More pronounced ischemia in LVSD (+) patients was also evidenced by a higher incidence of anterior wall location, reciprocal ST-segment depression ≥1 mm and grade 3 according to Sclarovsky-Birnbaum ischemia grading system at baseline. In post-PCI ECG assessment, lower incidence and degree of ST-segment resolution and longer duration of the QRS complex were associated with the presence of LVSD after 6 months. A detailed comparison of ECG parameters is reported in Table 4. As shown in Figure 1, we also found visual variability and a linear trend toward an increasing rate of LVSD at 6 months with an increasing duration of the QRS complex on admission (OR for the upper vs. combined lower and middle terciles 1.59; 95% CI 0.80–3.17; $p = 0.180$) and after PCI (OR for the upper vs. combined lower and middle terciles 3.42; 95% CI 1.76–6.66; $p < 0.001$). We also noticed significantly lower values of LVEF in the highest tercile of baseline and post-PCI QRS duration, compared with the lowest and middle terciles (see Figure 1).

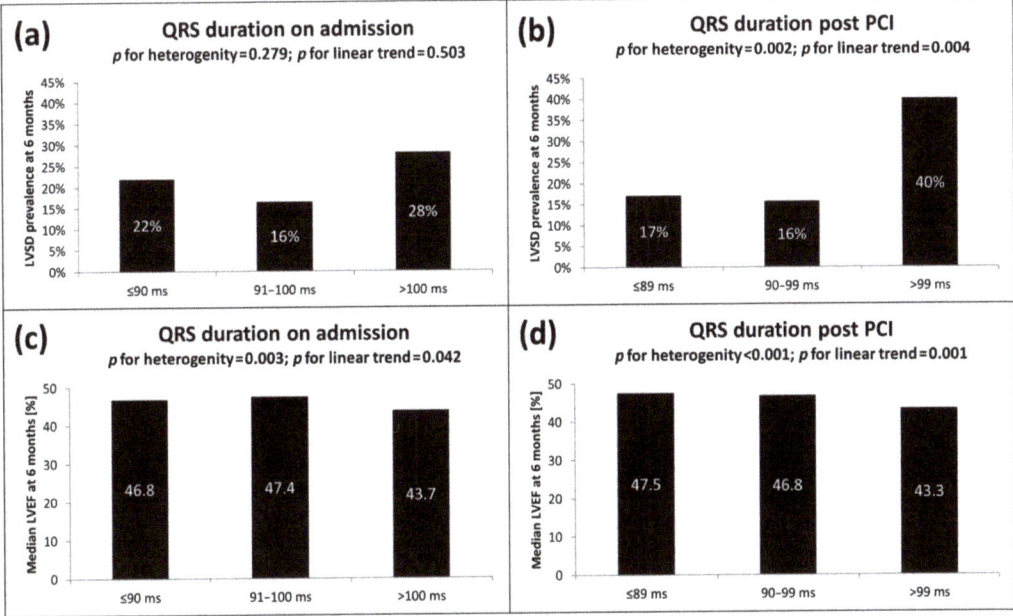

Figure 1. LVSD prevalence 6 months after STEMI according to terciles of QRS duration (**a**) on admission and (**b**) post PCI. Median LVEF 6 months after STEMI according to increasing terciles of QRS duration (**c**) on admission and (**d**) post PCI. LVEF, left ventricular ejection fraction; LVSD, left ventricular systolic dysfunction; ms, milliseconds; PCI, percutaneous coronary intervention; STEMI, ST-segment elevation myocardial infarction.

3.7. Predictors of the Presence of LVSD 6 Months after Discharge from Hospital

Initially, we performed a univariate regression analysis, including electrocardiographic parameters and the variables from Table 1, to identify possible predictors of LVSD after 6 months. Unadjusted models are summarized in Figure 2. Our results indicate strong association of LVSD after 6 months with the majority of electrocardiographic parameters assessed at the time of presentation to hospital and post PCI. Only baseline QRS duration did not show statistical significance. Of note, reciprocal ST-segment depression ≥ 1mm at baseline pointed to a lower likelihood of LVSD after 6 months.

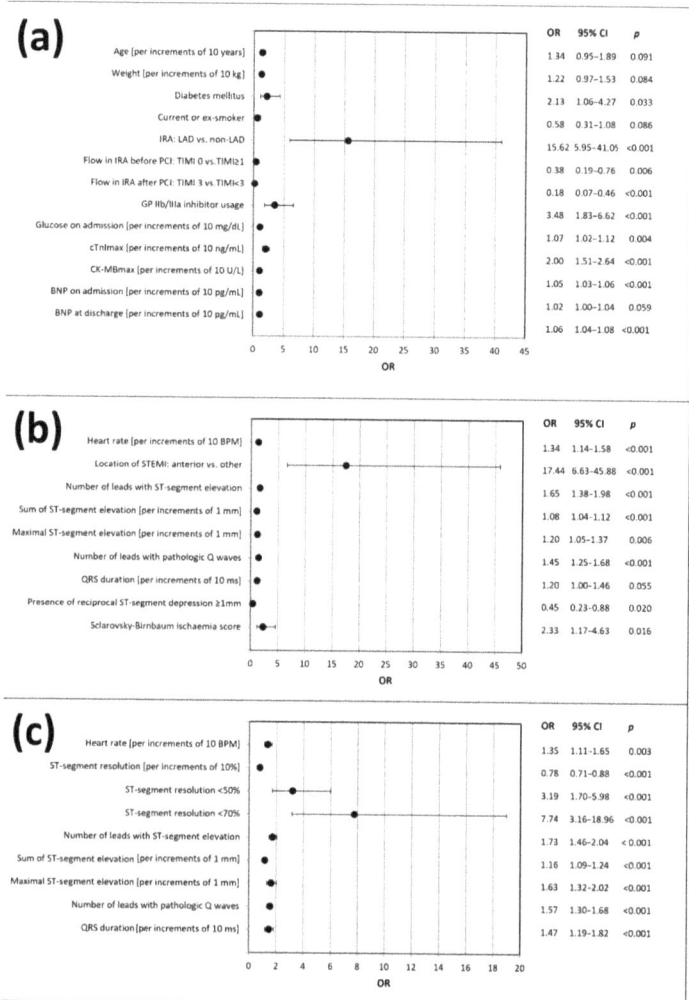

Figure 2. Predictors of LVSD occurrence after 6 months of follow-up according to the univariate logistic regression analysis: (**a**) demographic, clinical, angiographic and biochemical variables; (**b**) baseline electrocardiographic variables; (**c**) post-PCI electrocardiographic variables. BNP, B-type natriuretic peptide; CK-MBmax, maximal activity of isoenzyme MB of creatinine kinase; cTnImax, maximal concentration of troponin I; CI, confidence interval; IRA, infarct-related artery; LAD, left anterior descending artery; LVSD, left ventricular systolic dysfunction; ms, milliseconds; OR, odds ratio; PCI, percutaneous coronary intervention; STEMI, ST-segment elevation myocardial infarction; TIMI, thrombolysis in myocardial infarction score.

Among the analyzed angiographic variables, LAD as the IRA and usage of GP IIb/IIIa inhibitor were identified as predictors of LVSD occurrence, while TIMI 0 flow before PCI and TIMI 3 flow post PCI were associated with a lower incidence of LVSD after 6 months. The biochemical variables predicting LVSD occurrence included glucose concentration on admission, maximal cardiac troponin I concentration and CK-MB activity, as well as BNP concentration at discharge from hospital. The only clinical variable predictive of LVSD was the presence of diabetes mellitus.

Next, in order to determine possible independent predictors of LVSD after 6 months, a multivariate logistic regression analysis was performed. We identified anterior location of STEMI, longer post-PCI QRS duration and impaired post-PCI flow in the IRA as the independent predictors of LVSD 6 months after STEMI (Figure 3).

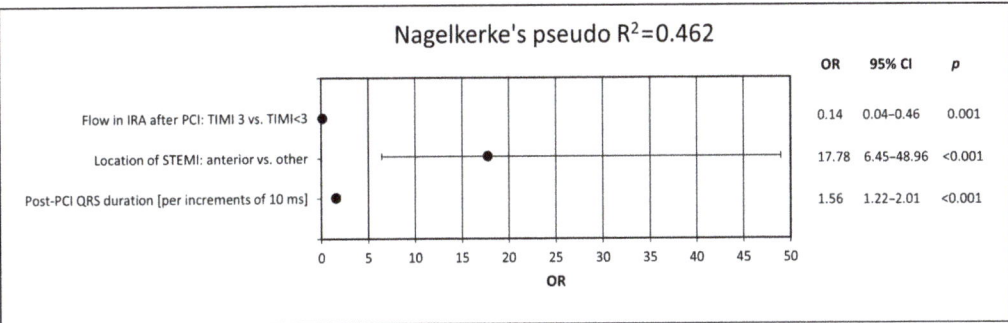

Figure 3. Predictors of LVSD presence after 6 months of follow-up. The model was created using multivariate logistic regression analysis by adding all electrocardiographic variables to the demographic, clinical, angiographic and biochemical data. CI, confidence interval; IRA, infarct-related artery; LVSD, left ventricular systolic dysfunction; ms, milliseconds; OR, odds ratio; PCI, percutaneous coronary intervention; STEMI, ST-segment elevation myocardial infarction, TIMI, thrombolysis in myocardial infarction score.

3.8. Determinants of LVEF Deterioration

In an attempt to more thoroughly explore the relationship between ECG parameters and LVEF, multiple linear regression analysis with a backward elimination was applied (Table 5). We found that anterior location of STEMI, longer post-PCI QRS duration, higher baseline number of pathological Q-waves and higher baseline Sclarovsky-Birnbaum ischemia score, together with impaired post-PCI flow in the IRA, higher values of body mass index and glucose concentration on admission, were independently associated with lower values of LVEF at 6 months.

Table 5. Impact of demographic, clinical, angiographic, biochemical and electrocardiographic variables on left ventricular ejection fraction (LVEF) 6 months after STEMI. The model was obtained using multiple regression by adding all electrocardiographic variables to the demographic, clinical and angiographic data.

Variable	Beta Coefficient	Beta Coefficient Standard Error	Direction Component Beta	Direction Component Beta Standard Error	p
Model characteristics: R = 0.682; R^2 = 0.464; corrected R^2 = 0.448; p < 0.00001					
Intercept			70.49	3.71	<0.0001
BMI [kg/m^2]	−0.10	0.05	−0.20	0.10	0.0461
Glucose on admission [per increments of 10 mg/dL]	−0.16	0.05	−0.21	0.07	0.0021
IRA TIMI 3 flow after PCI	0.12	0.05	−3.20	1.36	0.0196
Anterior location of STEMI	−0.36	0.05	−5.45	0.83	<0.0001
QRS duration on admission [per increments of 10 ms]	−0.28	0.05	−1.36	0.25	<0.0001
Number of leads with pathologic Q waves on admission	−0.24	0.05	−0.82	0.18	<0.0001
Sclarovsky-Birnbaum ischemia score [grade 3 vs. grade 2]	−0.12	0.05	−2.33	0.94	0.0137

BMI, body mass index; IRA, infarct-related artery; PCI, percutaneous coronary intervention; STEMI, ST-segment elevation myocardial infarction; TIMI, thrombolysis in myocardial infarction score.

4. Discussion

4.1. General Findings and Study Strengths

According to our results, the majority of the analyzed electrocardiographic parameters measured at baseline and directly after PCI were associated with LVSD 6 months after STEMI. However, when we considered demographic, clinical, angiographic and biochemical characteristics of our study participants, among all assessed ECG parameters, only anterior location of STEMI and longer post-PCI QRS duration remained independent predictors of post-MI LVSD. Additionally, in our study, anterior location of STEMI, longer post-PCI QRS duration, higher baseline number of pathological Q-waves and higher baseline Sclarovsky-Birnbaum ischemia score, together with impaired post-PCI flow in the IRA, higher values of body mass index and glucose concentration on admission, were independently associated with lower LVEF at 6 months.

All electrocardiographic parameters selected for our analysis have been described in the literature to have some predictive value towards LVEF and LVSD. However, many of these reports come from the thrombolysis era and from inhomogeneous cohorts of patients. Our study cohort is characterized by homogeneity concerning the form of acute coronary syndrome presentation (exclusively patients with a first STEMI), reperfusion therapy (exclusively primary PCI) and subsequent pharmacotherapy [18]. This uniformity in study cohort profile, in conjunction with appropriate inclusion and exclusion criteria, allowed us to avoid many potential confounders and enables the extrapolation of these results to the majority of contemporary patients with a first STEMI. Importantly, besides multiple ECG parameters, we examined the impact of numerous demographic, clinical, angiographic and biochemical variables on LVSD occurrence.

4.2. Heart Rate

Increased heart rate is a well-recognized risk factor for all-cause and cardiovascular mortality in the general population [29–35], as well as in patients with stable coronary disease [36–40], heart failure [41–45] and MI [46–48]. In STEMI patients, heart rate > 70 bpm recorded at hospital discharge was associated with 2-fold higher 1 year and 4 year mortality rates, while a 5 bpm increment of heart rate was considered to enhance 1 year and 4 year mortality by 29% and 24%, respectively [49]. As reflected by a U-shaped curve, extreme heart rate values (both high and low) are associated with increased mortality [50].

However, we have not found any relevant reports in the literature on the relation of heart rate in the early phase of STEMI with LVEF and the development of post-MI LVSD.

4.3. STEMI Location

Anterior wall location of STEMI is a strong independent predictor of bad prognosis, including death [51] and the occurrence of cardiogenic shock in the course of STEMI [52,53], even in the era of primary PCI for STEMI. Associations between anterior location of STEMI and more common development of LVSD [10,11] and left ventricular remodeling [54] have also been reported; however, they were not seen in all studies [55].

4.4. ST-Segment-Elevation-Related Parameters

We also evaluated three parameters related to ST-segment elevation (number of leads with ST-segment elevation, sum of ST-segment elevations in all leads, maximal ST-segment elevation in a single lead). According to Rodríguez-Palomares et al., the first two of the three parameters measured in pre-PCI ECG correlated with the size of myocardium at risk [56]. In research by Manes et al., the sum of ST-segment elevation, maximal ST-segment elevation and the number of leads with ST-segment elevation ≥ 1 mm in predischarge ECG in patients with anterior STEMI predicted a lower probability of recovery of left ventricular function after 90 days [17]. The 3 ST-segment-related parameters have been shown to predict post-STEMI mortality [50,57]. The amplitude of ST-segment elevation was found to be an independent predictor of post-MI 30-day mortality, particularly for total amplitudes ≥ 15 mm [58], and a marker of coronary microcirculation obstruction, performing even superior to ST-segment resolution [59]. It also predicted lack of improvement in left ventricular systolic function after STEMI in 6-month follow-up [60].

4.5. ST-Segment Resolution

Resolution of ST-segment elevation of ≥50% is considered a reliable indicator of patency of the IRA. However, restoration of myocardial tissue perfusion occurs only when complete (≥70%) ST-elevation resolution is achieved. Complete (≥70%) resolution of ST-segment elevation predicts lower 1–3 year mortality and lower rates of cardiovascular adverse events [61–63] and was associated with better preservation of left ventricular function in comparison with partial (30–70%) or no (<30%) ST-segment resolution. The beneficial outcome of early complete resolution of ST-segment elevation can be seen even after successful primary PCI, with early (i.e., directly after PCI) assessment being more precise in terms of predicting cardiovascular adverse events than assessment after 90 min [64–67]. Additionally, patients with such early ST-segment resolution also had higher LVEF in comparison to those who achieved ST-segment resolution after 90 min [64]. Failure to achieve complete ST-segment resolution also determined higher peak creatine kinase levels and more common prevalence of significant LVSD [68].

4.6. Reciprocal ST-Segment Depression

Besides ECG changes recorded in leads overlying the area of STEMI, the presence of reciprocal ST-segment depressions at baseline may also hold prognostic value. In literature reports it reflected larger infarct area and multivessel coronary artery disease and was associated with increased mortality and higher rates of heart failure, cardiogenic shock and second- and third-degree heart block in a manner proportional to their extent and amplitude [69,70]. Additionally, sustained ST-segment depressions after PCI are predictive of increased mortality after STEMI [71]. We have found no literature reports concerning associations of reciprocal ST-segment depressions with LVSD.

4.7. Pathological Q-Waves

The number of leads with pathological Q-waves is another well-recognized predictor of post-MI mortality. It successfully predicted lack of recovery of left ventricular systolic function (defined as absolute LVEF improvement by <10%) within 6 months after STEMI [60]. The presence of pathological Q-waves on the admission ECG is predictive of increased mortality, heart failure and cardiogenic shock after STEMI [3,4,72]. According to Lopez-Castillo et al., the sum of Q-wave depth at discharge performs better than the number of leads with pathological Q-waves as an independent predictor of LVSD development [73].

4.8. Sclarovsky-Birnbaum Ischemia Score

Based on the morphology of the terminal portion of the QRS complex and the relative magnitude of ST-segment elevation, the score identifies three grades of ischemia, with grade 3 reflecting most severe ischemia [74] and being an independent predictor of no-reflow phenomenon [67] and mortality [75,76]. Compared with grade 2, it indicates a more extensive infarction area and a higher rate of mortality, heart failure and reinfarction [67,76–84]. In terms of left ventricular systolic function, grade 3 of ischemia was associated with lower LVEF [82,85] and a higher incidence of LVSD [67].

4.9. QRS Duration

Prolonged QRS duration is another well-established predictor of increased mortality in STEMI patients [86–88]. The detrimental effects can already be seen with QRS duration of ≥100 ms [89]. An increase in 30-day mortality was even found for prolongation of QRS duration still within normal ranges (100 ms vs. 80 ms) [50]. Literature reports documenting the relation between QRS duration and LVSD are much scarcer; however, they point to prolonged QRS duration, and even QRS duration of ≥100 ms, as a predictor of LVSD [16,90].

4.10. Detailed Analysis of the Study Results

As one can surmise from the above review of the prognostic value of the electrocardiographic parameters, the majority of the literature concerns their association with mortality, while there is a scarcity of data concerning associations with LVSD or LVEF. This fact precludes direct comparison of our results with the cited investigations. However, recognizing LVSD as a surrogate for cardiovascular mortality, the results of our investigation support the prognostic value of ECG regarding prognosis assessment following STEMI.

The results of our investigation basically support the data from the literature. Our study participants who presented with LVSD 6 months after STEMI, in comparison to those without LVSD, had significantly higher values of heart rate, number of leads with ST-segment elevation and pathological Q-waves, sum of ST-segment elevation and maximal ST-segment elevation on admission to hospital and directly after PCI. They also showed a higher prevalence of anterior STEMI and considerably wider QRS after PCI, while QRS duration measurement at baseline showed no significant difference. Additionally, patients presenting with LVSD after 6 months showed more severe ischemia on admission, as assessed with Sclarovsky-Birnbaum ischemia score, smaller reciprocal ST-segment depression at baseline and less profound ST-segment resolution post PCI.

In univariate analysis, all but one of the ECG parameters predicted LVSD occurrence 6 months after STEMI, the most powerful being anterior location of STEMI (OR 17.44; 95% CI 6.63–45.88). Our analysis also indicates good predictive value of ST-segment resolution and grade 3 according to the Sclarovsky-Birnbaum ischemia score, which came in as the second and third most powerful LVSD predictors. However, it is important to remember that some of the remaining parameters were reported per increments, which means that their actual final impact potentiates when the increments are multiplied in measurements. The only exception was QRS duration at baseline, which did not show statistical significance. In contrast to literature data, in our investigation, the presence of reciprocal ST-segment depressions diminished the likelihood of LVSD occurrence 6 months after STEMI. Whether this could be a consequence of shorter time-to-balloon delay in this group, compared with patients without reciprocal ST-segment depressions, remains a matter of speculation and requires verification in a larger group since the difference in time-to-balloon between patients with and without LVSD was not statistically significant.

In the model adjusted for demographic, clinical, biochemical and angiographic variables, however, the majority of the ECG parameters did not maintain statistical significance. The only two parameters contributing to the multivariate regression model and thus recognized as independent predictors of LVSD in 6-month follow-up were anterior location of STEMI (OR 17.78; 95% CI 6.45–48.96; $p < 0.001$) and post-PCI QRS duration (OR 1.56; 95% CI 1.22–2.00; $p < 0.001$) expressed per increment of 10 ms. The highest tercile of post-PCI QRS duration (i.e., ≥100 ms) was associated with the highest prevalence of LVSD after 6 months and therefore appears to have the best discriminative value. The highest terciles of baseline and post-PCI QRS duration were also associated with significantly lower values of LVEF, compared with lower terciles.

4.11. Study Limitations

There are some limitations of this study to be mentioned. First, the study population is a fraction of the original cohort of patients recruited between 2005 and 2008. The time that had elapsed from patient recruitment to the onset of the project and clinical practice modifications implemented over that time could possibly impact the results. Second, LVSD, used as the endpoint in our investigation, is a well-documented prognostic factor in post-STEMI patients; however, it is still a surrogate of clinical endpoints. The choice of LVSD as an endpoint was dictated by lack of power of this study to evaluate clinical endpoints. Third, the duration of follow-up in our research was restricted to 6 months. It seems likely that extending this period might render more favorable results in terms of predictive capabilities of ECG. Forth, the relatively moderate left ventricular systolic function impairment and the applied exclusion criteria noticeably blunting the risk of death and the rate of adverse cardiovascular outcomes in our study group, together with the relatively short time to reperfusion, limit the applicability of our results to all STEMI patients. This warrants further research in non-uniform STEMI cohorts before unrestricted extrapolation of our findings to the general population is feasible. Fifth, enhanced precision of evaluation of left ventricular systolic function, size of myocardial necrosis and patency of the coronary microcirculation could possibly be achieved by employing magnetic resonance imaging. Sixth, we routinely used neither fractional flow reserve measurement nor intravascular ultrasound for the assessment of non-culprit lesions. Seventh, non-critical, non-culprit coronary lesions (stenoses 70–90%) were revascularized electively (within 1 month of the index hospital admission). This fact might have some impact on the study findings. Eighth, in a substantial number of our study participants, maximal concentration of cardiac troponin I exceeded 50 ng/mL. These serum samples were not further diluted, preventing precise estimation of the biochemical infarct size. Ninth, patients with left bundle branch block, isolated posterior myocardial infarction, isolated right ventricular myocardial infarction or permanent atrial fibrillation were excluded from the study. Therefore, the study findings may not to be attributable to such patients. Finally, post-reperfusion ECG parameters in time points other than directly after PCI were not assessed.

5. Conclusions

According to our study, baseline and post-PCI ECG parameters possess a modest predictive value for LVSD occurrence within 6 months of a first STEMI.

Author Contributions: Conceptualization, M.K. (Marek Koziński) and J.K.; data curation, T.F.; formal analysis, M.K. (Michał Kasprzak); investigation, T.F.; methodology, T.F. and M.K. (Marek Koziński); project administration, J.K.; supervision, M.K. (Marek Koziński) and J.K.; visualization, M.K. (Michał Kasprzak); writing—original draft, T.F. and M.K. (Michał Kasprzak); writing—review and editing, M.K. All authors have read and agreed to the published version of the manuscript.

Funding: This study was supported by the financial resources of the Polish Ministry of Science and Higher Education for Science, 2008–2011 (Research Project No. N402179534).

Institutional Review Board Statement: The study was conducted according to the guidelines of the Declaration of Helsinki and approved by the Ethics Committee of Collegium Medicum, Nicolaus Copernicus University (protocol code KB 440/2004, date of approval 5 August 2004).

Informed Consent Statement: Informed consent was obtained from all subjects involved in the study.

Data Availability Statement: Data sharing is not applicable to this article.

Acknowledgments: We are grateful to the staff of the Echocardiography Laboratory, particularly Iwona Świątkiewicz, for performing echocardiographic examinations. We would also like to thank the residents and nurses for their important contribution in participant enrolment, blood sampling and data collection.

Conflicts of Interest: The authors declare that there is no conflict of interest. The funders had no role in the design of the study; in the collection, analyses, or interpretation of data; in the writing of the manuscript, or in the decision to publish the results.

References

1. Fye, W.B. A history of the origin, evolution, and impact of electrocardiography. *Am. J. Cardiol.* **1994**, *73*, 937–949. [CrossRef]
2. Herring, N.; Paterson, D.J. ECG diagnosis of acute ischaemia and infarction: Past, present and future. *QJM* **2006**, *99*, 219–230. [CrossRef] [PubMed]
3. Siha, H.; Das, D.; Fu, Y.; Zheng, Y.; Westerhout, C.M.; Storey, R.F.; James, S.; Wallentin, L.; Armstrong, P.W. Baseline Q waves as a prognostic modulator in patients with ST segment elevation: Insights from the PLATO trial. *CMAJ* **2012**, *184*, 1135–1142. [CrossRef] [PubMed]

4. Kaul, P.; Fu, Y.; Westerhout, C.M.; Granger, C.B.; Armstrong, P.W. Relative prognostic value of baseline Q wave and time from symptom onset among men and women with ST-elevation myocardial infarction undergoing percutaneous coronary intervention. *Am. J. Cardiol.* **2012**, *110*, 1555–1560. [CrossRef]
5. Weir, R.A.; McMurray, J.J. Epidemiology of heart failure and left ventricular dysfunction after acute myocardial infarction. *Curr. Heart Fail. Rep.* **2006**, *3*, 175–180. [CrossRef]
6. Sutton, M.G.; Sharpe, N. Left ventricular remodeling after myocardial infarction: Pathophysiology and therapy. *Circulation* **2000**, *101*, 2981–2988. [CrossRef]
7. Minicucci, M.F.; Azevedo, P.S.; Polegato, B.F.; Paiva, S.A.; Zornoff, L.A. Heart failure after myocardial infarction: Clinical implications and treatment. *Clin. Cardiol.* **2011**, *34*, 410–414. [CrossRef]
8. Cohn, J.N.; Ferrari, R.; Sharpe, N. Cardiac remodeling—Concepts and clinical implications: A consensus paper from an international forum on cardiac remodeling. Behalf of an International Forum on Cardiac Remodeling. *J. Am. Coll. Cardiol.* **2000**, *35*, 569–582. [CrossRef]
9. Weir, R.A.; McMurray, J.J.; Velazquez, E.J. Epidemiology of heart failure and left ventricular systolic dysfunction after acute myocardial infarction: Prevalence, clinical characteristics, and prognostic importance. *Am. J. Cardiol.* **2006**, *97*, 13F–25F. [CrossRef]
10. Velazquez, E.J.; Francis, G.S.; Armstrong, P.W.; Aylward, P.E.; Diaz, R.; O'Connor, C.M.; White, H.D.; Henis, M.; Rittenhouse, L.M.; Kilaru, R.; et al. An international perspective on heart failure and left ventricular systolic dysfunction complicating myocardial infarction: The VALIANT registry. *Eur. Heart J.* **2004**, *25*, 1911–1919. [CrossRef]
11. Świątkiewicz, I.; Magielski, P.; Woźnicki, M.; Gierach, J.; Jabłoński, M.; Fabiszak, T.; Koziński, M.; Sukiennik, A.; Bronisz, A.; Kubica, J. Occurrence and predictors of left ventricular systolic dysfunction at hospital discharge and in long-term follow-up after acute myocardial infarction treated with primary percutaneous coronary intervention. *Kardiol. Pol.* **2012**, *70*, 329–340. [PubMed]
12. Nicod, P.; Gilpin, E.; Dittrich, H.; Chappuis, F.; Ahnve, S.; Engler, R.; Henning, H.; Ross, J., Jr. Influence on prognosis and morbidity of left ventricular ejection fraction with and without signs of left ventricular failure after acute myocardial infarction. *Am. J. Cardiol.* **1988**, *61*, 1165–1171. [CrossRef]
13. Ottervanger, J.P.; Ramdat Misier, A.R.; Dambrink, J.H.; de Boer, M.J.; Hoorntje, J.C.; Gosselink, A.T.; Suryapranata, H.; Reiffers, S.; van 't Hof, A.W.J. Mortality in patients with left ventricular ejection fraction ≤30% after primary percutaneous coronary intervention for ST-elevation myocardial infarction. *Am. J. Cardiol.* **2007**, *100*, 793–797. [CrossRef] [PubMed]
14. Daneault, B.; Généreux, P.; Kirtane, A.J.; Witzenbichler, B.; Guagliumi, G.; Paradis, J.M.; Fahy, M.P.; Mehran, R.; Stone, G.W. Comparison of Three-year outcomes after primary percutaneous coronary intervention in patients with left ventricular ejection fraction <40% versus ≥40% (from the HORIZONS-AMI trial). *Am. J. Cardiol.* **2013**, *111*, 12–20. [CrossRef] [PubMed]
15. Marenzi, G.; Moltrasio, M.; Assanelli, E.; Lauri, G.; Marana, I.; Grazi, M.; Rubino, M.; De Metrio, M.; Veglia, F.; Bartorelli, A.L. Impact of cardiac and renal dysfunction on inhospital morbidity and mortality of patients with acute myocardial infarction undergoing primary angioplasty. *Am. Heart J.* **2007**, *153*, 755–762. [CrossRef] [PubMed]
16. Murkofsky, R.L.; Dangas, G.; Diamond, J.A.; Mehta, D.; Schaffer, A.; Ambrose, J.A. A prolonged QRS duration on surface electrocardiogram is a specific indicator of left ventricular dysfunction. *J. Am. Coll. Cardiol.* **1998**, *32*, 476–482. [CrossRef]
17. Manes, C.; Pfeffer, M.A.; Rutherford, J.D.; Greaves, S.; Rouleau, J.L.; Arnold, J.M.; Menapace, F.; Solomon, S.D. Value of the electrocardiogram in predicting left ventricular enlargement and dysfunction after myocardial infarction. *Am. J. Med.* **2003**, *114*, 99–105. [CrossRef]
18. Kasprzak, M.; Fabiszak, T.; Koziński, M.; Kubica, J. Diagnostic Performance of Selected Baseline Electrocardiographic Parameters for Prediction of Left Ventricular Remodeling in Patients with ST-Segment Elevation Myocardial Infarction. *J. Clin. Med.* **2021**, *10*, 2405. [CrossRef] [PubMed]
19. Thygesen, K.; Alpert, J.S.; White, H.D. on behalf of the Joint ESC/ACCF/AHA/WHF Task Force for the Redefinition of Myocardial Infarction. Universal definition of myocardial infarction. *Eur. Heart J.* **2007**, *28*, 2525–2538.
20. Raymond, I.; Mehlsen, J.; Pedersen, F.; Dimsits, J.; Jacobsen, J.; Hildebrandt, P.R. The prognosis of impaired left ventricular systolic function and heart failure in a middle-aged and elderly population in an urban population segment of Copenhagen. *Eur. J. Heart Fail.* **2004**, *6*, 653–661. [CrossRef]
21. Krumholz, H.M.; Chen, J.; Chen, Y.T.; Wang, Y.; Radford, M.J. Predicting one-year mortality among elderly survivors of hospitalization for an acute myocardial infarction: Results from the Cooperative Cardiovascular Project. *J. Am. Coll. Cardiol.* **2001**, *38*, 453–459. [CrossRef]
22. Rott, D.; Behar, S.; Hod, H.; Feinberg, M.S.; Boyko, V.; Mandelzweig, L.; Kaplinsky, E.; Gottlieb, S.; Argatroban in Acute Myocardial Infarction-2 (ARGAMI-2) Study Group. Improved survival of patients with acute myocardial infarction with significant left ventricular dysfunction undergoing invasive coronary procedures. *Am. Heart J.* **2001**, *141*, 267–276. [CrossRef] [PubMed]
23. Swiatkiewicz, I.; Kozinski, M.; Magielski, P.; Gierach, J.; Fabiszak, T.; Kubica, A.; Sukiennik, A.; Navarese, E.P.; Odrowaz-Sypniewska, G.; Kubica, J. Usefulness of C-reactive protein as a marker of early post-infarct left ventricular systolic dysfunction. *Inflamm. Res.* **2012**, *61*, 725–734. [CrossRef] [PubMed]
24. Møller, J.E.; Brendorp, B.; Ottesen, M.; Køber, L.; Egstrup, K.; Poulsen, S.H.; Torp-Pedersen, C. Congestive heart failure with preserved left ventricular systolic function after acute myocardial infarction: Clinical and prognostic implications. *Eur. J. Heart Fail.* **2003**, *5*, 811–819. [CrossRef]

25. McDonagh, T.A.; Metra, M.; Adamo, M.; Gardner, R.S.; Baumbach, A.; Böhm, M.; Burri, H.; Butler, J.; Čelutkienė, J.; Chioncel, O.; et al. 2021 ESC Guidelines for the diagnosis and treatment of acute and chronic heart failure. *Eur Heart J.* **2021**, *42*, 3599–3726. [CrossRef]
26. Ibanez, B.; James, S.; Agewall, S.; Antunes, M.J.; Bucciarelli-Ducci, C.; Bueno, H.; Caforio, A.L.P.; Crea, F.; Goudevenos, J.A.; Halvorsen, S.; et al. 2017 ESC Guidelines for the management of acute myocardial infarction in patients presenting with ST-segment elevation: The Task Force for the management of acute myocardial infarction in patients presenting with ST-segment elevation of the European Society of Cardiology (ESC). *Eur. Heart J.* **2018**, *39*, 119–177.
27. Lang, R.; Bierig, M.; Devereux, B.; Flachskampf, F.A.; Foster, E.; Pellikka, P.A.; Picard, M.H.; Roman, M.J.; Seward, J.; Shanewise, J.; et al. Recommendations for chamber quantification. *Eur. J. Echocardiogr.* **2006**, *7*, 79–108. [CrossRef]
28. Schiller, N.; Shah, P.; Crawford, M.; DeMaria, A.; Devereux, R.; Feigenbaum, H.; Gutgesell, H.; Reichek, N.; Sahn, D.; Schnittger, I.; et al. Recommendations for quantitation of the left ventricle by two-dimensional echocardiography. *J. Am. Soc. Echocardiogr.* **1989**, *2*, 358–367. [CrossRef]
29. Kannel, W.B. Risk stratification in hypertension: New insights from the Framingham Study. *Am. J. Hypertens.* **2000**, *13*, 3S–10S. [CrossRef]
30. Hori, M.; Okamoto, H. Heart rate as a target of treatment of chronic heart failure. *J. Cardiol.* **2012**, *60*, 86–90. [CrossRef]
31. Perret-Guillaume, C.; Joly, L.; Benetos, A. Heart rate as a risk factor for cardiovascular disease. *Prog. Cardiovasc. Dis.* **2009**, *52*, 6–10. [CrossRef] [PubMed]
32. Palatini, P.; Thijs, L.; Staessen, J.A.; Fagard, R.H.; Bulpitt, C.J.; Clement, D.L.; de Leeuw, P.W.; Jaaskivi, M.; Leonetti, G.; Nachev, C.; et al. Predictive value of clinic and ambulatory heart rate for mortality in elderly subjects with systolic hypertension. *Arch. Intern. Med.* **2002**, *162*, 2313–2321. [CrossRef] [PubMed]
33. Reunanen, A.; Karjalainen, J.; Ristola, P.; Heliövaara, M.; Knekt, P.; Aromaa, A. Heart rate and mortality. *J. Intern. Med.* **2000**, *247*, 231–239. [CrossRef]
34. Jensen, M.T.; Marott, J.L.; Allin, K.H.; Nordestgaard, B.G.; Jensen, G.B. Resting heart rate is associated with cardiovascular and all-cause mortality after adjusting for inflammatory markers: The Copenhagen City Heart Study. *Eur. J. Prev. Cardiol.* **2012**, *19*, 102–108. [CrossRef]
35. Jouven, X.; Empana, J.P.; Schwartz, P.J.; Desnos, M.; Courbon, D.; Ducimetière, P. Heart-rate profile during exercise as a predictor of sudden death. *N. Engl. J. Med.* **2005**, *352*, 1951–1958. [CrossRef] [PubMed]
36. Diaz, A.; Bourassa, M.G.; Guertin, M.C.; Tardif, J.C. Long-term prognostic value of resting heart rate in patients with suspected or proven coronary artery disease. *Eur. Heart J.* **2005**, *26*, 967–974. [CrossRef] [PubMed]
37. Shaper, A.G.; Wannamethee, G.; Macfarlane, P.W.; Walker, M. Heart rate, ischaemic heart disease, and sudden cardiac death in middle-aged British men. *Br. Heart J.* **1993**, *70*, 49–55. [CrossRef]
38. Kolloch, R.; Legler, U.F.; Champion, A.; Cooper-Dehoff, R.M.; Handberg, E.; Zhou, Q.; Pepine, C.J. Impact of resting heart rate on outcomes in hypertensive patients with coronary artery disease: Findings from the INternationalVErapamil-SR/trandolapril STudy (INVEST). *Eur. Heart J.* **2008**, *29*, 1327–1334. [CrossRef]
39. O'Riordan, M. High Heart Rate Linked with Increased Mortality in Stable Coronary Heart Disease. Medscape 2010. Available online: http://www.medscape.com/viewarticle/731449 (accessed on 14 October 2021).
40. Lonn, E.M.; Rambihar, S.; Gao, P.; Custodis, F.F.; Sliwa, K.; Teo, K.K.; Yusuf, S.; Böhm, M. Heart rate is associated with increased risk of major cardiovascular events, cardiovascular and all-cause death in patients with stable chronic cardiovascular disease: An analysis of ONTARGET/TRANSCEND. *Clin. Res. Cardiol.* **2014**, *103*, 149–159. [CrossRef]
41. MERIT-HF Study Group. Effect of metoprolol CR/XL in chronic heart failure: Metoprolol CR/XL Randomised Intervention Trial in Congestive Heart Failure (MERIT-HF). *Lancet* **1999**, *353*, 2001–2007. [CrossRef]
42. Gullestad, L.; Wikstrand, J.; Deedwania, P.; Hjalmarson, A.; Egstrup, K.; Elkayam, U.; Gottlieb, S.; Rashkow, A.; Wedel, H.; Bermann, G.; et al. What resting heart rate should one aim for when treating patients with heart failure with a beta-blocker? Experiences from the Metoprolol Controlled Release/Extended Release Randomized Intervention Trial in Chronic Heart Failure (MERIT-HF). *J. Am. Coll. Cardiol.* **2005**, *45*, 252–259. [CrossRef] [PubMed]
43. Lechat, P.; Hulot, J.S.; Escolano, S.; Mallet, A.; Leizorovicz, A.; Werhlen-Grandjean, M.; Pochmalicki, G.; Dargie, H. Heart rate and cardiac rhythm relationships with bisoprolol benefit in chronic heart failure in CIBIS II Trial. *Circulation* **2001**, *103*, 1428–1433. [CrossRef] [PubMed]
44. Böhm, M.; Swedberg, K.; Komajda, M.; Borer, J.S.; Ford, I.; Dubost-Brama, A.; Dubost-Brama, A.; Lerebours, G.; Tavazzi, L. Heart rate as a risk factor in chronic heart failure (SHIFT): The association between heart rate and outcomes in a randomised placebo-controlled trial. *Lancet* **2010**, *376*, 886–894. [CrossRef]
45. Swedberg, K.; Komajda, M.; Böhm, M.; Borer, J.S.; Ford, I.; Dubost-Brama, A.; Lerebours, G.; Tavazzi, L. Ivabradine and outcomes in chronic heart failure (SHIFT): A randomised placebo-controlled study. *Lancet* **2010**, *376*, 875–885. [CrossRef]
46. Berton, G.S.; Cordiano, R.; Palmieri, R.; Gheno, G.; Mormino, P.; Palatini, P. Heart rate during myocardial infarction: Relationship with one-year global mortality in men and women. *Can. J. Cardiol.* **2002**, *18*, 495–502. [PubMed]
47. Hjalmarson, A.; Gilpin, E.A.; Kjekshus, J.; Schieman, G.; Nicod, P.; Henning, H.; Ross, J., Jr. Influence of heart rate on mortality after acute myocardial infarction. *Am. J. Cardiol.* **1990**, *65*, 547–553. [CrossRef]
48. Zuanetti, G.; Hernandez-Bernal, F.; Rossi, A.; Comerio, G.; Paolucci, G.; Maggioni, A.P. Relevance of heart rate as a prognostic factor in patients with acute myocardial infarction: The GISSI experience. *Eur. Heart J.* **1999**, *1*, H52–H57.

49. Antoni, M.L.; Boden, H.; Delgado, V.; Boersma, E.; Fox, K.; Schalij, M.J.; Bax, J.J. Relationship between discharge heart rate and mortality in patients after acute myocardial infarction treated with primary percutaneous coronary intervention. *Eur. Heart J.* **2012**, *33*, 96–102. [CrossRef]
50. Hathaway, W.R.; Peterson, E.D.; Wagner, G.S.; Granger, C.B.; Zabel, K.M.; Pieper, K.S.; Clark, K.A.; Woodlief, L.H.; Califf, R.M. Prognostic significance of the initial electrocardiogram in patients with acute myocardial infarction. GUSTO-I Investigators. Global Utilization of Streptokinase and t-PA for Occluded Coronary Arteries. *JAMA* **1998**, *279*, 387–391. [CrossRef]
51. Harjai, K.J.; Mehta, R.H.; Stone, G.W.; Boura, J.A.; Grines, L.; Brodie, B.R.; Cox, D.A.; O'Neill, W.W.; Grines, C.L. Does proximal location of culprit lesion confer worse prognosis in patients undergoing primary percutaneous coronary intervention for ST elevation myocardial infarction? *J. Interv. Cardiol.* **2006**, *19*, 285–294. [CrossRef]
52. Conde-Vela, C.; Moreno, R.; Hernández, R.; Pérez-Vizcayno, M.J.; Alfonso, F.; Escaned, J.; Sabaté, M.; Bañuelos, C.; Macaya, C. Cardiogenic shock at admission in patients with multivessel disease and acute myocardial infarction treated with percutaneous coronary intervention: Related factors. *Int. J. Cardiol.* **2007**, *123*, 29–33. [CrossRef]
53. Jarai, R.; Huber, K.; Bogaerts, K.; Sinnaeve, P.R.; Ezekowitz, J.; Ross, A.M.; Zeymer, U.; Armstrong, P.W.; Van de Werf, F.J. Prediction of cardiogenic shock using plasma B-type natriuretic peptide and the N-terminal fragment of its pro-hormone [corrected] concentrations in ST elevation myocardial infarction: An analysis from the ASSENT-4 Percutaneous Coronary Intervention Trial. *Crit. Care Med.* **2010**, *38*, 1793–1801. [CrossRef] [PubMed]
54. Bolognese, L.; Neskovic, A.N.; Parodi, G.; Cerisano, G.; Buonamici, P.; Santoro, G.M.; Antoniucci, D. Left ventricular remodeling after primary coronary angioplasty: Patterns of left ventricular dilation and long-term prognostic implications. *Circulation* **2002**, *106*, 2351–2357. [CrossRef] [PubMed]
55. Mattichak, S.J.; Harjai, K.J.; Dutcher, J.R.; Boura, J.A.; Stone, G.; Cox, D.; Brodie, B.R.; O'Neill, W.W.; Grines, C.L. Left ventricular remodeling and systolic deterioration in acute myocardial infarction: Findings from the Stent-PAMI Study. *J. Interv. Cardiol.* **2005**, *18*, 255–260. [CrossRef]
56. Rodríguez-Palomares, J.F.; Figueras-Bellot, J.; Descalzo, M.; Moral, S.; Otaegui, I.; Pineda, V.; Del Blanco, B.G.; González-Alujas, M.T.; Evangelista Masip, A.; García-Dorado, D. Relation of ST-segment elevation before and after percutaneous transluminal coronary angioplasty to left ventricular area at risk, myocardial infarct size, and systolic function. *Am. J. Cardiol.* **2014**, *113*, 593–600. [CrossRef] [PubMed]
57. Mauri, F.; Franzosi, M.G.; Maggioni, A.P.; Santoro, E.; Santoro, L. Clinical value of 12-lead electrocardiography to predict the long-term prognosis of GISSI-1 patients. *J. Am. Coll. Cardiol.* **2002**, *39*, 1594–1600. [CrossRef]
58. Sejersten, M.; Ripa, R.S.; Maynard, C.; Wagner, G.S.; Andersen, H.R.; Grande, P.; Mortensen, L.S.; Clemmensen, P. Usefulness of quantitative baseline ST-segment elevation for predicting outcomes after primary coronary angioplasty or fibrinolysis (results from the DANAMI-2 trial). *Am. J. Cardiol.* **2006**, *97*, 611–616. [CrossRef]
59. Husser, O.; Bodí, V.; Sanchis, J.; Núñez, J.; Mainar, L.; Rumiz, E.; López-Lereu, M.P.; Monmeneu, J.; Chaustre, F.; Trapero, I.; et al. The sum of ST-segment elevation is the best predictor of microvascular obstruction in patients treated successfully by primary percutaneous coronary intervention. Cardiovascular magnetic resonance study. *Rev. Esp. Cardiol.* **2010**, *63*, 1145–1154. [CrossRef]
60. Bigi, R.; Mafrici, A.; Colombo, P.; Gregori, D.; Corrada, E.; Alberti, A.; De Biase, A.; Orrego, P.S.; Fiorentini, C.; Klugmann, S. Relation of terminal QRS distortion to left ventricular functional recovery and remodeling in acute myocardial infarction treated with primary angioplasty. *Am. J. Cardiol.* **2005**, *96*, 1233–1236. [CrossRef]
61. Van der Zwaan, H.B.; Stoel, M.G.; Roos-Hesselink, J.W.; Veen, G.; Boersma, E.; von Birgelen, C. Early versus late ST-segment resolution and clinical outcomes after percutaneous coronary intervention for acute myocardial infarction. *Neth. Heart J.* **2010**, *18*, 416–422. [CrossRef]
62. Farkouh, M.E.; Reiffel, J.; Dressler, O.; Nikolsky, E.; Parise, H.; Cristea, E.; Baran, D.A.; Dizon, J.; Merab, J.P.; Lansky, A.J.; et al. Relationship between ST-segment recovery and clinical outcomes after primary percutaneous coronary intervention: The HORIZONS-AMI ECG substudy report. *Circ. Cardiovasc. Interv.* **2013**, *6*, 216–223. [CrossRef] [PubMed]
63. Vaturi, M.; Birnbaum, Y. The use of the electrocardiogram to identify epicardial coronary and tissue reperfusion in acute myocardial infarction. *J. Thromb. Thrombolysis* **2000**, *10*, 137–147. [CrossRef] [PubMed]
64. Kumar, S.; Sivagangabalan, G.; Hsieh, C.; Ryding, A.D.; Narayan, A.; Chan, H.; Burgess, D.C.; Ong, A.T.; Sadick, N.; Kovoor, P. Predictive value of ST resolution analysis performed immediately versus at ninety minutes after primary percutaneous coronary intervention. *Am. J. Cardiol.* **2010**, *105*, 467–474. [CrossRef] [PubMed]
65. Matetzky, S.; Novikov, M.; Gruberg, L.; Freimark, D.; Feinberg, M.; Elian, D.; Novikov, I.; Di Segni, E.; Agranat, O.; Har-Zahav, Y.; et al. The significance of persistent ST elevation versus early resolution of ST segment elevation after primary PTCA. *J. Am. Coll. Cardiol.* **1999**, *34*, 1932–1938. [CrossRef]
66. Buller, C.E.; Fu, Y.; Mahaffey, K.W.; Todaro, T.G.; Adams, P.; Westerhout, C.M.; White, H.D.; van 't Hof, A.W.; Van de Werf, F.J.; Wagner, G.S.; et al. ST-segment recovery and outcome after primary percutaneous coronary intervention for ST-elevation myocardial infarction: Insights from the Assessment of Pexelizumab in Acute Myocardial Infarction (APEX-AMI) trial. *Circulation* **2008**, *118*, 1335–1346. [CrossRef]
67. Wolak, A.; Yaroslavtsev, S.; Amit, G.; Birnbaum, Y.; Cafri, C.; Atar, S.; Gilutz, H.; Ilia, R.; Zahger, D. Grade 3 ischemia on the admission electrocardiogram predicts failure of ST resolution and of adequate flow restoration after primary percutaneous coronary intervention for acute myocardial infarction. *Am. Heart J.* **2007**, *153*, 410–417. [CrossRef] [PubMed]

68. Schröder, R.; Wegscheider, K.; Schröder, K.; Dissmann, R.; Meyer-Sabellek, W. Extent of early ST segment elevation resolution: A strong predictor of outcome in patients with acute myocardial infarction and a sensitive measure to compare thrombolytic regimens. A substudy of the International Joint Efficacy Comparison of Thrombolytics (INJECT) trial. *J. Am. Coll. Cardiol.* **1995**, *26*, 1657–1664. [PubMed]
69. Peterson, E.D.; Hathaway, W.R.; Zabel, K.M.; Pieper, K.S.; Granger, C.B.; Wagner, G.S.; Topol, E.J.; Bates, E.R.; Simoons, M.L.; Califf, R.M. Prognostic significance of precordial ST segment depression during inferior myocardial infarction in the thrombolytic era: Results in 16,521 patients. *J. Am. Coll. Cardiol.* **1996**, *28*, 305–312. [CrossRef]
70. Birnbaum, Y.; Herz, I.; Sclarovsky, S.; Zlotikamien, B.; Chetrit, A.; Olmer, L.; Barbash, G.I. Prognostic significance of precordial ST segment depression on admission electrocardiogram in patients with inferior wall myocardial infarction. *J. Am. Coll. Cardiol.* **1996**, *28*, 313–318. [CrossRef]
71. Kozuch, M.; Dobrzycki, S.; Nowak, K.; Prokopczuk, P.; Kralisz, P.; Bachorzewska-Gajewska, H.; Kaminski, K.; Kozieradzka, A.; Korecki, J.; Poniatowski, B.; et al. Lack of ST-segment depression normalization after PCI is a predictor of 5-year mortality in patients with ST-elevation myocardial infarction. *Circ. J.* **2007**, *71*, 1851–1856. [CrossRef] [PubMed]
72. Armstrong, P.W.; Fu, Y.; Westerhout, C.M.; Hudson, M.P.; Mahaffey, K.W.; White, H.D.; Todaro, T.G.; Adams, P.X.; Aylward, P.E.; Granger, C.B. Baseline Q-wave surpasses time from symptom onset as a prognostic marker in ST-segment elevation myocardial infarction patients treated with primary percutaneous coronary intervention. *J. Am. Coll. Cardiol.* **2009**, *53*, 1503–1509. [CrossRef]
73. López-Castillo, M.; Aceña, Á.; Pello-Lázaro, A.M.; Viegas, V.; Merchán Muñoz, B.; Carda, R.; Franco-Peláez, J.; Martín-Mariscal, M.L.; Briongos-Figuero, S.; Tuñón, J. Prognostic value of initial QRS analysis in anterior STEMI: Correlation with left ventricular systolic dysfunction, serum biomarkers, and cardiac outcomes. *Ann. Noninvasive Electrocardiol.* **2021**, *26*, e12791. [CrossRef]
74. Birnbaum, Y.; Sclarovsky, S. The grades of ischemia on the presenting electrocardiogram of patients with ST elevation acute myocardial infarction. *J. Electrocardiol.* **2001**, *34*, 17–26. [CrossRef] [PubMed]
75. Garcia-Rubira, J.C.; Perez-Leal, I.; Garcia-Martinez, J.T.; Molano, F.; Hidalgo, R.; Gómez-Barrado, J.J.; Cruz, J.M. The initial electrocardiographic pattern is a strong predictor of outcome in acute myocardial infarction. *Int. J. Cardiol.* **1995**, *51*, 301–305. [CrossRef]
76. Birnbaum, Y.; Herz, I.; Sclarovsky, S.; Zlotikamien, B.; Chetrit, A.; Olmer, L.; Barbash, G.I. Admission clinical and electrocardiographic characteristics predicting an increased risk for early reinfarction after thrombolytic therapy. *Am. Heart J.* **1998**, *135*, 805–812. [CrossRef]
77. Birnbaum, Y.; Herz, I.; Sclarovsky, S.; Zlotikamien, B.; Chetrit, A.; Olmer, L.; Barbash, G.I. Prognostic significance of the admission electrocardiogram in acute myocardial infarction. *J. Am. Coll. Cardiol.* **1996**, *27*, 1128–1132. [CrossRef]
78. Birnbaum, Y.; Goodman, S.; Barr, A.; Gates, K.B.; Barbash, G.I.; Battler, A.; Barbagelata, A.; Clemmensen, P.; Sgarbossa, E.B.; Granger, C.B.; et al. Comparison of primary coronary angioplasty versus thrombolysis in patients with ST-segment elevation acute myocardial infarction and grade II and grade III myocardial ischemia on the enrollment electrocardiogram. *Am. J. Cardiol.* **2001**, *88*, 842–847. [CrossRef]
79. Birnbaum, Y.; Kloner, R.; Sclarovsky, S.; Cannon, C.P.; McCabe, C.H.; Davis, V.G.; Zaret, B.L.; Wackers, F.J.; Braunwald, E. Distortion of the terminal portion of the QRS on the admission electrocardiogram in acute myocardial infarction and correlation with infarct size and long term prognosis (Thrombolysis in Myocardial Infarction 4 Trial). *Am. J. Cardiol.* **1996**, *78*, 396–403. [CrossRef]
80. Birnbaum, Y.; Maynard, C.; Wolfe, S.; Mager, A.; Strasberg, B.; Rechavia, E.; Gates, K.; Wagner, G.S. Terminal QRS distortion on admission is better than ST-segment measurements in predicting final infarct size and assessing the Potential effect of thrombolytic therapy in anterior wall acute myocardial infarction. *Am. J. Cardiol.* **1999**, *84*, 530–534. [CrossRef]
81. Birnbaum, Y.; Criger, D.A.; Wagner, G.S.; Strasberg, B.; Mager, A.; Gates, K.; Granger, C.B.; Ross, A.M.; Barbash, G.I. Prediction of the extent and severity of left ventricular dysfunction in anterior acute myocardial infarction by the admission electrocardiogram. *Am. Heart J.* **2001**, *141*, 915–924. [CrossRef] [PubMed]
82. Lee, C.W.; Hong, M.K.; Yang, H.S.; Choi, S.W.; Kim, J.J.; Park, S.W.; Park, S.J. Determinants and prognostic implications of terminal QRS complex distortion in patients treated with primary angioplasty for acute myocardial infarction. *Am. J. Cardiol.* **2001**, *88*, 210–213. [CrossRef]
83. Valle-Caballero, M.J.; Fernández-Jiménez, R.; Díaz-Munoz, R.; Mateos, A.; Rodríguez-Álvarez, M.; Iglesias-Vázquez, J.A.; Saborido, C.; Navarro, C.; Dominguez, M.L.; Gorjón, L.; et al. QRS distortion in pre-reperfusion electrocardiogram is a bedside predictor of large myocardium at risk and infarct size (a METOCARD-CNIC trial substudy). *Int. J. Cardiol.* **2016**, *202*, 666–673. [CrossRef] [PubMed]
84. Fernandez-Jimenez, R.; Valle-Caballero, M.J.; Diaz-Munoz, R.; Pizarro, G.; Fernandez-Friera, L.; Garcia-Ruiz, J.M.; Garcia-Alvarez, A.; Fuster, V.; Garcia-Rubira, J.C.; Ibanez, B. Terminal QRS distortion is an independent predictor of large area at risk and infarct size in patients with anterior STEMI. *J. Am. Coll. Cardiol.* **2015**, *65*, A196. [CrossRef]
85. Tamura, A.; Nagase, K.; Watanabe, T.; Nasu, M. Relationship between terminal QRS distortion on the admission and the time course of left ventricular wall motion in anterior wall acute myocardial infarction. *Jpn. Circ. J.* **2001**, *65*, 63–66. [CrossRef]
86. Iuliano, S.; Fisher, S.G.; Karasik, P.E.; Fletcher, R.D.; Singh, S.N. QRS duration and mortality in patients with congestive heart failure. *Am. Heart J.* **2002**, *143*, 1085–1091. [CrossRef] [PubMed]

87. Oikarinen, L.; Nieminen, M.S.; Viitasalo, M.; Toivonen, L.; Sverker, J.; Dahlöf, B.; Devereux, R.B.; Okin, P.M. QRS Duration and QT Interval Predict Mortality in Hypertensive Patients With Left Ventricular Hypertrophy. The Losartan Intervention for Endpoint Reduction in Hypertension Study. *Hypertension* **2004**, *43*, 1029–1034. [CrossRef] [PubMed]
88. Bauer, A.; Watanabe, M.A.; Barthel, P.; Schneider, R.; Ulm, K.; Schmidt, G. QRS duration and late mortality in unselected post-infarction patients of the revascularization era. *Eur. Heart J.* **2006**, *27*, 427–433. [CrossRef] [PubMed]
89. Nwakile, C.; Purushottam, B.; Yun, J.; Bhalla, V.; Morris, D.L.; Figueredo, V.M. QRS duration predicts 30 day mortality following ST elevation myocardial infarction. *Int. J. Cardiol. Heart Vasc.* **2014**, *5*, 42–44. [PubMed]
90. Olesen, L.L.; Andersen, A. ECG as a first step in the detection of left ventricular systolic dysfunction in the elderly. *ESC Heart Fail.* **2016**, *3*, 44–52. [CrossRef]

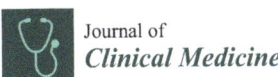

Article

Preoperative Predictors of Adverse Clinical Outcome in Emergent Repair of Acute Type A Aortic Dissection in 15 Year Follow Up

Miriam Freundt [1,2,*,†], Philipp Kolat [1,†], Christine Friedrich [1], Mohamed Salem [1], Matthias Gruenewald [3], Gunnar Elke [3], Thomas Pühler [1], Jochen Cremer [1] and Assad Haneya [1]

1. Department of Cardiovascular Surgery, University Medical Center Schleswig-Holstein, Campus Kiel, Arnold-Heller-Straße 3, 24105 Kiel, Germany; Philipp.Kolat@uksh.de (P.K.); Christine.Friedrich@uksh.de (C.F.); Mohamed.Salem@uksh.de (M.S.); Thomas.Puehler@uksh.de (T.P.); Jochen.Cremer@uksh.de (J.C.); assad.haneya@uksh.de (A.H.)
2. Heart and Vascular Institute, Intensive Care Unit, Penn State Health Milton S. Hershey Medical Center, Hershey, PA 23538, USA
3. Department of Anaesthesiology and Intensive Care Medicine, University Medical Center Schleswig-Holstein, Campus Kiel, Arnold-Heller-Str. 3 Haus R3, 24105 Kiel, Germany; Matthias.Gruenewald@uksh.de (M.G.); Gunnar.Elke@uksh.de (G.E.)
* Correspondence: mfreundt@psu.edu
† These authors contributed equally.

Abstract: Background: Acute type A aortic dissection (AAAD) has high mortality. Improvements in surgical technique have lowered mortality but postoperative functional status and decreased quality of life due to debilitating deficits remain of concern. Our study aims to identify preoperative conditions predictive of undesirable outcome to help guide perioperative management. Methods: We performed retrospective analysis of 394 cases of AAAD who underwent repair in our institution between 2001 and 2018. A combined endpoint of parameters was defined as (1) 30-day versus hospital mortality, (2) new neurological deficit, (3) new acute renal insufficiency requiring postoperative renal replacement, and (4) prolonged mechanical ventilation with need for tracheostomy. Results: Total survival/ follow-up time averaged 3.2 years with follow-up completeness of 94%. Endpoint was reached by 52.8%. Those had higher EuroSCORE II (7.5 versus 5.5), higher incidence of coronary artery disease (CAD) (9.2% versus 3.2%), neurological deficit (ND) upon presentation (26.4% versus 11.8%), cardiopulmonary resuscitation (CPR) (14.4% versus 1.6%) and intubation (RF) before surgery (16.9% versus 4.8%). 7-day mortality was 21.6% versus 0%. Hospital mortality 30.8% versus 0%. Conclusions: This 15-year follow up shows, that unfavorable postoperative clinical outcome is related to ND, CAD, CPR and RF on arrival.

Keywords: predictor; adverse outcome; emergent surgical repair; acute type A dissection

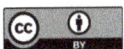

1. Introduction

Acute type A aortic dissection (AAAD) is a catastrophic event in which the inner layer of the ascending aorta tears and separates from the middle layer. Blood surges into the false lumen, which can result in multiple organ damage due to hypoperfusion. The condition can quickly deteriorate into shock, hemodynamic instability and death. Emergent surgical repair remains the gold standard of care. Due to acuity of the illness preoperative evaluation is limited, immediate decisions have to be made by surgeons and postoperative adverse clinical outcome remains oftentimes of concern [1–8]. Without treatment mortality increases dramatically by the hour and has been reported as high as 1 to 3% per hour during the first 24 h, 30% after one week, 80% after two weeks, and 90% at one year [9]. About 20% of patients with AAAD die before even reaching the hospital [9]. A recent multi-institutional study across all emergency rooms in Berlin, Germany from 2006 to 2016 showed an incidence of AAAD of 5.24 cases in 100,000 visits per year but based on the city's autopsy results 50% of AAAD had remained undetected [10]. Even with surgical repair mortality is high and ranges up to 16–27% within 30-days [11–13]. We may be able to reduce mortality with advances in surgical strategies and perioperative critical care, but functional status and quality of life (QoL) in survivors are becoming an increasing concern since simply surviving surgery but then ending up in an overall devastating condition must not be a goal. Alterations in lifestyle and emotional state are common in survivors of AAAD and many patients are unable to return to their previous occupation [14]. Previous studies investigating the survival of AAAD patients have been published. But there is only scarce data on the effect of preoperative risk factors on clinical outcome of these patients. Hence, the aim of this study was to associate obvious preoperative conditions with a combined endpoint of undesirable adverse clinical outcome, that might guide clinicians in future decision-making.

2. Materials and Methods

2.1. Study Design and Patient Population

We performed a retrospective analysis of our Aortic Dissection Register, which included all consecutive 394 cases of AAAD who underwent emergent repair in moderate hypothermic cardiac arrest (MHCA) in our institution between 2001 and 2018. AAAD was defined as dissection of the aortic wall that involved the ascending aorta with extension to the arch or descending aorta, regardless of the site of the primary intimal tear. Variants with aortic intramural hematoma and intimal tears without hematoma as well as penetrating atherosclerotic ulcers were included. Diagnosis was generally established with emergent computed tomographic (CT) angiography of the chest, abdomen, and pelvis. Bedside transthoracic echocardiography was used to assess the presence of pericardial effusion and overall left ventricular function and in addition patients routinely underwent transesophageal echocardiography after induction of general anesthesia and endotracheal intubation in the operating room to evaluate heart valves for need for concomitant procedures. A combined endpoint of four clinical outcome parameters was defined as (1) 30-day versus hospital mortality, (2) new neurological deficit, (3) new acute renal insufficiency requiring postoperative renal replacement therapy, and (4) prolonged mechanical ventilation with need for tracheostomy. Follow-up was conducted in May 2020 and long-term survival was evaluated by information given by the registry office.

2.2. Operative Technique and Postoperative Management

All cases were performed by experienced senior surgeons under general anesthesia in supine position with standard hemodynamic monitoring. All patients underwent median sternotomy and longitudinal pericardiotomy with cardiopulmonary bypass (CPB) in MHCA. The temperature probe was positioned in the nasopharynx and goal temperature was kept between 20 to 24 °C. From 2001 to 2010 arterial cannulation was achieved either by echocardiogram guided direct cannulation of the distal ascending aorta, the aortic arch, the apex, or either through the femoral or subclavian artery after surgical cut down. Starting in 2010 we gradually changed our standard approach for arterial cannulation to trans-atrial cannulation of the left ventricle via the right upper pulmonary vein [15]. The standard approach for venous drainage was cavoatrial cannulation with a common two-stage single venous cannula. Alternatively, we used echo guided cannulation of the femoral vein with a cannula extending into the right atrium or bicaval cannulation. Generally, we used retrograde injection of cold blood cardioplegic solution for myocardial protection after cross-clamping of the aorta. Bilateral antegrade cerebral perfusion with oxygenated cold blood (18 °C) was introduced through a balloon catheter inserted into the arch vessels with controlled flow pressure of 50–60 mmHg.

The origin and extend of the intimal tear determined the need for supracoronary ascending aortic replacement, partial versus total arch replacement with reimplantation of head and neck arteries, frozen elephant trunk, need for associated coronary artery bypass grafting or Conduit/Bentall procedure with reimplantation of coronary arteries versus David operation. After suturing of the distal anastomosis, the perfusion cannula was directly inserted into the graft. The aortic air was removed by resuming retrograde perfusion via the venous cannula followed by slow antegrade perfusion and then CPB was restarted. Continuous CO_2 insufflation was used in addition. After the establishment of the proximal anastomosis, transesophageal echocardiography was done to rule out remaining intracardiac air. After primary hemostasis was achieved, the chest was closed, and the patient was brought to the cardiac intensive care unit (ICU) for standard postoperative care.

Patients were assessed for neurological deficit routinely every hour while in the ICU and every eight hours after transfer to the floor. In case of a new deficit, CT head was performed followed by formal neurological evaluation and magnetic resonance imaging of the brain to confirm the diagnosis. Kidney function was assessed every hour while in the ICU and every eight hours on the floor. In case of acute renal insufficiency renal replacement therapy was initiated after evaluation by a nephrologist or in case of severe electrolyte disturbances emergently. Mechanical ventilation was weaned per standard postoperative protocol with a goal for liberation as soon as possible. Tracheostomy was performed if weaning from mechanical ventilation and extubation was not possible within 10–12 days postoperatively.

2.3. Statistics

Normally distributed continuous variables were presented as mean ± standard deviation and compared by unpaired t-test. Categorical data were summarized as absolute (n) and relative (%) frequencies and compared by Chi^2-test or Fisher's exact test. Pre- and intraoperative variables were assessed for association with the combined endpoint by univariate analysis. 15-year survival was estimated by Kaplan-Meier curves. All tests were conducted 2-sided and a p-value of ≤ 0.05 was considered statistically significant. Data were analyzed with IBM SPSS Statistics for Windows (Version 24.0).

3. Results

Total survival/ follow-up time averaged 3.2 years with follow-up completeness of 94%. Follow-up was significantly shorter in the group who reached the combined endpoint, with 2.1 years versus 4.3 years, $p < 0.001$.

3.1. Preoperative Characteristics

The combined endpoint was reached by 52.8%. Patients who reached the endpoint had a significantly higher EuroSCORE II (7.5 versus 5.5, $p < 0.001$), higher incidence of coronary artery disease with previous percutaneous intervention (9.2% versus 3.2%, $p = 0.016$), higher incidence of neurological deficit upon presentation (26.4% versus 11.8%, $p < 0.001$), higher incidence of preoperative cardiopulmonary resuscitation (14.4% versus 1.6%, $p < 0.001$) and higher incidence of intubation before surgery (16.9% versus 4.8%, $p < 0.001$). There were no further significant differences with regard to clinical presentations between the groups. Table 1 shows detailed demographic and clinical characteristics of the study population.

3.2. Intraoperative Characteristics

Intraoperative characteristics are shown in Table 2. Patients who reached the combined endpoint also had significantly longer surgery duration (288 versus 256 min, $p = 0.001$), longer cardiopulmonary bypass times (180 versus 159 min, $p < 0.001$), longer cross-clamp time (96 versus 84 min, $p = 0.010$), and longer circulatory arrest (39 versus 32 min, $p < 0.001$). The requirement for intraoperative transfusion of blood products was higher in the group who reached the combined endpoint (number of units of red blood cells 4 versus 2, $p < 0.001$, number of units of fresh frozen plasma 1.5 versus 0, $p = 0.031$, number of pools of platelets 2 (ranging from 5 to 0) versus 2 (ranging from 4 to 0), $p = 0.002$). The need for total arch replacement was significantly higher in the group who reached the endpoint (21.2% versus

8.1%, $p < 0.001$). There were no differences between groups for all other surgical procedures such as single supracoronary replacement of the ascending aorta, partial arch replacement, Bentall operation, David Operation, Elephant trunk, associated coronary artery bypass grafting or cannulation site.

Table 1. Demographic and clinical characteristics of the study population.

KERRYPNX	All Patients (n = 394)	Combined Endpoint = 0 (n = 186/47.2%)	Combined Endpoint = 1 (n = 208/52.8%)	p-Value
Age, years	62.5 ± 13.0	61.7 ± 14.0	63.2 ± 11.9	0.567
	63.0 (53.0;73.0)	63.0 (53.0;71.3)	63.5 (53.3;73.0)	
Male gender	256 (65.0%)	112 (60.2%)	144 (69.2%)	0.061
DeBakey classification,				0.108
DeBakey I	292 (78.5%)	131 (74.9%)	161 (81.7%)	
DeBakey II	80 (21.5%)	44 (25.1%)	36 (18.3%)	
Logistic EuroSCORE I	28.7 (18.1; 43.6)	24.6 (16.1; 39.7)	31.8 (18.7; 47.9)	0.018
EuroSCORE II	6.6 (3.8; 13.3)	5.5 (3.6; 10.3)	7.5 (4.0; 15.9)	<0.001
Body mass index [kg/m^2]	26.2 (23.9; 29.3)	26.3 (24.0; 29.4)	26.1 (23.8; 29.2)	0.933
Body mass index > 30 [kg/m^2]	79 (20.1%)	36 (19.4%)	43 (20.8%)	0.726
Arterial hypertension	263 (66.8%)	125 (67.2%)	138 (66.3%)	0.857
Pulmonary hypertension	7 (1.8%)	4 (2.2%)	3 (1.4%)	0.712
Type 2 Diabetes mellitus	20 (5.1%)	7 (3.8%)	13 (6.3%)	0.262
Insulin dependent	6 (1.5%)	3 (1.6%)	3 (1.4%)	1.000
Hyperlipoproteinaemia	42 (10.7%)	22 (11.8%)	20 (9.6%)	0.477
Creatinine at admission > 200 [µmol/L]	17 (4.6%)	6 (3.4%)	11 (5.8%)	0.270
Chronic renal insufficiency	46 (11.7%)	16 (8.6%)	30 (14.4%)	0.072
Decompensated renal insufficiency	9 (2.3%)	3 (1.6%)	6 (2.9%)	0.510
Renal replacement therapy ("chron Dialyse")	7 (1.8%)	4 (2.2%)	3 (1.4%)	0.712
COPD	26 (6.6%)	13 (7.0%)	13 (6.3%)	0.768
Peripheral vascular disease	15 (3.8%)	7 (3.8%)	8 (3.8%)	0.966
Smoking	75 (19.1%)	37 (19.9%)	38 (18.4%)	0.699
Coronary heart disease	68 (17.3%)	25 (13.4%)	43 (20.7%)	0.058
Heart rhythm				
Sinus rhythm	328 (83.2%)	159 (85.5%)	169 (81.3%)	0.261
Atrial fibrillation	54 (13.7%)	22 (11.8%)	32 (15.4%)	0.305
LVEF (%),	60 (55; 70)	60 (56; 70)	60 (55; 70)	0.200
Previous PCI	25 (6.4%)	6 (3.2%)	19 (9.2%)	0.016
Previous cardiac surgery	36 (9.1%)	21 (11.3%)	15 (7.2%)	0.161
Previous CABG	12 (3.0%)	5 (2.7%)	7 (3.4%)	0.696
IABP/ECLS	5 (1.3%)	0 (0.0%)	5 (2.4%)	0.063
Pericardial tamponade	71 (18.1%)	29 (15.6%)	42 (20.3%)	0.227
Marfan syndrome	11 (2.8%)	7 (3.8%)	4 (1.9%)	0.272
Bicuspid aortic valve	18 (4.7%)	8 (4.4%)	10 (4.9%)	0.849
Aortic valve vitium				0.987
Aortic valve stenosis	10 (2.6%)	5 (2.7%)	5 (2.5%)	1.000
Aortic valve insufficiency	133 (35.1%)	65 (35.7%)	68 (34.5%)	0.807
Combined Aortic valve vitium at Aortic valve replacement	6 (1.6%)	3 (1.6%)	3 (1.5%)	1.000
Neurological deficits	77 (19.5%)	22 (11.8%)	55 (26.4%)	<0.001

Table 1. Cont.

KERRYPNX	All Patients (n = 394)	Combined Endpoint = 0 (n = 186/47.2%)	Combined Endpoint = 1 (n = 208/52.8%)	p-Value
Clinical presentation				
Acute myocardial infarction (≤48 h)	14 (3.6%)	4 (2.2%)	10 (4.8%)	0.155
Cardiogenic shock	30 (7.6%)	10 (5.4%)	20 (9.7%)	0.110
CPR (≤48 h)	33 (8.4%)	3 (1.6%)	30 (14.4%)	<0.001
Transfer from intensive care unit	47 (11.9%)	16 (8.6%)	31 (14.9%)	0.054
Intubated at admission	44 (11.2%)	9 (4.8%)	35 (16.9%)	<0.001

Table 2. Operative data.

	All Patients (n = 394)	Combined Endpoint = 0 (n = 186/47.2%)	Combined Endpoint = 1 (n = 208/52.8%)	p-Value
Length of surgery [min]	275 (227; 340)	256 (218; 311)	288 (233; 358)	0.001
Cardiopulmonary bypass time [min]	167 (136; 212)	159 (130; 199)	180 (140; 228)	<0.001
Cross-clamp time [min]	92 (71; 132)	84 (65; 130)	96 (75; 134)	0.010
Circulatory arrest [min]	35 (26; 50)	32 (24; 42)	39 (28; 60)	<0.001
Number of packed red blood cells, unit	2.5 (0–16)	2 (0–16)	4 (0–16)	<0.001
Number of fresh frozen plasma, unit	0 (0–21)	0 (0–16)	1.5 (0–21)	0.031
Number of platelets, unit	2 (0–5)	2 (0–4)	2 (0–5)	0.002
Surgical procedure				
Single supracoronary replacement of the ascending aorta	187 (47.5%)	87 (46.8%)	100 (48.1%)	0.796
Partial arch replacement	94 (23.9%)	50 (27.0%)	44 (21.2%)	0.173
Total arch replacement	59 (15.0%)	15 (8.1%)	44 (21.2%)	<0.001
Conduit/Bentall operation	72 (18.3%)	35 (18.8%)	37 (17.8%)	0.792
David operation	24 (6.1%)	15 (8.1%)	9 (4.3%)	0.121
Elephant-trunk	9 (2.3%)	2 (1.1%)	7 (3.4%)	0.181
Associated with Aortic valve replacement	65 (16.5%)	30 (16.1%)	35 (16.8%)	0.852
Associated with CABG	29 (7.4%)	9 (4.8%)	20 (9.6%)	0.070
TEVAR(EVAR)	27 (6.9%)	10 (5.4%)	17 (8.2%)	0.267
Arterial cannulation				0.612
Femoral artery	62 (15.7%)	30 (16.1%)	32 (15.4%)	0.839
Ascending aorta	83 (21.1%)	33 (17.7%)	50 (24.0%)	0.126
Aortic arch	9 (2.3%)	4 (2.2%)	5 (2.4%)	1.000
Subclavian artery	1 (0.3%)	0 (0.0%)	1 (0.5%)	1.000
Apex	5 (1.3%)	2 (1.1%)	3 (1.4%)	1.000
Pulmonary vein	234 (59.4%)	117 (62.9%)	117 (56.3%)	0.179
Venous cannulation				
Right atrium	382 (97.2%)	183 (98.4%)	199 (96.1%)	0.328
Bicaval	3 (0.8%)	0 (0.0%)	3 (1.4%)	0.177
Femoral vein	8 (2.0%)	3 (1.6%)	5 (2.4%)	0.727

3.3. Postoperative Data and Outcome

Postoperative data and outcomes are shown in Table 3. Mortality was higher and complications were more common in the group who reached the combined end point. 7-day mortality was 21.6% versus 0%, $p < 0.001$. Hospital mortality was 30.8% versus 0%, $p < 0.001$. Causes of death were cardiac 53%, multiple organ failure in 43%, cerebral 9%, and sepsis 3%. The group who reached the endpoint had a significantly longer stay in the intensive care unit (10 days versus 4 days, $p < 0.001$), larger amount of postoperative drainage loss (1030 mL versus 750 mL, $p < 0.001$, greater need for postoperative blood transfusions (83.7% versus 64.5% of patients, $p < 0.001$), fresh frozen plasma transfusions (60.1% versus 40.3%, $p < 0.001$) and platelet transfusions (55.9% versus 37.6%, $p < 0.001$), as well as higher incidence of re-thoracotomy (26.9% versus 8.1%, $p < 0.001$). They also had a greater need for postoperative balloon pump and/or extracorporeal life support (5.1% versus 0.5%, $p = 0.008$), reintubation (27.9% versus 5.9%, $p < 0.001$), prolonged mechanical ventilation (189 h versus 24 h, $p < 0.001$) with need for tracheostomy (47.6% versus 0%, $p < 0.001$), readmission to the intensive care unit (13.5% versus 4.3%, $p = 0.002$), bacteremia/sepsis (8.7% versus 0.5%, $p < 0.001$), bronchopulmonary infection (22.1% versus 6.5%, $p < 0.001$), cardiac arrest (11.1% versus 2.2%, $p < 0.001$), new neurological deficit consistent with TIA/stroke (45.2% versus 0%, $p < 0.001$), myocardial infarction (2.9% versus 0%, $p = 0.032$), and acute renal insufficiency with need for renal replacement therapy (41.3% versus 0%, $p < 0.001$). While several parameters were less common in the group that reached the endpoint, they showed no statistical significance. Those were postoperative delirium (15.9% versus 21.1%), sternal wound infections (1.0% versus 2.2%) and atrial fibrillation (10.7% versus 10.2%).

Table 3. Postoperative data and outcomes.

	All Patients (n = 394)	Combined Endpoint = 0 (n = 186/47.2%)	Combined Endpoint = 1 (n = 208/52.8%)	p-Value
48 h-drainage loss [mL]	900 (500; 1513)	750 (350; 1200)	1030 (650; 1878)	<0.001
Postoperative blood transfusion	290 (74.6%)	120 (64.5%)	170 (83.7%)	<0.001
Postoperative fresh frozen plasma	197 (50.6%)	75 (40.3%)	122 (60.1%)	<0.001
Postoperative platelets	183 (47.2%)	70 (37.6%)	113 (55.9%)	<0.001
24 h-Number of packed red blood cells, unit,	1 (0–17)	0 (0–17)	1 (0–15)	0.029
24 h-Number of fresh frozen plasma, unit,	0 (0–24)	0 (0–24)	0.5 (0–23)	<0.001
24 h-Number of platelets, unit,	0 (0–10)	0 (0–5)	0 (0–10)	<0.001
Total number of packed red blood cells, unit	4 (0–56)	2 (0–38)	6 (0–56)	<0.001
Total number of fresh frozen plasma, unit	1 (0–76)	0 (0–36)	4 (0–76)	<0.001
Total number of platelets, unit	0 (0–20)	0 (0–9)	1 (0–20)	<0.001
IABP/ECLS	11 (2.9%)	1 (0.5%)	10 (5.1%)	0.008
Reintubation	69 (17.5%)	11 (5.9%)	58 (27.9%)	<0.001
Tracheotomy	99 (25.1%)	0 (0.0%)	99 (47.6%)	<0.001
Re-admission to the ICU	36 (9.2%)	8 (4.3%)	28 (13.5%)	0.002
Postoperative delirium	72 (18.4%)	39 (21.1%)	33 (15.9%)	0.190
Postoperative myocardial infarction	6 (1.5%)	0 (0.0%)	6 (2.9%)	0.032
TIA/Stroke	94 (23.9%)	0 (0.0%)	94 (45.2%)	<0.001
CPR	27 (6.9%)	4 (2.2%)	23 (11.1%)	<0.001
Bronchopulmonary infection	58 (14.7%)	12 (6.5%)	46 (22.1%)	<0.001
Bacteriaemia/sepsis	19 (4.8%)	1 (0.5%)	18 (8.7%)	<0.001
Rethoracotomy	71 (18.0%)	15 (8.1%)	56 (26.9%)	<0.001
Sternal wound infection/VAC revision	6 (1.5%)	4 (2.2%)	2 (1.0%)	0.431
New –onset of Hemodialysis	85 (21.7%)	0 (0.0%)	85 (41.3%)	<0.001
Atrial fibrillation	41 (10.5%)	19 (10.2%)	22 (10.7%)	0.881
Ventilation time [h]	69 (20; 209)	24 (15; 57)	189 (81; 387)	<0.001
ICU time [d]	6 (2; 12)	4 (2; 6)	10 (4; 18)	<0.001
Postoperative days	10 (7; 19)	9 (7; 13)	13 (7; 23)	<0.001
7 d-Mortality	45 (11.4%)	0 (0.0%)	45 (21.6%)	<0.001
Hospital Mortality	64 (16.2%)	0 (0.0%)	64 (30.8%)	<0.001
Cardiac death	34 (53.1%)	0 (0.0%)	34 (53.1%)	—
Cerebral death	6 (9.4%)	0 (0.0%)	6 (9.4%)	—
Sepsis	2 (3.1%)	0 (0.0%)	2 (3.1%)	—
MOF	22 (34.4%)	0 (0.0%)	22 (34.4%)	—

3.4. Risk Factors for Combined Endpoint

Independent preoperative risk factors to reach the combined endpoint of mortality, new neurological deficit, prolonged mechanical ventilation with need for tracheostomy and acute renal insufficiency with need for renal replacement therapy were assessed with multivariable logistic regression analysis as shown in Table 4. Significant were coronary heart disease ($p = 0.021$, OR 2.122, CI 1.1–4.0), presence of a neurological deficit ($p < 0.001$, OR 3.6, CI 1.98–6.5), preoperative need for cardiopulmonary resuscitation ($p = 0.001$, OR 8.99, CI 2.5–32.3) and need for intubation on admission ($p = 0.033$, OR 2.5, CI 1.1–5.9).

Table 4. Multivariable analysis of risk factors for the combined endpoint.

Variable	p	Odds Ratio	Confidence Interval
Coronary heart disease	0.021	2.122	1.118–4.028
Neurological deficits	<0.001	3.598	1.985–6.521
CPR	0.001	8.993	2.501–32.343
Intubated at admission	0.033	2.512	1.077–5.861

3.5. Survival Curve

Figure 1 shows the Kaplan-Meier survival curve of patients who did and did not reach the combined endpoint with a follow-up time of 15 years. The group who reached the endpoint had significantly decreased 15-year survival, however, it is notable that curves are almost parallel, after the first 30-days, indicating that the highest rate of death occurs in the immediate postoperative period.

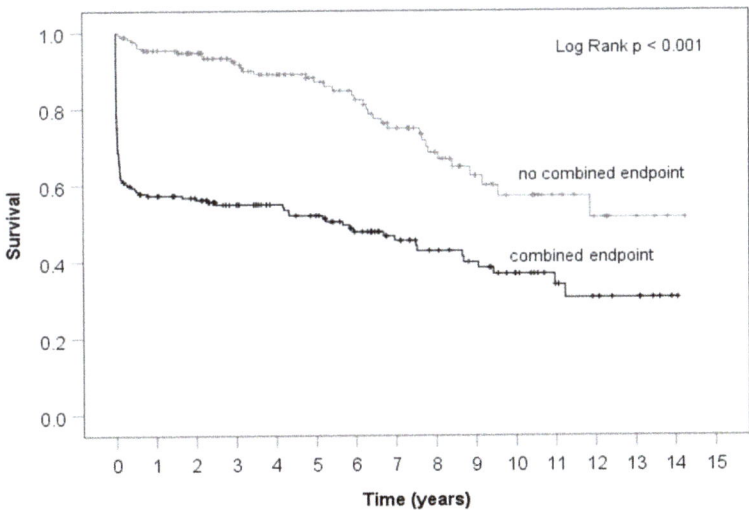

Figure 1. Survival curves of patients with and without reaching the combined endpoint.

4. Discussion

It seems remarkable that the majority of patients who had complications did not just have one but multiple. Taken all facts into account, 52.8% of the patients in our population had an undesirable outcome.

Many previous studies have already evaluated risk factors for postoperative survival [9,16–19], but the universal ethical question remains in which high risk cases withholding surgery would provide less harm than performing it, since over 50% of survivors may have to tolerate devastating conditions on long term ventilation with tracheostomy, long-term dialysis and a severe neurological deficit. IRAD data indicated a mortality of 58% among those not receiving surgery, typically because of advanced age and comorbidity [20].

The intention of this study was to assess if undesirable post-operative outcome was associated with certain parameters present on presentation, to help eventually develop a strategy to know for which patient surgery is likely harmful. Accordingly, we chose a combination of severe debilitating complications as endpoint.

A common assumption is that patients with multiple underlying medical conditions such as hypertension, diabetes, hyperlipidemia, chronic kidney disease, smoking or previous cardiac surgery have adverse outcome [2]. However, in our study, the group who reached the combined endpoint had no higher incidence of such diagnoses, despite a higher EuroSCORE II. Therefore, the proposal is, that risk factors for developing aortic dissection are not applicable for suffering poor post-operative outcome. According to data from the Swedish National Diabetes Register patients with type 2 diabetes actually had significantly less risk of aortic aneurysm, dissection and reduced mortality after hospitalization compared to matched healthy controls. The authors hypothesized that glycated cross-links in aortic tissue may play a protective role in the progression of aortic diseases [21]. The previously published analysis of our database suggested that mortality was multifactorial and especially age, previous cardiac surgery, preoperative cardiopulmonary resuscitation, blood transfusion, and postoperative renal failure were considered risk factors [6].

According to our current data, the clinical condition in which the patient arrives preoperatively is predictive of poor outcome. Other authors showed as well that in-hospital adverse outcome was associated with the presence of lower limb hypoperfusion symptoms prior to surgery [2]. Since time is such an essential part, prompt diagnosis and referral to immediate surgical repair remain the main goal. Michael DeBakey once stated: "no physician can diagnose a condition he never thinks about". An analysis from the International Registry of Acute Aortic Dissection (IRAD) indicates that the median time from emergency department presentation to definitive diagnosis of acute aortic dissection is 4.3 h, with an additional 4 h between diagnosis and surgical intervention for type A patients [22].

The response time for emergency medical services is legally regulated in Germany and should not exceed 12 min from alarm to arrival in our federal state [23], but even in densely populated areas averages 8–10 min. Emergency physicians ride on the ambulance and can make an immediate assessment. If AAAD is suspected, the physician alarms the emergency room personnel to have imaging available immediately on arrival, as well as the cardiovascular surgeon on stand-by. Despite these seemingly ideal conditions, analysis of the German Registry for Acute Aortic Dissection Type A including 2137 patients by Boening et al., revealed an overall 30-day mortality of 16.9% and new neurologic dysfunction postoperatively in 9.5% [11]. While our mortality coincides well with the national level, our rate of neurological complications seems to be higher ranging up to 23.9%. In another single center retrospective analysis by Haldenwang et al., the 30-day mortality rate was 16.4%. In their population 33.6% suffered transient neurological dysfunction and 16.4% had a postoperative stroke [5]. They also looked at a combined adverse outcome defined as stroke and 30-day mortality and found high body mass index, preoperative hypoperfusion syndrome, and left ventricular ejection fraction <50% to be independent predictors. Our results indicate a higher incidence of cardiopulmonary resuscitation within 48 h before surgery and preoperative mechanical ventilation in the combined endpoint group, but there was no higher incidence in the presence of IABP/ ECLS, cardiogenic shock, pericardial tamponade or decompensated renal insufficiency. There was also no higher prevalence of Marfan Syndrome or difference in average left ventricular ejection fraction.

Current risk assessment scores don't seem to provide an accurate answer in AAAD, especially EuroSCORE II appears to underestimate mortality. Our current analysis does not evaluate postoperative QoL in such circumstances. A previous investigation within our group found however, that the QoL scores were lower one year after emergent surgery for AAAD compared to the general, age-matched population in Germany especially regarding pain score and social functioning [3].

With growing socioeconomic and financial pressure in hospitals and healthcare systems, early identification of patients at risk for prolonged length of hospital stay with needs for advanced therapies is also essential. It was no surprise that patients who reached the combined endpoint had significantly longer stays on the ventilator, in the intensive care unit as well as in the hospital compared to those who did not reach the endpoint.

Our results stress again the importance of early diagnosis of AAAD and immediate referral to a facility capable to operate immediately, since the clinical condition on arrival plays such an important role as prognostic marker.

This study is designed as single-center retrospective review of an internal database and not a randomized prospective trial. Information was obtained from our institutional database. Data were entered by staff physicians during the patients' hospitalizations. Therefore, data may be subject to bias. From our data it remains unclear if and how our change of strategy regarding atrial canulation may have influenced the outcome.

5. Conclusions

We showed, in 15-year follow up, that relevant risk factors for adverse postoperative clinical outcome are rather related to the clinical condition in which the patient arrives preoperatively, than preexisting medical illnesses widely assumed to be responsible for poor outcome. This supports prioritizing immediate surgical attention to patients, before they may otherwise progress to hemodynamic instability and hypoperfusion even if they have underlying medical conditions or advanced age. The ethical dilemma arises when patients arrive at the hospital with already existing hypoperfusion, ongoing cardiopulmonary resuscitation or even intubation. In those cases, our data suggest that physicians may recommend either non-surgical treatment due to extremely poor chances for acceptable outcome or have a detailed discussion with patient and families of what to expect.

Author Contributions: Conceptualization, A.H. and J.C.; methodology, C.F.; software, T.P.; validation, M.G., G.E. and M.S.; formal analysis, C.F.; investigation, P.K., A.H.; resources, M.F.; data curation, C.F.; writing—original draft preparation, M.F.; writing—review and editing, A.H.; visualization, C.F.; supervision, J.C.; All authors have read and agreed to the published version of the manuscript.

Funding: This research received no external funding.

Institutional Review Board Statement: This study was approved by the Local Ethics Committee (Christian-Albrechts-University Kiel, Schwanenweg 20, D-24105 Kiel, Referral number: D417/17XXX).

Informed Consent Statement: Patient consent to participate in this study was waived due to the retrospective design. However, written informed consent for surgery was obtained from all surviving patients included into this study.

Conflicts of Interest: The authors declare no conflict of interest.

References

1. Di Eusanio, M.; Trimarchi, S.; Patel, H.J.; Hutchison, S.; Suzuki, T.; Peterson, M.D.; di Bartolomeo, R.; Folesani, G.; Pyeritz, R.E.; Braverman, A.C.; et al. Clinical presentation, management, and short-term outcome of patients with type A acute dissection complicated by mesenteric malperfusion: Observations from the International Registry of Acute Aortic Dissection. *J. Thorac. Cardiovasc. Surg.* **2013**, *145*, 385–390.e1. [CrossRef]
2. Wei, J.; Chen, Z.; Zhang, H.; Sun, X.; Qian, X.; Yu, C. In-hospital major adverse outcomes of acute Type A aortic dissection. *Eur. J. Cardio Thorac. Surg.* **2019**, *55*, 345–350. [CrossRef] [PubMed]
3. Jussli-Melchers, J.; Panholzer, B.; Friedrich, C.; Broch, O.; Renner, J.; Schöttler, J.; Rahimi, A.; Cremer, J.; Schoeneich, F.; Haneya, A. Long-term outcome and quality of life following emergency surgery for acute aortic dissection type A: A comparison between young and elderly adults. *Eur. J. Cardio Thorac. Surg.* **2016**, *51*, 465–471. [CrossRef]
4. Friedrich, C.; Salem, M.A.; Puehler, T.; Hoffmann, G.; Lutter, G.; Cremer, J.; Haneya, A. Sex-specific risk factors for early mortality and survival after surgery of acute aortic dissection type a: A retrospective observational study. *J. Cardiothorac. Surg.* **2020**, *15*, 1–12. [CrossRef]
5. Haldenwang, P.L.; Wahlers, T.; Himmels, A.; Wippermann, J.; Zeriouh, M.; Kröner, A.; Kuhr, K.; Strauch, J.T. Evaluation of risk factors for transient neurological dysfunction and adverse outcome after repair of acute type A aortic dissection in 122 consecutive patients. *Eur. J. Cardio Thorac. Surg.* **2012**, *42*, e115–e120. [CrossRef]

6. Salem, M.; Friedrich, C.; Thiem, A.; Huenges, K.; Puehler, T.; Cremer, J.; Haneya, A. Risk Factors for Mortality in Acute Aortic Dissection Type A: A Centre Experience Over 15 Years. *Thorac. Cardiovasc. Surg.* **2021**, *69*, 322–328. [CrossRef]
7. Conzelmann, L.O.; Weigang, E.; Mehlhorn, U.; Abugameh, A.; Hoffmann, I.; Blettner, M.; Etz, C.D.; Czerny, M.; Vahl, C.F. Mortality in patients with acute aortic dissection type A: Analysis of pre- and intraoperative risk factors from the German Registry for Acute Aortic Dissection Type A (GERAADA). *Eur. J. Cardio Thorac. Surg.* **2016**, *49*, e44–e52. [CrossRef] [PubMed]
8. Caus, T.; Frapier, J.M.; Giorgi, R.; Aymard, T.; Riberi, A.; Albat, B.; Chaptal, P.A.; Mesana, T. Clinical outcome after repair of acute type A dissection in patients over 70 years-old. *Eur. J. Cardio Thorac. Surg.* **2002**, *22*, 211–217. [CrossRef]
9. Tsai, T.T.; Evangelista, A.; Nienaber, C.A.; Trimarchi, S.; Sechtem, U.; Fattori, R.; Myrmel, T.; Pape, L.; Cooper, J.V.; Smith, D.E.; et al. Long-Term Survival in Patients Presenting with Type A Acute Aortic Dissection: Insights from the International Registry of Acute Aortic Dissection (IRAD). *J. Circ.* **2006**, *114*, I-350–I-356. [CrossRef] [PubMed]
10. Wundram, M.; Falk, V.; Eulert-Grehn, J.-J.; Herbst, H.; Thurau, J.; Leidel, B.A.; Göncz, E.; Bauer, W.; Habazettl, H.; Kurz, S.D. Incidence of acute type A aortic dissection in emergency departments. *Sci. Rep.* **2020**, *10*, 1–6. [CrossRef]
11. Karck, M.; Conzelmann, L.; Easo, J.; Krüger, T.; Rylski, B.; Weigang, E.; Boening, A. German Registry for Acute Aortic Dissection Type A: Structure, Results, and Future Perspectives. *Thorac. Cardiovasc. Surg.* **2016**, *65*, 077–084. [CrossRef] [PubMed]
12. Easo, J.; Weigang, E.; Hölzl, P.P.; Horst, M.; Hoffmann, I.; Blettner, M.; Dapunt, O.E. Influence of operative strategy for the aortic arch in DeBakey type I aortic dissection: Analysis of the German Registry for Acute Aortic Dissection Type A. *J. Thorac. Cardiovasc. Surg.* **2012**, *144*, 617–623. [CrossRef] [PubMed]
13. Rylski, B.; Hoffmann, I.; Beyersdorf, F.; Suedkamp, M.; Siepe, M.; Nitsch, B.; Blettner, M.; Borger, M.; Weigang, E. Acute Aortic Dissection Type A: Age-related management and outcomes reported in the german registry for acute aortic dissection type a (GERAADA) of over 2000 patients. *Ann. Surg.* **2014**, *259*, 598–604. [CrossRef]
14. Chaddha, A.; Kline-Rogers, E.; Braverman, A.C.; Erickson, S.R.; Jackson, E.A.; Franklin, B.A.; Bs, E.M.W.; Jabara, J.T.; Ms, D.G.M.; Eagle, K.A. Survivors of Aortic Dissection: Activity, Mental Health, and Sexual Function. *Clin. Cardiol.* **2015**, *38*, 652–659. [CrossRef]
15. Rahimi-Barfeh, A.; Grothusen, C.; Haneya, A.; Schöttler, J.; Eide, A.M.; Erdmann, M.; Friedrich, C.; Hoffmann, G.; Cremer, J.; Schoeneich, F. Transatrial Cannulation of the Left Ventricle for Acute Type A Aortic Dissection: A 5-Year Experience. *Ann. Thorac. Surg.* **2016**, *101*, 1753–1758. [CrossRef] [PubMed]
16. Mehta, R.H.; Suzuki, T.; Hagan, P.G.; Bossone, E.; Gilon, D.; Llovet, A.; Maroto, L.C.; Cooper, J.V.; Smith, D.E.; Armstrong, W.F.; et al. Predicting Death in Patients with Acute Type A Aortic Dissection. *J. Circ.* **2002**, *105*, 200–206. [CrossRef]
17. Bossone, E.; Rampoldi, V.; Nienaber, C.; Trimarchi, S.; Ballotta, A.; Cooper, J.V.; Smith, D.; Eagle, K.; Mehta, R.H. Usefulness of pulse deficit to predict in-hospital complications and mortality in patients with acute type A aortic dissection. *Am. J. Cardiol.* **2002**, *89*, 851–855. [CrossRef]
18. Rampoldi, V.; Trimarchi, S.; Eagle, K.A.; Nienaber, C.A.; Oh, J.K.; Bossone, E.; Myrmel, T.; Sangiorgi, G.; De Vincentiis, C.; Cooper, J.V.; et al. Simple Risk Models to Predict Surgical Mortality in Acute Type A Aortic Dissection: The International Registry of Acute Aortic Dissection Score. *Ann. Thorac. Surg.* **2007**, *83*, 55–61. [CrossRef]
19. Yang, G.; Zhou, Y.; He, H.; Pan, X.; Li, X.; Chai, X. A nomogram for predicting in-hospital mortality in acute type A aortic dissection patients. *J. Thorac. Dis.* **2020**, *12*, 264–275. [CrossRef] [PubMed]
20. Hagan, P.G.; Nienaber, C.A.; Isselbacher, E.M.; Bruckman, D.; Karavite, D.J.; Russman, P.L.; Evangelista, A.; Fattori, R.; Suzuki, T.; Oh, J.K.; et al. The International Registry of Acute Aortic Dissection (IRAD). *JAMA* **2000**, *283*, 897–903. [CrossRef]
21. Avdic, T.; Franzén, S.; Zarrouk, M.; Acosta, S.; Nilsson, P.; Gottsäter, A.; Svensson, A.; Gudbjörnsdottir, S.; Eliasson, B. Reduced Long-Term Risk of Aortic Aneurysm and Aortic Dissection Among Individuals with Type 2 Diabetes Mellitus: A Nationwide Observational Study. *J. Am. Hear. Assoc.* **2018**, *7*, e007618. [CrossRef] [PubMed]
22. Lloyd-Jones, D.M. Cardiovascular health and protection against CVD: More than the sum of the parts? *J. Circ.* **2014**, *130*, 1671–1673. [CrossRef] [PubMed]
23. Gesetze-Rechtsprechung Schleswig-Holstein RettDGDV SH 2019 | Landesnorm Schleswig-Holstein | Gesamtausgabe | Landesverordnung zur Durchführung des Schleswig-Holsteinischen Rettungsdienstgesetzes (SHRDG-DVO) vom 4. Dezember 2018 | Gültig von: 01.01.2019 Gültig bis: 31.12.2023. Available online: http://www.gesetze-rechtsprechung.sh.juris.de/jportal/?quelle=jlink&query=RettDGDV+SH&psml=bsshoprod.psml&max=true&aiz=true (accessed on 8 September 2020).

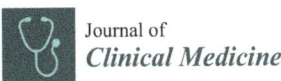

Article

Predicting Mortality in Patients with Atrial Fibrillation and Obstructive Chronic Coronary Syndrome: The Bialystok Coronary Project

Łukasz Kuźma [1], Anna Tomaszuk-Kazberuk [2,*], Anna Kurasz [1], Sławomir Dobrzycki [1], Marek Koziński [3], Bożena Sobkowicz [2] and Gregory Y. H. Lip [4,5]

[1] Department of Invasive Cardiology, Medical University of Białystok, 15-089 Białystok, Poland; kuzma.lukasz@gmail.com (Ł.K.); annaxkurasz@gmail.com (A.K.); slawek_dobrzycki@yahoo.com (S.D.)
[2] Department of Cardiology, Medical University of Białystok, 15-089 Białystok, Poland; sobkowic@wp.pl
[3] Department of Cardiology and Internal Medicine, Medical University of Gdańsk, 81-519 Gdynia, Poland; marek.kozinski@gumed.edu.pl
[4] Liverpool Centre for Cardiovascular Science, University of Liverpool and Liverpool Heart & Chest Hospital, Liverpool L14 3PE, UK; gregory.lip@liverpool.ac.uk
[5] Aalborg Thrombosis Research Unit, Department of Clinical Medicine, Aalborg University, 9220 Aalborg, Denmark
* Correspondence: a.tomaszuk@poczta.fm; Tel.: +48-600-044-992

Abstract: Over the next decades, the prevalence of atrial fibrillation (AF) is estimated to double. Our aim was to investigate the causes of the long-term mortality in relation to the diagnosis of atrial fibrillation (AF) and chronic coronary syndrome (CCS). The analysed population consisted of 7367 consecutive patients referred for elective coronary angiography enrolled in a large single-centre retrospective registry, out of whom 1484 had AF and 2881 were diagnosed with obstructive CCS. During follow-up (median = 2029 days), 1201 patients died. The highest all-cause death was seen in AF(+)/CCS(+) [194/527; 36.8%], followed by AF(+)/CCS(−) [210/957; 21.9%], AF(−)/CCS(+) [(459/2354; 19.5%)] subgroups. AF ([HR]$_{AC}$ = 1.48, 95%CI, 1.09–2.01; HR$_{CV}$ = 1.34, 95%CI, 1.07–1.68) and obstructive CCS (HR$_{AC}$ = 1.90, 95%CI, 1.56–2.31; HR$_{CV}$ = 2.27, 95%CI, 1.94–2.65) together with age, male gender, heart failure, obstructive pulmonary disease, diabetes were predictors of both all-cause and CV mortality. The main findings are as follow among patients referred for elective coronary angiography, both AF and obstructive CCS are strong and independent predictors of the long-term mortality. Mortality of AF without CCS was at least as high as non-AF patients with CCS. CV deaths were more frequent than non-CV deaths in AF patients with CCS compared to those with either AF or CCS alone.

Keywords: atrial fibrillation; chronic coronary syndrome; coronary artery disease; mortality; AF-CAD study

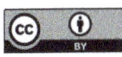

1. Introduction

The prevalence of atrial fibrillation (AF) in adults varies from 2% to 4%, but about one of three cases remains undetected [1–3]. Over the next few years, the prevalence of AF is estimated to double, associated with the aging of the population and the increasing incidence of hypertension, diabetes, heart failure, mitral valve defects, and chronic coronary syndromes (CCS). Indeed, one in five patients with CCS have coexisting AF, leading to a worsening of the patient's prognosis [4]. The risk of ischemic stroke and heart failure in AF patients with CCS, as well as reduced life expectancy, is greater than in the CCS population without the AF [5–7].

In the LIFE-Heart Study, there were no associations between AF and location of coronary stenosis among patients with single-vessel coronary artery disease (CAD) and, in comparison to patients with single-vessel CAD, the risk for AF was lower in those with double and triple CAD [8]. In our Białystok Coronary Project of patients undergoing elective coronary angiography, AF was associated with a lack of obstructive coronary lesions [9]. The reason for these findings might be multifactorial, such as AF symptoms may mimic CCS symptoms, computed tomography scan and stress tests are difficult to interpret in AF patients.

AF is associated with high morbidity and mortality, placing a significant burden on the patients themselves as well as the health care system [10,11]. The presence of AF alone independently increases the risk of death [12,13]. However, there is a paucity of data regarding a possible association between the diagnosis of AF and/or CCS and long-term mortality. When considering this potential relationship, numerous questions arise (e.g., whether coexisting AF and CCS independently contribute to unfavourable prognosis, whether AF (+)/CCS (−) patients have similar long-term mortality as AF (−)/CCS (+) patients, whether causes of death differ in relation to the diagnosis of AF and/or CCS).

The objectives of this study are to investigate the causes of the long-term mortality in patients referred for elective coronary angiography in relation to the diagnosis of AF and/or CCS, and second, to identify the factors that predispose to death in these patients.

2. Materials and Methods

2.1. Study Design

The Bialystok Coronary Project is a retrospective cohort study of consecutive patients with confirmed or suspected obstructive CCS conducted in the Department of Invasive Cardiology of the Medical University of Bialystok, Poland.

Patients were recruited between 2007 and 2016. In total, we screened 26,985 patients from Białystok, the largest city in north-eastern Poland. We excluded patients with acute coronary syndromes (ACS), Takotsubo cardiomyopathy, and a history of ischemic heart disease, as well as those referred for coronary angiography before heart valve surgery. Prior heart valve replacement was also an exclusion criterion. The final sample of the Bialystok Coronary Project consisted of 8288 patients referred for elective coronary angiography. Study details and outcomes have been presented previously [9].

We conducted a two-step follow-up examination. In the first stage, the general type of medication prescribed at discharge and planned revascularization treatment was evaluated. In the second stage, data on all-cause mortality was collected from the National Statistical Office in Poland. The exact collection date was 1 January 2019. The median duration of follow-up was 2029 (1283–3059) days. The records included information on the date and causes of death. The first aim of the present study was to investigate the relationship between long-term mortality and the diagnosis of AF and/or CCS. As shown in Figure 1, we divided our cohort into four subgroups, as follows: AF (+)/CCS (+), AF (+)/CCS (−), AF (−)/CCS (+), and AF (−)/CCS (−). Second, we investigated the predictors of the long-term all-cause and cardiovascular (CV) mortality in particular in the overall study population and the above-listed subgroups.

The study protocol conformed to the ethical guidelines of the Declaration of Helsinki and STROBE guidelines [14]. Additionally, it was approved by the local bioethics committee of the Medical University of Bialystok (Approval No. R-1-002/18/2019) and registered in the database of clinical studies www.clinicaltrials.gov (accessed on 23 October 2021) (Identifier: NCT04541498).

2.2. Study Parameters and Definitions

The CCS diagnosis was established according to the European guidelines in force at that time [15]. A significant stenosis of the coronary vessel (obstructive stenosis) was defined as stenosis of 50% or more of the diameter of the left main stem coronary artery or stenosis of 70% or more of the diameter of the rest of the arteries. We classified patients not fulfilling this criterion as CCS (−). In the group of patients with an obstructive coronary lesion, we classified CCS as single-, double-, or multi-vessel disease (MVD) defined as a triple-vessel disease and/or significant left main stem stenosis. A decision regarding optimal CCS management in our study participants (i.e., percutaneous coronary interventions (PCI), conservative management, or coronary bypass grafting surgery (CABG)) was performed by the attending international cardiologist and if required by the members of our Heart Team according to the guidelines current at the time of hospitalization.

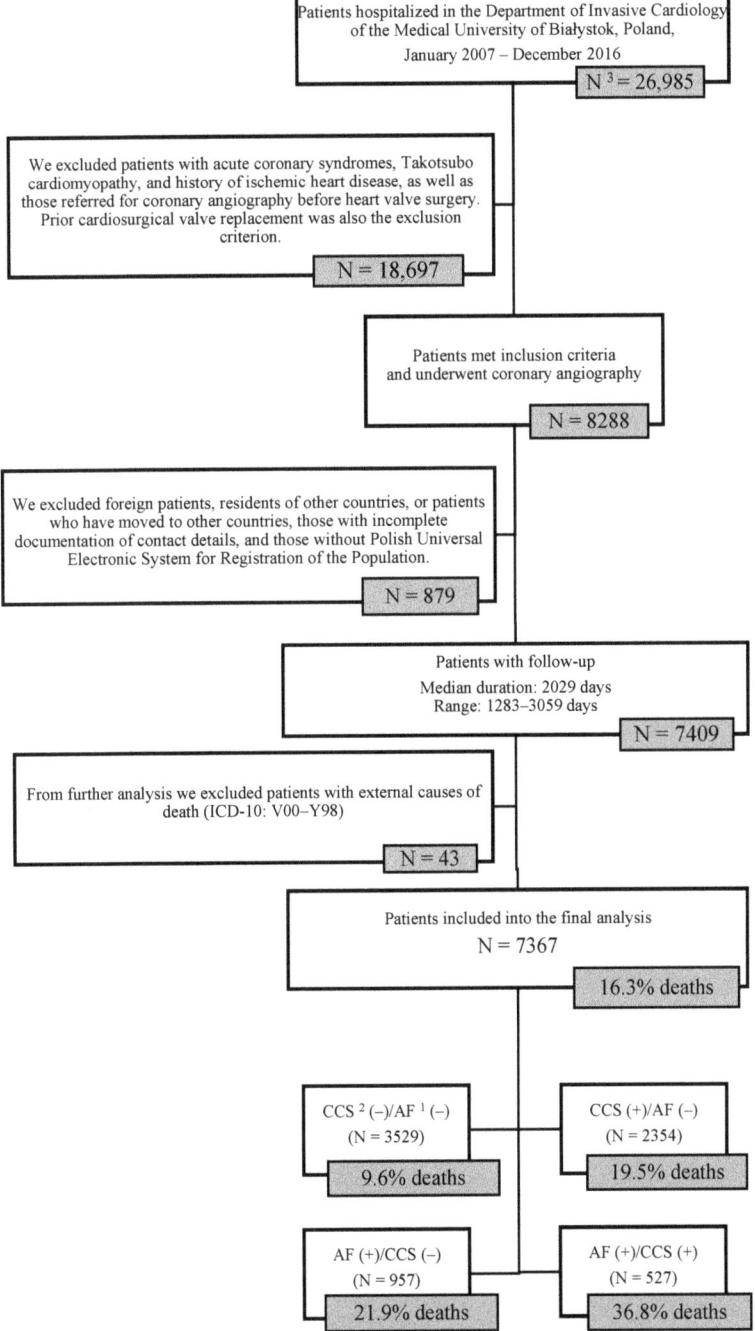

Figure 1. Selection of the study population. [1] AF, atrial fibrillation; [2] CCS, chronic coronary syndrome; [3] N, number.

We based diagnoses and AF classification on physician-assigned diagnoses in medical records corresponding to ICD-10-CM codes for AF at the hospital discharge or outpatient databases. The diagnoses were made based on the medical history, 24-h ECG monitoring, and standard 12-lead ECG performed on admission. AF was subclassified into paroxysmal, persistent, or permanent.

Left ventricular ejection fraction (LVEF) was assessed in the routine transthoracic echocardiography using the modified biplane Simpson's method, following the European Society of Echocardiography recommendations [16]. The estimated glomerular filtration rate (eGFR) using the CKD-EPI formula and chronic kidney disease (CKD) was accessed according to the KDIGO 2012 Clinical Practice Guideline for the Evaluation and Management of Chronic Kidney Disease [17]. Obesity was defined as a body mass index ≥ 30 kg/m^2. The diagnosis of other coexisting conditions was made based on medical history, physical examination results, and additional tests by the attending physician; it was not re-examined at the time of inclusion into the study.

The medications prescribed at discharge were divided into seven groups: acetylsalicylic acid (ASA), dual antiplatelet therapy (DAPT), vitamin K antagonists (VKAs), direct oral anticoagulants (DOACs), angiotensin-converting-enzyme inhibitors/angiotensin II receptor blockers (ACEI/ARB), beta-adrenergic antagonists (BB), and statins. Dual antiplatelet therapy (DAPT) was defined as taking acetylsalicylic acid (ASA) with clopidogrel, a platelet P2Y$_{12}$ receptor inhibitor. The group of DOACs includes dabigatran, rivaroxaban, and apixaban.

2.3. Long-Term Mortality Data

The records collected from the National Statistical Office included information on the date and the causes of deaths recorded (codes in the International Classification of Diseases (ICD)—10th Revision). According to codes, we extracted the data for CV-related mortality (ICD-10 codes from I00 to I99).

2.4. Statistical Analysis

Data were collected and analysed using MS Excel (Microsoft, 2020, version 16.40). We used the Kolmogorov–Smirnov test to assess the distribution of continuous variables. None of the continuous variables followed the Gaussian distribution. Data were presented as medians (Me) and interquartile range (IQR) for not normally distributed continuous variables, and as the number (N) of cases and percentage (%) for categorical variables.

Statistical significance of differences between two groups were determined using the χ^2 and Mann–Whitney U tests when appropriate. To compare multiple subgroups for non-normally distributed variables, we applied Kruskal–Wallis test with multiple pairwise comparisons using the Steel–Dwass–Critchlow–Fligner procedure, whereas for the comparison of categorical variables χ^2 test was used.

The associations between parameters and mortality risk were estimated by Cox proportional hazard regression univariate and multivariate models. The multivariate analysis included variables with a p value < 0.1 in the univariate analysis. The results are presented as hazard ratio (HR) and 95% confidence intervals (CI). Kaplan–Meier curves were used for graphical assessment of time-dependent mortality according to the presence of AF and/or CCS. Multiple comparisons between groups were performed by the Dunn–Sidak method. For all analyses, we set the level of statistical significance at $p < 0.05$.

All analyses were performed using XL Stat (Addinsoft, 2020, version 2020.03.01, New York, NY, USA), Stata (StataCorp LLC, 2020, version 17, Lakeway Drive, TX, USA), and MS Excel (Microsoft, 2020, version 16.40, Redmond, WA, USA).

3. Results

3.1. Participant Characteristics

The final analyzed population consisted of 7367 patients (54% men, median (IQR) age: 65 (58–73) years), out of whom 1484 (20.1%) had AF and 2881 (39.1%) were diagnosed with obstructive CCS. During the median follow-up of 2029 (range 1283–3059) days, 1201 (16.3%) study participants died (Figure 1). Patients who died during the follow-up were older, more likely to be male gender, had lower body mass index and left ventricular ejection fraction, significantly more often presented with AF, obstructive CCS, advanced CAD (i.e., multi-vessel coronary artery disease and/or left main stem stenosis), diabetes, CKD and chronic obstructive pulmonary disease (COPD). Patients who died were less likely to be diagnosed with hypertension and hyperlipidemia but had higher values of CHA_2DS_2-VASc score (Table 1).

Table 1. Baseline characteristics in the whole cohort, and alive and dead participants at follow-up.

	All Study Participants (N = 7367)	Alive Participants (N = 6166)	Dead Participants (N = 1201)	p Value for the Comparison between Alive and Dead Study Participants
Age, years; Me [13] (IQR [11])	65 (58–73)	64 (57–72)	71 (62–77)	<0.001
Male; % (N [14])	54 (3978)	51.4 (3168)	67.4 (810)	<0.001
BMI [5]; Me (IQR)	29 (26–32)	29 (26–32)	28 (25–31)	<0.001
Obesity; % (N)	35.0 (2582)	36.1 (2225)	29.7 (357)	<0.001
Atrial fibrillation; % (N)	20.1 (1484)	17.5 (1080)	33.6 (404)	<0.001
Paroxysmal atrial fibrillation; % (N)	8.9 (656)	8.5 (525)	10.9 (131)	0.02
Persistent atrial fibrillation; % (N)	8.8 (649)	6.8 (417)	19.3 (232)	
Permanent atrial fibrillation; % (N)	2.4 (179)	2.2 (138)	3.4 (41)	
Hypertension; % (N)	82.8 (6103)	83.3 (5134)	80.7 (969)	0.03
Diabetes mellitus; % (N)	25.5 (1878)	24.2 (1492)	32.1 (386)	<0.001
Hyperlipidaemia; % (N)	88.6 (6526)	89.3 (5505)	85.0 (1021)	<0.001
Low-density lipoprotein cholesterol, mg/dL; Me (IQR)	100 (78–128)	100 (79–128)	100 (77–127)	0.35
High-density lipoprotein cholesterol, mg/dL; Me (IQR)	46 (39–56)	47 (39–56)	44 (37–53)	<0.001
Chronic heart failure; % (N)	18.3 (1345)	14.3 (884)	38.4 (461)	<0.001
LVEF [12], %; Me (IQR)	55 (43–60)	55 (48–60)	45 (30–55)	<0.001
Chronic kidney disease; % (N)	20 (1471)	16.6 (1021)	37.5 (450)	<0.001
eGFR [10], mL/min/1.73 m^2; Me (IQR)	79 (65–91)	81 (68–92)	71 (54–86)	<0.001
COPD [7], % (N)	4.5 (335)	3.4 (211)	10.3 (124)	<0.001
Obstructive CCS [6]; % (N)	39.1 (2881)	36.1 (2228)	54.4 (653)	<0.001
Single-vessel CCS; % (N)	17.2 (1270)	16.1 (993)	23.1 (277)	<0.001
Double-vessel CCS; % (N)	9.6 (710)	9.0 (555)	12.9 (155)	
Multi-vessel CCS; % (N)	21.9 (1611)	20.0 (1235)	31.3 (376)	
Significant stenosis; % (N)				
• Left main	3 (220)	2.7 (166)	4.5 (54)	<0.001
• Left anterior descending artery	24.9 (1837)	23.2 (1428)	34.1 (409)	<0.001
• Diagonal artery	8.9 (654)	8.1 (501)	12.7 (153)	<0.001
• Circumflex artery	13.3 (976)	12.1 (747)	19.1 (229)	<0.001
• Left marginal artery	8.6 (634)	8.0 (492)	11.2 (142)	<0.001
• Right coronary artery	19.1 (1405)	16.8 (1037)	30.6 (368)	<0.001

Table 1. Cont.

	All Study Participants (N = 7367)	Alive Participants (N = 6166)	Dead Participants (N = 1201)	p Value for the Comparison between Alive and Dead Study Participants
Chronic total occlusion; % (N)	8.1 (596)	7.3 (451)	12.1 (145)	<0.001
• Left main	0.4 (32)	0.4 (23)	0.7 (9)	0.61
• Left anterior descending artery	5.6 (414)	5.0 (306)	9.0 (108)	0.03
• Diagonal artery	1.8 (133)	1.6 (99)	2.8 (34)	0.51
• Circumflex artery	3.0 (222)	2.5 (154)	5.7 (68)	0.004
• Left marginal artery	2.2 (163)	2.0 (123)	3.3 (40)	0.45
• Right coronary artery	5.3 (391)	4.7 (289)	8.5 (102)	0.96
Patients treated with sucessful PCI, % (N)				
• Left main	0.6 (41)	0.4 (27)	1.2 (14)	0.52
• Left anterior descending artery	13.1 (965)	12.6 (779)	15.5 (186)	0.02
• Diagonal artery	3.9 (285)	3.5 (218)	5.6 (67)	0.91
• Circumflex artery	6.5 (479)	6.2 (380)	8.2 (99)	0.44
• Left marginal artery	3.3 (244)	3.3 (205)	3.2 (39)	0.94
• Right coronary artery	8.5 (628)	7.9 (489)	11.6 (139)	0.02
Unsuccessful PCI	0.9 (64)	0.9 (55)	0.7 (9)	0.64
Medication prescribed at discharge; % (N)				
• ASA [3]	81.1 (5976)	81.8 (5046)	77.4 (930)	<0.001
• DAPT [8]	21.7 (1599)	21.1 (1300)	24.9 (299)	0.003
• DOAC [9]	4.3 (316)	4.5 (277)	3.3 (39)	0.051
• VKA [15]	12.4 (914)	10.4 (643)	22.6 (271)	<0.001
• ACEI [1]/ARB [2]	87.4 (6438)	86.8 (5353)	90.4 (1085)	<0.001
• BB [4]	89.5 (6595)	89.0 (5486)	92.4 (1109)	<0.001
• Statin	83.9 (6184)	84.5 (5208)	81.3 (976)	0.006
CHA_2DS_2-VASc score; Me (IQR)	3 (2–4)	3 (2–4)	4 (3–5)	<0.001

[1] ACEI, angiotensin-converting-enzyme inhibitor; [2] ARB, angiotensin receptor blocker; [3] ASA, acetylsalicylic acid; [4] BB, beta adrenergic receptor antagonist; [5] BMI, body mass index; [6] CCS, chronic coronary syndrome; [7] COPD, chronic obstructive pulmonary disease; [8] DAPT, dual antiplatelet therapy; [9] DOAC, direct oral anticoagulant; [10] eGFR, estimated glomerular filtration rate; [11] IQR, interquartile range; [12] LVEF, left ventricular ejection fraction; [13] Me, median; [14] N, number; [15] VKA, vitamin K antagonist.

Comparing two CCS (+) subgroups, the subgroup with AF was significantly less likely to have a multi-vessel obstructive CCS and chronic total occlusion than the subgroup without AF (Table 2). The latter subgroup was less often diagnosed with COPD.

3.2. Mortality Analysis in the Subgroups

As shown in Figure 2, the all-cause death was highest in the AF (+)/CCS (+) subgroup, followed by AF (+)/CCS (−), AF (−)/CCS (+) and AF (−)/CCS (−) patients. The crude all-cause mortality rate was higher in AF (+)/CCS (−) vs. AF (−)/CCS (+) patients (21.9% (210/957) vs. 19.5% (459/2354); $p < 0.01$). Similar results were evident for CV mortality (Table 3 and Supplementary Figure S1). CV deaths were more frequent than non-CV deaths in all subgroups except AF (−)/CCS (−) patients (Table 3).

Table 2. Differences in the characteristic of study participants according to the presence of atrial fibrillation and obstructive chronic coronary syndrome.

	AF (+)/CCS (+) [a] (N = 527)	AF (+)/CCS (−) [b] (N = 957)	AF (−)/CCS (+) [c] (N = 2354)	AF (−)/CCS (−) [d] (N = 3529)	p Value for the Comparison among Sub-Groups
Age, years; Me (IQR)	71 (66–77)	68 (60–74)	66 (59–73)	63 (56–71)	<0.001
Male; % (N)	68.7 (362)	57.2 (547)	66.7 (1570)	42.5 (1499)	<0.001 [1]
Obesity; % (N)	36.1 (190)	42.3 (405)	31.7 (747)	35.1 (1240)	<0.001 [2]
MVD; % (N)	45.5 (241)	N/A	58.2 (1370)	N/A	<0.001
Chronic total occlusion; % (N)	15.9 (84)	N/A	21.8 (512)	N/A	<0.001
Hypertension; % (N)	83.9 (442)	79.6 (762)	86.8 (2042)	81 (2857)	<0.001 [3]
Diabetes mellitus; % (N)	32.1 (169)	26.3 (252)	29.9 (704)	21.3 (753)	<0.001 [4]
Hyperlipidaemia; % (N)	89.9 (474)	79.9 (765)	96.2 (2265)	85.6 (3022)	<0.001
Chronic heart failure; % (N)	42.1 (222)	39.5 (378)	14.5 (341)	11.4 (404)	<0.001 [5]
Chronic kidney disease; % (N)	41.0 (216)	28.4 (272)	20.2 (475)	14. (508)	<0.001
COPD, % (N)	7.2 (38)	6.6 (63)	4.0 (94)	4.0 (140)	<0.001 [6]
Conservative management, % (N)	13.3 (70)	N/A	11.7 (275)	N/A	<0.001
Patients sucessfully treated with PCI, % (N)	46.2 (233)	N/A	50.1 (1180)	N/A	
Unsuccessful PCI, %, (N)	2.7 (14)	N/A	2.1 (50)	N/A	
Patients qualified for CABG, % (N)	39.9 (210)	N/A	36.1 (849)	N/A	
DOACs prescribed at discharge, % (N)	15.7 (83)	22.3 (213)	0.2 (5)	0.4 (15)	<0.001 [7]
VKAs prescribed at discharge, % (N)	56.4 (297)	57.3 (548)	0.8 (21)	1.3 (48)	<0.001 [6]
CHA$_2$DS$_2$-VASc score; Me (IQR)	5 (4–5)	4 (3–5)	4 (3–5)	3 (2–4)	<0.001

[1] no significant differences between the [a] vs. [c] groups. [2] no significant differences between the [a] vs. [d] and [a] vs. [c] groups. [3] no significant differences between the [a/b] vs. [d] and [b/c] vs. [a] groups. [4] no significant differences between the [b/c] vs. [a] and [b] vs. [c] groups. [5] no significant differences between the [a] vs. [b] groups. [6] no significant differences between the [a] vs. [b] and [c] vs. [d] groups. [7] no significant differences between the [c] vs. [d] groups. AF, atrial fibrillation; CABG; coronary artery bypass grafting; CCS; chronic coronary syndrome; COPD, chronic obstructive pulmonary disease; IQR, interquartile range; Me, median; MVD, multivessel disease (CCS with significant triple-vessel and/or left main stem stenosis); N/A, not applicable; N, number.

CV mortality in the AF (+)/CCS (+) subgroup (70.1%, N = 136) was higher than in the AF (−)/CCS (+) patients (53.2% (N = 244; $p < 0.001$)). Coronary heart disease was a more common cause of death in the AF (+)/CCS (+) subgroup than in the AF (−)/CCS (+) subgroup (33.0% (*N = 64) vs. 21.8% (N = 100); $p < 0.001$), as well as in the AF (+)/CCS (−) subgroup compared to the AF (−)/CCS (−) one (27.6% (N = 58) vs. 14.8% (N = 50); $p < 0.001$). When comparing patients without CCS, more patients with AF than without AF died due to intracerebral haemorrhage (5.7% (N = 12) vs. 1.5% (N = 5); $p = 0.005$), see Table 3.

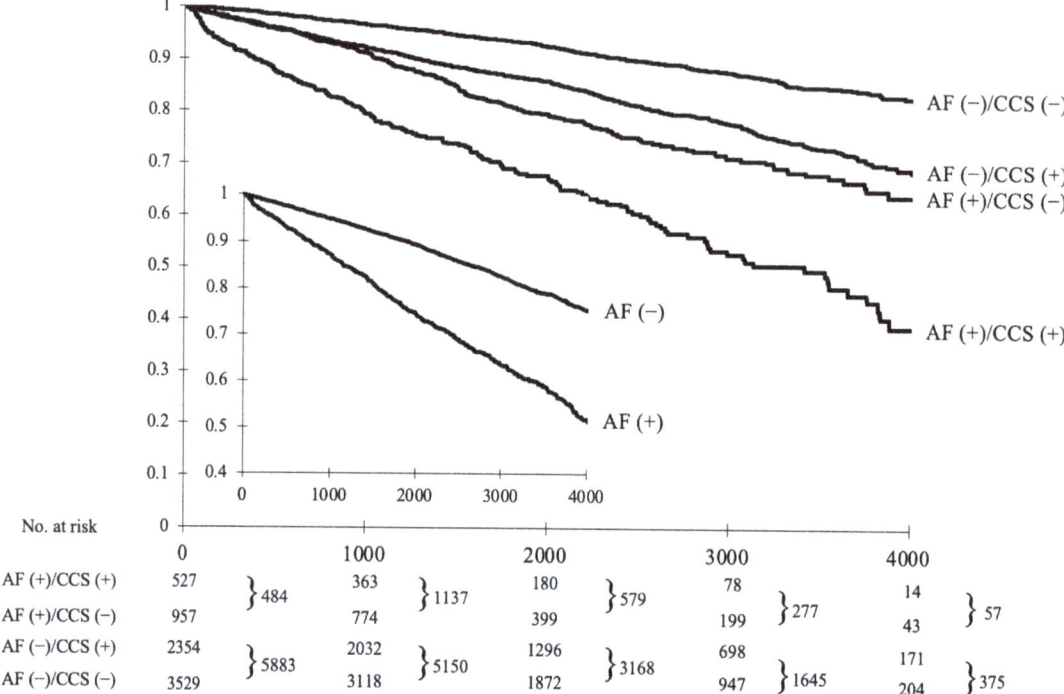

Figure 2. Kaplan–Meier survival analysis of all-cause mortality in relation of the diagnosis of atrial fibrillation and obstructive chronic coronary syndrome (large graph). The inner graph represents the comparison between patients with and without atrial fibrillation independently of the diagnosis of obstructive chronic coronary syndrome. All differences between curves are statistically significant (adjusted p values < 0.01 for all tests). AF, atrial fibrillation; CCS, chronic coronary syndrome.

3.3. Predictors of Mortality

Significant predictors found on univariate analysis are presented in Supplementary Table S1. Variables with a p value <0.1 in the univariate analysis were incorporated in the multivariate analysis. Figure 3 shows the predictors of all-cause and CV mortality in multivariate Cox proportional hazards models: AF and obstructive CCS together with increasing age, male gender, chronic heart failure, chronic obstructive pulmonary disease, diabetes mellitus, and lower values of red blood cells were independent predictors of both all-cause and CV mortality. Chronic kidney disease increased, but statin therapy decreased, the risk of all-cause mortality.

The presence of obstructive CCS increased all-cause and CV mortality risk by 2-fold and 3-fold, respectively. As shown in Figure 4, other independent predictors of total mortality in the AF subgroups were increasing age, chronic heart failure, COPD, and lower values of red blood cells, whereas male sex, chronic heart failure, diabetes mellitus, and lower values of red blood cells were associated with CV mortality. Increasing age was found to be a significant predictor of all-cause mortality in all subgroups, but was associated with CV mortality only in the AF (−)/CCS (+) and AF (−)/CCS (−) patients (Table 4). Male sex was associated with CV mortality in all subgroups and with all-cause mortality in all subgroups except the AF (+)/CCS (+) patients. Baseline diagnosis of chronic heart failure predicted both all-cause and CV mortality in all subgroups, especially in AF (−)/CCS (−) patients.

Table 3. Causes of deaths in the study participants.

All Deaths, % (N)	Total 16.3 (1201)	AF (+)/CCS (+) [a] 36.8 (194)	AF (+)/CCS (−) [b] 21.9 (210)	AF (−)/CCS (+) [c] 19.5 (459)	AF (−)/CCS (−) [d] 9.6 (338)	p Value for the Comparison among Subgroups
Cardiovascular deaths, % * (N)	53.5 (643)	70.1 (136)	58.6 (123)	53.2 (244)	41.4 (140)	<0.001 [1]
Non-cardiovascular deaths, % (N)	46.5 (558)	20.9 (58)	52.4 (87)	46.8 (215)	58.6 (198)	<0.001 [1]
Neoplasm deaths, % (N)	25.6 (307)	14.9 (29)	20 (42)	27.9 (128)	32 (108)	<0.001 [2]
Other deaths, % (N)	20.9 (251)	14.9 (29)	21.4 (45)	19 (87)	26.6 (90)	0.01 [3]
Leading causes of death						
Coronary heart disease, % (N)	22.6 (272)	33 (64)	27.6 (58)	21.8 (100)	14.8 (50)	<0.001 [4]
Lung cancer, % (N)	7.2 (87)	4.1 (8)	3.3 (7)	8.3 (38)	10.1 (34)	0.006 [5]
Cardiomyopathy, % (N)	3.2 (38)	2.1 (4)	4.3 (9)	1.1 (5)	5.9 (20)	0.001 [6]
Cerebral infarction, % (N)	5.1 (61)	6.7 (13)	7.6 (16)	4.8 (22)	3 (10)	0.07
Myocardial infarction, % (N)	5 (60)	6.2 (12)	1.9 (4)	6.3 (29)	4.4 (15)	0.08
Instantaneous death, % (N)	4.9 (59)	4.1 (8)	6.2 (13)	4.6 (21)	5 (17)	0.77
Heart failure, % (N)	4.5 (54)	6.7 (13)	4.3 (9)	4.1 (19)	3.8 (13)	0.44
Pneumonia, % (N)	3 (36)	0.5 (1)	3.8 (8)	3.1 (14)	3.8 (13)	0.14
Intracerebral haemorrhage, % (N)	2.3 (28)	2.1 (4)	5.7 (12)	1.5 (7)	1.5 (5)	0.005 [7]
Prostate cancer, % (N)	2.2 (27)	1 (2)	3.3 (7)	2.6 (12)	1.8 (6)	0.38
Colon cancer, % (N)	2 (24)	2.6 (5)	2.4 (5)	2 (9)	1.5 (5)	0.81
COPD, % (N)	1.8 (22)	0.5 (1)	1.4 (3)	1.3 (6)	3.6 (12)	0.06
Hypertensive heart disease, % (N)	1.7 (20)	0.5 (1)	0.5 (1)	2 (9)	2.7 (9)	0.13
Diabetes mellitus, % (N)	1.6 (19)	3.1 (6)	0.5 (1)	1.7 (8)	1.2 (4)	0.18
Gastric cancer, % (N)	1.5 (18)	1 (2)	0 (0)	1.7 (8)	2.4 (8)	0.15
Atherosclerosis, % (N)	1.3 (16)	2.6 (5)	1 (2)	1.7 (8)	0.3 (1)	0.12
Pancreatic cancer, % (N)	1.2 (14)	0 (0)	0.5 (1)	1.5 (7)	1.8 (6)	0.2
Brain tumour, % (N)	1.2 (14)	0.5 (1)	1 (2)	1.1 (5)	1.8 (6)	0.6
Intestinal ischemia, % (N)	1.2 (14)	1 (2)	1 (2)	1.1 (5)	1.5 (5)	0.94
Aortic valve disorders, % (N)	1.1 (13)	2.6 (5)	0.5 (1)	1.3 (6)	0.3 (1)	0.07
Pulmonary hypertension, % (N)	1 (12)	0.5 (1)	1 (2)	0.9 (4)	1.5 (5)	0.72
Other, % (N)	23.6 (283)	17 (33)	21.9 (46)	24.2 (111)	27.5 (93)	<0.001

* percentage of deaths. [1] no significant differences between the [a/c] vs. [b] groups. [2] no significant differences between the [a/c] vs. [b] and [c] vs. [d] groups. [3] no significant differences between the [a/c/d] vs. [b] and [a] vs. [c] groups. [4] no significant differences between the [a/c] vs. [b] and [d] vs. [c] groups. [5] significant differences between the [d] vs. [b] groups. [6] significant differences between the [b/d] vs. [c] groups. [7] significant differences between the [c/d] vs. [b] groups. AF, atrial fibrillation; CCS; chronic coronary syndrome; COPD, chronic obstructive pulmonary disease; N, number.

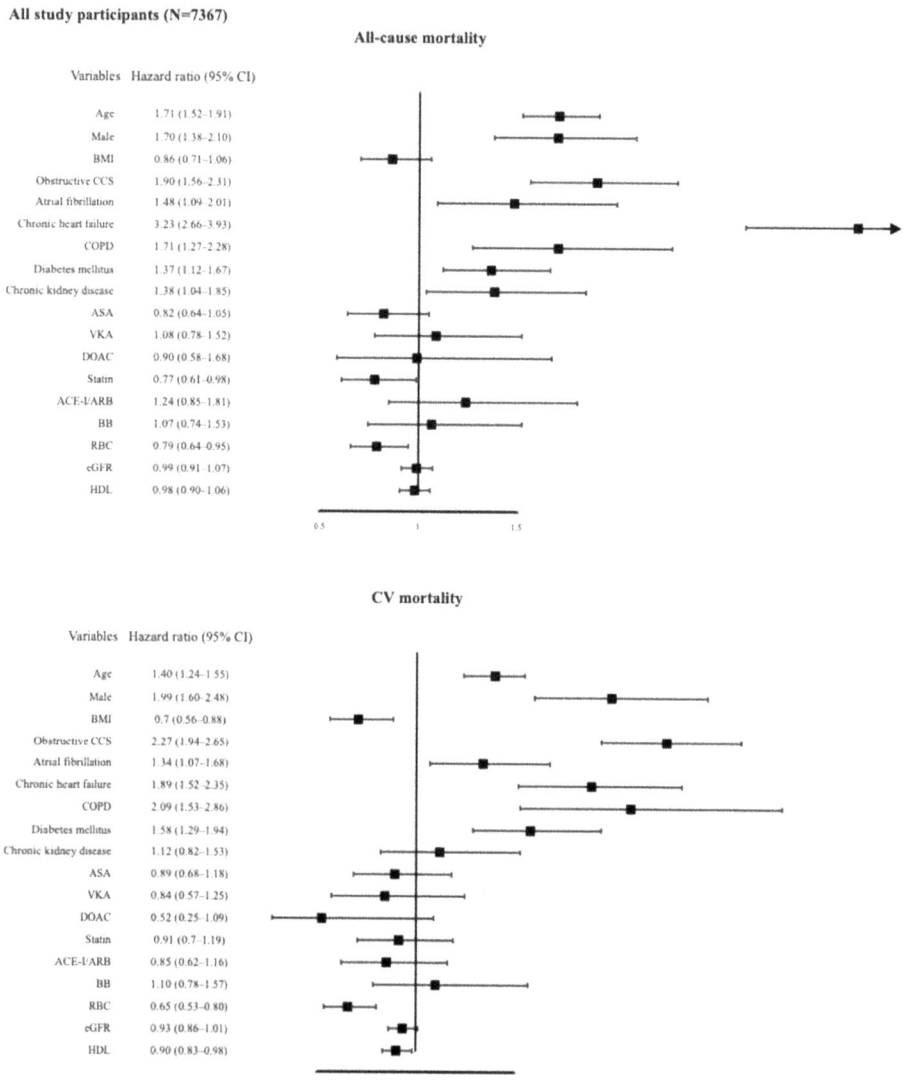

Figure 3. Predictors of all-cause and cardiovascular mortality in all study participants using multivariate analysis. ACEI, angiotensin-converting-enzyme inhibitor; ARB, angiotensin receptor blocker; ASA, acetylsalicylic acid; BB, beta adrenergic receptor antagonist; BMI, body mass index; CCS, chronic coronary syndrome; COPD, chronic obstructive pulmonary disease; CV, cardiovascular; DOAC, direct oral anticoagulant; eGFR, estimated glomerular filtration rate; HDL, high-density lipoprotein cholesterol; RBC, red blood cells; VKA, vitamin K antagonist.

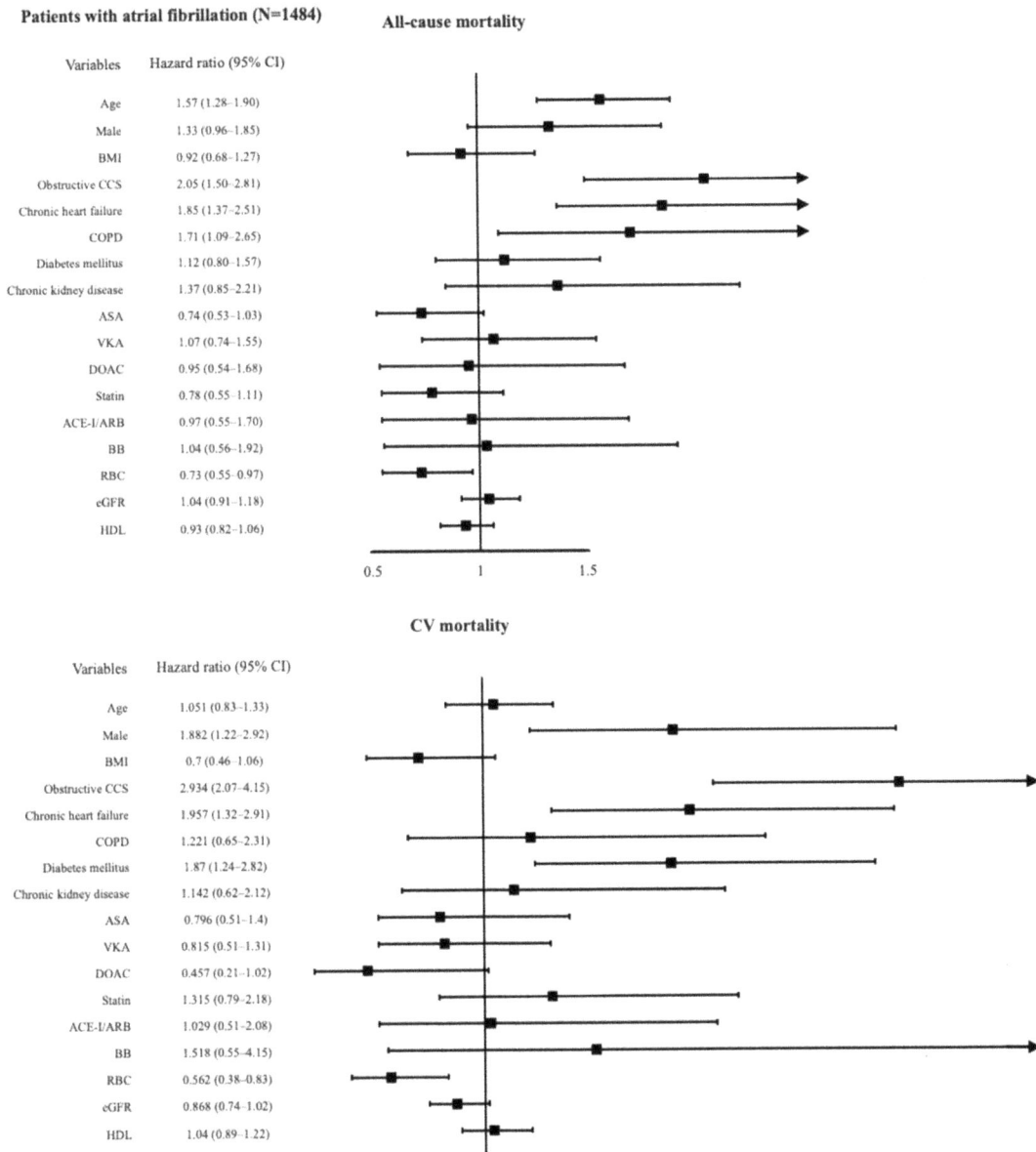

Figure 4. Predictors of all-cause and cardiovascular mortality in patients with atrial fibrillation using multivariate analysis. ACEI, angiotensin-converting-enzyme inhibitor; ARB, angiotensin receptor blocker; ASA, acetylsalicylic acid; BB, beta adrenergic receptor antagonist; BMI, body mass index; CCS, chronic coronary syndrome; COPD, chronic obstructive pulmonary disease; CV, cardiovascular; DOAC, direct oral anticoagulant; eGFR, estimated glomerular filtration rate; HDL, high-density lipoprotein cholesterol; RBC, red blood cells; VKA, vitamin K antagonist.

Table 4. Predictors of all-cause and cardiovascular mortality in the subgroups according to the presence of atrial fibrillation and obstructive chronic coronary syndromes. Multivariate analysis using Cox proportional hazards models. Results are shown as hazard ratios with 95% confidence intervals and corresponding p values.

Variables		AF (+)/CCS (+) [a] (N = 527)	AF (+)/CCS (−) [b] (N = 957)	AF (−)/CCS (+) [c] (N = 2354)	AF (−)/CCS (−) [d] (N = 3529)	p Value for the Comparison among Subgroups
Age, (for a 10-year increase)	All-cause mortality	1.68 (1.24–2.24) $p < 0.001$	1.55 (1.17–2.04) $p < 0.001$	1.79 (1.51–2.14) $p < 0.001$	1.64 (1.32–2.06) $p < 0.001$	$p = 0.67$
	CV mortality	1.21 (0.83–1.77) $p = 0.32$	0.95 (0.69–1.29) $p = 0.73$	1.38 (1.16–1.64) $p < 0.001$	1.64 (1.37–1.97) $p < 0.001$	$p = 0.04$ [1]
Male	All-cause mortality	0.92 (0.58–1.44) $p = 0.71$	1.93 (1.18–3.16) $p = 0.01$	1.45 (1.03–2.05) $p = 0.03$	2.76 (1.76–4.33) $p < 0.001$	$p = 0.03$ [2]
	CV mortality	2.44 (1.13–5.30) $p = 0.02$	1.77 (1.03–3.07) $p = 0.04$	1.52 (1.05–2.21) $p = 0.03$	2.57 (1.81–3.64) $p < 0.001$	$p = 0.045$ [3]
Chronic heart failure	All-cause mortality	1.65 (1.08–2.53) $p = 0.02$	2.32 (1.47–3.65) $p < 0.001$	3.64 (2.69–4.92) $p < 0.001$	6.55 (4.33–9.91) $p < 0.001$	$p = 0.024$ [4]
	CV mortality	2.23 (1.18–4.24) $p = 0.01$	1.99 (1.17–3.39) $p = 0.01$	1.83 (1.27–2.63) $p < 0.001$	1.93 (1.30–2.87) $p < 0.001$	$p = 0.77$
Diabetes mellitus	All-cause mortality	1.31 (0.82–2.07) $p = 0.26$	0.94 (0.57–1.56) $p = 0.82$	1.44 (1.07–1.95) $p = 0.02$	1.59 (1.03–2.46) $p = 0.04$	$p = 0.43$
	CV mortality	2.86 (1.47–5.55) $p < 0.001$	1.75 (1.00–3.07) $p = 0.05$	1.33 (0.96–1.84) $p = 0.09$	1.76 (1.24–2.51) $p < 0.001$	$p = 0.04$ [5]
Statin	All-cause mortality	0.90 (0.51–1.60) $p = 0.73$	0.77 (0.49–1.22) $p = 0.27$	0.81 (0.49–1.33) $p = 0.4$	0.87 (0.53–1.43) $p = 0.58$	$p = 0.81$
	CV mortality	0.88 (0.37–2.1) $p = 0.78$	1.52 (0.81–2.84) $p = 0.19$	1.15 (0.63–2.09) $p = 0.65$	0.62 (0.43–0.91) $p = 0.01$	$p = 0.02$ [6]
ACEI/ARB at discharge	All-cause mortality	1.51 (0.59–3.84) $p = 0.39$	0.57 (0.27–1.19) $p = 0.14$	0.93 (0.53–1.64) $p = 0.8$	3.27 (1.01–10.59) $p = 0.05$	$p = 0.01$ [7]
	CV mortality	2.60 (0.73–9.34) $p = 0.14$	0.86 (0.36–2.08) $p = 0.74$	0.95 (0.53–1.68) $p = 0.85$	0.72 (0.46–1.13) $p = 0.15$	$p = 0.42$
RBC, (for a $10^6/mm^3$ increase)	All-cause mortality	0.75 (0.52–1.10) $p = 0.14$	0.68 (0.44–1.05) $p = 0.08$	0.77 (0.56–1.05) $p = 0.1$	1.27 (0.84–1.91) $p = 0.26$	$p = 0.04$ [7]
	CV mortality	0.45 (0.25–0.82) $p = 0.01$	0.63 (0.36–1.11) $p = 0.11$	0.70 (0.50–0.99) $p = 0.05$	0.62 (0.43–0.88) $p = 0.01$	$p = 0.55$
HDL (for a 10 mg/dL increase)	All-cause mortality	1.01 (0.83–1.22) $p = 0.94$	0.88 (0.72–1.06) $p = 0.18$	0.92 (0.81–1.05) $p = 0.24$	1.13 (0.9–1.31) $p = 0.11$	$p = 0.048$ [8]
	CV mortality	0.90 (0.68–1.17) $p = 0.42$	1.16 (0.95–1.42) $p = 0.15$	0.85 (0.74–0.98) $p = 0.02$	0.89 (0.78–1.01) $p = 0.07$	$p = 0.03$ [1]

[1] significant difference between the [b] vs. [c/d] groups. [2] significant differences between the [d] vs. [a/c] and [a] vs. [b] groups. [3] significant differences between the [b] vs. [c] groups. [4] no significant differences between the [b] vs. [a/c] groups. [5] significant differences between the [a] vs. [c] groups. [6] significant differences between the [a] vs. [b] groups. [7] significant differences between the [b] vs. [d] groups. [8] significant differences between the [d] vs. [b/c] groups. ACEI, angiotensin-converting-enzyme inhibitor; ARB, angiotensin receptor blocker; CV, cardiovascular; HDL, high-density lipoprotein cholesterol; RBC, red blood cells.

4. Discussion

In this large analysis from the Bialystok Coronary Project, our principal findings are as follows: (I) both AF and obstructive CCS were strong and independent predictors of the long-term all-cause and CV mortality; (II) mortality of AF patients without CCS was at least as high as non-AF patients with CCS; and (III) CV deaths were more frequent than non-CV deaths in AF patients with CCS compared to those with either AF or CCS alone. Our study not only highlights the fact that the diagnosis of AF remains a strong predictor of long-term mortality, but also clearly demonstrates that coexistence of AF with obstructive CCS further reduces the survival.

Specific causes of death are frequently not reported in studies exploring long-term mortality in AF patients. Similar to our data, Lee et al. found that among 15,411 AF patients from the Korean registry, CV mortality was more frequent than cancer-related mortality [18]. Additionally, AF patients had a 4-fold increased risk of all-cause mortality compared with the general population. In contrast to our study cohort, Lee et al. found that cerebral infarction (but not coronary heart disease) was the most common cause of death [18]. In Europe, Fauchier et al. analysed patients diagnosed with AF in four hospitals, and demonstrated that the majority of deaths were of CV origin [19], most commonly heart failure (29%), infection (18%), and cancer (12%), while fatal stroke or fatal bleeding each accounted for 7% of all deaths. These findings are concordant with our results in the overall population of the Białystok Coronary Project, with CV deaths more frequent than non-CV deaths in all subgroups except for the AF (−)/CCS (−) patients.

An increased short- and long-term mortality in ACS patients with coexisting AF remains a well-known phenomenon [7,20–23]. We hypothesize that pre-existing AF in ACS patients may be a marker of prior myocardial disease, while new-onset AF may be associated with more extensive myocardial injury in the course of ACS. Nonetheless, data from ACS studies do not necessarily apply to CCS patients. Of note, ACS patients were excluded from the present study.

Our findings correspond with the results of a Spanish study including 17,100 patients aged at least 50 years with known or suspected CCS who underwent exercise electrocardiography (N = 11,911) or exercise echocardiography (N = 5189) [24]. The highest long-term mortality in patients with AF and a positive stress test result when compared with other subgroups. In addition, the diagnosis of AF remained an independent predictor of all-cause mortality, but not of nonfatal myocardial infarction or coronary revascularization [24]. In an Austrian single-centre registry including 1434 patients with CCS and 1456 patients with ACS, patients undergoing elective or urgent coronary revascularization and suffering from AF had a 2-fold increased adjusted relative risk of death after a mean follow-up of 4.8 years [25]. Similar to our data, CKD, CCS, and diabetes were independent predictors of 1-year all-cause mortality in patients with both AF and chronic heart failure with reduced ejection fraction [26].

Another main finding of our work is that patients with AF but without obstructive CCS have a reduced survival when compared with those with obstructive CCS but without concomitant AF. In a cohort of patients referred for exercise stress testing for myocardial ischemia, Bouzas-Mosquera et al. demonstrated a higher long-term all-cause mortality in AF patients with negative stress testing compared to patients without AF [24]. However, patients with AF have coexisting obstructive CCS more often than those with sinus rhythm [27]. Given that the prevalence of obstructive CCS in patients with AF may be as high as 46.5%, it is possible that at the time of inclusion to the study the lesions in their epicardial coronary arteries were not yet so advanced so as to be considered significant at coronary angiography [6,28]. In addition, coronary atherosclerosis tends to progress over time and the co-occurrence of AF and obstructive CCS worsens the patients' prognosis even when they are carefully treated [7,28].

We observed that AF (+)/CCS (−) vs. AF (−)/CCS (+) patients had a higher proportion of deaths due to intracerebral haemorrhage. This may be associated with an under-use of DOACs, which are not refundable in Poland, unlike the VKAs. A large study from various European countries from 2011–2016—overlapping with our study period—showed that out of patients taking oral anticoagulants, 67% were on VKAs and only 33% on DOACs [29].

Our study has limitations. First, our follow-up includes only mortality, there are no data on the condition of patients' health and nonfatal clinical events after inclusion into the study. Second, our findings were obtained in a retrospective single-center study and should be verified in a prospective multicenter study. Third, our observations are restricted to elective patients as those with ACS were excluded from the study. Fourth, fractional flow reserve measurements were not performed on regular basis in our study participants and therefore assessment of the significance of coronary stenoses might have been inaccurate in some of our patients. Fifth, we were not able to obtain reliable data on AF ablation procedures, smoking status, and diabetes therapy in our study participants which may be a confounder in our analysis. Sixth, due to the high count of garbage codes in total mortality in Poland, case-specific mortality is likely to be underestimated. Finally, many of AF patients in our study also suffered from heart failure and vice versa. Additionally, heart failure was a common cause of mortality in our study. These facts might affect our findings.

5. Conclusions

Among patients referred for elective coronary angiography, both AF and obstructive CCS are strong and independent predictors of the long-term all-cause and CV mortality. Mortality of AF without CCS was at least as high as non-AF patients with CCS. CV deaths were more frequent than non-CV deaths in AF patients with CCS compared to those with either AF or CCS alone. Therefore, we recommend a careful clinical follow-up of AF patients, with a particular emphasis on stroke prevention and modification of CV risk factors.

Supplementary Materials: The following are available online at https://www.mdpi.com/2077-0383/10/21/4949/s1, Figure S1: Kaplan–Meier survival analysis of cardiovascular mortality in relation of the diagnosis of atrial fibrillation and chronic coronary syndromes (multiple comparisons: adjusted p value < 0.01 for all tests); Table S1: Predictors of all-cause and cardiovascular mortality in all study participants according to the univariate analysis using Cox proportional hazards models.

Author Contributions: Conceptualization, Ł.K. and A.T.-K.; methodology, Ł.K.; validation, A.T.-K., M.K. and G.Y.H.L.; formal analysis, Ł.K.; investigation, Ł.K.; writing—original draft preparation, Ł.K., A.K. and M.K.; writing—review and editing, M.K. and G.Y.H.L.; visualization, Ł.K. and M.K.; supervision, G.Y.H.L., S.D. and B.S. All authors have read and agreed to the published version of the manuscript.

Funding: This research received no external funding.

Institutional Review Board Statement: The study was conducted according to the guidelines of the Declaration of Helsinki, approved by the ethics committees of the Medical University of Bialystok (R-1-002/18/2019), and registered in the database of clinical studies www.clinicaltrials.gov (accessed on 23 October 2021) (Identifier: NCT04541498).

Informed Consent Statement: Informed consent was obtained from all subjects involved in the study.

Data Availability Statement: The data presented in this study are available on request from the corresponding author.

Conflicts of Interest: The authors declare no conflict of interest.

References

1. Benjamin, E.J.; Muntner, P.; Alonso, A.; Bittencourt, M.S.; Callaway, C.W.; Carson, A.P.; Chamberlain, A.M.; Chang, A.R.; Cheng, S.; Das, S.R.; et al. Heart Disease and Stroke Statistics-2019 Update: A Report from the American Heart Association. *Circulation* **2019**, *139*, e56–e528. [CrossRef] [PubMed]
2. Krijthe, B.P.; Kunst, A.; Benjamin, E.J.; Lip, G.Y.; Franco, O.H.; Hofman, A.; Witteman, J.C.; Stricker, B.H.; Heeringa, J. Projections on the number of individuals with atrial fibrillation in the European Union, from 2000 to 2060. *Eur. Heart J.* **2013**, *34*, 2746–2751. [CrossRef]

3. Kornej, J.; Börschel, C.S.; Benjamin, E.J.; Schnabel, R.B. Epidemiology of Atrial Fibrillation in the 21st Century: Novel Methods and New Insights. *Circ. Res.* **2020**, *127*, 4–20. [CrossRef] [PubMed]
4. Virani, S.S.; Alonso, A.; Benjamin, E.J.; Bittencourt, M.S.; Callaway, C.W.; Carson, A.P.; Chamberlain, A.M.; Chang, A.R.; Cheng, S.; Delling, F.N.; et al. Heart Disease and Stroke Statistics-2020 Update: A Report From the American Heart Association. *Circulation* **2020**, *141*, e139–e596. [CrossRef] [PubMed]
5. Lloyd-Jones, D.M.; Wang, T.J.; Leip, E.P.; Larson, M.G.; Levy, D.; Vasan, R.S.; D'Agostino, R.B.; Massaro, J.M.; Beiser, A.; Wolf, P.A.; et al. Lifetime risk for development of atrial fibrillation: The Framingham Heart Study. *Circulation* **2004**, *110*, 1042–1046. [CrossRef] [PubMed]
6. Patel, N.J.; Patel, A.; Agnihotri, K.; Pau, D.; Patel, S.; Thakkar, B.; Nalluri, N.; Asti, D.; Kanotra, R.; Kadavath, S.; et al. Prognostic impact of atrial fibrillation on clinical outcomes of acute coronary syndromes, heart failure and chronic kidney disease. *World J. Cardiol.* **2015**, *7*, 397–403. [CrossRef] [PubMed]
7. Pilgrim, T.; Kalesan, B.; Zanchin, T.; Pulver, C.; Jung, S.; Mattle, H.; Carrel, T.; Moschovitis, A.; Stortecky, S.; Wenaweser, P.; et al. Impact of atrial fibrillation on clinical outcomes among patients with coronary artery disease undergoing revascularisation with drug-eluting stents. *EuroIntervention* **2013**, *8*, 1061–1071. [CrossRef]
8. Kornej, J.; Henger, S.; Seewöster, T.; Teren, A.; Burkhardt, R.; Thiele, H.; Thiery, J.; Scholz, M. Prevalence of atrial fibrillation dependent on coronary artery status: Insights from the LIFE-Heart Study. *Clin. Cardiol.* **2020**, *43*, 1616–1623. [CrossRef]
9. Tomaszuk-Kazberuk, A.; Koziński, M.; Kuźma, Ł.; Bujno, E.; Łopatowska, P.; Rogalska, E.; Dobrzycki, S.; Sobkowicz, B.; Lip, G.Y.H. Atrial fibrillation is more frequently associated with nonobstructive coronary lesions: The Bialystok Coronary Project. *Pol. Arch. Intern. Med.* **2020**, *130*, 1029–1036. [CrossRef] [PubMed]
10. Chugh, S.S.; Havmoeller, R.; Narayanan, K.; Singh, D.; Rienstra, M.; Benjamin, E.J.; Gillum, R.F.; Kim, Y.H.; McAnulty, J.H., Jr.; Zheng, Z.J.; et al. Worldwide epidemiology of atrial fibrillation: A Global Burden of Disease 2010 Study. *Circulation* **2014**, *129*, 837–847. [CrossRef]
11. Kuźma, Ł.; Tomaszuk-Kazberuk, A.; Kurasz, A.; Zalewska-Adamiec, M.; Bachórzewska-Gajewska, H.; Dobrzycki, S.; Kwiatkowska, M.; Małyszko, J. Atrial Fibrillation and Chronic Kidney Disease—A Risky Combination for Post-Contrast Acute Kidney Injury. *J. Clin. Med.* **2021**, *10*, 4140. [CrossRef] [PubMed]
12. Hindricks, G.; Potpara, T.; Dagres, N.; Arbelo, E.; Bax, J.J.; Blomström-Lundqvist, C.; Boriani, G.; Castella, M.; Dan, G.A.; Dilaveris, P.E.; et al. 2020 ESC Guidelines for the diagnosis and management of atrial fibrillation developed in collaboration with the European Association for Cardio-Thoracic Surgery (EACTS): The Task Force for the diagnosis and management of atrial fibrillation of the European Society of Cardiology (ESC) Developed with the special contribution of the European Heart Rhythm Association (EHRA) of the ESC. *Eur. Heart J.* **2021**, *42*, 373–498. [CrossRef] [PubMed]
13. Kirchhof, P.; Auricchio, A.; Bax, J.; Crijns, H.; Camm, J.; Diener, H.C.; Goette, A.; Hindricks, G.; Hohnloser, S.; Kappenberger, L.; et al. Outcome parameters for trials in atrial fibrillation: Recommendations from a consensus conference organized by the German Atrial Fibrillation Competence NETwork and the European Heart Rhythm Association. *Europace* **2007**, *9*, 1006–1023. [CrossRef] [PubMed]
14. von Elm, E.; Altman, D.G.; Egger, M.; Pocock, S.J.; Gøtzsche, P.C.; Vandenbroucke, J.P.; STROBE Initiative. The Strengthening the Reporting of Observational Studies in Epidemiology (STROBE) Statement: Guidelines for reporting observational studies. *Int. J. Surg.* **2014**, *12*, 1495–1499. [CrossRef]
15. Knuuti, J.; Wijns, W.; Saraste, A.; Capodanno, D.; Barbato, E.; Funck-Brentano, C.; Prescott, E.; Storey, R.F.; Deaton, C.; Cuisset, T.; et al. ESC Scientific Document Group. 2019 ESC Guidelines for the diagnosis and management of chronic coronary syndromes. *Eur. Heart J.* **2020**, *41*, 407–477. [CrossRef] [PubMed]
16. Lang, R.M.; Badano, L.P.; Mor-Avi, V.; Afilalo, J.; Armstrong, A.; Ernande, L.; Flachskampf, F.A.; Foster, E.; Goldstein, S.A.; Kuznetsova, T.; et al. Recommendations for cardiac chamber quantification by echocardiography in adults: An update from the American Society of Echocardiography and the European Association of Cardiovascular Imaging. *J. Am. Soc. Echocardiogr.* **2015**, *28*, 1–39.e14. [CrossRef] [PubMed]
17. Stevens, P.E.; Levin, A.; Kidney Disease: Improving Global Outcomes Chronic Kidney Disease Guideline Development Work Group Members. Evaluation and management of chronic kidney disease: Synopsis of the kidney disease: Improving global outcomes 2012 clinical practice guideline. *Ann. Intern. Med.* **2013**, *158*, 825–830. [CrossRef] [PubMed]
18. Lee, E.; Choi, E.K.; Han, K.D.; Lee, H.; Choe, W.S.; Lee, S.R.; Cha, M.J.; Lim, W.H.; Kim, Y.J.; Oh, S. Mortality and causes of death in patients with atrial fibrillation: A nationwide population-based study. *PLoS ONE* **2018**, *13*, e0209687. [CrossRef] [PubMed]
19. Fauchier, L.; Villejoubert, O.; Clementy, N.; Bernard, A.; Pierre, B.; Angoulvant, D.; Ivanes, F.; Babuty, D.; Lip, G.Y. Causes of Death and Influencing Factors in Patients with Atrial Fibrillation. *Am. J. Med.* **2016**, *129*, 1278–1287. [CrossRef] [PubMed]
20. Rathore, S.S.; Berger, A.K.; Weinfurt, K.P.; Schulman, K.A.; Oetgen, W.J.; Gersh, B.J.; Solomon, A.J. Acute myocardial infarction complicated by atrial fibrillation in the elderly: Prevalence and outcomes. *Circulation* **2000**, *101*, 969–974. [CrossRef] [PubMed]
21. Crenshaw, B.S.; Ward, S.R.; Granger, C.B.; Stebbins, A.L.; Topol, E.J.; Califf, R.M. Atrial fibrillation in the setting of acute myocardial infarction: The GUSTO-I experience: Global Utilization of Streptokinase and TPA for Occluded Coronary Arteries. *J. Am. Coll. Cardiol.* **1997**, *30*, 406–413. [CrossRef]
22. Lopes, R.D.; Pieper, K.S.; Horton, J.R.; Al-Khatib, S.M.; Newby, L.K.; Mehta, R.H.; Van de Werf, F.; Armstrong, P.W.; Mahaffey, K.W.; Harrington, R.A.; et al. Short- and long-term outcomes following atrial fibrillation in patients with acute coronary syndromes with or without ST-segment elevation. *Heart* **2008**, *94*, 867–873. [CrossRef] [PubMed]

23. Al-Khatib, S.M.; Pieper, K.S.; Lee, K.L.; Mahaffey, K.W.; Hochman, J.S.; Pepine, C.J.; Kopecky, S.L.; Akkerhuis, M.; Stepinska, J.; Simoons, M.L.; et al. Atrial fibrillation and mortality among patients with acute coronary syndromes without ST-segment elevation: Results from the PURSUIT trial. *Am. J. Cardiol.* **2001**, *88*, 76–79. [CrossRef]
24. Bouzas-Mosquera, A.; Peteiro, J.; Broullón, F.J.; Alvarez-García, N.; Mosquera, V.X.; Casas, S.; Pérez, A.; Méndez, E.; Castro-Beiras, A. Effect of atrial fibrillation on outcome in patients with known or suspected coronary artery disease referred for exercise stress testing. *Am. J. Cardiol.* **2010**, *105*, 1207–1211. [CrossRef] [PubMed]
25. Rohla, M.; Vennekate, C.K.; Tentzeris, I.; Freynhofer, M.K.; Farhan, S.; Egger, F.; Weiss, T.W.; Wojta, J.; Granger, C.B.; Huber, K. Long-term mortality of patients with atrial fibrillation undergoing percutaneous coronary intervention with stent implantation for acute and stable coronary artery disease. *Int. J. Cardiol.* **2015**, *184*, 108–114. [CrossRef] [PubMed]
26. Horodinschi, R.N.; Diaconu, C.C. Comorbidities Associated with One-Year Mortality in Patients with Atrial Fibrillation and Heart Failure. *Healthcare* **2021**, *9*, 830. [CrossRef] [PubMed]
27. Weijs, B.; Pisters, R.; Haest, R.J.; Kragten, J.A.; Joosen, I.A.; Versteylen, M.; Timmermans, C.C.; Pison, L.; Blaauw, Y.; Hofstra, L.; et al. Patients originally diagnosed with idiopathic atrial fibrillation more often suffer from insidious coronary artery disease compared to healthy sinus rhythm controls. *Heart Rhythm.* **2012**, *9*, 1923–1929. [CrossRef]
28. Kralev, S.; Schneider, K.; Lang, S.; Süselbeck, T.; Borggrefe, M. Incidence and severity of coronary artery disease in patients with atrial fibrillation undergoing first-time coronary angiography. *PLoS ONE* **2011**, *6*, e24964. [CrossRef] [PubMed]
29. Amara, W.; Larsen, T.B.; Sciaraffia, E.; Hernández Madrid, A.; Chen, J.; Estner, H.; Todd, D.; Bongiorni, M.G.; Potpara, T.S.; Dagres, N.; et al. Patients' attitude and knowledge about oral anticoagulation therapy: Results of a self-assessment survey in patients with atrial fibrillation conducted by the European Heart Rhythm Association. *Europace* **2016**, *18*, 151–155. [CrossRef]

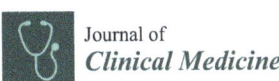

Journal of Clinical Medicine

Article

Impact of Bundle Branch Block on Permanent Pacemaker Implantation after Transcatheter Aortic Valve Implantation: A Meta-Analysis

Justine M. Ravaux [1,*,†], Michele Di Mauro [1,†], Kevin Vernooy [2,3,4], Silvia Mariani [1], Daniele Ronco [1,5], Jorik Simons [1], Arnoud W. Van't Hof [2,3], Leo Veenstra [2], Suzanne Kats [1], Jos G. Maessen [1,3] and Roberto Lorusso [1,3]

1. Department of Cardio-Thoracic Surgery, Heart and Vascular Centre, Maastricht University Medical Centre (MUMC), 6202 AZ Maastricht, The Netherlands; mdimauro1973@gmail.com (M.D.M.); s.mariani1985@gmail.com (S.M.); daniele.ronco@LIVE.IT (D.R.); Jorik_Simons@hotmail.com (J.S.); suzanne.kats@mumc.nl (S.K.); j.g.maessen@mumc.nl (J.G.M.); roberto.lorussobs@gmail.com (R.L.)
2. Department of Cardiology, Maastricht University Medical Centre (MUMC), 6202 AZ Maastricht, The Netherlands; kevin.vernooy@mumc.nl (K.V.); arnoud.vant.hof@mumc.nl (A.W.V.H.); l.veenstra@mumc.nl (L.V.)
3. Cardiovascular Research Institute Maastricht (CARIM), Maastricht University Medical Center, 6202 AZ Maastricht, The Netherlands
4. Department of Cardiology, Radboud University Medical Center (Radboudumc), 6525 GA Nijmegen, The Netherlands
5. Department of Medicine and Surgery, Circolo Hospital, University of Insubria, 21100 Varese, VA, Italy
* Correspondence: jmravaux@hotmail.com
† Co-author, equally contributors.

Abstract: Data regarding the impact of infra-Hisian conduction disturbances leading to permanent pacemaker implantation (PPI) after transcatheter aortic valve implantation (TAVI) remain limited. The aim of this study was to determine the impact of right and/or left bundle branch block (RBBB/LBBB) on post-TAVI PPI. We performed a systematic literature review to identify studies reporting on RBBB and/or LBBB status and post-TAVI PPI. Study design, patient characteristics, and the presence of branch block were analyzed. Odds ratios (ORs) with 95% CI were extracted. The final analysis included 36 studies, reporting about 55,851 patients. Data on LBBB were extracted from 33 studies. Among 51,026 patients included, 5503 showed pre-implant LBBB (11.9% (10.4%–13.8%)). The influence of LBBB on post-TAVI PPI was not significant OR 1.1474 (0.9025; 1.4588), $p = 0.2618$. Data on RBBB were extracted from 28 studies. Among 46,663 patients included, 31,603 showed pre-implant RBBB (9.2% (7.3%–11.6%)). The influence of RBBB on post-TAVI PPI was significant OR 4.8581 (4.1571; 5.6775), $p < 0.0001$. From this meta-analysis, the presence of RBBB increased the risk for post-TAVI PPI, independent of age or LVEF, while this finding was not confirmed for patients experimenting with LBBB. This result emphasizes the need for pre-operative evaluation strategies in patient selection for TAVI.

Keywords: transcatheter aortic valve implantation; right bundle branch block; left bundle branch block; permanent pacemaker implantation

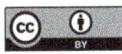

1. Introduction

Atrio-ventricular conduction disturbances and subsequent permanent pacemaker implantation (PPI) represent frequent complication after transcatheter aortic valve implantation (TAVI) [1,2]. Notably, infra-Hisian conductions' desynchrony such as left bundle branch block (LBBB) and right bundle branch block (RBBB) remain an ongoing issue in TAVI [3,4], especially considering TAVI as well-established therapeutic approach for patients with aortic stenosis at high surgical risk [5], while considerable advances in procedural techniques tend to extend TAVI indications to patients with a lower surgical risk [6].

Mechanical stress on the aortic valve annulus, deterioration of the ventricular septum, and local edema may all injury the atrio-ventricular conduction during the TAVI procedures [1,3]. In patients with pre-existing conduction system impairments, such additional procedural-related factors may contribute to a higher post-TAVI PPI rate. Consequently, complications such as PPI thus remain a substantial barrier to extending this technique to operable patients who would otherwise undergo surgery [7]. Therefore, better patient selection and identification of pre-operative risk factors for progression of conduction disturbances, and subsequently PPI, are decisive [8]. Current data about the clinical impact of bundle branch block on post-TAVI PPI remain controversial [9,10]. Left bundle branch block (LBBB) occurs in 5 to 65% in TAVI patients and leads to PPI in 15 of 20% of cases [11]. Pre-operative right bundle branch block (RBBB) is present in 10 to 21% of patients and results in up to 40% of post-operative PPI, making pre-operative RBBB the most important patient-related factor [2,12]. However, the prognostic value on pre-existing infra-Hisian conduction disturbances on post-TAVI PPI remains unclear [10–12].

We aim to investigate the clinical impact of pre-operative RBBB/LBBB on PPI after TAVI.

2. Materials and Methods

2.1. Research Strategy

This meta-analysis was performed in accordance with the Preferred Reporting Items for Systematic Reviews and Meta-Analyses (PRISMA) and the research strategy was developed according to available guidance from the Cochrane Collaboration. A broad, computerized literature search was performed to identify all relevant studies from Embase, Cochrane database, and PubMed exploring Medical Subject Heading (MeSH) terms related to pre-operative RBBB or pre-operative/new-onset LBBB in TAVI population. The PubMed database was searched entering the following key words: "Pacemaker, Artificial" [Mesh] OR pacemaker implantation AND "Transcatheter Aortic Valve Replacement" [Mesh] OR transcatheter aortic valve replacement AND "Bundle-Branch Block" [Mesh]. We restricted the research to English publications. Last access to the database was on 1 November 2020. The search was limited to studies in human.

2.2. Eligibility Criteria and Studies Selection

Studies were included in the final analyses if patients were >18 years (I); >250 patients were included in the main analysis, in order to provide data interpretation of the most consistent clinical series (II); and studies provided a description of pacemaker status of the population (III). Furthermore, articles with no possible extraction of the presence of RBBB/LBBB were excluded. Pre-operative RBBB/LBBB and new-onset RBBB/LBBB were both included in the present analysis. Systematic review and meta-analyses were not taken in account. Studies describing cardiac surgery procedures were also left out. The selected articles underwent extensive evaluation at title and abstract level by two independent researchers (J.R. and M.D.M.) to assess the potential inclusion in the meta-analysis. Discrepancies were solved by consensus with the intervention of a third reviewer (R.L.). There were no duplicate data.

2.3. Statistical Analysis

Calculation of an overall proportion from studies reporting a single proportion was performed using a meta-analytic approach by means of metaprop function of meta package in R. A logit-transformation was performed as suggested by Warton & Hui [13] to calculate confidence intervals (CIs) for individual study results. A Clopper–Pearson approach and a DerSimonian–Laird estimator were used to estimate the between-study variance [14]. Total proportion with 95% CI was reported. Funnel plot and Egger's test were used for estimation of publication bias. The primary endpoint was 30-day or in-hospital PPI after TAVI, so odds ratios (OR) with 95% CI were extracted from 36 studies. Statistical pooling of OR was performed using a random effect model with 95% CI. Forest plots were used to plot the effect size, either for each study or overall. We calculated the I2 statistics (0%~100%) to explain the between-study heterogeneity, with I2 ≤ 25% suggesting more homogeneity, 25% < I2 ≤ 75% suggesting moderate heterogeneity, and I2 > 75% suggesting high heterogeneity [15,16]. If the null hypothesis was rejected, a random effects model was used to calculate pooled effect estimations. If the null hypothesis was not rejected, a fixed effects model was used to calculate pooled effect estimations [14]; 95% CI was also reported. Forest plots were used to plot the effect size, either for each study or overall. Publication bias was evaluated by graphical inspection of funnel plot; estimation of publication bias was quantified by means of Egger's linear regression test [17]. In the case of moderate or high heterogeneity, influence analysis was performed with different approaches: Baujat plot [18] and a leave-one-out sensitivity analysis were performed by iteratively removing one study at a time to confirm that our findings were not driven by any single study. Meta-regression analysis was performed, reporting results as regression coefficient (i.e., Beta) and *p*-value. One removed analysis was performed as a sensitivity analysis. "Meta package" in R-studio version 1.1.463 (2009–2018) was used. Because this study was a systematic review and meta-analysis based on published articles, ethical approval was waived by the institutional review board of the University Hospital of Maastricht.

3. Results

3.1. Study Inclusion

Our search yielded 877 records initially screened at the title and abstract level, with 222 papers fully reviewed for eligibility. There were no duplicate data. Ultimately, 36 studies were identified and provided data for the research analysis (Supplementary Figure S1).

3.2. Baseline Characteristics of Included Patients and Permanent Pacemaker Implantation Details

Table 1 shows the baseline characteristics of the included studies. The 36 studies included a total of 55,851 patients in the final analysis, from 2005 to 2018 [19–54]. The mean age of the patients was 81.9 years, with a mean STS score of 8.3. Only five studies were prospective in nature [35,40,41,44,51]. The PPI details in the included studies are reported in Table 2. The overall incidence of PPI reached 15.2%, ranging from 4.3% to 32%.

Table 1. Baseline characteristics of included studies (n = 36). TAVI, transcatheter aortic valve implantation.

Study	Year	Study Design (Nr Centers)	Sample Size	Age (Years)	STS-Score (%)	Inclusion Period	Valve Type	Follow-Up (Months) *	Approach for TAVI	Mortality at 30 Days
De Carlo et al. [19]	2012	Retrospective (3)	275	82.4	na	Sep 2007–Jul 20120	100% MCV	12	na	3%
Gensas et al. [20]	2014	Retrospective (18)	353	82	14.4	Jan 2008–Feb 2012	85.8% SE 14.2% BE	60	na	na
Mouillet et al. [21]	2015	Retrospective (29)	833	82	14.1	Jan 2010–Oct 2011	100% SE	8	na	9.3%
Nazif et al. [22]	2015	Retrospective (21)	1973	84.5	11.4	May 2007–Sept 2011	100% BE	12	na	6.6%
Rodriguez-Olivares et al. [23]	2016	Retrospective (1)	302	81	na	Nov 2005–Jan 2015	67.2% SE 21.2% BE 11.6% ME	na	na	na
Gonska et al. [24]	2017	Retrospective (1)	283	79.9	6.7	na	100% ES3	na	na	na
Raelson et al. [25]	2017	Retrospective (1)	578	85.5	Na	Mar 2009–Dec 2014	21% SE 79% BE	1	na	na
Dumonteil et al. [26]	2017	Retrospective (14)	250	84	6.3	Oct 2012–May 2014	100% ME	12	100% TF	4%
Monteiro et al. [27]	2017	Retrospective (22)	670	81.8	10.7	Jan 2008–Jan 2015	74% MCV 26% ES	na	96% TF 4% others	na
Pellegrini et al. [28]	2018	Retrospective (3)	283	80.8	6	Jan 2014–Jan 2016	100% SE	12	100% TF	na
De-Torres-Alba et al. [29]	2018	Retrospective (1)	606	81.6	na	Jan 2014–Jan 2017	100% BE	na	na	na
Mangieri et al. [30]	2018	Retrospective (1)	611	84.4	6.9	Oct 2007–Jul 2015	51.7% BE 33.7% SE	12	na	na
Bhardwaj et al. [31]	2018	Retrospective (1)	383	83	9	Jan 2012–July 2016	82% BE 18% SE	9	84% TF	na
Pellegrini et al. [32]	2018	Retrospective (3)	709	81	na	Jan 2014–Jan 2016	100% BE	na	100% TF	1.6%
Gaede et al. [33]	2018	Retrospective (1)	1025	81.9	na	2010–2015	na	2.4	na	na
Nadeem et al. [34]	2018	Retrospective (1)	672	81.4	7.4	2011–2017	na	12	na	na
Chamandi et al. [35]	2018	Prospective (9)	1629	81.5	10.9	May 2009–Feb 2015	50.3% BE 49.7% SE	48	na	42.3%
Doshi et al. [36]	2018	Retrospective (na)	8148	82.5	na	Jan 2012–Dec 2014	na	na	na	na

Table 1. Cont.

Study	Year	Study Design (Nr Centers)	Sample Size	Age (Years)	STS-Score (%)	Inclusion Period	Valve Type	Follow-Up (Months) *	Approach for TAVI	Mortality at 30 Days
Vejpongsa et al. [37]	2018	Retrospective (na)	18,400	81.2	na	Jan 2012–Dec 2013	na	na	TF 75.5% 24.5% TA	na
Cresse et al. [38]	2019	Retrospective (1)	386	83	na	Apr 2008–Jun 2017	na	na	na	na
Dolci et al. [39]	2019	Retrospective (1)	266	80	na	Feb 2014–Feb 2018	100% BE	12	84% TF 16% TA	na
Costa et al. [40]	2019	Prospective (1)	1116	82	4.4	June 2007–Feb 2018	61.8% SE 27.2% BE 0.5% ME 10.5% Others	72	97% TF 3% others	3.9%
Meduri et al. [41]	2019	Prospective (1)	704	82.5	6.6	na	34% SE 66% ME	12	na	na
Du et al. [42]	2020	Retrospective (1)	256	76.5	7.1	Mar 2013–Oct 2018	na	12	Na	3.3%
Shivamurthy et al. [43]	2020	Retrospective (1)	917	80	na	Nov 2011–Feb 2017	na	na	89.7% TF 10.3% TA	na
Studies reporting only on RBBB status in pacemaker population (n = 3)										
Watanabe et al. [44]	2016	Prospective (9)	749	85	6.9	Oct 2013–Aug 2015	100% BE	16.4	78.5% TF 18.8% TA 2.7% T iliac	4%
Auffret et al. [45]	2017	Retrospective (na)	3527	82	na	na	55.8% BE 44.2% SE	23	79.6% TF 16.4% TA 1.9% T aortic 2.1% TS	7.2%
Maeno et al. [46]	2019	Retrospective (1)	659	83	na	Jan 2013–Dec 2015	85% BE 15% SE	19.1	na	2.6%
Studies reporting only on LBBB status in pacemaker population (n = 8)										
Testa et al. [47]	2013	Retrospective (na)	818	82	na	Oct 2007–Apr 2011	100% SE	9	88.6% TF 11.4% TS	5.5%
Schymik et al. [48]	2014	Retrospective (1)	624	82	na	May 2008–Apr 2012	80.8% BE 19.2% SE	12	na	na
Urena et al. [49]	2014	Retrospective (4)	668	79.5	na	na	100% BE	13	2.8% TAortic 42.9% TA 54.3% TF	na

Table 1. Cont.

Study	Year	Study Design (Nr Centers)	Sample Size	Age (Years)	STS-Score (%)	Inclusion Period	Valve Type	Follow-Up (Months) *	Approach for TAVI	Mortality at 30 Days
Nazif et al. [50]	2014	Retrospective (21)	1151	84	11.2	Mar 2007–Mar 2009	100% BE	12	57% TF 43% TA	3.6%
Fischer et al. [51]	2018	Prospective (18)	3404	81.5	5.9	Feb 2005–Oct 2017	46% SE 54% BE	22	82.2% TF 2.2% TS 14.2% TA 1.4% T aortic	5.7%
Chamandi et al. [52]	2019	Retrospective (9)	1020	80.5	6.6	May 2007–Feb 2015	48% BE 52% SE	36	84% TF 11% TA 2% Taortic 3% TS	na
Nazif et al. [53]	2019	Retrospective (51)	1179	81.2	5.5	Dec 2011–Nov 2013	100% BE	24	83.5% TF 16.5% Tthoracic	1.3%
Hamandi et al. [54]	2020	Retrospective (1)	424	82	7.6	Jan 2012–Mar 2016	87% SE 13% BE	12	85% TF 13% TA 3% TAortic	1.3%

Values are n (%), mean = SD, or median (interquartile range) as appropriate. * Follow-up is reported as mean or median as given by the authors. LBBB = left bundle branch block; RBBB = right bundle branch block; SE = self-expandable; BE = balloon-expandable; ME = mechanically-expandable; TF = trans-femoral; TS = trans-subclavian; TA = trans-apical; T iliac = trans-iliac; T aortic = trans-aortic.

Table 2. Pacemaker-related details in included studies. PPI, pacemaker implantation.

Studies Reporting on RBBB and LBBB Status in Pacemaker Population (n = 25)

Study	AVB/SSS/others		%					Predictors	Outcomes
De Carlo et al. [19]	70% AVB 3% SSS 27% others	4	24%	32	37	15	9	* lower MCV implantation below aortic annulus * RBBB * left anterior hemiblock * longer PR interval	na
Gensas et al. [20]	na	na	25.2%	41	50	22	10	* pre-existing RBBB * balloon pre-dilatation * CoreValve use	na
Mouillet et al. [21]	na	na	30.3%	115	106	60	24	na	na
Nazif et al. [22]	79% AVB 17.3% SSS	3	8.8%	312	174	82	12	* Pre-existing RBBB * Prosthesis to LV outflow tract diameter ratio * LV-end diastolic diameter	* longer duration of hospitalization * higher rates of repeat hospitalization and mortality or repeat hospitalization at 1 year
Rodriguez-Olivares et al. [23]	na	na	22.5%	28	32	13	5	na	*more LVOT oversizing associated with higher PPI
Gonska et al. [24]	94.2% AVB 3.8% B 2% others	4,3	18.4%	22	74	13	6	* baseline AV1B * preprocedural complete RBBB	na
Raelson et al. [25]	82% AVB	3	9%	65	50	19	3	na	na
Dumonteil et al. [26]	88.9% AVB 5.9% others	3	32%	26	145	20	14	* baseline RBBB * LV outflow tract overstretch >10%	* trend lower PPI rate at 30 days with shallower (<=5mm) implant depth
Monteiro et al. [27]	na	na	20.1%	71	93	36	15	* previous RBBB * mean aortic gradient >50mmHg * MCV	na

Table 2. *Cont.*

Study	Indication								
Pellegrini et al. [28]	71.5% AVB 3.5% SSS 25% B	na	10%	22	25	6	4	* higher EuroSCORE	na
De-Torres-Alba et al. [29]	96% AVB 1.4% B 2.6% others	na	12.5%	20	74	7	11	na	na
Mangieri et al. [30]	84% AVB 8.4% B	0,3	8.8%	37	61	7	5	na	na
Bhardwaj et al. [31]	na	na	11.5%	50	39	11	3	* PPI with short-term reduction in QoL without long-term implications	na
Pellegrini et al. [32]	71.3% AVB 5.2% SSS 23.5% B	na	16.2%	63	41	30	4	* increase in prosthesis oversizing	na
Gaede et al. [33]	90% AVB 8% SSS 2% B	4	14.7%	98	107	31	17	* pre-existing RBBB * CoreValve prosthesis	Predictors of lack of recovery of AVB * prior RBBB * higher mean aortic valve gradient * post-dilatation of the prosthesis
Nadeem et al. [34]	na	na	21.7%	113	51	65	4	na	* PPI more likely to have heart failure admissions * PPI trend toward increased mortality
Chamandi et al. [35]	76.7% AVB 5.6% SSS 3.1% B 14.6% others	2	19.8%	169	179	84	37	na	* PPI higher rates of rehospitalization due to heart failure and combined endpoint of mortality or heart failure rehospitalization * PPI lesser improvement in LVEF over time, particularly in patients with reduced LVEF before TAVI
Doshi et al. [36]	na	na	24%	220	724	96	253	* female sex * AF * LBBB * AVB	na

Table 2. Cont.

Study									
Vejpongsa et al. [37]	na	2	9.9%	715	1670	265	390	na	na
Cresse et al. [38]	na	4	6.7%	14	97	6	12	na	* RBBB, LBBB, △PR >40 ms associated with PPI
Dolci et al. [39]	80% AVB 11% B 9% others	4	13%	29	41	12	3	* baseline RBBB * QRS width immediately after TAVI	na
Costa et al. [40]	84.8% AVB 4.1% SSS 11% Others	na	13%	92	99	39	8	na	* PPI associated with increased 6 years mortality * baseline RBBB higher chance of being dependent at follow-up
Meduri et al. [41]	90% AVB 6% B 4% others	2	28.4%	85	56	68	20	* baseline RBBB * mean depth of valve implantation	* medically-treated diabetes mellitus in LOTUS valve patients
Du et al. [42]	89.5% AVB	8.7	14.8%	20	19	6	3	na	na
Shivamurthy et al. [43]	na	na	9.8%	130	79	38	9	na	na
Studies reporting only on RBBB status in pacemaker population (n = 3)									
Watanabe et al. [44]	na	na	4.9%	108	na	18	na	na	na
Auffret et al. [45]	na	na	16.5%	362	na	137	na	na	na
Maeno et al. [46]	77.9% AVB 11.5% SSS 10.6%	na	15.8%	101	na	38	na	na	na
Studies reporting only on LBBB status in pacemaker population (n = 8)									
Testa et al. [47]	na	na	17.4%	na	224	na	41	na	* LBBB associated with higher short-term PPI
Schymik et al. [48]	na	na	10.8%	na	197	na	28	* chronic AF * baseline RBBB * MCV	na

Table 2. *Cont.*

Urena et al. [49]	55.5% AVB SSS 20.7% 24.1% B	365	4.3%	na	128	na	11	na	na
Nazif et al. [50]	na	na	5.1%	na	121	na	12	* LBBB with higher PPI and failure of LVEF	na
Fischer et al. [51]	na	na	15.5%	na	398	na	84	* pre-existing LBBB increase risk of death but not late PPI	* pre-existing LBBB associated with lower pre-operative LVEF
Chamandi et al. [52]	na	na	7.2%	na	212	na	29	na	na
Nazif et al. [53]	na	na	4.8%	na	179	na	9	na	* LBBB associated with PPI and repeat hospitalizations
Hamandi et al. [54]	na	na	18%	na	52	na	6	na	na

Values are *n* (%), mean = SD, or median (interquartile range) as appropriate. * Follow-up is reported as mean or median as given by the authors. PPI = permanent pacemaker implantation; AVB = atrio-ventricular block; SSS = Sick Sinus Syndrom; B = bradycardia; AV = atrio-ventricular; LVEF = left ventricle ejection fraction; VVI = single chamber device; DDD = dual chamber device; MCV = Medtronic CoreValve; RBBB = right bundle branch block; LVF = left ventricle function; BMI = body mass index; QoL = quality of life; AF = atrial fibrillation; LBBB = left bundle branch block; TAVI = trans-catheter aortic valve implantation; na = not available.

3.3. Influence of LBBB on PPI

Data on LBBB were extracted from 33 studies [19–43,47–54]; among the 51,026 patients included in the analysis, there were 5503 showing pre-implant LBBB. The cumulative proportion of LBBB was 11.9% (10.4%–13.8%) (Supplementary Figure S2). Heterogeneity was high (I^2 96.4% [95.6%; 97.0%]). No publication bias was found ($p = 0.2921$). The cumulative proportion of LBBB in a subset of 7315 patients with post-TAVI PPI was 13.0% (10.6%–15.8%) with high heterogeneity (I^2 87.7% [83.7%; 90.6%]) and no publication bias ($p = 0.3856$) (Supplementary Figure S3). The cumulative proportion of LBBB in a subset of 43,650 patients without post-TAVI PPI was 12.3% (10.5%–14.4%) with high heterogeneity (I^2 96.5% [95.8%; 97.1%]) and no publication bias ($p = 0.6200$) (Supplementary Figure S4).

The influence of LBBB on post-TAVI PPI was not significant OR 1.1474 (0.9025; 1.4588, $p = 0.2618$) with high heterogeneity $I^2 = 86.2\%$ [81.7%; 89.6%] and no publication bias ($p = 0.7100$) (Figure 1). The baujat plot (Supplementary Figure S5) shows that the study by Vejpongsa et al. [37] may impact high heterogeneity, even if the sensitivity analysis does not confirm this hypothesis, as no influence of LBBB on post-TAVI PPI rate was evidenced at the leave-one out analysis (Figure 2). Meta-regression failed to identify some modifiers: age ($r = -0.0592$, $p = 0.4292$), left ventricular ejection fraction (LVEF, $r = 0.0754$, $p = 0.1741$), and year of the study ($r = -0.0008$, $p = 0.9893$) did not show any influence on the meta-analytic results (Supplementary Figures S6–S8).

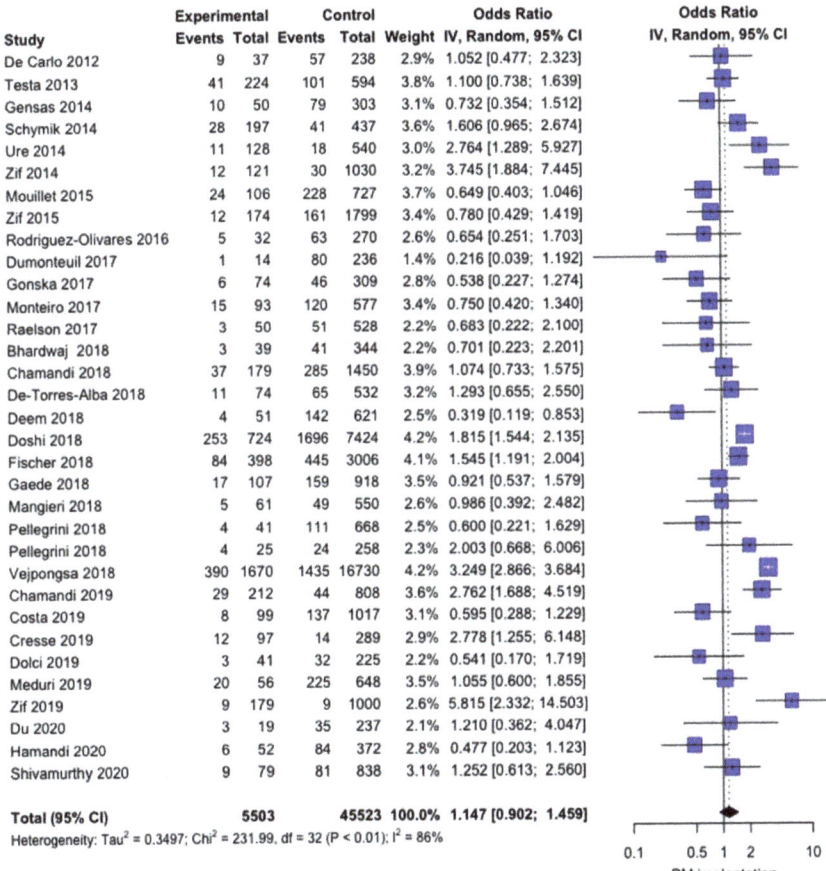

Figure 1. Forest plot comparing the effect of LBBB on the rate of post-TAVI PPI. IV= interval variable; 95% CI = confidence interval.

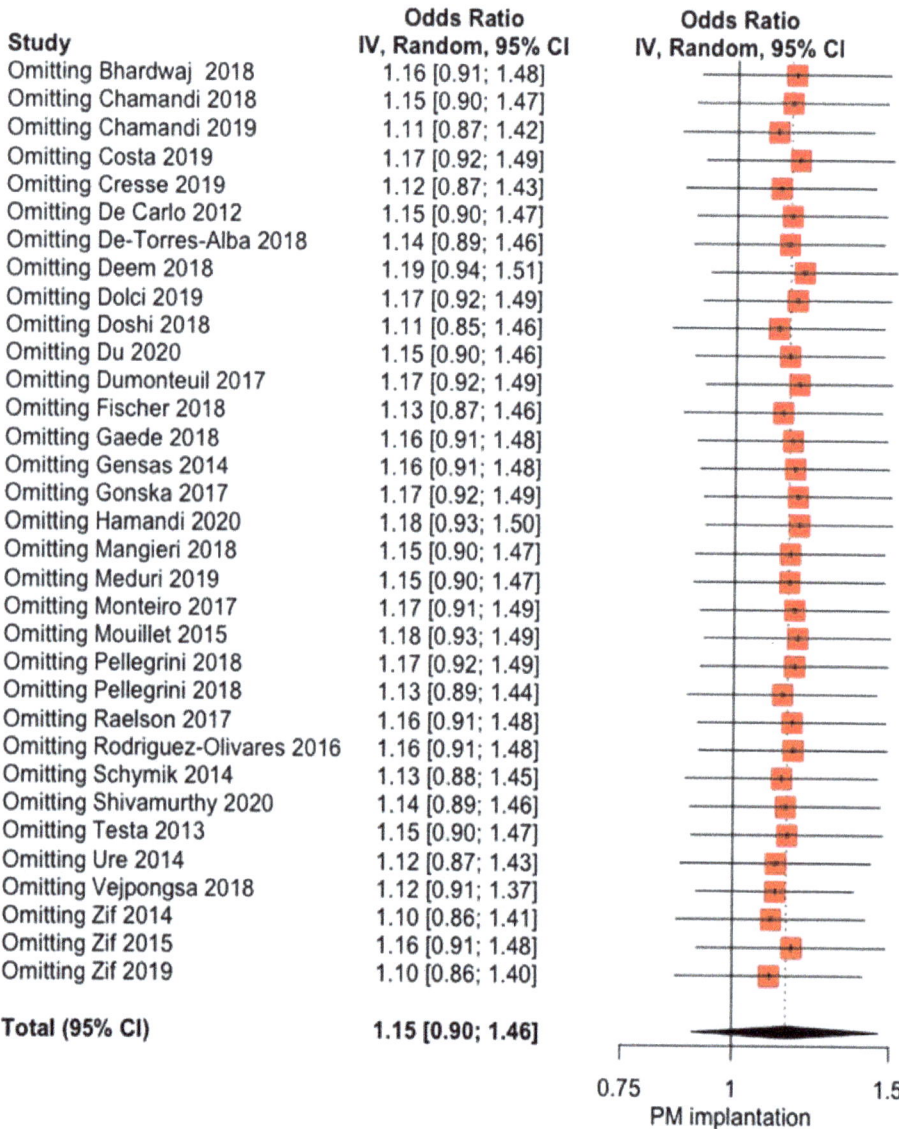

Figure 2. Forest plot leave one-out analysis comparing the effect of the presence of LBBB on the rate of post-TAVI PPI. IV= interval variable; 95% CI= confidence interval.

3.4. Influence of RBBB on PPI

Data on RBBB were extracted from 28 studies (19–46); among the 46,663 patients included in the analysis, there were 31,603 showing pre-implant RBBB. The cumulative proportion of RBBB was 9.2% (7.3%–11.6%) (Supplementary Figure S9). Heterogeneity was high (97.8% [97.3%; 98.1%]). No publication bias was found ($p = 0.1112$). The cumulative proportion of RBBB in a subset of 6932 patients with post-TAVI PPI was 24.7% (19.6%–30.6%) with high heterogeneity (94.6% [93.2%; 95.8%]) and no publication bias ($p = 0.1023$) (Supplementary Figure S10). The cumulative proportion of RBBB in a subset of 39,670 patients without post-TAVI PPI was 6.3% (4.9%–8.1%) with high heterogeneity (I^2 96.6% [95.9%; 97.3%]) and no publication bias ($p = 0.2659$) (Supplementary Figure S11).

The influence of RBBB on post-TAVI PPI was significant, with OR 4.8581 (4.1571; 5.6775), $p < 0.0001$ with moderate heterogeneity $I^2 = 63.4\%$ [45.1%; 75.6%] and no publication bias ($p = 0.937$) (Figure 3). The baujat plot (Supplementary Figure S12) shows that two studies [36,37] may impact the heterogeneity. Sensitivity analysis confirms the impact of RBBB on the post-TAVI PPI rate even at the leave-one out analysis (Figure 4). Meta-regression failed to identify some modifiers: age ($r = -0.0592$; $p = 0.4292$), left ventricular ejection fraction (LVEF, $r = 0.0246$, $p = 0.3755$), and year of the study ($r = 0.0489$, $p = 0.3038$) did not show any influence on meta-analytic results (Supplementary Figures S13–S15).

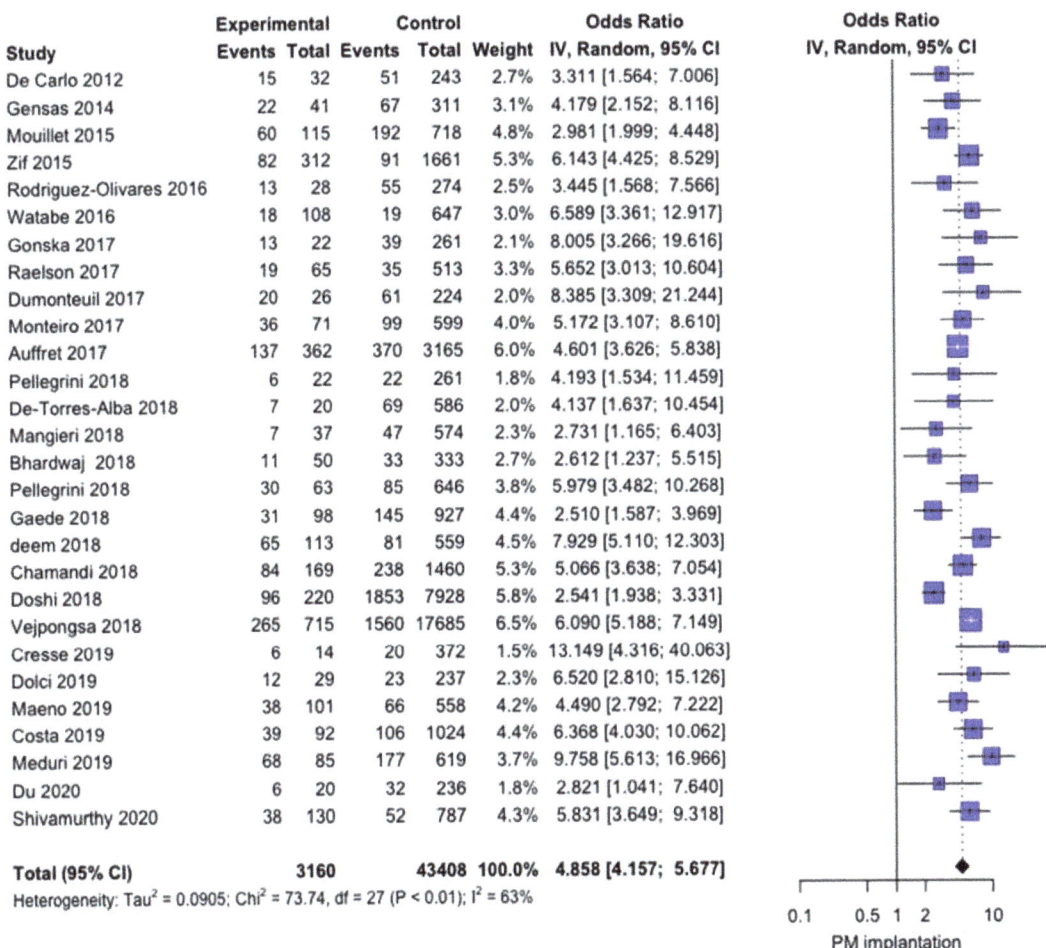

Figure 3. Forest plot comparing the effect of RBBB on the rate of post-TAVI PPI.

post-TAVI PPI.

IV = interval variable; 95%CI = confidence interval.

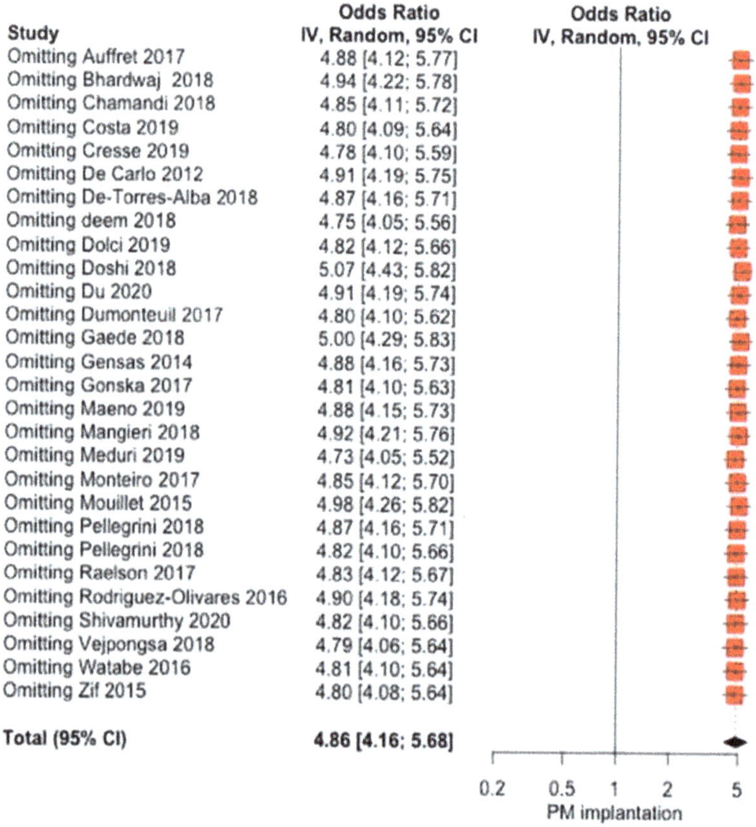

Study	Odds Ratio IV, Random, 95% CI
Omitting Auffret 2017	4.88 [4.12; 5.77]
Omitting Bhardwaj 2018	4.94 [4.22; 5.78]
Omitting Chamandi 2018	4.85 [4.11; 5.72]
Omitting Costa 2019	4.80 [4.09; 5.64]
Omitting Cresse 2019	4.78 [4.10; 5.59]
Omitting De Carlo 2012	4.91 [4.19; 5.75]
Omitting De-Torres-Alba 2018	4.87 [4.16; 5.71]
Omitting deem 2018	4.75 [4.05; 5.56]
Omitting Dolci 2019	4.82 [4.12; 5.66]
Omitting Doshi 2018	5.07 [4.43; 5.82]
Omitting Du 2020	4.91 [4.19; 5.74]
Omitting Dumonteuil 2017	4.80 [4.10; 5.62]
Omitting Gaede 2018	5.00 [4.29; 5.83]
Omitting Gensas 2014	4.88 [4.16; 5.73]
Omitting Gonska 2017	4.81 [4.10; 5.63]
Omitting Maeno 2019	4.88 [4.15; 5.73]
Omitting Mangieri 2018	4.92 [4.21; 5.76]
Omitting Meduri 2019	4.73 [4.05; 5.52]
Omitting Monteiro 2017	4.85 [4.12; 5.70]
Omitting Mouillet 2015	4.98 [4.26; 5.82]
Omitting Pellegrini 2018	4.87 [4.16; 5.71]
Omitting Pellegrini 2018	4.82 [4.10; 5.66]
Omitting Raelson 2017	4.83 [4.12; 5.67]
Omitting Rodriguez-Olivares 2016	4.90 [4.18; 5.74]
Omitting Shivamurthy 2020	4.82 [4.10; 5.66]
Omitting Vejpongsa 2018	4.79 [4.06; 5.64]
Omitting Watabe 2016	4.81 [4.10; 5.64]
Omitting Zif 2015	4.80 [4.08; 5.64]
Total (95% CI)	**4.86 [4.16; 5.68]**

Figure 4. Forest plot leave one-out analysis comparing the effect of the presence of RBBB on the rate of post-TAVI PPI.

4. Discussion

Our meta-analysis demonstrates the impact of bundle branch block on post-TAVI PPI. Our study is derived from 36 studies reporting clinical outcomes in 55,851 patients receiving TAVI and presenting bundle branch conduction disturbances. The main results of this study can be assumed as follows: (i) the presence of LBBB does not influence post-TAVI PPI; (ii) the presence of RBBB has a significant impact on post-TAVI PPI.

The prevalence of LBBB in TAVI candidates is closed to 10% according to previous studies [45,55,56] and new-onset LBBB occurs in ≅30% after TAVI, depending on the type of prosthesis [9,57]. In the present study, the cumulative proportion of LBBB was 11.9%, including pre-operative LBBB and new-onset LBBB after TAVI. This rate is thus in accordance with previously published data [4,58]. The impact of LBBB on post-TAVI PPI remains controversial [49,50,59]. Data from the PARTNER experience [50,53] suggested that new-onset LBBB increases the rate of post-TAVI PPI. Moreover, an analysis at a national registry level as the prospective open TAVI Karlsruhe registry [48] identified slightly more PPI in patients with persistent new-onset LBBB. However, current data do not promote prophylactic PPI in patients presenting new-onset LBBB after TAVI [60] and some studies failed to identify LBBB as predictors for post-TAVI PPI [58,61]. In our study, the influence of LBBB on post-TAVI PPI was not significant. These controversial results can be related to various definitions of LBBB according to the degree of QRS prolongation defining the LBBB [58,61–63] or to the high heterogeneity among the current studies [64]. Moreover, only three studies [22,50,53] quantified LBBB as left anterior fascicular or left posterior fascicular block, which may underestimate the impact of LBBB on post-TAVI PPI. As development of high-degree atrio-ventricular block is shown to be a common complication in patients with pre-existing LBBB (or RBBB) after TAVI [65], we shared the view of Waksman and colleagues [66] emphasizing the need for routine electrophysiology evaluation in patients undergoing TAVI in order to limit post-TAVI PPI. Electrophysiology testing differentiates the supra-nodal conduction disturbances from the infra-nodal ones by analyzing the atrial-His and the His-ventricular intervals. By integrating these values into the baseline electrocardiogram, we may be able to predict the evolution of the atrio-ventricular conduction in high-grade atrio-ventricular block. Such data may help the clinicians to choose between an aggressive strategy of early post-TAVI PPI or, on the contrary, an expectative strategy, avoiding some unnecessary post-TAVI PPI. The results of current ongoing trials investigating the use of electrophysiology-based algorithmic approaches with HV measurements as a guide for PPI, particularly in patients with LBBB (Clinical Monitoring Strategy vs. EP-Guided Algorithmic in LBBB Patients Post-TAVR (NCT03303612); The MARE Study (NCT02153307); Prospective Validation of a Pre-Specified algorithm for the management of conduction disturbances following transcatheter aortic valve replacement PROMOTE (NCT04139616)), are expected with impatience.

Pre-existing RBBB has been demonstrated in 6.9% [67] up to 13.6% [44] of patients undergoing TAVI and is a common underlying conduction disturbance in TAVI patients [10]. In this study, the cumulative proportion of RBBB among the included studies reached 9.2%, also in accordance with the studies of Auffret and colleagues [45], reporting a prevalence of RBBB of 10.3% in TAVI candidates. Several studies have already highlighted the role of pre-existing RBBB in the development of atrioventricular conduction, leading to post-TAVI PPI [2,3,22,26,33,39,41]. Our findings confirm the impact of such a condition on post-TAVI PPI, without the influence of age or LVEF. As previous studies emphasized the higher all-cause mortality and the poorer clinical outcomes in patients with pre-existing RBBB [10,45], bradyarrhythmia events may participate in the poorer outcomes of these patients. However, this analysis does not provide the cause of such discrepancies between RBBB and LBBB. The fragility of the right bundle branch during minor trauma or procedures may partially explain its highest incidence in the general population and, consequently, the more important impact of RBBB in post-TAVI PPI [68]. We look forward to having definitive data and guidelines to determine the optimal management and monitoring of patients with RBBB undergoing TAVI [60].

The current guidelines with respect to post-TAVI PPI [69] do not specify the adequate timing for post-TAVI PPI. Previously, the 2013 European Society Guidelines [70] recommended a clinical rhythm observation period of 7 days in the presence of high-grade trio-ventricular block before proceeding to post-TAVI PPI. In the current meta-analysis, the range of timing for PPI varied from day 0 to 1 year, also emphasizing the need for PPI after discharge and the influence of atrio-ventricular conduction in the long term [49]. This hypothetical observation period may be shortened or lengthened according to patient-related factors and electrical findings. Once again, electrophysiological study may identify some high-risk patients for the development of high-grade atrio-ventricular disturbances and, thereby, adjust the observation rhythm period in such patients [71].

As the definitive impact of infra-Hisian conduction disturbances on post-TAVI PPI has not definitively been clarified yet, specific recommendations for the type of valves used in such patients must be done with caution. However, some studies investigated the impact of the valves used on post-TAVI conduction disturbances [3,44,49,61]. Indeed, Franzoni and colleagues [61] found a higher incidence of LBBB when using a Medtronic CoreRevalving System with respect to the Edwards Sapien Valve. A more intra-ventricular implantation of the stent valve frame may result in higher rate of post-TAVI PPI [49]. Furthermore, the gap between the lower edge of the coronary cusp and the end of the frame of the prosthetics valve has been shown to be greater in patients with new-onset LBBB than in patients with post-operative conduction disturbances [61], emphasizing the role of the prosthesis placement in the development of post-operative conduction disturbances. Nevertheless, the requirement for post-TAVI PPI is multifactorial and studies incorporating electrophysiological findings with procedural data are mandatory [72].

Study Limitations

This meta-analysis has several limitations to be acknowledged. First, this meta-analysis possesses all the inherent bias associated with this investigation technique. Second, including pre-operative LBBB and new-onset LBBB in the analysis may be considered as a limitation for the interpretation of the final results, as the pre-operative LBBB can be related to other cardiovascular conditions and the new-onset LBBB can be related to procedural/interventional aspects. However, as our primary outcome was 30-day or in-hospital PPI, we can afford to compare both LBBB as conduction disturbances present after TAVI, which can lead to PPI, independently of the chronic or acute apparition of the LBBB. Third, distinction of LBBB in left anterior fascicular or left posterior fascicular block was lacking in the majority of the included studies, thereby not providing enough information to perform in-depth analysis. Further research in this respect is currently needed. Finally, analysis of individual patient-level data may provide further understandings.

5. Conclusions

This meta-analysis found that patients with the presence of RBBB have higher risk for post-TAVI PPI, with no influence of age or LVEF. This finding has not been confirmed for patients experimenting with LBBB. Pre-operative evaluation strategies, including electrophysiological characteristics, are crucial in further extending patient selection for TAVI.

Supplementary Materials: The following are available online at https://www.mdpi.com/2077-0383/10/12/2719/s1, Figure S1. Flowsheet of the included studies, Figure S2. Forest plot pooling the proportion of LBBB in 33 studies, Figure S3. Forest plot pooling the proportion of LBBB in subset of 7315 patients with post-TAVI PPI, Figure S4. Forest plot pooling the proportion of LBBB in subset of 43,650 patients without post-TAVI PPI, Figure S5. Baujat plot: impact of the studies on overall heterogeneity in studies reporting on LBBB status, Figure S6. Bubble plots: influence of age on risk for post-TAVI PPI in patients with LBBB, Figure S7. Bubble plots: influence of LVEF on risk for post-TAVI PPI in patients with LBBB, Figure S8. Bubble plots: influence of the year of the study on risk for post-TAVI PPI in patients with LBBB, Figure S9. Forest plot pooling the proportion of RBBB in 28 studies, Figure S10. Forest plot pooling the proportion of RBBB in subset of 6932 patients with post-TAVI PPI, Figure S11. Forest plot pooling the proportion of RBBB in subset of 39,670 patients without post-TAVI PPI, Figure S12. Baujat plot: impact of the studies on overall heterogeneity in studies reporting on RBBB status, Figure S13. Bubble plots: influence of age on risk for post-TAVI PPI in patients with RBBB, Figure S14. Bubble plots: influence of LVEF on risk for post-TAVI PPI in patients with RBBB, Figure S15. Bubble plots: influence of the year of the study on risk for post-TAVI PPI in patients with RBBB.

Author Contributions: Conceptualization, J.M.R., M.D.M. and R.L.; methodology, J.M.R., M.D.M. and R.L.; software, M.D.M.; validation, K.V., S.M., A.W.V.H., S.K. and L.V.; formal analysis, J.M.R. and M.D.M.; investigation, J.M.R. and M.D.M.; resources, S.M., D.R. and J.S.; data curation, J.M.R. and M.D.M.; writing—original draft preparation, J.M.R. and M.D.M.; writing—review and editing, J.M.R., M.D.M. and R.L.; visualization, J.M.R., M.D.M., K.V., S.M., D.R., J.S., A.W.V.H., L.V., S.K., J.G.M. and R.L.; supervision, S.K. and R.L.; project administration, J.M.R., M.D.M. and R.L.; funding acquisition, none. All authors have read and agreed to the published version of the manuscript.

Funding: This research received no external funding.

Institutional Review Board Statement: Because this study was a systematic review and meta-analysis based on published articles, ethical approval was waived by the institutional review board of the University Hospital of Maastricht.

Informed Consent Statement: Patient consent was waived due to the systematic review and meta-analytic nature of this study.

Data Availability Statement: No new data were created or analyzed in this study. Data sharing is not applicable to this article.

Conflicts of Interest: The authors declare no conflict of interest.

References

1. Erkapic, D.; De Rosa, S.; Kelava, A.; Lehmann, R.; Fichtlscherer, S.; Hohnloser, S.H. Risk for permanent pacemaker after transcatheter aortic valve implantation: A comprehensive analysis of the literature. *J. Cardiovasc. Electrophysiol.* **2012**, *23*, 391–397. [CrossRef]
2. Siontis, G.C.; Jüni, P.; Pilgrim, T.; Stortecky, S.; Büllesfeld, L.; Meier, B.; Wenaweser, P.; Windecker, S. Predictors of permanent pacemaker implantation in patients with severe aortic stenosis undergoing TAVR: A meta-analysis. *J. Am. Coll. Cardiol.* **2014**, *64*, 129–140. [CrossRef] [PubMed]
3. Van Gils, L.; Tchetche, D.; Lhermusier, T.; Abawi, M.; Dumonteuil, N.; Rodriguez-Olivares, R.; Molina-Martin, D.N.J.; Stella, P.R.; Carrié, D.; De Jaegere, P.P.; et al. Transcatheter Heart Valve Selection and Permanent Pacemaker Implantation in Patients with Pre-Existent Right Bundle Branch Block. *J. Am. Heart Assoc.* **2017**, *6*, e005028. [CrossRef]
4. Lopez-Aguilera, J.; Saint-Gerons, J.M.S.; Bellido, F.M.; Suarez, D.L.H.D.T.J.; Pineda, S.O.; Alvarez-Ossorio, M.P.; Angel, R.M.M.; Pavlovic, D.; Suarez, D.L.C.C.J. Effect of New-Onset Left Bundle Branch Block After Transcatheter Aortic Valve Implantation (CoreValve) on Mortality, Frequency of Re-Hospitalization, and Need for Pacemaker. *Am. J. Cardiol.* **2016**, *118*, 1380–1385. [CrossRef]
5. Rodès-Cabau, J. Transcatheter aortic valve implantation: Current and future approaches. *Nat. Rev. Cardiol.* **2012**, *9*, 15–29. [CrossRef] [PubMed]
6. Waksman, R.; Rogers, T.; Torguson, R.; Gordon, P.; Ehsan, A.; Wilson, S.R.; Goncalves, J.; Levitt, R.; Hahn, C.; Parikh, P.; et al. Transcatheter Aortic Valve Replacement in Low-Risk Patients with Symptomatic Severe Aortic Stenosis. *J. Am. Coll. Cardiol.* **2018**, *72*, 2095–2105. [CrossRef] [PubMed]
7. Finkelstein, A.; Rozenbaum, Z.; Halkin, A.; Banai, S.; Bazan, S.; Barbash, I.; Segev, A.; Fefer, P.; Maor, E.; Danenberg, H.; et al. Outcomes of Transcatheter Aortic Valve Implantation in Patients with Low Versus Intermediate to High Surgical Risk. *Am. J. Cardiol.* **2019**, *123*, 644–649. [CrossRef]
8. Voigtländer, L.; Seiffert, M. Expanding TAVI to Low and Intermediate Risk Patients. *Front. Cardiovasc. Med.* **2018**, *5*, 92. [CrossRef] [PubMed]
9. Regueiro, A.; Abdul-Jawad, A.O.; Del Trigo, M.; Campelo-Parada, F.; Puri, R.; Urena, M.; Philippon, F.; Rodès-Cabau, J. Impact of New-Onset Left Bundle Branch Block and Periprocedural Permanent Pacemaker Implantation on Clinical Outcomes in Patients Undergoing Transcatheter Aortic Valve Replacement: A systematic Review and Meta-Analysis. *Circ. Cardiovasc. Interv.* **2016**, *9*, e003635. [CrossRef] [PubMed]
10. Croix, G.R.S.; Spencer, C.; Hrachian, H.L.; Beohar, N. Clinical Impact of Preexisting Right Bundle Branch Block after Transcatheter Aortic Valve Replacement: A Systematic Review and Meta-Analysis. *J. Interv. Cardiol.* **2020**, *2020*, 1789516.
11. Massouillé, G.; Bordachar, P.; Ellenbogen, K.A.; Souteyrand, G.; Jean, F.; Combaret, N.; Vorilhon, C.; Clerfond, G.; Farhat, M.; Ritter, P.; et al. New-onset left bundle branch block induced by transcutaneous aortic valve implantation. *Am. J. Cardiol.* **2016**, *117*, 867–873. [CrossRef] [PubMed]
12. Rivard, L.; Schram, G.; Asgar, A.; Khairy, P.; Andrade, J.G.; Bonan, R.; Dubuc, M.; Guerra, P.G.; Ibrahim, R.; Macle, L.; et al. Electrocardiographic and electrophysiological predictors of atrioventricular block after transcatheter aortic valve replacement. *Heart Rhythm.* **2015**, *12*, 321–329. [CrossRef] [PubMed]
13. Warton, D.I.; Hui, F.K.C. The arcsine is asinine: The analysis of proportions in ecology. *Ecology* **2011**, *92*, 3–10. [CrossRef] [PubMed]
14. DerSimonian, R.; Laird, N. Meta-analysis in clinical trials revisited. *Contemp. Clin. Trials* **2015**, *45 Pt A*, 139–145. [CrossRef]
15. Bowden, J.; Tierney, J.F.; Copas, A.J.; Burdett, S. Quantifying, displaying and accounting for heterogeneity in the meta-analysis of RCTs using standard and generalized Q statistics. *BMC Med. Res. Methodol.* **2011**, *11*, 41–52. [CrossRef]
16. Huedo-Medina, T.B.; Sanchez-Meca, J.; Marin-Martinez, F.; Botella, J. Assessing heterogeneity in meta-analysis: Q statistic or I2 index? *Psychol. Methods* **2006**, *11*, 193–206. [CrossRef] [PubMed]
17. Begg, C.B.; Mazumdar, M. Operating characteristics of a rank correlation test for publication bias. *Biometrics* **1994**, *50*, 1088–1101. [CrossRef] [PubMed]
18. Baujat, B.; Mahé, C.; Pignon, J.-P.; Hill, C. A graphical method for exploring heterogeneity in meta-analyses: Application to a meta-analysis of 65 trials. *Stat. Med.* **2002**, *21*, 2641–2652. [CrossRef] [PubMed]

19. De Carlo, M.; Giannini, C.; Bedogni, F.; Klugmann, S.; Brambilla, N.; De Marco, F.; Zuchelli, G.; Testa, L.; Oreglia, J.; Petronio, A.S. Safety of a conservative strategy of permanent pacemaker implantation after transcatheter aortic CoreValve implantation. *Am. Heart J.* **2012**, *163*, 492–499. [CrossRef] [PubMed]
20. Gensas, C.S.; Caixeta, A.; Siqueira, D.; Carvalho, L.A.; Sarmento-Leite, R.; Mangione, J.A.; Lemos, P.A.; Colafranceschi, A.S.; Caramori, P.; Ferreira, M.C.; et al. Brazilian Registry in Transcatheter Aortic Valve Implantation Investigators. Predictors of permanent pacemaker requirement after transcatheter aortic valve implantation: Insights from a Brazilian registry. *Int. J. Cardiol.* **2014**, *175*, 248–252. [CrossRef]
21. Mouillet, G.; Lellouche, N.; Yamamoto, M.; Oguri, A.; Dubois-Rande, J.L.; Van Belle, E.; Gilard, M.; Laskar, M.; Teiger, E. Outcomes following pacemaker implantation after transcatheter aortic valve implantation with CoreValve (®) devices: Results from the FRANCE 2 Registry. *Catheter. Cardiovasc. Interv.* **2015**, *86*, E158–E166. [CrossRef] [PubMed]
22. Nazif, T.M.; Dizon, J.M.; Hahn, R.T.; Xu, K.; Babaliaros, V.; Douglas, P.S.; El-Chami, M.F.; Herrmann, H.C.; Mack, M.; Makkar, R.R.; et al. Predictors and clinical outcomes of permanent pacemaker implantation after transcatheter aortic valve replacement: The PARTNER (Placement of AoRtic TraNscathertER Valves) trial and registry. *JACC Cardiovasc. Interv.* **2015**, *8 Pt A*, 60–69. [CrossRef]
23. Rodríguez-Olivaresa, R.; van Gils, L.; El Faquir, N.; Rahhab, Z.; Di Martino, L.F.M.; van Weenen, S.; de Vriesa, J.; Galema, T.W.; Geleijnse, M.L.; Budde, R.P.; et al. Importance of the left ventricular outflow tract in the need for pacemaker implantation after transcatheter aortic valve replacement. *Int. J. Cardiol.* **2016**, *216*, 9–15. [CrossRef]
24. Gonska, B.; Seeger, J.; Keßler, M.; Von Keil, A.; Rottbauer, W.; Wöhrle, J. Predictors for permanent pacemaker implantation in patients undergoing transfemoral aortic valve implantation with the Edwards Sapien 3 valve. *Clin. Res. Cardiol.* **2017**, *106*, 590–597. [CrossRef] [PubMed]
25. Raelson, C.A.; Gabriels, J.; Ruan, J.; Ip, J.E.; Thomas, G.; Liu, C.F.; Cheung, J.W.; Lerman, B.B.; Patel, A.; Markowitz, S.M. Recovery of atrioventricular conduction in patients with heart block after transcatheter aortic valve replacement. *J. Cardiovasc. Electrophysiol.* **2017**, *28*, 1196–1202. [CrossRef]
26. Dumonteil, N.; Meredith, I.T.; Blackman, D.J.; Tchétché, D.; Hildick-Smith, D.; Spence, M.S.; Walters, D.L.; Harnek, J.; Worthley, S.G.; Rioufol, G.; et al. Insights into the need for permanent pacemaker following implantation of the repositionable LOTUS valve for transcatheter aortic valve replacement in 250 patients: Results from the REPRISE II trial with extended cohort. *Euro Interv.* **2017**, *13*, 796–803. [CrossRef]
27. Monteiro, C.; Di Leoni, F.A.; Caramori, P.R.; Carvalho, L.A.F.; Siqueira, D.A.; Sao, T.L.E.K.; Perin, M.; De Lima, V.C.; Guérios, E.; Brito, F.S.D., Jr.; et al. Permanent Pacing After Transcatheter Aortic Valve Implantation: Incidence, Predictors and Evolution of Left Ventricular Function. *Arq. Bras. Cardiol.* **2017**, *109*, 550–559. [CrossRef] [PubMed]
28. Pellegrini, C.; Kim, W.K.; Holzamer, A.; Walther, T.; Mayr, N.P.; Michel, J.; Rheude, T.; Nuñez, J.; Kasel, A.M.; Trenkwalder, T.; et al. Multicenter Evaluation of Prosthesis Oversizing of the SAPIEN 3 Transcatheter Heart Valve Impact on Device Failure and New Pacemaker Implantations. *Rev. Esp. Cardiol.* **2019**, *72*, 641–648. [CrossRef] [PubMed]
29. De-Torres-Alba, F.; Kaleschke, G.; Vormbrock, J.; Orwat, S.; Radke, R.; Feurle, M.; Diller, G.P.; Reinecke, H.; Baumgartner, H. Delayed pacemaker requirement after transcatheter aortic valve implantation with a new-generation balloon expandable valve: Should we monitor longer? *Int. J. Cardiol.* **2018**, *273*, 56–62. [CrossRef] [PubMed]
30. Mangieri, A.; Lanzillo, G.; Bertoldi, L.; Jabbour, R.J.; Regazzoli, D.; Ancona, M.B.; Tanaka, A.; Mitomo, S.; Garducci, S.; Montalto, C.; et al. Predictors of Advanced Conduction Disturbances Requiring a Late (≥48 h) Permanent Pacemaker Following Transcatheter Aortic Valve Replacement. *JACC Cardiovasc. Interv.* **2018**, *11*, 1519–1526. [CrossRef]
31. Bhardwaj, A.; Ramanan, T.; Sawant, A.C.; Sinibaldi, E.; Pham, M.; Khan, S.; Qureshi, R.; Agrawal, N.; Khalil, C.; Hansen, R.; et al. Quality of life outcomes in transcatheter aortic valve replacement patients requiring pacemaker implantation. *J. Arrhythm.* **2018**, *34*, 441–449. [CrossRef] [PubMed]
32. Pellegrini, C.; Husser, O.; Kim, W.K.; Holzamer, A.; Walther, T.; Rheude, T.; Mayr, N.P.; Trenkwalder, T.; Joner, M.; Michel, J.; et al. Predictors of Need for Permanent Pacemaker Implantation and Conduction Abnormalities With a Novel Self-expanding Transcatheter Heart Valve. *Rev. Esp. Cardiol.* **2019**, *72*, 145–153. [CrossRef]
33. Gaede, L.; Kim, W.K.; Liebetrau, C.; Dörr, O.; Sperzel, J.; Blumenstein, J.; Berkowitsch, A.; Walther, T.; Hamm, C.; Elsässer, A.; et al. Pacemaker implantation after TAVI: Predictors of AV block persistence. *Clin. Res. Cardiol.* **2018**, *107*, 60–69. [CrossRef] [PubMed]
34. Nadeem, F.; Tsushima, T.; Ladas, T.P.; Thomas, R.B.; Patel, S.M.; Saric, P.; Patel, T.; Lipinski, J.; Li, J.; Costa, M.A.; et al. Impact of Right Ventricular Pacing in Patients Who Underwent Implantation of Permanent Pacemaker After Transcatheter Aortic Valve Implantation. *Am. J. Cardiol.* **2018**, *122*, 1712–1717. [CrossRef] [PubMed]
35. Chamandi, C.; Barbanti, M.; Munoz-Garcia, A.; Latib, A.; Nombela-Franco, L.; Gutiérrez-Ibanez, E.; Veiga-Fernandez, G.; Cheema, A.N.; Cruz-Gonzalez, I.; Serra, V.; et al. Long-Term Outcomes in Patients with New Permanent Pacemaker Implantation Following Transcatheter Aortic Valve Replacement. *JACC Cardiovasc. Interv.* **2018**, *11*, 301–310. [CrossRef] [PubMed]
36. Doshi, R.; Decter, D.H.; Meraj, P. Incidence of arrhythmias and impact of permanent pacemaker implantation in hospitalizations with transcatheter aortic valve replacement. *Clin. Cardiol.* **2018**, *41*, 640–645. [CrossRef]
37. Vejpongsa, P.; Zhang, X.; Bhise, V.; Kitkungvan, D.; Shivamurthy, P.; Anderson, H.V.; Balan, P.; Nguyen, T.C.; Estrera, A.L.; Dougherty, A.H.; et al. Risk Prediction Model for Permanent Pacemaker Implantation after Transcatheter Aortic Valve Replacement. *Struct. Heart* **2018**, *2*, 328–335. [CrossRef]

38. Cresse, S.; Eisenberg, T.; Alfonso, C.; Cohen, M.G.; DeMarchena, E.; Williams, D.; Carrillo, R. Cardiac conduction abnormalities associated with pacemaker implantation after transcatheter aortic valve replacement. *Pacing Clin. Electrophysiol.* **2019**, *42*, 846–852. [CrossRef] [PubMed]
39. Dolci, G.; Vollema, E.M.; Van Der Kley, F.; De Weger, A.; Marsa, N.A.; Delgado, V.; Bax, J.J. One-Year Follow-Up of Conduction Abdormalities After Transcatheter Aortic Valve Implantation with the SAPIEN 3 Valve. *Am. J. Cardiol.* **2019**, *124*, 1239–1245. [CrossRef] [PubMed]
40. Costa, G.; Zappulla, P.; Barbanti, M.; Cirasa, A.; Todaro, D.; Rapisarda, G.; Picci, A.; Platania, F.; Tosto, A.; Di Grazia, A.; et al. Pacemaker dependency after transcatheter aortic valve implantation: Incidence, predictors and long-term outcomes. *EuroIntervention* **2019**, *15*, 875–883. [CrossRef]
41. Meduri, C.U.; Kereiakes, D.J.; Rajagopal, V.; Makkar, R.R.; O'Hair, D.; Linke, A.; Waksman, R.; Babliaros, V.; Stoler, R.C.; Mishkel, G.J.; et al. Pacemaker Implantation and Dependency After Transcatheter Aortic Valve Replacement in the REPRISE III Trial. *J. Am. Heart Assoc.* **2019**, *8*, e012594. [CrossRef] [PubMed]
42. Du, F.; Zhu, Q.; Jiang, J.; Chen, H.; Liu, X.; Wang, J. Incidence and Predictors of Permanent Pacemaker Implantation in Patients Who Underwent Transcatheter Aortic Valve Replacement: Observation of a Chinese Population. *Cardioliology* **2019**, *145*, 27–34. [CrossRef] [PubMed]
43. Shivamurthy, P.; Vejpongsa, P.; Gurung, S.; Jacob, R.; Zhao, Y.; Anderson, H.V.; Balan, P.; Nguyen, T.C.; Estrera, A.L.; Dougherty, A.H.; et al. Validation of Scoring System Predicting Permanent Pacemaker Implantation after Transcatheter Aortic Valve Replacement. *Pacing Clin. Electrophysiol.* **2020**, *43*, 479–485. [CrossRef] [PubMed]
44. Watanabe, Y.; Kozuma, K.; Hioki, H.; Kawashima, H.; Nara, Y.; Kataoka, A.; Nagura, F.; Nakashima, M.; Shirai, S.; Tada, N.; et al. Pre-Existing Right Bundle Branch Block Increases Risk for Death After Transcatheter Aortic Valve Replacement with a Balloon-Expandable Valve. *JACC Cardiovasc. Interv.* **2016**, *9*, 2210–2216. [CrossRef] [PubMed]
45. Auffret, V.; Webb, J.G.; Eltchaninoff, H.; Munoz-Garcia, A.J.; Himbert, D.; Tamburino, C.; Nombela-Franco, L.; Nietlispach, F.; Moris, C.; Ruel, M.; et al. Clinical Impact of Baseline Right Bundle Branch Block in Patients Undergoing Transcatheter Aortic Valve Replacement. *JACC Cardiovasc. Interv.* **2017**, *10*, 1564–1574. [CrossRef]
46. Maeno, Y.; Abramowitz, Y.; Israr, S.; Yoon, S.-H.; Kubo, S.; Nomura, T.; Miyasaka, H.; Kawamori, H.; Kazuno, Y.; Takahashi, N.; et al. Prognostic impact of Permanent Pacemaker Implantation in Patients with Low Left Ventricular Ejection Fraction Following Transcatheter Aortic Valve Replacement. *J. Invasive Cardiol.* **2019**, *31*, E15–E22.
47. Testa, L.; Latib, A.; De Marco, F.; De Carlo, M.; Agnifili, M.; Latino, R.A.; Petronio, A.S.; Ettori, F.; Poli, A.; De Servi, S.; et al. Clinical Impact of persistent left bundle-branch block after transcatheter aortic valve implantation with CoreValve Revalving System. *Circulation* **2013**, *127*, 1300–1307. [CrossRef] [PubMed]
48. Schymik, G.; Tzamalis, P.; Bramlage, P.; Heimeshoff, M.; Würth, A.; Wondraschek, R.; Gonska, B.-D.; Posival, H.; Schmitt, C.; Schröfel, H.; et al. Clinical impact of a new left bundle branch block following TAVI implantation: 1-year results of the TAVIK cohort. *Clin. Res. Cardiol.* **2014**, *104*, 351–362. [CrossRef] [PubMed]
49. Urena, M.; Webb, J.G.; Cheema, A.; Serra, V.; Toggweiler, S.; Barbanti, M.; Cheung, A.; Ye, J.; Dumont, E.; DeLarochellière, R.; et al. Impact of New-Onset Persistent Left Bundle Branch Block on Late Clinical Outcomes in Patients Undergoing Transcatheter Aortic Valve Implantation with a Balloon-Expandable Valve. *JACC Cardiovasc. Interv.* **2014**, *7*, 128–136. [CrossRef] [PubMed]
50. Nazif, T.M.; Williams, M.R.; Hahn, R.T.; Kapadia, S.; Babaliaros, V.; Rodés-Cabau, J.; Szeto, W.Y.; Jilaihawi, H.; Fearon, W.F.; Dvir, D.; et al. Clinical implications of new-onset left bundle branch block after transcatheter aortic valve replacement: Analysis of the PARTNER experience. *Eur. Heart J.* **2014**, *35*, 1599–1607. [CrossRef] [PubMed]
51. Fischer, Q.; Himbert, D.; Webb, J.G.; Eltchaninoff, H.; Munoz-Garcia, A.J.; Tamburino, C.; Nombela-Franco, L.; Nietlispach, F.; Moris, C.; Ruel, M.; et al. Impact of Preexisting Left Bundle Branch Block in Transcatheter Aortic Valve Replacement Recipients. *Circ. Cardiovasc. Interv.* **2018**, *11*, e006927. [CrossRef] [PubMed]
52. Chamandi, C.; Barbanti, M.; Munoz-Garcia, A.; Latib, A.; Nombela-Franco, L.; Guttiérrez-Ibanez, E.; Veiga-Fernandez, G.; Cheema, A.N.; Cruz-Gonzales, I.; Serra, V.; et al. Long-term Outcomes in Patients with New-Onset Persistent Left Bundle Branch Block Following TAVR. *JACC Cardiovasc. Interv.* **2019**, *12*, 1175–1184. [CrossRef] [PubMed]
53. Nazif, T.M.; Chen, S.; George, I.; Dizon, J.M.; Hahn, R.T.; Crowley, A.; Alu, M.C.; Babaliaros, V.; Thourani, V.H.; Herrmann, H.C.; et al. New-onset left bundle branch block after transcatheter aortic valve replacement is associated with adverse long-term clinical outcomes in intermediate-risk patients: An analysis from the PARTNER II trial. *Eur. Heart J.* **2019**, *40*, 2218–2227. [CrossRef] [PubMed]
54. Hamandi, M.; Tabachnick, D.; Lanfear, A.T.; Baxter, R.; Shin, K.; Zingler, B.; Mack, M.J.; DiMaio, J.M.; Kindsvater, S. Effect of new and persistent left bundle branch block after transcatheter aortic valve replacement on long-term need for pacemaker implantation. *Bayl. Univ. Med. Cent. Proc.* **2020**, *33*, 157–162. [CrossRef]
55. Urena, M.; Webb, J.G.; Eltchaninoff, H.; Munoz-Garcia, A.J.; Bouleti, C.; Tamburino, C.; Nombela-Franco, L.; Nietlispach, F.; Moris, C.; Ruel, M.; et al. Late cardiac death in patients undergoing transcatheter aortic valve replacement: Incidence and predictors of advanced heart failure and sudden cardiac death. *J. Am. Coll. Cardiol.* **2015**, *65*, 437–448. [CrossRef] [PubMed]
56. Erkapic, D.; Kim, W.-K.; Weber, M.; Möllmann, H.; Berkowitsch, A.; Zaltsberg, S.; Pajitnev, D.J.; Rixe, J.; Neumann, T.; Kuniss, M.; et al. Electrocardiographic and further predictors for permanent pacemaker requirement after transcatheter aortic valve implantation. *Europace* **2010**, *12*, 1188–1190. [CrossRef] [PubMed]

57. Van der Boon, R.M.; Nuis, R.J.; Van Mieghem, N.M.; Jordaens, L.; Rodès-Cabau, J.; Van Domburg, R.T.; Seruys, P.W.; Anderson, R.H.; De Jaegere, P.P.T. New conduction abnormalities after TAVI-frequency and causes. *Nat. Rev. Cardiol.* **2012**, *9*, 454–463. [CrossRef]
58. Sasaki, K.; Izumo, M.; Kuwata, S.; Ishibashi, Y.; Kamijima, R.; Watanabe, M.; Kaihara, T.; Okuyama, K.; Koga, M.; Nishikawa, H.; et al. Clinical Impact of New-Onset Left Bundle-Branch Block After Transcatheter Aortic Valve Implantation in the Japanese Population. *Circ. J.* **2020**, *84*, 1012–1019. [CrossRef] [PubMed]
59. Keßler, M.; Gonska, B.; Seeger, J.; Rottbauer, W.; Wöhrle, J. Long-term clinical outcome of persistent left bundle branch block after transfemoral aortic valve implantation. *Catheter. Cardiovasc. Interv.* **2018**, *93*, 538–544. [CrossRef] [PubMed]
60. Muntané-Carol, G.; Guimaraes, L.; Ferreira-Neto, A.N.; Wintzer-Wehekind, J.; Junquera, L.; Del Val, D.; Faroux, L.; Philippon, F.; Rodés-Cabau, J. How does new-onset left bundle branch block affect the outcomes of transcatheter aortic valve repair? *Expert Rev. Med. Devices* **2019**, *16*, 589–602. [CrossRef]
61. Franzoni, I.; Latib, A.; Maisano, F.; Costopoulos, C.; Testa, L.; Figini, F.; Giannini, F.; Basavarajaiah, S.; Mussardo, M.; Slavich, M.; et al. Comparison of Incidence and Predictors of Left Bundle Branch Block After Transcatheter Aortic Valve Implantation Using the CoreValve Versus the Edwards Valve. *Am. J. Cardiol.* **2013**, *112*, 554–559. [CrossRef]
62. Urena, M.; Mok, M.; Serra, V.; Dumont, E.; Nombela-Franco, L.; DeLarochellière, R.; Doyle, D.; Igual, A.; Larose, E.; Amat-Santos, I.; et al. Predictive factors and long-term clinical consequences of persistent left bundle branch block following transcatheter aortic valve implantation with a balloon expandable valve. *J. Am. Coll. Cardiol.* **2012**, *60*, 1743–1752. [CrossRef]
63. Vernooy, K.; Verbeek, X.A.; Peschar, M.; Crijns, H.J.G.M.; Arts, T.; Cornelussen, R.N.M.; Prinzen, F.W. Left bundle branch block induces ventricular remodeling and functional septal hypoperfusion. *Eur. Heart J.* **2005**, *26*, 91–98. [CrossRef] [PubMed]
64. Shoar, S.; Batra, S.; Gulraiz, I.W.; Javed, M.; Hosseini, F.; Naderan, M.; Shoar, N.; John, J.; Modukuru, V.R.; Sharma, S.K. Effect of pre-existing left bundle branch block on post-procedural outcomes of transcatheter aortic valve replacement: A meta-analysis of comparative studies. *Am. J. Cardiovasc. Dis.* **2020**, *10*, 294–300. [PubMed]
65. Egger, F.; Nürnberg, M.; Rohla, M.; Weiss, T.W.; Unger, G.; Smetana, P.; Geppert, A.; Gruber, S.C.; Bambazek, A.; Falkensammer, J.; et al. High-degree atrioventricular block in patients with preexisting bundle branch block or bundle branch block occurring during transcatheter aortic valve implantation. *Heart Rhythm.* **2014**, *11*, 2176–2182. [CrossRef] [PubMed]
66. Waksman, R.; Khan, J.M. Left Bundle Branch Block After TAVR. Buddle or Trouble? *JACC Cardiovasc. Interv.* **2019**, *12*, 1185–1187. [CrossRef] [PubMed]
67. Husser, O.; Pellegrini, C.; Kim, W.-K.; Holzamer, A.; Pilgrim, T.; Toggweiler, S.; Schäfer, U.; Blumenstein, J.; Deuschl, F.; Rheude, T.; et al. Transcatheter Valve SELECTion in Patients with Right Bundle Branch Block and Impact on Pacemaker Implantation. *J. Am. Coll. Cardiol. Interv.* **2019**, *12*, 1781–1793. [CrossRef] [PubMed]
68. Kumpuris, A.G.; Casale, T.B.; Mokotoff, D.M.; Miller, R.R.; Luchi, R.J. Right bundle-branch block. Occurrence following nonpenetrating chest trauma without evidence of cardiac contusion. *JAMA* **1979**, *242*, 172–173. [CrossRef] [PubMed]
69. Kusumoto, F.M.; Schoenfeld, M.H.; Barrett, C.; Edgerton, J.R.; Ellenbogen, K.A.; Gold, M.R.; Goldschlager, N.F.; Hamilton, R.M.; Joglar, J.A.; Kim, R.J.; et al. 2018 ACC/AHA/HRS Guideline on the Evaluation and Management of Patients with Bradycardia and Cardiac Conduction Delay: A Report of the American College of Cardiology/American Heart Association Task Force on Clinical Practice Guidelines and the Heart Rhythm Society. *Circulation* **2019**, *140*, e382–e482. [PubMed]
70. Brignole, M.; Auricchio, A.; Baron-Esquivias, G.; Bordachar, P.; Boriani, G.; Breithardt, O.-A.; Cleland, J.; Deharo, J.-C.; Delgado, V.; Elliott, P.M.; et al. 2013 ESC Guidelines on cardiac pacing and cardiac resynchronization therapy. *Eur. Heart J.* **2013**, *34*, 2281–2329. [CrossRef] [PubMed]
71. Knecht, S.; Schaer, B.; Reichlin, T.; Spies, F.; Madaffari, A.; Vischer, A.; Fahrni, G.; Jeger, R.; Kaiser, C.; Osswald, S.; et al. Electrophysiology Testing to Stratify Patients with Left Bundle Branch Block After Transcatheter Aortic Valve Implantation. *J. Am. Heart Assoc.* **2020**, *9*, e014446. [CrossRef] [PubMed]
72. Sandhu, A.; Tzou, W.; Ream, K.; Valle, J.; Tompkins, C.; Nguyen, D.T.; Sauer, J.D.; Messenger, J.; Aleong, R.G. Heart Block After Discharge in Patients Undergoing TAVR with Latest-Generation Valves. *J. Am. Coll. Cardiol.* **2018**, *71*, 577–578. [CrossRef] [PubMed]

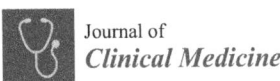

Journal of Clinical Medicine

Article

Patients with Non-Obstructive Coronary Artery Disease Require Strict Control of All Cardiovascular Risk Factors: Results from the Polish Local Population Medical Records

Jarosław Hiczkiewicz [1,2,†], Paweł Burchardt [2,3,4,†], Jan Budzianowski [1,2,*], Konrad Pieszko [1,2], Dariusz Hiczkiewicz [1,2], Bogdan Musielak [1,2], Anna Winnicka-Zielińska [2], Daria M. Keller [5], Wojciech Faron [2] and Janusz Rzeźniczak [4]

1. Department of Interventional Cardiology, Collegium Medicum, University of Zielona Góra, 65-046 Zielona Góra, Poland; jhiczkiewicz@uz.zgora.pl (J.H.); kpieszko@uz.zgora.pl (K.P.); dhiczkiewicz@uz.zgora.pl (D.H.); bmusielak@uz.zgora.pl (B.M.)
2. Department of Cardiology, Nowa Sól Multidisciplinary Hospital, 67-100 Nowa Sól, Poland; pburchardt@ump.edu.pl (P.B.); awinnik@tlen.pl (A.W.-Z.); wfaron@poczta.onet.pl (W.F.)
3. Department of Hypertension, Angiology, and Internal Medicine, Poznan University of Medical Sciences, 61-848 Poznań, Poland
4. Department of Cardiology, J. Strus Hospital, 61-285 Poznań, Poland; syngo@wp.pl
5. 1st Department of Cardiology, Poznan University of Medical Sciences, 61-848 Poznań, Poland; daria.keller@skpp.edu.pl
* Correspondence: jbudzianowski@uz.zgora.pl
† Equal contribution.

Abstract: The aim of the project was to compare patients treated with percutaneous transluminal coronary angioplasty (PTCA), who also had undergone PTCA in the past, with a group of people who had had no angiographic stenosis in the lumen of the coronary arteries in the past, and who also required PTCA during index hospitalization. The secondary aim was to compare the obtained data with the characteristics of a group of people who had undergone angiography twice and for whom no significant stenosis had been found in their coronary arteries. The study used registry data concerning 3085 people who had undergone at least two invasive procedures. Acute coronary syndrome (ACS) was significantly more often observed (Non-ST-segment elevation myocardial infarction (NSTEMI) OR 2.76 [1.91–3.99] and ST-segment elevation myocardial infarction (STEMI) OR 2.35 [1.85–2.99]) in patients with no significant coronary stenosis in the past (who required coronary angioplasty at the time of the study), compared to patients who had already had PTCA. They also demonstrated more frequent occurrence of 'multivessel disease'. This was probably most likely caused by inadequate control of cardiovascular risk factors, as determined by higher total cholesterol levels ([mg/dL] 193.7 ± 44.4 vs. 178.2 ± 43.7) and LDL (123.4 ± 36.2 vs. 117.7 ± 36.2). On the other hand, patients in whom no significant stenosis was found in two consecutive angiographies were more likely to be burdened with chronic obstructive pulmonary disease, atrial fibrillation and chronic kidney disease.

Keywords: subsequent percutaneous coronary intervention; no obstructive coronary artery disease; coronary angiography

1. Introduction

In the 20th century, significant medical advances improved the treatment methods of coronary artery disease (CAD), which is the most common cause of death. The etiopathogenesis of CAD, which determines the main risk factors, was successfully defined. Additionally, the possibility of diagnostic visualization of coronary arteries was achieved, and various techniques were finally developed to perform revasularization. Numerous literature reports confirm that the performance of percutaneous transluminal coronary angioplasty (PTCA) or the diagnosis of atherosclerosis also determines further optimal medical treatment (OMT), the effectiveness of which depends on the compliance with medical recommendations and the use of pharmacotherapy [1]. The more we know about the disease itself and the methods of treating it, the more narrow areas of investigation or intricate not fully studied issues appear. Indeed, they all pose many scientific questions and simply arouse curiosity. One of them is, for example, the clinical characteristics of patients who have been qualified to undergo narrowed vessel angioplasty, and who had angiography performed in the past with no significant stenosis found. This is why, in this study, the patients who underwent angioplasty of a narrowed coronary artery during index hospitalization were split into two groups: the patients in which PTCA was also performed in the past and the ones which had no significant stenoses in the lumen of coronary arteries in the past. The two groups were compared with each other.

It was also scientifically intriguing to compare the clinical characteristics of patients who had undergone coronary angiographies several times (with no significant narrowing lesions in the lumen of the arteries found) with the patients who had undergone coronary angioplasty. This was the secondary goal of the project.

2. Materials and Methods

2.1. Study Population

The study included recorded data from 3085 people (2445 included in the coronary artery disease group + 640 subjects in the control group) who underwent hospitalization at the Cardiology Department, Multidisciplinary Hospital Nowa Sól, between 1 January 2009 and 15 May 2015. The study was retrospective, carried out in accordance with the principles of the Helsinki Declaration and did not require separate approval of the bioethics committee.

The study was carried out on the subjects who had undergone at least two invasive procedures, while the data collected during the second procedure constituted the analyzed 'output data'. Of the subjects, 2445 patients underwent angioplasty of all significantly narrowed coronary arteries during index hospitalization. Stenosis was measured by quantitative coronary angiography (QCA), and those arteries with a diameter reduced by more than 70% (according to current standards) were regarded as significant. In questionable cases, fractional flow reserve (FFR) was undertaken according to the European Society of Cardiology (ESC) guidelines; however, these were sporadic. Regrettably, it was not possible to perform FFR in all the cases given the limited availability of the procedure in Poland in 2009–2015—the time when the project was carried out.

The patients from the CAD groups were divided into the following subgroups with respect to the history of coronary angioplasty and myocardial infarction:

Subgroup A included 1328 patients who underwent coronary angiography in the past (no significant lesions were found there) and PTCA during index hospitalization.

Subgroup B comprised 434 patients. Previously, they had PTCA performed given a negative myocardial infarction (MI) history. Another PTCA was performed during index hospitalization.

Subgroup C included 683 patients. Previously, they had PTCA for MI performed and another PTCA was carried out during index hospitalization.

The remaining 640 patients made up the control group (CG), which was described in our previous project [2]. Previously, no significant coronary artery stenoses during angiography were found in the past, nor during index hospitalization.

The data obtained from patients during index hospitalization were analyzed in light of specific anatomical and morphological features found in the coronary angiograms, the type of techniques used during interventional procedures and the presence of particular clinical features.

The mean observation time between procedures in subgroup A was 1281 days, 230 days in subgroup B and 944 days in subgroup C.

The exclusion criteria in the study were as follows:

- history of coronary artery bypass graft (CABG) or qualification for this procedure during the observation period;
- significant stenosis of the left main coronary artery;
- coexisting heart defects;
- concomitant severe NYHA III/IV heart failure.

The study flow chart is presented in Figure 1.

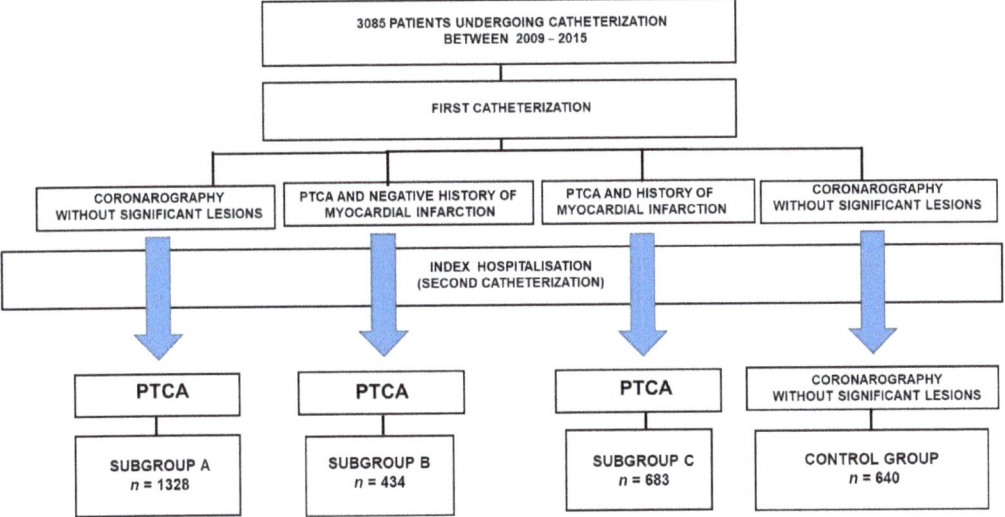

Figure 1. Flow chart of the study. PTCA—Percutaneous transluminal coronary angioplasty.

2.2. Laboratory Assessments

Although blood was collected at each intervention, laboratory tests relied on the material obtained during the second angiography. In the analyses, peripheral blood count was measured with CELL-DYN Ruby (Abbott Diagnostics, Santa Clara CA, USA). TnT was measured with a Cobas 6000 device (Roche Diagnostics GmbH, Mannheim, Germany) with a cut-off value of 14 pg/L. Creatinine, total cholesterol, triglycerides and high-density lipoproteins were analyzed by means of a photometric test (Roche Diagnostics GmbH, Mannheim, Germany).

2.3. Statistical Analysis

The analysis focused on interval and nominal scale data. Interval data, i.e., laboratory results, were presented as mean and standard deviation. Comparisons were made between more than two groups; one-way analysis of variance (ANOVA) was used together with Tukey's post hoc test or the Shapiro–Wilk test as well as Levene's test; the Kruskal–Wallis test and post hoc Dunn's test were employed as an alternative. Subsequently, one-dimensional logistic regression models were applied, followed by multi-dimensional logistic regression models. The results obtained were presented as an odds ratio (OR) with a 95% confidence interval (CI). The survival analysis results are presented graphically as Kaplan–Meier curves. Statistical analysis was performed using STATA15.1 software (College Station, TX, USA). All tests were analyzed at alpha significance level = 0.05.

The study was retrospective, carried out in accordance with the principles of the Helsinki Declaration, and did not require separate consent of the bioethics committee.

The data concerning a 60-month survival period were collected prospectively using updated electronic data from the national health care system.

3. Results

3.1. Characteristics of the Studied Groups and Differences between the CAD Group and the CG

The characteristics of the coronary artery group and the control group, together with the differences between the groups, are presented in Tables 1 and 2. Although the coronary artery disease (CAD) group and the control group (CG) were described previously in [2], the context of the description was completely different.

The characteristics are provided in Tables 1 and 2.

Table 1. Characteristics of the studied group.

Parameter	Coronary Artery Disease Group $n = 2445$	Control Group $n = 640$	p-Value
Age [years]	64.8 ± 9.8	66.6 ± 8.9	$p = 0.0005$
Male sex [%]	68	61.7	$p = 0.0081$
Hypertension (AH) [%]	92.7	82	$p = 0.0000$
Diabetes (DM) [%]	24	21	$p = 0.1639$
Heart failure by NYHA I/II [%]	10	15	$p = 0.0013$
Chronic kidney disease (CKD) [%]	3	15	$p < 0.0001$
Chronic obstructive pulmonary disease (COPD) [%]	4	12	$p < 0.0001$
Claudication	6	12.8	$p < 0.0001$
Dyslipidaemia [%]	26	40	$p < 0.0001$
Stroke [%]	4.7	2.3	$p = 0.0214$
Smoking [%]	11.6	15	$p = 0.0081$

Table 2. Results of one-dimensional logistic regression for CAD vs. CG (where the CAD group was the reference).

Parameter	OR	95% CI
Age during procedure	1.02	[1.01; 1.03]
Male sex	0.73	[0.59; 0.89]
Hypertension	0.36	[0.27; 0.48]
Insulin-dependent DM	0.17	[0.09; 0.31]
CKD	2.83	[2.1; 3.81]
COPD	2.3	[1.67; 3.18]
Intermittent claudication	1.49	[1.09; 2.01]
Ischemic stoke	0.48	[0.25; 0.92]
Sinus rhythm	0.45	[0.34; 0.59]
AF	3.02	[2.25; 4.07]
Lack of R progression in ECG	4.37	[3.43; 5.57]

Abbreviations: AF—atrial fibrillation; CKD—chronic kidney disease; COPD—chronic obstructive pulmonary disease; DM—diabetes mellitus; type 2 diabetes; AH—arterial hypertension; ECG—electrocardiography; OR—odds ratio; CI—confidence interval.

3.2. Characteristics of Patients without Previous Cardiovascular Intervention vs. Patients with History of PTCA and MI

Subgroup A: 1328 patients without MI who had undergone coronary angiography and who underwent PTCA during index hospitalization.

Subgroup B: 434 patients with a history of PTCA and negative history of myocardial infarction. Another PTCA was performed during index hospitalization.

Subgroup C: 683 patients with past MI and PTCA, who had their second PTCA performed during index hospitalization.

In comparison to subgroup A, arterial hypertension was observed significantly more often in subgroups B and C. A similar percentage of diabetes was observed in A, B and C as well as in the CG, except for insulin-dependent diabetes. Heart failure (NYHA I and II) was slightly more frequent in C (patients after MI), i.e., 16.0% vs. 12.3% in A and 8.7% in B ($p < 0.002$). In the CG, incidence of heart failure was 15.0%. With respect to COPD, A, B and C did not differ significantly and the highest risk of its occurrence was observed in the CG (Tables 3 and 4). Additionally, A, B and C demonstrated no significant differences in terms of history of stroke; the percentages were, respectively 4.7%, 3.2% and 5.2%.

The percentage of cigarette smokers was clearly lower in B and C compared to A.

Further characteristics are provided in Tables 3 and 4.

Table 3. Patient characteristics: history of cardiovascular interventions vs. history of PTCA and myocardial infarction.

Parameter \ Group	A	B	C	p-Value
Age [years]	64.8 ± 9.8 [a,b]	65.8 ± 9.8 [b]	64.4 ± 9.8 [a]	p = 0.0464
Male sex %	65 [a]	70.5 [b]	76.1 [b]	p < 0.0001
Stroke %	4.7	3.2	5.2	p = 0.1812
TC [mg/dL]	193.7 ± 44.4 [b]	173.6 ± 49.4 [a,b]	178.2 ± 43.7 [a]	p = 0.0015
LDL [mg/dL]	123.4 ± 36.2 [b]	110.3 ± 38.8 [a,b]	117.7 ± 36.2 [a]	p = 0.0023
HDL [mg/dL]	44.1 ± 14.1	44.3 ± 11.2	45.2 ± 14.1	p = 0.6810
TG [mg/dL]	146.1 ± 95.6	142.3 ± 75.0	131.5 ± 95.7	p = 0.2200
Creatinine	1.03 ± 0.44	1.13 ± 0.78	1.07 ± 0.5	p = 0.180
EF%	45.8 ± 12.3 [b]	44.9 ± 12.2 [a,b]	42.1 ± 12.6 [a]	p = 0.0413

[a,b,c]—groups followed by the same letter do not differ significantly at significance level α = 0.05. Abbreviations: TC—total cholesterol, LDL—low-density lipoprotein, HDL—high-density lipoprotein, TG—triglycerides, EF—ejection fraction.

Table 4. Results of one-dimensional logistic regression for subgroups A vs. B + C (B + C as a reference).

Parameter	OR	95% CI
Number of procedures (3 and more)	1.32	[1.13; 1.54]
Restenosis	0.26	[0.18; 0.37]
Male sex	0.65	[0.56; 0.76]
NSTEMI	2.76	[1.91; 3.99]
AH	0.51	[0.38; 0.67]
DM	0.79	[0.64; 0.97]
Smoking habit	1.36	[1.01; 1.82]
Occlusion in LAD	0.73	[1.51; 1.98]
Occlusion in D	1.66	[1.31; 2.12]
Occlusion in RCA	1.39	[1.21; 1.59]
Number of critically narrowed arteries		
1	1	-
2	1.6	[1.36; 1.88]
3	2.04	[1.59; 2.61]
Thrombectomy	7.56	[3.92; 14.57]
BMS	2.15	[1.88; 2.48]
POBA	0.39	[0.29; 0.52]
Direct stenting	1.16	[1.02; 1.34]
Sinus rhythm	0.72	[0.55; 0.93]
AF	1.47	[1.09; 1.99]
ST elevation	2.35	[1.85; 2.99]
ST depression	1.46	[1.22; 1.76]
Negative T wave	0.83	[0.71; 0.97]
Absence of R progression	0.73	[0.57; 0.94]
Troponin > upper limit of normal (ULN)	1.75	[1.37; 2.24]
Troponin 3x > ULN	1.73	[1.34; 2.22]
Troponin 5x > ULN	1.63	[1.26; 2.09]
TC	1.008	[1.003; 1.013]
LDL	1.009	[1.003; 1.015]
EF	1.02	[1.01; 1.04]

Abbreviations: AF—atrial fibrillation, BMS—bare metal stent, D—diagonal, DM—type 2 diabetes, EF—ejection fraction, AH—arterial hypertension, LAD—left anterior descending, LDL—low-density lipoprotein, NSTEMI—non-ST elevation myocardial infarction, POBA—plain old balloon angioplasty, RCA—right coronary artery, TC—total cholesterol.

3.3. Multivariate Regression Results

The results of multivariate regression analysis carried out with the parameters which significantly differentiated groups A vs. B and C in the univariate analysis are shown in Figure 2.

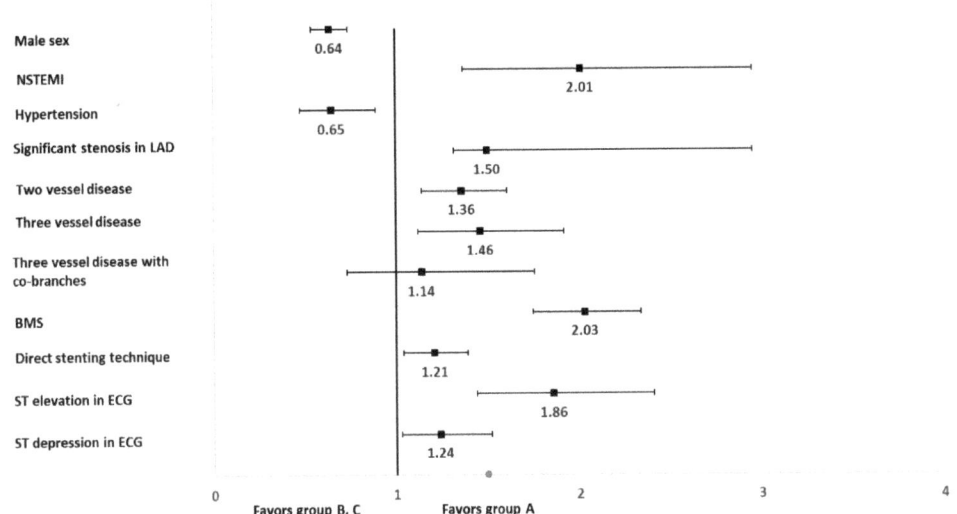

Figure 2. The results of multivariate regression analysis carried out with the parameters which significantly differentiated groups A vs. B and C in the univariate analysis. Abbreviations: NSTEMI—Non-ST-segment elevation myocardial infarction; LAD—left artery descending; BMS—bare metal stent; ECG—electrocardiography.

3.4. Analysis of Baseline Coronary Angiography (Second Invasive Procedure)

The risk of significant left anterior descending (LAD) narrowing in coronary angiography performed during index hospitalization was lower by half in B and C when compared to A, with ORs at 0.5 and 0.63, respectively. The incidence of significantly narrowed left circumplex (LCx) was almost identical in the three groups and amounted to 28–29%. The risk of significantly constricted right coronary artery (RCA) was 38% and 13% lower in B and C compared to A. The respective estimated ORs were 0.62 and 0.87.

3.5. Analysis of the Initial Electrocardiography Record (Second Invasive Procedure)

Atrial fibrillation was significantly less common in all the patients with CAD compared to CG. ST segment elevation (regardless of location) was several-fold less frequent in B and C vs. A. Similarly, ST segment depression occurred considerably less frequently in B and C vs. A. Negative T wave was observed significantly more often in CG and C (patients after myocardial infarction) compared to B and A. Pathological Q wave was most often observed in group C (19.3%), with lower percentages in B (4.6%) and A (6.3%), resulting in statistically significant differences ($p < 0.001$).

In the CG, heart rate was significantly higher compared to patients from subgroups A, B and C: 82/min vs. 73/min, 69/min, 71/min, respectively ($p < 0.001$).

3.6. Analysis of Data from Initial Echocardiography (Second Invasive Procedure)

Interpretable echocardiographic data were obtained from 793 patients, i.e., 23.3% of the entire population. Ejection fraction (EF) in A, B and C was 45.8%, 44.9% and 42.1%, respectively ($p < 0.041$). In the CG, EF was 54.4% ($n = 180$). Contractility abnormalities were assessed in two anterolateral anatomical regions with an interventricular septum and a posterolateral septum. Hypokinesis and/or akinesis on the anterolateral and posterolateral walls were detected significantly more often in C vs. A and B, $p < 0.05$.

3.7. Assessment of Total Mortality

During the follow-up period, the absolute number of deaths was significantly greater in A (13.5%) and C (13.0%) compared to B (8.1%), with $p < 0.0026$. Survival calculated from

Kaplan–Meier curves following 60 months of observation in subgroups A, B and C was 88%, 92% and 87%, respectively ($p < 0.01$) (Figure 3).

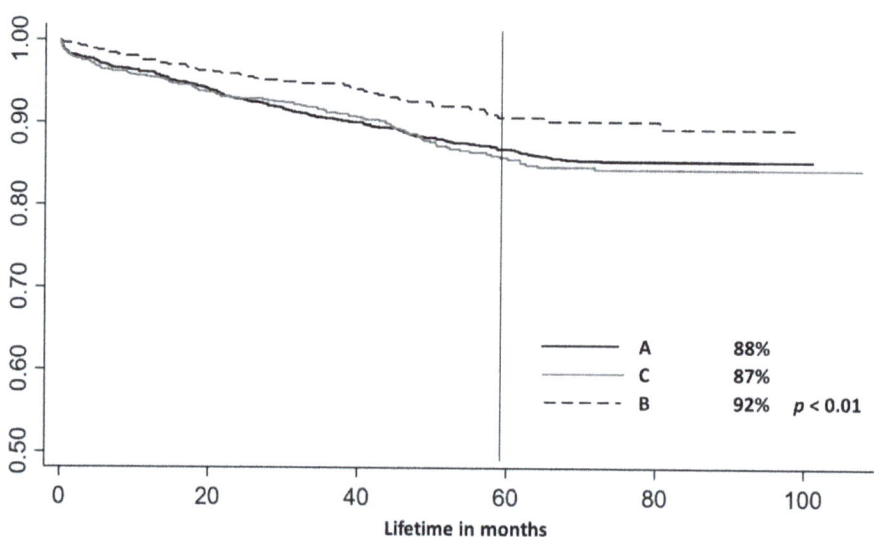

Figure 3. Survival curves for subgroups: 60-month survival in respective subgroups. Legend: Subgroup A—patients without MI who had undergone coronary angiography in the past and who underwent PTCA during the second hospitalization. Subgroup B—patients who had a history of PTCA but did not have a history of myocardial infarction (MI). During the index hospitalization, they had a second PTCA. Subgroup C—patients with past MI and PTCA, who had their second PTCA performed during index hospitalization.

4. Discussion

Every year, about 4 million coronary angiography procedures are performed in Europe and the USA, but in as many as 50% of subjects, no significant stenosis is found in the lumen of the coronary arteries [3]. The cause of their clinical symptoms in those cases is most likely coronary microcirculation disease and/or vasospastic angina [3]. Patients with stable CAD are classified into a generally defined non-obstructive coronary artery disease (INOCA) group, distinguished in a manner similar to those presenting myocardial infarction with non-obstructive coronary arteries (MINOCAs), who are admitted to hospitals as acute coronary syndrome (ACS) cases. There are more and more clinical observations dedicated to these patients [3–7]. It is also acknowledged that in patients in whom coronary angiography showed no significant changes, symptoms of angina are reduced by nearly a half [8,9]. Regrettably, the pertinent literature offers no accurate data on the implementation of the prescribed pharmacological treatment (adherence and compliance) in these particular population groups of patients, while data on the their subsequent fate are considerably limited [10,11].

One must also remember that insignificant hemodynamic lesions in the coronary lumen arteries may also be the cause of future ACS or, after several years of stable disease progression, may cause symptoms of ischemia requiring further intervention. Our results seem to confirm this hypothesis, which is a spectacular result of this project.

Our study included the patients who underwent angioplasty for the first time but, importantly, no significant narrowing lesions were found in the coronary angiography they had had in the past. Compared to the patients with previous PTCA, ACS (Non-ST-segment elevation myocardial infarction (NSTEMI) and ST-segment elevation myocardial infarction

(STEMI)) was observed significantly more often in this group; multivessel disease occurred more often as well, while TC and LDL levels were elevated. We may only speculate that adherence to OMT recommendations had been insufficient or completely neglected in those patients, which did not inhibit the natural progress of atherosclerosis and as a result caused it to be more advanced than in the other studied groups. Another aspect seems to confirm this observation, namely the interval between invasive procedures: 1,281 days among the patients from subgroup A, compared to 230 days in B and 844 days in C. As can be seen, the patients whose first angiography showed no significant lesions had another intervention after 3.5 years. The delay in performing the next examination in this group of people seems to contradict the hypothesis of accelerated progression of atherosclerosis, and appears to provide evidence for its natural course.

It may be conjectured that unlike the patients with previous PTCA, the individuals from that particular group would present less advanced atherosclerotic lesions, but the obtained results yet again contradict such a premise. Thus, the group of people who underwent PTCA five times during the follow-up comprised as much as 64% of those who had not demonstrated significant stenosis in the lumen of the coronary arteries during the first angiography. In addition, they also had a higher number of critically altered coronary arteries observed during index hospitalization (unpublished data). Apart from the aforementioned inadequate therapeutic management in those groups, incorrect assessment of atherosclerotic lesions in the coronary arteries during the first angiography may also account for such a result. The phenomenon in question is reported in the literature [12–15].

In the group of patients with normal angiographic images from the first coronary angiography, critically altered LAD and multivessel disease were observed more often during index hospitalization in comparison to the group of subjects with a history of both PTCA and MI. This is consistent with the few pertinent scientific reports, which observe that among those with insignificant changes in coronary arteries, patients with a diameter narrowed by 20 to 50% are most exposed to CAD progression when compared to people with narrowing lesions below 20% [16–18].

Given that our team did not have access to such accurate angiographic data, an analysis of this kind was not performed as part of this project.

Nevertheless, patients with insignificant coronary stenosis or no evidence of atherosclerotic plaques in the vascular bed should be methodically and closely monitored, with a view to maintaining rigorous control of cardiovascular risk factors, as well as ensuring adherence to and compliance with OMT against CAD.

In the present clinical conditions, further invasive diagnostic procedures such as coronary fraction reserve (CFR), FFR and acetylocholine (ACH) tests are also performed in these patients to determine microvascular angina (MVA) or vascular spasm angina (VSA) features [3]. This did not take place as part of our observation study and certainly represents a significant limitation of the project. That particular group should be also diagnosed with other causes of their conditions, as our study demonstrated that atrial fibrillation (AF) or chronic obstructive pulmonary disease (COPD) can also play a role in this respect.

Patients after coronary stent implantation are more likely to take medications as well as to cooperate better with their physicians. Nevertheless, the EuroAspire V study shows that only about 29% achieve therapeutic goals for lipid concentration, approximately 58% achieve proper blood pressure values and only 54% reach the glycated hemoglobin goal [19]. It may be interesting to note that although about 75% of all patients declare full adherence and compliance, the actual failure to comply observed in this group of subjects is responsible for 9% of all cardiovascular events in Europe [19].

Nevertheless, these unsatisfactory data still translate into a better clinical course of coronary artery disease in these patients in comparison to those with angiographically implicit CAD, which indirectly follows from our analysis.

Limitations of the Study

In this study, the patients with severe heart failure (NYHA III/IV), left main stenosis, extensive atherosclerotic lesions qualified for CABG, concomitant heart defects and primary myocardial diseases were excluded. The criterion of significant lumen narrowing (>70% in diameter) was adopted as a guideline (the analysis did not take into account the fate (observation of survival) of the patients with atherosclerotic lesions in the range of 30–70%, not requiring stenting according to current standards [1,2]). The study was a single-center retrospective analysis and we had no data regarding, e.g., the number of patients with implanted peacemakers.

The population included patients with both ACS and stable coronary artery disease. However, the control group was not homogeneous regarding the standards of ambulatory care, i.e., the frequency of follow-up visits, as well as the type of pharmacotherapy. The group of people with insignificant coronary artery stenosis was referred to general practitioners' (GP) care. Most of them had their next cardiac catheterization due to acute coronary syndrome.

5. Conclusions

In the patients with no significant coronary stenosis in the past, who subsequently required coronary angioplasty during index hospitalization, angiographic advancement of atherosclerosis was greater compared to those who had PTCA in the past (as well as required repeated PTCA during index hospitalization). This may be related to a better control of the disease risk factors and significantly better adherence to treatment among those with angiographically proven CAD. On the other hand, those who did not demonstrate significant stenosis in two consecutive angiographies were more likely to be burdened with COPD, AF and CKD, which could be misconstrued as CAD.

Author Contributions: Conceptualization and methodology: J.H., P.B., J.B., K.P. and J.R.; validation: J.H., P.B., J.B. and J.R. formal analysis: J.H., P.B., J.B., K.P., D.M.K. and J.R. investigation: J.H., P.B., J.B., K.P., D.H., B.M., A.W.-Z., D.M.K. and W.F.; writing—original draft preparation, J.H., P.B., J.B., K.P. and J.R.; writing—review and editing: J.H., P.B., J.B., K.P., D.H., B.M., A.W.-Z., D.M.K., W.F. and J.R.; statistical analysis: P.B. and K.P.; supervision: J.H., P.B. and J.R. Each author has made substantial contributions to the conception or design of the work and accepts accountability for the overall work. All authors have read and agreed to the published version of the manuscript.

Funding: This research received no external funding.

Institutional Review Board Statement: The study was retrospective, carried out in accordance with the principles of the Helsinki Declaration and did not require separate consent of the bioethics committee.

Informed Consent Statement: Not applicable, because this is a retrospective study with anonymized data.

Data Availability Statement: The data presented in this study are available on request from the corresponding author.

Conflicts of Interest: The authors declare no conflict of interest.

References

1. Knuuti, J.; Wijns, W.; Saraste, A.; Capodanno, D.; Barbato, E.; Funck-Brentano, C.; Prescott, E.; Storey, R.F.; Deaton, C.; Cuisset, T.; et al. ESC Scientific Document Group, 2019 ESC Guidelines for the diagnosis and management of chronic coronary syndromes: The Task Force for the diagnosis and management of chronic coronary syndromes of the European Society of Cardiology (ESC). *Eur. Heart J.* **2020**, *14*, 407–477. [CrossRef] [PubMed]
2. Hiczkiewicz, J.; Burchardt, P.; Pieszko, K.; Budzianowski, J.; Hiczkiewicz, D.; Musielak, B.; Winnicka-Zielińska, A.; Adamczak, D.; Faron, W.; Rzeźniczak, J. The risk for subsequent coronary interventions in a local Polish population. *Adv. Interv. Cardiol.* **2020**, *16*, 429–435.
3. Ford, T.J.; Berry, C. How to Diagnose and Manage Angina Without Obstructive Coronary Artery Disease: Lessons from the British Heart Foundation CorMicA Trial. *Interv. Cardiol.* **2019**, *14*, 76–82. [CrossRef] [PubMed]
4. Cook, S.; Walker, A.; Hugli, O.; Togni, M.; Meier, B. Percutaneous coronary interventions in Europe. *Clin. Res. Cardiol.* **2007**, *96*, 375–382. [CrossRef] [PubMed]

5. Patel, M.R.; Peterson, E.D.; Dai, D.; Brennan, J.M.; Redberg, R.F.; Anderson, H.V.; Brindis, R.G.; Douglas, P.S. Low diagnostic yield of elective coronary angiography. *N. Engl. J. Med.* **2010**, *362*, 886–895. [CrossRef] [PubMed]
6. Ford, T.J.; Corcoran, D.; Sidik, N.; Rocchiccioli, P.; McEntegart, M.; Berry, C. MINOCA: Requirement for definitive diagnostic work-up. *Heart Lung Circ.* **2019**, *28*, e4–e6. [CrossRef] [PubMed]
7. Stone, G.W.; Hochman, J.S.; Williams, D.O.; Boden, W.E.; Ferguson, T.B.; Harrington, R.A.; Maron, D.J. Medical Therapy With Versus Without Revascularization in Stable Patients With Moderate and Severe Ischemia. *J. Am. Coll. Cardiol.* **2016**, *67*, 81–99. [CrossRef] [PubMed]
8. Rajkumar, C.A.; Nijjer, S.S.; Cole, G.D.; Al-Lamee, R.; Francis, D.P. "Faith Healing" and "Subtraction Anxiety" in Unblinded Trials of Procedures. *Circ. Cardiovasc. Qual. Outcomes* **2018**, *11*, e004665. [CrossRef] [PubMed]
9. Stone, G.W.; Maehara, A.; Lansky, A.J.; De Bruyne, B.; Cristea, E.; Mintz, G.S.; Mehran, R.; McPherson, J.; Farhat, N.; Marso, S.P.; et al. A prospective natural-history study of coronary atherosclerosis. *N. Engl. J. Med.* **2011**, *364*, 226–235. [CrossRef] [PubMed]
10. Ahmadi, A.; Leipsic, J.; Blankstein, R.; Taylor, C.; Hecht, H.; Stone, G.W.; Narula, J. Do plaques rapidly progress prior to myocardial infarction? The interplay between plaque vulnerability and progression. *Circ. Res.* **2015**, *117*, 99–104. [CrossRef]
11. Fernández-Friera, L.; Fuster, V.; López-Melgar, B.; Oliva, B.; García-Ruiz, J.M.; Mendiguren, J.; Bueno, H.; Pocock, S.; Ibanez, B.; Fernández-Ortiz, A.; et al. Normal LDL-Cholesterol Levels Are Associated With Subclinical Atherosclerosis in the Absence of Risk Factors. *J. Am. Coll. Cardiol.* **2017**, *70*, 2979–2991. [CrossRef] [PubMed]
12. Nambi, V.; Bhatt, D.L. Primary Prevention of Atherosclerosis: Time to Take a Selfie? *J. Am. Coll. Cardiol.* **2017**, *70*, 2992–2994. [CrossRef]
13. Gerber, Y.; Weston, S.A.; Enriquez-Sarano, M.; Manemann, S.M.; Chamberlain, A.M.; Jiang, R.; Roger, V.L. Atherosclerotic Burden and Heart Failure After Myocardial Infarction. *JAMA Cardiol.* **2016**, *1*, 156–162. [CrossRef]
14. Maddox, T.M.; Ho, P.M.; Roe, M.; Dai, D.; Tsai, T.T.; Rumsfeld, J.S. Utilization of secondary prevention therapies in patients with nonobstructive coronary artery disease identified during cardiac catheterization: Insights from the National Cardiovascular Data Registry Cath-PCI Registry. *Circ. Cardiovasc. Qual. Outcomes* **2010**, *3*, 632–641. [CrossRef]
15. Dwyer, J.P.; Redfern, J.; Freedman, S.B. Low utilisation of cardiovascular risk reducing therapy in patients with acute coronary syndromes and non-obstructive coronary artery disease. *Int. J. Cardiol.* **2008**, *129*, 394–398. [CrossRef] [PubMed]
16. Libby, P.; Theroux, P. Pathophysiology of coronary artery disease. *Circulation* **2005**, *111*, 3481–3488. [CrossRef] [PubMed]
17. Little, W.C.; Constantinescu, M.; Applegate, R.J.; Kutcher, M.A.; Burrows, M.T.; Kahl, F.R.; Santamore, W.P. Can coronary angiography predict the site of a subsequent myocardial infarction in patients with mild-to-moderate coronary artery disease? *Circulation* **1988**, *78*, 1157–1166. [CrossRef] [PubMed]
18. Maddox, T.M.; Stanislawski, M.A.; Grunwald, G.K.; Bradley, S.M.; Ho, P.M.; Tsai, T.T.; Rumsfeld, J.S. Nonobstructive coronary artery disease and risk of myocardial infarction. *JAMA* **2014**, *312*, 1754–1763. [CrossRef] [PubMed]
19. Kotseva, K.; De Backer, G.; De Bacquer, D.; Rydén, L.; Hoes, A.; Grobbee, D.; Maggioni, A.; Marques-Vidal, P.; Jennings, C.; Abreu, A.; et al. EUROASPIRE Investigators*. Lifestyle and impact on cardiovascular risk factor control in coronary patients across 27 countries: Results from the European Society of Cardiology ESC-EORP EUROASPIRE V registry. *Eur. J. Prev. Cardiol.* **2019**, *26*, 824–835. [CrossRef] [PubMed]

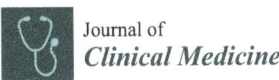

Article

Predictors of Early-Recurrence Atrial Fibrillation after Catheter Ablation in Women and Men with Abnormal Body Weight

Jan Budzianowski [1,2,*], Jarosław Hiczkiewicz [1,2], Katarzyna Łojewska [1], Edyta Kawka [3], Rafał Rutkowski [3] and Katarzyna Korybalska [3]

1. Department of Cardiology, Nowa Sól Multidisciplinary Hospital, 67-100 Nowa Sól, Poland; jhiczkiewicz@uz.zgora.pl (J.H.); katarzyna.lojewska@poczta.onet.pl (K.Ł.)
2. Collegium Medicum, University of Zielona Góra, 65-046 Zielona Góra, Poland
3. Department of Pathophysiology, Poznan University of Medical Sciences, 60-806 Poznań, Poland; ekawka@ump.edu.pl (E.K.); rrutkowski@ump.edu.pl (R.R.); koryb@ump.edu.pl (K.K.)
* Correspondence: jbudzianowski@uz.zgora.pl

Abstract: Our study aimed to select factors that affect the rate of early recurrence (up to 3 months) of atrial fibrillation (AF) (ERAF) following pulmonary veins isolation (PVI) in obese women and men. The study comprised 114 patients: 54 women (age: 63.8 ± 6.3, BMI 31 ± 4 kg/m^2), and 60 men (age: 60.7 ± 6.7; BMI 31 ± 3 kg/m^2) with paroxysmal, persistent and long-standing persistent AF. They had been scheduled to undergo cryoballoon (men n = 30; women n = 30) and radiofrequency (RF) ablation (men n = 30; women n = 24) using the CARTO-mapping. The blood was collected at baseline and 24 h after ablation. The rate of ERAF was comparable after cryoballoon and RF ablation and constituted 18% in women and 22% in men. Almost 70 parameters were selected to perform univariate and multivariate analysis and to create a multivariate logistic regression (MLR) model of ERAF in the obese men and women. The MLR analysis was performed by forward stepwise logistic regression with three variables. It was only possible to create the MLR model for the group of obese men. It revealed a poor predictive value with an unsatisfactory sensitivity of 31%. Men with ERAF: smokers (OR 39.25, 95% CI 1.050–1467.8, p = 0.0021), with a higher ST2 elevation (OR 1.68, 95% CI 1.115–2.536, p = 0.0021) who received dihydropyridine calcium channel blockers (OR 0.042, 95% CI 0.002–1.071, p = 0.0021) less frequently. Our results indicate a complex pathogenesis of ERAF dependent on the patients' gender.

Keywords: catheter ablation; atrial fibrillation; obesity; early recurrence; biomarkers

1. Introduction

It is estimated that ERAF occurs in up to 20–50% of patients after ablation procedures and is considered to be a strong predictor of late recurrence of atrial fibrillation (LRAF) [1,2]. The mechanism of ERAF in patients with obesity is not fully explained in the literature. Nowadays, the origin of this disorder can be explained by: a transient acute inflammation caused by the application of the cryoenergy and radiofrequency (RF) current, a temporary imbalance in the functioning of the autonomic nervous system, a delayed effect of RF current application due to the scar maturation after ablation [1]. Furthermore, the initially incomplete pulmonary vein (PV) isolation is considered as the cause of ERAF [1]. Consequently, obese patients experience electrophysiological and structural atrial changes, the so-called atrial remodeling [1]. In addition, obesity is accompanied by subclinical inflammation and the adipose tissue itself is a source of inflammatory mediators [3]. The epidemiological data suggest a strong correlation between obesity, the impaired left ventricular diastolic function and AF. The increased left atrial (LA) pressure and dimension in obese patients are associated with a longer refraction duration in LA and PVs [1].

Taking into account the increasing number of obese men and women with cardiovascular complications, we decided to select the predictors that affect the rate of ERAF (up to 3 months) following PVs cryoballoon and RF ablation.

2. Materials and Methods

2.1. Study Population

The study group of 114 patients: 60 men (age 60.7 ± 6.7 years; BMI 30.9 ± 2.7 kg/m^2) and 54 women (age 63.8 ± 6.3 years; BMI 31.4 ± 4.3 kg/m^2) with abnormal body weights (BMI > 25 < 40 kg/m^2; mean BMI 31 ± 3 kg/m^2, min 29.8, max 38.7, median 32.5), age (>18 and <80; mean age 62 ± 7 years), with documented symptomatic paroxysmal, persistent and long-standing persistent AF, who were scheduled to undergo cryoballoon and RF ablation using the CARTO-mapping at the Cardiology Department in the Multidisciplinary Hospital in Nowa Sól, Poland. The first PVs isolation was performed in 77 patients. The same procedure was performed for the second time in the case of 34 patients and for the third time in the case of 3 patients. Obesity is defined as having a BMI of >25 kg/m^2 <40 kg/m^2.

The exclusion criteria in this study were as follows: thrombus located in the LA appendage, acute or chronic infection, diabetes, antibiotic therapy, malignancies, heart failure exacerbation or cardiac surgery, stroke and acute coronary syndromes over the past 3 months.

All the patients studied first underwent a detailed interview with an assessment of arrhythmia symptoms (EHRA scale), comorbidities and current medication. A thorough physical examination was carried out (height, body mass, temperature and blood pressure). The BMI index was calculated as a person's weight in kilograms divided by their height in metres squared. Waist circumference (WC) was measured midway between the lower rib margin and the iliac crest. Pre-procedural transthoracic and transoesophageal echocardiography (TEE) were performed in all the patients prior to ablation.

The study protocol was approved by the Medical Ethics Committee at the Poznań University of Medical Sciences (Approval 44/16) while all the patients signed a written consent for participation. The study was carried out between May 2016 and March 2018. All the participants fulfilled the criteria and completed the study. The study flow chart is presented in Figure 1.

Statistical methods estimate that the total sample size required for the study is 93 patients to ensure the power of the test is 90% at 5% level of significance. The presentation of the subgroups of men and women resulted from the fact that the studied groups were homogenous in terms of the number of patients undergoing RF and cryoablation (60 vs. 54) and comparable representation of men compared to women both undergoing only cryoablation (30 vs. 30) and only RF ablation (30 vs. 24). There was a lower number of women undergoing RF ablation (24). Initially, we planned 30 vs. 30, but some women did not qualify for the study.

2.2. Radiofrequency Ablation

RF ablation was performed point-by-point in accordance with the guidelines [1]. PV isolation was performed using the focal ablation strategy guided by the CARTO 3-D mapping system (Biosense Webster, Diamond Bar, CA, USA). All the procedures were performed under conscious sedation with local anasthetic. The double transseptal puncture was performed following the fluoroscopic guidelines. Immediately after the puncture, intravenous unfractioned heparin (UFH) was administered to maintain the target activated clotting time of 300–350 s. PV isolation was performed using 7F Navistar ThermoCool and 8F ThermoCool SmartTouch SF (Biosense Webster). In five patients RF ablation was performed using the "ablation index" algorithm.

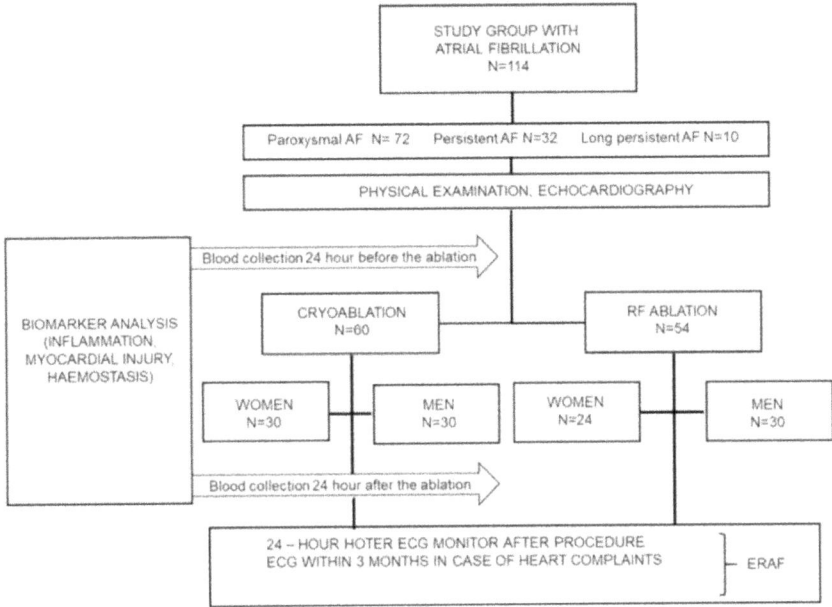

Figure 1. Flowchart of the study.

2.3. Cryoballoon Ablation

Cryoablation was performed as previously reported [2]. The second generation 28 mm cryoballoon (Arctic Front Advance, Medtronic, Minneapolis, MN, USA) was used. The venous delivery of the cryoballoon was managed using a 15F steerable sheath (FlexCath Advance, Medtronic). The correct position of the cryoballoon was confirmed by contrast retention in the PVs. The cryoapplication process lasted 180–240 s per vein and was verified by the circular mapping catheter (CMC, Achieve™; Medtronic, Minneapolis, MN, USA) to confirm electrical isolation. During the application in the right veins, the diaphragmatic nerve was constantly stimulated (30/min) to avoid its paralysis.

2.4. Biochemical Analyses

The venous blood was collected at baseline and 24 h after ablation. All routine biochemical analyses (D-dimer, fibrinogen, INR, aPTT, hsTnT, CK, CKMB, CRP) were performed immediately in a central hospital laboratory. In the analysis the peripheral blood count was marked with CELL-DYN Ruby (Abbott Diagnostics, Santa Clara CA, USA USA). D-dimer, fibrinogen, INR and aPTT were tested using STACompact Max (Diagnostica Stago, Parsippany, NJ, USA). High sensitivity TnT (hsTnT) was marked with a Cobas c601 device (Roche Diagnostics GmbH, Mannheim, Germany). CK was analyzed using a kinetic serum test while CKMB was analyzed with CKMB immunoassay concentrations. CRP was inspected with an immunoturbimetric latex CRP assay (Roche Diagnostics GmbH Mannheim, Germany).

The additional samples of serum were aliquoted and stored at −80 °C until assayed. The following parameters were measured using DuoSet Immunoassay Development Kits (R&D Systems, Minneapolis, MN, USA) according to the manufacturer's instructions: hsIL-6, pentraxin (PTX), von Willebrand factor (vWF), thrombomodulin (TM), sICAM-1, sVCAM-1, t-PA, PAI-1, ST2, leptin, adiponectin. The sensitivities of the assays are presented in Table S1.

2.5. Post-Ablation Management and Follow-Up

The patients were monitored for the first 24 h after ablation using a 24-h Holter monitoring in an outpatient clinic to evaluate ERAF within 3 months after ablation (Mortara Instrument, Milwaukee, WI, USA). Additionally, a 12-lead electrocardiogram (ECG) was recommended for the patients with symptoms of arrhythmia. Antiarrhythmic drugs (AAD) were not routinely used after ablation except for the highly symptomatic patients with ERAF. Oral anticoagulants were continued for at least 2 months. The decision to continue anticoagulation was based on an individual's stroke risk determined by the CHA_2DS_2-VASc score.

2.6. Echocardiogram

Transthoracic echocardiography (TTE) (iE33, Philips Medical Systems, Andover, MA, USA), was performed with a two-dimensional Doppler assessment in typical projections in accordance with the American Echocardiographic Society and the European Association of Cardiovascular Imaging [4]. The left ventricle ejection fraction was assessed by a modified Simpson's rule. The LA volume index was calculated using the disk summation technique.

2.7. Statistical Analysis

Statistical analysis was performed using Statistica 12.0 software (StatSoft, Tulsa, OK, USA) and GraphPad PrismTM 6.00 (GraphPad Software Inc., La Jolla, CA, USA). The student's t-test was used to test the significance of the assessed parameters before and after the procedure. For variables not normally distributed, a Wilcoxon signed rank test was used to compare the patients within a group and a Mann-Whitney test was used to compare the groups with each other. The normal distribution of continuous variables was tested with the Shapiro–Wilk and the D'Agostino & Pearson tests. Pearson and Spearman correlation analysis was used for assessing the correlation depending on the data distribution. Contingency was analyzed with a Chi-square test.

Multivariate logistic regression (MLR) analysis was performed to identify the logistic regression model of ERAF predictors. The MLR model was built using the forward stepwise logistic regression method. Only a limited number of variables (out of 66 available variables) was used to create the MLR model in accordance with statistical rules. The variables that could potentially be associated with the occurrence of ERAF were used based on the literature and clinical experience. A p-value < 0.05 was considered significant. Continuous parameters were expressed as means standard deviation and categorical variables as numbers and percentages.

3. Results

3.1. Patient Characteristics

A total of 114 patients with abnormal body weight and symptomatic, refractory AF treated with cryoablation (60 patients; 30 women, 30 men) and RF ablation (54 patients; 24 women, 30 men) participated in the study. The baseline characteristics of all the women and men have been summarised in Table 1. The study flow chart is presented in Figure 1. As demonstrated in Table 1 persistent AF was significantly more frequent in the group of men (19% vs. 37%). Other parameters relevant to the procedure were comparable in both groups (EHRA score, HAS-BLED, LA Volume, LAVI, EF), except for the CHA_2DS_2-VASC score.

The patients were matched according to their age and BMI, but the men tended to have a higher body weight, WC, and a five times lower leptin concentration than the women. Dyslipidemia was more pronounced in the female group which is a consequence of the (i) abnormal body weight, (ii) higher incidence of hypothyroidism (significant increase in TSH in women) and (iii) menopause. The male group was characterized by higher morbidity due to coronary artery disease (CAD), which resulted in higher ST2, hs-TnT and vWF levels. The group of women was slightly older than the group of men, which probably resulted in their lowered GFR.

Table 1. Baseline characteristics of the studied patients.

Parameter	Females (n = 54)	Males (n = 60)	p Value
Age (years)	63.8 ± 6.3	60.7 ± 6.7	p = 0.0660
BMI (kg/m^2)	31.4 ± 4.3	30.9 ± 2.7	p = 0.3827
WC (cm)	97.9 ± 12.8	104.8 ± 10.8	p = 0.0017
Leptin, ng/mL	30.7 ± 20.6	6.2 ± 6.0	p < 0.0001
CRP, µg/mL	0.25 ± 0.24	0.24 ± 0.19	p = 0.7764
INR	1.83 ± 0.77	1.53 ± 0.66	p = 0.0253
Fibrinogen, mg/dL	399 ± 86	367 ± 74	p = 0.0308
PLT, 10^3/mL	235 ± 67	197 ± 48	p = 0.0008
Haemoglobin, g/dL	14.1 ± 1.1	15.5 ± 1.4	p < 0.0001
Glucose, mg/dL	100.8 ± 9.9	102.3 ± 11.1	p = 0.3615
Cholesterol, mg/dL	197.0 ± 37.3	173.9 ± 38.4	p = 0.0005
LDL, mg/dL	124.7 ± 35.6	111.2 ± 33.9	p = 0.0406
HDL, mg/dL	65.5 ± 14.15	54.0 ± 9.8	p < 0.0001
GFR, mL/min	67.9 ± 14.7	80.5 ± 14.9	p < 0.0001
TSH µU/mL	2.6 ± 2.4	1.6 ± 1.6	p = 0.0081
hs-TnT, ng/L	9.1 ± 10.0	9.3 ± 5.0	p = 0.0422
vWF, ng/mL	1.81 ± 0.66	2.24 ± 1.01	p = 0.0083
ST2, ng/mL	1.5 ± 1.4	1.8 ± 1.9	p = 0.0314
Paroxysmal AF, no, (%)	39 (72)	33 (55)	p = 0.0854
Persistent AF, no, (%)	10 (19)	22 (37)	p = 0.0313
Long-standing persistent AF, no, (%)	5 (9)	5 (8)	p = 0.8615
EHRA 1, n (%)	0 (0)	2 (3)	p = 0.1759
EHRA 2a, n (%)	8 (15)	18 (30)	p = 0.0537
EHRA 2b, n (%)	24 (44)	19 (32)	p = 0.1599
EHRA 3, n (%)	20 (37)	20 (33)	p = 0.6791
EHRA 4, n (%)	2 (4)	1 (2)	p = 0.4975
Left atrial volume	93.9 ± 25.2	96.4 ± 34.4	p = 0.6258
LAVI, mL/m^2	47.8 ± 11.8	44.1 ± 14.5	p = 0.1464
LVEF, %	58.1 ± 3.1	56.7 ± 6.9	p = 0.7078
SBP	129 ± 14	126 ± 11	p = 0.1997
DBP	77 ± 10	81 ± 11	p = 0.0619
Mean CHA2DS2-VASC score	2.4 ± 1	1.5 ± 0.89	p < 0.0001
Mean HAS-BLED score	1.3 ± 0.80	1.1 ± 0.68	p = 0.0957
Comorbidities and Medications			
Hypertension, no, (%)	39 (72)	42 (70)	p = 0.7939
Coronary artery disease, no, (%)	3 (6)	11 (18)	p = 0.0379
Dyslipidemia, no, (%)	25 (46)	15 (25)	p = 0.0174
Heart Failure, no, (%)	1 (2)	4 (7)	p = 0.1431

Table 1. Cont.

Parameter	Females (n = 54)	Males (n = 60)	p Value
Thyroid disease, no, (%)	19 (35)	11 (18)	p = 0.0966
Beta-blocker, no, (%)	47 (87)	47 (78)	p = 0.2225
CCB, no, (%)	11 (20)	13 (22)	p = 0.8654
NOAC, no, (%)	33 (61)	47 (78)	p = 0.0448
VKA, no, (%)	21 (39)	13 (22)	p = 0.0264
Statins, no, (%)	23 (43)	25 (42)	p = 0.9204
Diuretics, no, (%)	16 (30)	19 (32)	p = 0.8139
ACE inhibitor, no, (%)	18 (33)	18 (30)	p = 0.7022
ARB, no, (%)	15 (28)	19 (32)	p = 0.6504
Anti-arrhythmic drugs, no, (%)	30 (56)	28 (47)	p = 0.3432

Continuous data are presented as means ± SD. Categorical data are presented as counts with their percentage values in brackets. BMI, body mass index; W, waist circumference; CRP, C-reactive protein; INR, international normalized ratio; PLT, platelets; GFR, glomerular filtration rate; hs-TnT, high-sensitive cardiac troponin T; vWF, von Willebrandt factor; AF, atrial fibrillation; EHRA, European Heart Rhythm Association; LAVI, left atrial volume index; LVEF, Left ventricle ejection fraction; SBP, Systolic blood pressure; DBP, Diastolic blood pressure; CHA2DS2-VASc, Congestive heart failure, Hypertension, Age ≥ 75, Diabetes, Stroke, Vascular disease, Age 65–74, Sex (female); HAS-BLED, Hypertension, Abnormal renal/liver function, Stroke, Bleeding history or predisposition, Labile INR, Elderly (>65 years), Drugs/alcohol concomitantly; CCB, calcium channel blockers; NOAC, non-vitamin K antagonist oral anticoagulants; VKA, vitamin K antagonist; ACE-I, angiotensin converting enzyme inhibitor; ARB, angiotensin II receptor blocker.

Physiologically females have a higher level of fibrinogen than males, which among many other factors, predisposes them to a higher risk of thromboembolism and a higher CHA$_2$DS$_2$-VASC score. The women were more frequently treated with vitamin K antagonists monitored by INR, which was higher in their group. The men used non-vitamin K antagonist oral anticoagulants more often than the women.

3.2. Ablation Procedure—Early and Late Recurrence of AF

As opposed to cryoablation, RF ablation was associated with a higher number of applications, significantly longer procedural and application time but shorter fluoroscopy duration (Table 2). ERAF occurred in 20% of all the treated patients (23 with ERAF out of 114). There were no differences between women and men in the rates of ERAF (18% vs. 22%) (Table 3). The percentage of ERAF was similar after cryoballoon and RF ablation (Table 2). Furthermore, the rate of paroxysmal ERAF was similar to the rate of persistent ERAF after both procedures (Table 2). The females treated with RF ablation were older than men (64 vs. 58 years) and had a higher BMI when treated with cryoablation (32.8 vs. 30.5; Table 2).

Table 2. Procedural characteristics and the type of ERAF after catheter ablation in obese females and obese males.

	Females (n = 54)		Males (n = 60)	
	Cryoablation (n = 30)	RF Ablation (n = 24)	Cryoablation (n = 30)	RF Ablation (n = 30)
Age, years	63 ± 5.8	## 64 ± 6.9	62 ± 5.5	58 ± 9.0 *
BMI, kg/m^2	# 32.8 ± 3.5	29.8 ± 4.6 **	31.0 ± 2.1	30.5 ± 3.0
Total procedure time, min	105.2 ± 30.2	196.9 ± 52.1 ****	98.6 ± 25.0	199.7 ± 37.7 ****
Fluoroscopy time, min	15.5 ± 5.9	8.3 ± 3.3 ****	14.3 ± 5.4	9.2 ± 4.5 ***
Application time, min	30.5 ± 8.7	54.9 ± 16.2 ****	28.2 ± 8.2	58.4 ± 17.5 ****

Table 2. Cont.

	Females (n = 54)		Males (n = 60)	
	Cryoablation (n = 30)	RF Ablation (n = 24)	Cryoablation (n = 30)	RF Ablation (n = 30)
Application number	8.2 ± 2.4	47.2 ± 50.9 ****	7.8 ± 2.3	25.2 ± 10.1 ****
ERAF, n (%)	5 (17)	5 (21)	5 (17)	8 (27)
Paroxysmal ERAF, n (%)	4 (13)	3 (12.5)	3 (10)	4 (13)
Persistent ERAF, n (%)	1 (3)	2 (8)	2 (7)	4 (13)

* Significant difference CB vs. RF ablation, # significance difference females vs. males. * $p < 0.05$, ** $p < 0.01$, *** $p < 0.001$, **** $p < 0.0001$; # $p < 0.05$, ## $p < 0.05$.

Table 3. Comparison of clinical and laboratory characteristics in obese females and obese males with and without ERAF following cryoballoon and RF ablation.

	Females		Males	
Parameter	(+) ERAF	(−) ERAF	(+) ERAF	(−) ERAF
n (%)	10 (18)	44 (82)	13 (22)	47 (78)
Age (years)	64.3 ± 7.7	63.7 ± 6.1	59.1 ± 9.9	60.5 ± 7.1
Smoking, n (%)	0 (0)	2 (2)	2 (15)	1 (2)
BMI, kg/m^2	30.4 ± 3.7	31.7 ± 4.4	31.3 ± 3.5	30.6 ± 2.3
WC, cm	96.1 ± 7.5	98.7 ± 13.3	107.3 ± 12.1	104.4 ± 10.0
leptin, ng/mL	29.9 ± 17.9	30.9 ± 21.4	6.8 ± 4.3	6.1 ± 6.4
	Ablation Procedure			
ERAF n, (%)	10 (18)	0 (0)	13 (22)	0 (0)
Procedure time, min	139.0 ± 64.4	147.5 ± 61.6	155.3 ± 59.8	147.4 ± 60.6
Cryoablation time, min	97.0 ± 32.1	106.8 ± 30.2	95.8 ± 21.1	99.2 ± 26.0
RF ablation time, min	181.0 ± 62.5	201.1 ± 50.1	192.5 ± 42.0	202.3 ± 36.7
Fluoroscopic time, min	11.4 ± 5.7	12.5 ± 6.2	11.3 ± 5.4	11.9 ± 5.6
Application time, min	35.1 ± 10.8	42.0 ± 18.2	45.2 ± 20.9	42.5 ± 20.4
Number of applications	23.0 ± 33.3	25.1 ± 39.5	17.1 ± 13.7	16.2 ± 10.9
Cryoablation, n (%)	5 (50)	25 (57)	5 (38)	25 (53)
RF ablation, n (%)	5 (50)	19 (43)	8 (62)	22 (47)
	Cardiovascular Parameters			
LA volume, mL	91.8 ± 27.2	94.3 ± 25.1	106.8 ± 30	93.9 ± 35.1
LAVI, mL/m^2	46.7 ± 11.4	48.7 ± 12.0	49.9 ± 15.0	42.8 ± 14.6
EF, %	58.1 ± 2.8	58.1 ± 3.2	57.2 ± 9.7	56.6 ± 6.2
CHA2DS2-VASC score, mean ± SD	2.4 ± 1.3	2.4 ± 1.0	1.6 ± 1.0	1.5 ± 0.9
HAS-BLED score, mean ± SD	1.3 ± 1.1	1.3 ± 0.7	1.1 ± 0.8	1.1 ± 06
SBP, mmHg	130 ± 14.6	129 ± 13.6	125 ± 11.9	127 ± 11.2
DBP, mmHg	78 ± 12.4	77 ± 9.3	83 ± 15.0	80 ± 9.5

Table 3. Cont.

	Females		Males	
Comorbidities and Medications				
Hypertension, n (%)	7 (70)	32 (59)	9 (69)	33 (70)
CAD, n (%)	1 (10)	2 (4)	1 (8)	10 (21)
Dyslipidemia, n (%)	4 (40)	21 (48)	2 (15)	13 (28)
Heart Failure, n (%)	0 (0)	1 (2)	1 (8)	10 (21)
Beta Blocker, n (%)	9 (90)	38 (86)	11 (85)	36 (77)
CCB, n (%)	0 (0)	11 (25)	1 (8)	12 (26)
NOAC, n (%)	7 (70)	26 (59)	12 (92)	35 (74)
VKA, n (%)	3 (30)	18 (41)	1 (8)	12 (26)
Statins, n (%)	5 (50)	18 (41)	5 (38)	20 (43)
Diuretics, n (%)	3 (30)	13 (29)	3 (23)	16 (34)
ACEI, n (%)	3 (30)	15 (34)	4 (31)	14 (30)
ARBs, n (%)	4 (40)	11 (25)	2 (15)	17 (36)
AAD, n (%)	5 (50)	25 (57)	6 (46)	23 (49)
Laboratory Findings				
Glucose, mg/dL	104.3 ± 8.2	100.0 ± 10.2	105.5 ± 12.7	101.4 ± 10.6
Cholesterol, mg/dL	187.1 ± 27.9	199.3 ± 39.1	165.9 ± 32.2	176.1 ± 39.9
LDL, mg/dL	118.5 ± 27.4	126.1 ± 37.3	104.8 ± 27.1	113.0 ± 35.6
eGFR, mL/min	72.3 ± 18.5	66.9 ± 13.7	81.2 ± 23.4	80.3 ± 11.9
Response to Ablation				
Parameter	delta	Delta	delta	delta
CRP, μg/mL	0.7 ± 0.5	0.8 ± 0.8	1.2 ± 1.6	0.6 ± 0.5
hsIL-6, pg/mL	20.0 ± 19.9	15.7 ± 15.8	14.6 ± 34.5	12.4 ± 14.3
PLT, 10^3/mL	−40.7 ± 36.6	−45.3 ± 30.5	−29.9 ± 29.8	−29.8 ± 18.7
Fibrinogen, mg/dL	−34.4 ± 47.9	−42.2 ± 87.2	19.7 ± 58.6	−14.7 ± 67.3
D-Dimer, mg/dL	0.5 ± 1.2	0.2 ± 0.6	0.07 ± 0.1	0.1 ± 0.3
Hs-TnT, ng/L	1.1 ± 0.5	1.3 ± 0.8	1.2 ± 0.6	1.2 ± 0.5
CPK, U/L	100.6 ± 85.3	139.1 ± 117.9	35.7 ± 96.4	111.2 ± 130.6
CK-MB, U/L	10.3 ± 10.2	15.9 ± 16.8	9.0 ± 10.8	16.2 ± 18.5
vWF, ng/mL	0.37 ± 0.65	0.11 ± 0.58	0.2 ± 0.5	0.06 ± 0.7
sICAM-1, ng/mL	0.8 ± 14.1 *	−22.2 ± 52.6 *	13.4 ± 73.7	0.03 ± 20.6
ST-2, ng/mL	1.9 ± 4.2	1.5 ± 2.4	2.5 ± 2.6 *	1.1 ± 1.9

Abbreviations: BMI, body mass index; WC, waist circumference; ERAF, early recurrence atrial fibrillation; RF, radiofrequency; LAVI, left atrial volume index; EF, ejection fraction; CHA$_2$DS$_2$-VASc, Congestive heart failure, Hypertension, Age ≥ 75 (doubled), Diabetes, Stroke (doubled), Vascular disease, Age 65–74, Sex (female); HAS-BLED, Hypertension, Abnormal renal/liver function, Stroke, Bleeding history or predisposition, Labile INR, Elderly (>65 years), Drugs/alcohol concomitantly; SBP, Systolic blood pressure; DBP, Diastolic blood pressure; CAD, coronary artery disease; CCB, calcium channel blockers; NOAC, non-vitamin K antagonist oral anticoagulant; VKA, vitamin K antagonist; ACE-I, angiotensin converting enzyme inhibitor; ARB, angiotensin II receptor blocker, AAD, anti-arrhythmic drugs; GFR, glomerular filtration rate; CRP, C-reactive protein; PLT, platelets; hs-TnT, high-sensitive cardiac troponin T; vWF, von Willebrandt factor; s-ICAM, intercellular adhesion molecul; Delta denotes the response to the ablation procedure. Delta was defined as the change in the biomarker concentration between two assays performed within 24-hour period (after ablation—before ablation). Significance difference ERAF(+) vs. ERAF (−) * $p < 0.05$.

Both methods of treatment triggered inflammation which was confirmed by the increased values of CRP inflammation markers (Figure 2A,B), hsIL-6 (Figure 2C,D), WBC (data not shown), and pentraxin (data not shown). There was no difference between the elevation of inflammatory parameters such as CRP in both procedures. Only the evaluation of high sensitivity parameters such as hsIL-6 did show that RF ablation generates more intense inflammation than cryoballoon ablation (Figure 2C,D). It was shown that the women treated with cryoballoon ablation developed greater inflammation resulting in higher hsIL-6 delta after the procedure (Figure 2D).

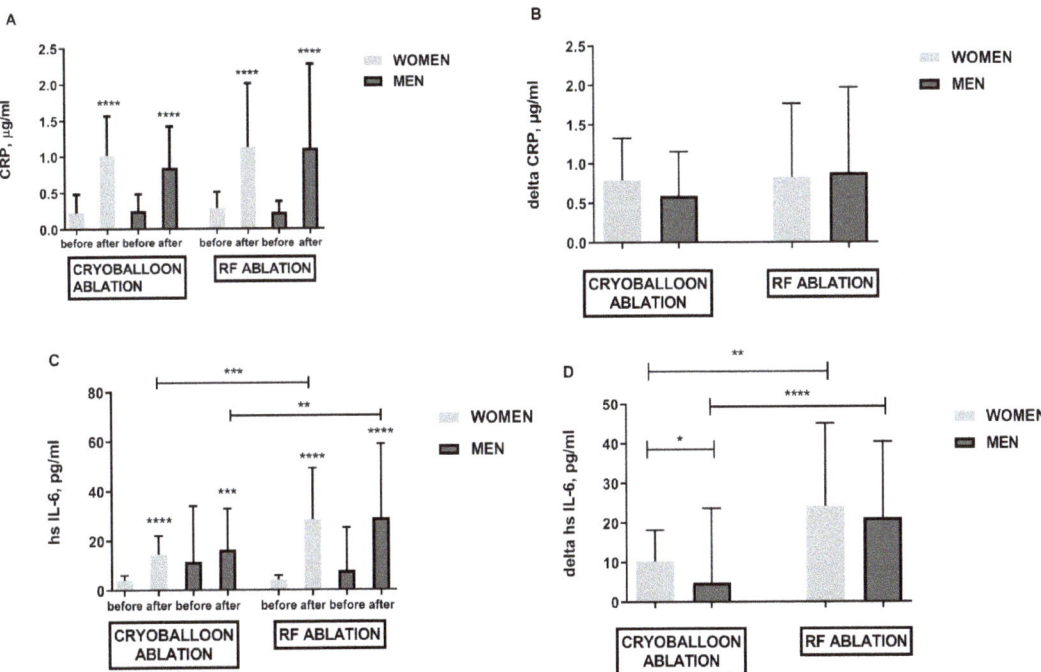

Figure 2. Biomarkers of inflammation in obese females and obese males following cryoballoon and RF ablation; panel (**A**)—CRP elevation in response to cryo and RF ablation; panel (**B**)—CRP difference before and after cryoballoon and RF ablation (delta); panel (**C**)—hs Il-6 elevation in response to cryoballoon and RF ablation; panel (**D**)—hs Il-6 difference before and after cryoballoon and RF ablation (delta). Asterisks represent a significant difference: * $p < 0.05$, ** $p < 0.01$, *** $p < 0.001$, **** $p < 0.0001$.

Both cryoballoon and RF ablations are inherently associated with cardiomyocyte damage and release of hs-TnT (Figure 3A), CPK (data not shown), and CK-MB (data not shown). However, RF ablation engenders greater cardiomyocyte damage (Figure 3A,B). When it comes to atrial myocardial injury and hs-TnT release, both are proportional to the hsIL-6 concentration regardless of gender (Figure 3C,D).

Out of 114 patients, 32 (28%) of them also experienced AF late recurrence (LRAF) assessed by a 24-h Holter monitoring at 6-, 9-, and 12-month intervals following ablation (authors' observation). The number of patients with ERAF was comparable to the number of patients with LRAF (ERAF 20% vs. LRAF 28%, $p = 0.1636$). Among 23 patients with ERAF, 16 of them (70%) also had LRAF (70% vs. 30%, $p = 0.008$) (data not shown).

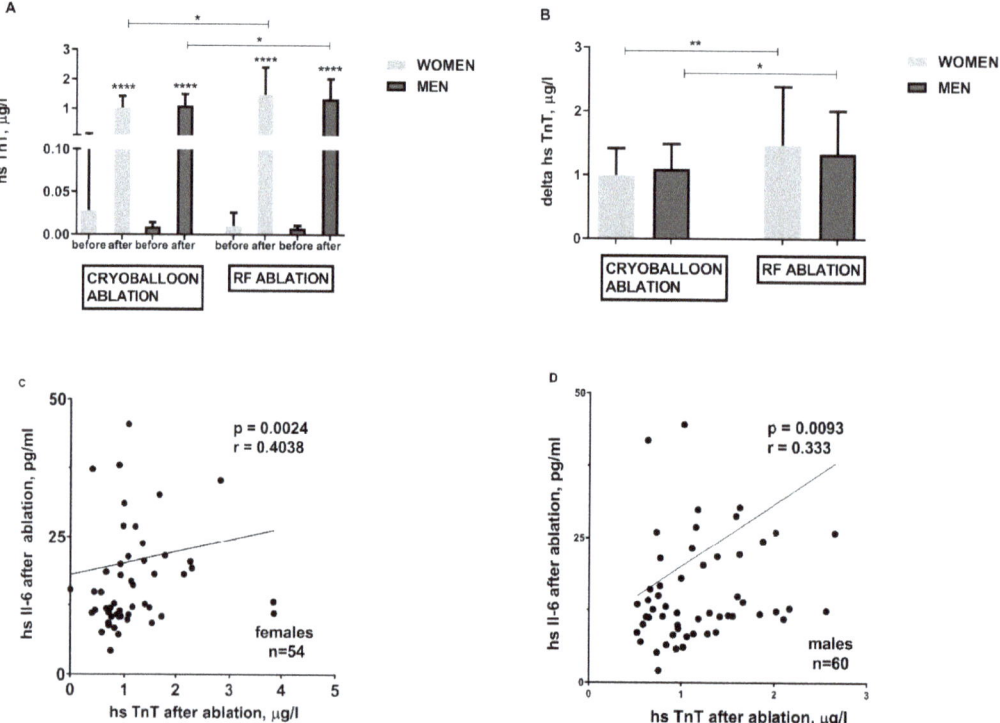

Figure 3. Troponin concentration before and after cryoballoon and RF ablation and its relationship with ablation-induced inflammatory process in obese females and obese males; panel (**A**)—hs TnT elevation in response to CB and RF ablation; panel (**B**)—hs TnT difference before and after cryoballoon and RF ablation (delta); The relationship between the degree of troponin release and the intensity of inflammation in the group of females panel (**C**) and males panel (**D**). Asterisks represent a significant difference: * $p < 0.05$, ** $p < 0.01$, **** $p < 0.0001$.

3.3. Predictors of ERA—Univariate Model

Since there was no difference in ERAF and its occurrence in both methods (Table 2) and in both groups of obese women and men (Tables 2 and 3), we decided to divide all the females and males into two groups (with and without ERAF) and compare them (Table 3), forming an univariate model. Among many analyzed parameters in both men and women with ERAF, only two parameters distinguished them from those without ERAF. In the group of men and women, it was always a higher response to the ablation procedure (delta). Also, a higher value of sICAM-1 characterized the group of women with ERAF while a higher value of ST-2 protein characterized the group of men (Table 3). Both procedures increased the ST2 concentration, but we also documented that higher ST2 levels were particularly characteristic of the men qualified for cryoablation. RF ablation was responsible for a higher ST2 protein production only in the women (data not shown). The obese women had higher sICAM–1 before the treatment than the obese men (data not shown). Therefore, sICAM-1 which characterizes inflammatory activation of endothelium in obesity, could be a determinate parameter for ERAF only in the group of women.

3.4. Predictors of ERAF—Multivariate Model

Out of 66 available variables (presented in Table S2) only a limited number of them was used in the MLR analysis, which was performed in several variants for the entire group of obese patients ($n = 114$) and separately for the group of obese women ($n = 54$) and obese men ($n = 60$). We only managed to create three MLR models in the group of men.

The model with the best results is presented in Table S3. The results demonstrated that the extent of ST2 protein elevation (OR 1.68, 95% CI, 1.115–2.536, $p = 0.011$), less frequent use of calcium channel blockers (CCB) (OR 0.042, 95% CI 0.002–1.071, $p < 0.05$) and smoking (OR 39.25, 95%CI, 1.050–1467.8, $p = 0.042$) were the independent predictors of ERAF in males. The proposed model of ERAF had a high specificity of 95.74%, and low sensitivity at 30.77%. Summing up, the MLR model is suitable for classifying obese men without ERAF (high specificity) while it is not satisfactory for detecting obese men with ERAF (low sensitivity).

4. Discussion

Due to the increasing number of obese patients suffering from an increased recurrence of atrial arrhythmias, we decided to recruit two groups of obese men and women who were qualified for cyoballoon and RF ablation and assess the treatments' effectiveness based on ERAF. In the examined group of 114 obese patients with matched age and BMI, ERAF occurred in 20% of them with the same frequency in both women and men following both types of ablation. Having two groups of patients, women and men, collecting 66 variables describing the patients' clinical condition required laboratory tests and ablation procedures. They enabled us to perform three MLR models to find the factor/factors conducive to ERAF three months after ablation. A separate analysis was done for the entire group of obese patients ($n = 114$), the group of obese women ($n = 54$), and obese men ($n = 60$). We only managed to create three MLR models in the group of obese men. As stated above, the results demonstrated that the extent of ST2 protein elevation, less frequent use of CCB and smoking were the independent predictors of ERAF in obese males. The proposed model of ERAF had a high specificity of 95.74%, which indicates that people without ERAF are correctly classified as patients with successful ablation (over 90%). Unfortunately, the model has a low sensitivity of 30.77%, which means that not all obese men with ERAF are detected.

The ST2 protein is associated with inflammation, fibrosis and myocardial overload. We noted a slightly higher concentration of ST2 protein before the procedure in men (probably due to higher CAD morbidity in this group) and its prominent elevation after both ablation methods. The higher ST2 concentration was particularly characteristic of the men qualified for cryoablation. The large population in the Framingham Heart Study also demonstrated higher ST2 levels in men [5]. The above trend may be related to sex hormones. It has been proven that in the group of postmenopausal women, without cardiovascular diseases, the concentration of ST2 was significantly lower when compared to the men of similar age [6]. In the study of Okar et al. [7], in MLR, the ST2 protein was an independent predictor of AF recurrence after cryoablation due to paroxysmal AF [7].

Smoking is a widely recognized factor leading to more than a two-fold increased risk of AF [8]. Smoking increases the incidence of nonPV triggers in patients with persistent AF. Smokers who had arrhythmia triggers located in the right atrium had a worse outcome after ablation [9].

The last MLR model seemed to be the most unexpected. It is linked to the less frequent use of CCBs dihydropyridine antihypertensive drugs in males with ERAF. Given the characteristics of the study group—elderly, obese patients with hypertension (71%), CAD (12%), and dyslipidemia (35%), this type of medication is commonly used. However, it is worth emphasizing that dihydropyridine CCBs lack an antiarrhythmic effect [10].

The results of ablation in women and men are inconclusive. Previous studies revealed that gender affects the recurrence rate of AF after catheter ablation. In large multicenter studies, female patients had a lower long-term efficacy than males [11,12]. However, Andrade et al., in the STOP AF trial, reported that the only significant factor associated with ERAF was the male sex [13]. Our MLR analysis performed on all 114 participants reveals that in obese patients, there is no relationship between gender and the recurrence rate of AF after catheter ablation.

Our study confirmed that the obese women had an 80% higher leptin concentration than the obese men. A higher leptin concentration in women results from a higher percentage of adipose tissue and greater secreted leptin per unit mass of adipose tissue. Leptin directly modulates atrial myocytes' electrophysiological basis by regulating calcium homeostasis in atrial myocytes, affecting atrial fibrosis and angiotensin II-induced AF [14]. Additionally, we observed a higher body weight and WC in the group of men, resulting from a different distribution of body fat in both sexes. Women had higher incidence of dyslipidemia. Demerath et al., showed a relationship between sICAM-1, sVCAM-1 and the concentration of total cholesterol and HDL cholesterol. This effect may be an explanation for the observed effect of higher concentration of these molecules in women due to observed dyslipidemia and physiologically higher concentration of HDL in women compared to men (Table 1) [15]. Men had higher concentrations of vWF. There is a relationship between vWF and the amount of visceral fat that produces adipokines responsible for endothelial dysfunction [16]. Moreover, the group of men suffered from CAD more frequently than the women (18% vs. 6%), which points at equally frequent atherosclerosis dominated by endothelial dysfunction.

Obesity is associated with a higher recurrence and greater impact of AF. The ESC-EHRA Atrial Fibrillation Ablation Long-Term Registry shows that BMI > 30 kg/m^2 can increase the recurrence rate of AF after ablation [17]. Nevertheless, no study so far has attempted to evaluate the parameters responsible for ERAF in overweight and obese patients.

The total procedural time, the number and duration of applications were longer in RF ablation than in cryoablation. RF ablation also generated more inflammation, which indicates the significant complexity of this method, the need to perform a precise map of LA and PVs using the CARTO electroanatomical system. However, CARTO practically limits the use of fluoroscopy.

Many authors emphasize that the frequency of ERAF is similar in RF and cryoballoon ablation [18,19], which is also confirmed by our research. The most common parameters that contribute to the recurrence of arrhythmia after ablation are: age [20], LA dimension [18,20], inflammatory markers [18], and reduced troponin levels [2,20]. The studies mentioned above indicate that LA inflammation and an increased LA dimension play an essential role in AF recurrence after ablation. In our study the differences in baseline characteristics could have an impact on clinical outcomes. First, the enrolled women were older and their GFR was lower than the men. Age-related fibrosis and lower GFR are common factors associated with AF recurrence after catheter ablation [20]. Second, a higher incidence of persistent AF in the male group is indeed associated with poor clinical outcomes [1].

Each ablation procedure causes damage to cardiomyocytes, more prominent in RF ablation, which is reflected in higher hs-TnT levels [2,20]. As we presented, the hs-TnT concentration increases proportionally to the inflammatory process both in men and women. We also showed a significantly higher concentration of hs-TnT before catheter ablation in the obese men, which may be associated with a higher incidence of CAD in this group [21].

In summary, we indicated the importance of structural remodeling by demonstrating the increasing ST2 protein concentrations associated with ERAF in obese men. Additionally, the CCB therapy and smoking also seemed to be the important factors contributing to ERAF in this group of patients. It was only possible to create MLR model in the group of the obese men due to the lack of statistical significance in the other two remaining groups (the obese women and the entire group of patients). The MLR model is suitable for classifying obese men without ERAF (high specificity) while not satisfactory for detecting obese men with ERAF (low sensitivity).

The poor predictive value of the MLR model may indicate the multifactorial nature of ERAF and the limited predictive value of biomarkers. The assessment of inflammation using highly sensitive markers such as sICAM-1, which characterizes the inflammation of the endothelium in obesity, may aid detecting patients more susceptible to ERAF. What is more, the evaluation of myocardial overload and fibrosis, such as the ST-2 protein, may help to select patients with more severe left atrial fibrosis who will potentially be at a higher risk of ERAF. Nevertheless, further research is required when it comes to the assessment of ERAF with more accurate methods of heart rhythm monitoring such as long- term rhythm monitoring and AF burden evaluation, which better reflect the outcomes that are clinically relevant [22].

Limitations of the Study

Our study was single-centred with a relatively small number of patients. The study group was heterogeneous in terms of the number of ablation procedures and RF ablation technique. ERAF was detected based on clinical symptoms, 12-lead ECG and 24-h Holter monitoring. Therefore, asymptomatic ERAF might have been missed. UFH could have modified the concentration of assessed biomarkers. Due to complex pharmacokinetics, UFH is theoretically absent in the blood collected 24 h after ablation. However, its earlier effect may be detected and it may change the concentration of some of the assessed parameters. Furthermore, the heparinized saline solution (0.9% NaCl) used during the procedure may have had an impact on the dilution of some biomarkers tested after ablation and thus also on their concentration 24 h after the procedure. The decision to collect blood 24 h after procedure was based on the expertise of the researchers who stated that during this time the severity of inflammation and myocardial injury after ablation is the highest [23]. Also, a specific limitation in the interpretation of myocardial injury biomarkers such as CPK and CK-MB occurred due to their thermal instability during RF ablation [21].

5. Conclusions

It was only possible to create the MLR model in the group of obese men, but not in the group of obese women. It revealed a poor predictive value with an unsatisfactory sensitivity of 31%, which indicates a poor classification of patients with ERAF following catheter ablation. The males with ERAF, who were smokers, had a higher level of ST2 cardiac stress biomarker in response to ablation. CCBs were less frequently administered in this group. The results demonstrate the multifactorial character of ERAF, which is determined by the gender of the obese patients.

Supplementary Materials: The following are available online at https://www.mdpi.com/2077-0383/10/12/2694/s1, Table S1: The sensitivities of the assays, Table S2: Variables used for multivariate logistic regression analysis, Table S3: Multivariate logistic regression model of early recurrence atrial fibrillation created in the group of men.

Author Contributions: Conceptualization, K.K. and J.B.; Methodology, K.K., E.K., R.R., K.Ł.; Validation, K.K., J.H.; Formal Analysis K.K., J.B.; Investigation, J.B., K.K., E.K., R.R., K.Ł.; Resources, K.K.; Data Curation, J.B.; Writing—Original Draft Preparation, J.B., K.K.; Writing—Review & Editing, J.B., K.K.; Visualization, J.B., K.K.; Supervision, K.K., J.H.; Funding Acquisition, K.K. All authors have read and agreed to the published version of the manuscript.

Funding: This research received no external funding.

Institutional Review Board Statement: The study was conducted according to the guidelines of the Declaration of Helsinki, and approved by the Ethics Committee of Poznan University of Medical Sciences (protocol code 44/16).

Informed Consent Statement: Informed consent was obtained from all subjects involved in the study.

Data Availability Statement: The data presented in this study are available in this article and supplementary material.

Acknowledgments: Special thanks for Natasza Czepulis and Joanna Łuczak for their contribution in samples preparation and laboratory assistance. We would like to thank Izabela Miechowicz for expert statistical analysis.

Conflicts of Interest: The authors declare no conflict of interest.

References

1. Calkins, H.; Hindricks, G.; Cappato, R.; Kim, Y.H.; Saad, E.B.; Aguinaga, L.; Akar, J.G.; Badhwar, J.; Brugada, J.; Camm, J.; et al. 2017 HRS/EHRA/ECAS/APHRS/SOLAECE expert consensus statement on catheter and surgical ablation of atrial fibrillation. *Europace* **2018**, *20*, e1–e160. [CrossRef] [PubMed]
2. Budzianowski, J.; Hiczkiewicz, J.; Burchardt, P.; Pieszko, K.; Rzeźniczak, J.; Budzianowski, P.; Korybalska, K. Predictors of atrial fibrillation early recurrence following cryoballoon ablation of pulmonary veins using statistical assessment and machine learning algorithms. *Heart Vessel.* **2019**, *34*, 352–359. [CrossRef] [PubMed]
3. Korybalska, K.; Luczak, J.; Swora-Cwynar, E.; Kanikowska, A.; Czepulis, N.; Kanikowska, D.; Skalisz, H.; Bręborowicz, A.; Grzymisławski, M.; Witowski, J. Weight loss-dependent and-independent effects of moderate calorie restriction on endothelial cell markers in obesity. *J. Physiol. Pharmacol.* **2017**, *68*, 597–608. [PubMed]
4. Lang, R.M.; Badano, L.P.; Mor-Avi, V.; Afilalo, J.; Armstrong, A.; Ernande, L.; Flachskampf, F.A.; Foster, E.; Goldstein, S.A.; Kuznetsova, T.; et al. Recommendations for cardiac chamber quantification by echocardiography in adults: An update from the American society of echocardiography and the European association of cardiovascular imaging. *Eur. Heart J. Cardiovasc. Imaging* **2015**, *16*, 233–271. [CrossRef]
5. Coglianese, E.E.; Larson, M.; Vasan, R.S.; Ho, J.E.; Ghorbani, A.; McCabe, E.L.; Cheng, S.; Fradley, M.G.; Kretschman, D.; Gao, W.; et al. Distribution and Clinical Correlates of the Interleukin Receptor Family Member Soluble ST2 in the Framingham Heart Study. *Clin. Chem.* **2012**, *58*, 1673–1681. [CrossRef]
6. Lew, J.; Sanghavi, M.; Ayers, C.R.; McGuire, D.K.; Omland, T.; Atzler, D.; Gore, M.O.; Neeland, I.; Berry, J.D.; Khera, A.; et al. Sex-Based Differences in Cardiometabolic Biomarkers. *Circulation* **2017**, *135*, 544–555. [CrossRef]
7. Okar, S.; Kaypakli, O.; Şahin, D.Y.; Koç, M. Fibrosis Marker Soluble ST2 Predicts Atrial Fibrillation Recurrence after Cryoballoon Catheter Ablation of Nonvalvular Paroxysmal Atrial Fibrillation. *Korean Circ. J.* **2018**, *48*, 920–929. [CrossRef]
8. Chamberlain, A.M.; Agarwal, S.K.; Folsom, A.R.; Duval, S.; Soliman, E.Z.; Ambrose, M.; Eberly, L.; Alonso, A. Smoking and incidence of atrial fibrillation: Results from the Atherosclerosis Risk in Communities (ARIC) Study. *Heart Rhythm.* **2011**, *8*, 1160–1166. [CrossRef]
9. Cheng, W.-H.; Lo, L.-W.; Lin, Y.-J.; Chang, S.-L.; Hu, Y.-F.; Hung, Y.; Chung, F.-P.; Chang, T.-Y.; Huang, T.-C.; Yamada, S.; et al. Cigarette smoking causes a worse long-term outcome in persistent atrial fibrillation following catheter ablation. *J. Cardiovasc. Electrophysiol.* **2018**, *29*, 699–706. [CrossRef]
10. Godfraind, T. Discovery and Development of Calcium Channel Blockers. *Front. Pharmacol.* **2017**, *8*, 286. [CrossRef] [PubMed]
11. Providência, R.; Adragão, P.; de Asmundis, C.; Chun, J.; Chierchia, G.; Defaye, P.; Anselme, F.; Creta, A.; Lambiase, P.D.; Schmidt, B.; et al. Impact of Body Mass Index on the Outcomes of Catheter Ablation of Atrial Fibrillation: A European Observational Multicenter Study. *J. Am. Heart Assoc.* **2019**, *8*, e012253. [CrossRef] [PubMed]
12. Ricciardi, D.; Arena, G.; Verlato, R.; Iacopino, S.; Pieragnoli, P.; Molon, G.; Manfrin, M.; Allocca, G.; Cattafi, G.; Sirico, G.; et al. Sex effect on efficacy of pulmonary vein cryoablation in patients with atrial fibrillation: Data from the multicenter real-world 1STOP project. *J. Interv. Card. Electrophysiol.* **2019**, *56*, 9–18. [CrossRef] [PubMed]
13. Andrade, J.G.; Khairy, P.; Macle, L.; Packer, D.L.; Lehmann, J.W.; Holcomb, R.G.; Ruskin, J.N.; Dubuc, M. Incidence and significance of early recurrences of atrial fibrillation after cryoballoon ablation: Insights from the multicenter Sustained Treatment of Paroxysmal Atrial Fibrillation (STOP AF) Trial. *Circ. Arrhythmia Electrophysiol.* **2014**, *7*, 69–75. [CrossRef]
14. Fukui, A.; Takahashi, N.; Nakada, C.; Masaki, T.; Kume, O.; Shinohara, T.; Teshima, Y.; Hara, M.; Saikawa, T. Role of Leptin Signaling in the Pathogenesis of Angiotensin II—Mediated Atrial Fibrosis and Fibrillation. *Circ. Arrhythmia Electrophysiol.* **2013**, *6*, 402–409. [CrossRef]
15. Demerath, E.; Towne, B.; Blangero, J.; Siervogel, R.M. The relationship of soluble ICAM-1, VCAM-1, P-selectin and E-selectin to cardiovascular disease risk factors in healthy men and women. *Ann. Hum. Biol.* **2001**, *28*, 664–678. [CrossRef]
16. Mertens, I.; Van der Planken, M.; Corthouts, B.; Van Gaal, L.F. Is visceral adipose tissue a determinant of von Willebrand factor in overweight and obese premenopausal women? *Metabolism* **2006**, *55*, 650–655. [CrossRef]
17. Glover, B.M.; Hong, K.L.; Dagres, N.; Arbelo, E.; Laroche, C.; Riahi, S.; Bertini, M.; Mikhaylov, E.; Galvin, J.; Kiliszek, M.; et al. Impact of body mass index on the outcome of catheter ablation of atrial fibrillation. *Heart* **2018**, *105*, 244–250. [CrossRef]
18. Miyazaki, S.; Taniguchi, H.; Nakamura, H.; Takagi, T.; Iwasawa, J.; Hachiya, H.; Iesaka, Y. Clinical Significance of Early Recurrence After Pulmonary Vein Antrum Isolation in Paroxysmal Atrial Fibrillation—Insight into the Mechanism. *Circ. J.* **2015**, *79*, 2353–2359. [CrossRef] [PubMed]
19. Gunawardene, M.A.; Hoffmann, B.A.; Schaeffer, B.; Chung, D.-U.; Moser, J.; Akbulak, R.O.; Jularic, M.; Eickholt, C.; Nuehrich, J.; Meyer, C.; et al. Influence of energy source on early atrial fibrillation recurrences: A comparison of cryoballoon vs. radiofrequency current energy ablation with the endpoint of unexcitability in pulmonary vein isolation. *Europace* **2016**, *20*, 43–49. [CrossRef] [PubMed]
20. Kızılırmak, F.; Gokdeniz, T.; Gunes, H.M.; Demir, G.G.; Cakal, B.; Guler, G.B.; Guler, E.; Olgun, F.E.; Kilicaslan, F. Myocardial injury biomarkers after radiofrequency catheter and cryoballoon ablation for atrial fibrillation and their impact on recurrence. *Kardiol. Pol.* **2017**, *75*, 126–134. [CrossRef]
21. Wójcik, M.; Janin, S.; Kuniss, M.; Berkowitsch, A.; Erkapic, D.; Zaltsberg, S.; Madlener, K.; Wysokiński, A.; Hamm, C.W.; Pitschner, H.F.; et al. Limitations of Biomarkers Serum Levels During Pulmonary Vein Isolation. *Rev. Esp. Cardiol.* **2011**, *64*, 127–132. [CrossRef] [PubMed]

22. Andrade, J.G.; Champagne, J.; Dubuc, M.; Deyell, M.W.; Verma, A.; Macle, L.; Leon-Sit, P.; Novak, P.; Badra-Verdu, M.; Sapp, J.; et al. Cryoballoon or radiofrequency ablation for atrial fibrillation assessed by continuous monitoring: A randomized clinical trial. *Circulation* **2019**, *140*, 1779–1788. [CrossRef] [PubMed]
23. Lim, H.S.; Schultz, C.; Dang, J.; Alasady, M.; Lau, D.H.; Brooks, A.G.; Wong, C.X.; Roberts-Thomson, K.C.; Young, G.D.; Worthley, M.I.; et al. Time Course of Inflammation, Myocardial Injury, and Prothrombotic Response After Radiofrequency Catheter Ablation for Atrial Fibrillation. *Circ. Arrhythmia Electrophysiol.* **2014**, *7*, 83–89. [CrossRef] [PubMed]

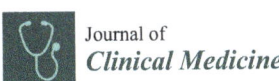

Journal of Clinical Medicine

Article

Holter-Derived Autonomic Function, Arrhythmias and Carbohydrate Metabolism in Patients with Class III Obesity Treated with Laparoscopic Sleeve Gastrectomy

Piotr Bienias [1,*], Zuzanna Rymarczyk [1], Justyna Domienik-Karłowicz [1], Wojciech Lisik [2], Piotr Sobieraj [3], Piotr Pruszczyk [1] and Michał Ciurzyński [1]

[1] Department of Internal Medicine and Cardiology, Medical University of Warsaw, 02-005 Warsaw, Poland; zmrymarczyk@gmail.com (Z.R.); jdomienik@o2.pl (J.D.-K.); piotr.pruszczyk@wum.edu.pl (P.P.); michal.ciurzynski@wum.edu.pl (M.C.)

[2] Department of General Surgery and Transplantology, Medical University of Warsaw, 02-005 Warsaw, Poland; wojciech.lisik@wum.edu.pl

[3] Department of Internal Medicine, Hypertension and Vascular Diseases, Medical University of Warsaw, 02-005 Warsaw, Poland; piotr.sobieraj@wum.edu.pl

* Correspondence: pbienias@mp.pl; Tel.: +48-225021144; Fax: +48-225022142

Citation: Bienias, P.; Rymarczyk, Z.; Domienik-Karłowicz, J.; Lisik, W.; Sobieraj, P.; Pruszczyk, P.; Ciurzyński, M. Holter-Derived Autonomic Function, Arrhythmias and Carbohydrate Metabolism in Patients with Class III Obesity Treated with Laparoscopic Sleeve Gastrectomy. *J. Clin. Med.* 2021, 10, 2140. https://doi.org/10.3390/jcm10102140

Academic Editor: Roberto De Ponti

Received: 15 April 2021
Accepted: 11 May 2021
Published: 15 May 2021

Publisher's Note: MDPI stays neutral with regard to jurisdictional claims in published maps and institutional affiliations.

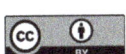

Copyright: © 2021 by the authors. Licensee MDPI, Basel, Switzerland. This article is an open access article distributed under the terms and conditions of the Creative Commons Attribution (CC BY) license (https://creativecommons.org/licenses/by/4.0/).

Abstract: The effects of weight loss following bariatric surgery on autonomic balance, arrhythmias and insulin resistance are still of interest. We prospectively investigated 50 patients with BMI > 40 kg/m^2, aged 36.5 (18–56) years who underwent laparoscopic sleeve gastrectomy. Among other examinations, all subjects had 24-h Holter monitoring with heart rate variability (HRV) and heart rate turbulence (HRT) evaluation. After a median of 15 months, BMI decreased from 43.9 to 29.7 kg/m^2, the incidence of hypertension decreased from 54 to 32% ($p = 0.04$) and any carbohydrate disorders decreased from 24 to 6% ($p = 0.02$). Fasting insulin concentration and insulin resistance index improved significantly ($p < 0.001$). Improvements in HRV parameters related to the sympathetic autonomic division were also observed ($p < 0.001$), while HRT evaluation was not conclusive. The enhancement of autonomic tone indices was correlated with reduction of BMI (SDNN-I r = 0.281 $p = 0.04$; SDNN r = 0.267 $p = 0.05$), but not with reduction of waist circumference, and it was also associated with decrease of mean heart rate (OR 0.02, 95%CI 0.0–0.1, $p < 0.001$). The incidence of arrhythmias was low and similar before and after follow-up. In conclusion, improvement of homeostasis of carbohydrate metabolism and autonomic function is observed in relatively young patients after weight loss due to laparoscopic sleeve gastrectomy.

Keywords: class III obesity; cardiac autonomic function; heart rate variability; arrhythmias; insulin resistance

1. Introduction

Morbid obesity may cause various cardiovascular complications, including hypertension, arrhythmias and cardiac autonomic nervous system (ANS) abnormality. Obesity is also associated with dysfunctional metabolic status including a higher incidence of various carbohydrate metabolism disorders and insulin resistance. In addition, some results suggest an association between hyperinsulinemia and insulin resistance in obesity and ANS imbalance [1–3].

Cardiac complications in obesity can be complex and result from left ventricular systolic or diastolic dysfunction, atrial dilatation and its electrical remodeling, myocyte hypertrophy, fibrosis and fatty infiltration. Many studies, including meta-analyses, suggest that weight loss after bariatric surgery is associated with significant improvements in cardiac morphology and function [1,4]. The effects of weight loss following various techniques of bariatric surgery on hyperinsulinemia, insulin resistance and obesity associated neuropathy are still of interest. Available data suggest that various techniques of bariatric surgery improve metabolic control, including glycemic homeostasis and increased insulin sensitivity [5–9]. However, limited recent results are available on assessment of the dynamics of fasting glucose, insulin levels, insulin resistance/sensitivity indices and also ANS indices in patients with class III obesity, who lost weight due to laparoscopic sleeve gastrectomy (LSG), especially at a relatively young age and without severe accompanying diseases. The available data often provide inconclusive and contradictory results too [7,10–13]. There is also no detailed evaluation of the impact of weight loss following bariatric surgery on the occurrence of various arrhythmias [14,15].

Therefore, we assessed patients with class III obesity in detail before LSG and after 12–18 months of follow-up. Our aim was to investigate the influence of weight loss on cardiac autonomic function and arrhythmias (primary endpoint) as well as selected parameters of carbohydrate metabolism (secondary endpoint) in relation to anthropometric measurements of obesity. Next to laboratory tests, we focused on detailed evaluation of Holter-derived time-domain heart rate variability (HRV) and heart rate turbulence (HRT), as they are established methods for assessing cardiac ANS function [16–18]. Both insulin resistance and HRV and HRT are also independent and important predictors of future cardiac, neurological and metabolic health. Other studies mainly assessed the metabolic status and ANS early after bariatric surgery; thus, we decided to check these conditions later, i.e., >12 months after surgery. Our research hypothesis was as follows: decreases in body mass index (BMI) and waist circumference (WC) after LSG due to class III obesity resulted in multi-profile improvements in cardiac ANS function, heart rhythm disturbances and carbohydrate metabolism.

2. Material and Methods

2.1. Study Population and Laboratory Tests

This is a single center, prospective cohort study. Fifty adult patients aged ≥ 18 years with initially BMI ≥ 40 kg/m^2 who underwent LSG were selected for the study evaluation. Patients were examined at the start of the study and after 12–18 months of follow-up. Our group was drawn from 81 individuals with class III obesity who were referred to LSG, as detailed in our previous publication (including also standard 12-lead electrocardiography and echocardiography) [19]. In this report, we present 50 patients who underwent LSG and underwent follow-up examination. Others were not finally qualified for surgery or did not report for a follow-up visit within the required period.

All subjects were stable outpatients who underwent 24-h Holter monitoring and basic laboratory tests, including insulin levels. On the basis of fasting glucose and insulin levels, the insulin resistance index (HOMA-IR, homeostatic model assessment to quantify insulin resistance, normal value ≤ 0.9) and also the insulin sensitivity index (QUICKI, Quantitative Insulin Sensitivity Check Index, normal value ≥ 0.34) were calculated according to widely available specific formulas.

To avoid the influence of various factors that are well known to strongly affect both cardiac ANS and arrhythmias, we did not include patients with various clinical or laboratory abnormalities, i.e., chronic coronary syndromes, heart failure with reduced ejection fraction <50%, significant heart valvular abnormalities, poorly controlled arterial hypertension, earlier confirmed by polysomnography obstructive sleep apnea syndrome, unexplained anemia (hemoglobin <12.0 g/l), uncontrolled thyroid dysfunction and reduction in glomerular filtration rate <60 mL/min, according to the Cockcroft–Gault equation. Since the assessment of cardiac ANS function based on Holter recording is possible only in people with sinus rhythm, and patients with persistent or permanent atrial fibrillation or flutter were also excluded. Studied patients cannot use anti-arrhythmic drugs class I–IV according to Vaughan Williams classification for any reasons (including beta-blockers or non-dihydropyridine calcium antagonists). Use of ≥ 2 antihypertensive medications at full doses was also an exclusion criterion. Patients with other acute or significant chronic diseases were not included either. All patients gave their written informed consent to participate in the study. This study was conducted in accordance with the amended Declaration of Helsinki. The protocol of the study was accepted by the Bioethics Committee of the Medical University of Warsaw, Poland (protocol no. AKBE/108/15).

2.2. 24-h Holter Monitoring

The Holter monitoring was recorded during normal everyday activity on a 3-channel digital device (Lifecard CF, Spacelabs Healthcare, Snoqualmie, WA, USA). An evaluation of heart rate, various arrhythmias and time-domain HRV was performed (Sentinel Impresario, Spacelabs Healthcare, WA, USA). According to European and American Task Force 6, indices of time-domain HRV were measured (full names and abbreviations in Table 1) [20]. The SDNN and HRV-Index estimated of overall HRV, SDANN estimated of long-term components of HRV and RMSSD and pNN50 estimated of short-term components of HRV. Two numerical HRT parameters after ventricular extrasystoles, e.g., turbulence onset and turbulence slope, were calculated using custom designed software based on the described methodology (details in our previous article) [19,21]. All HRV and HRT parameters were evaluated for the full 24 h without separation for the day and night periods. Holter recording was analyzed by the qualified cardiologist.

Table 1. Arrhythmias and heart rate variability parameters in 24-h Holter monitoring in patients before and after bariatric surgery.

Characteristic	Patients Before Bariatric Surgery (n = 50)	Patients After Bariatric Surgery (n = 50)	p Value
Heart rate [1]			
Mean heart rate (bpm)	80 ± 11	74 ± 10	<0.001
Minimal heart rate (bpm) *	58 (39–89)	51 (33–68)	<0.001
Maximal heart rate (bpm)	127 (100–181)	126 (105–167)	0.21
Supraventricular arrhythmias (no., %)			
Supraventricular extrasystoles >100/24 h	2 (4%)	3 (6%)	1.0
Non-sustained supraventricular tachycardia [2]	5 (10%)	15 (30%)	0.02
Ventricular arrhythmias (no., %)			
Ventricular extrasystoles >100/24 h	1 (2%)	3 (6%)	0.62
Non-sustained ventricular tachycardia [2]	0 (0%)	2 (4%)	0.49
Time-domain heart rate variability parameters [3]			
SDNN (ms) *	115 (73–225)	145 (83–282)	<0.001
SDNN-I (ms) *	41 (20–115)	45 (24–122)	<0.001
SDANN (ms) *	102 (68–181)	134 (78–264)	<0.001
RMSSD (ms) *	34 (15–122)	33 (16–112)	0.25
pNN50 (%) *	8.6 (0.3–44.1)	9.3 (0.4–50.8)	0.06
HRV-index *	16 (10–35)	22 (11–38)	<0.001
Heart rate turbulence parameters [4]			
Turbulence onset (%) *	−2.1 (−7.5–−0.6)	−3.6 (−8.6–1.2)	0.73
Turbulence slope (ms/RR) *	7.5 (−3.1–21.8)	8.6 (−3.1–43.8)	0.22
Abnormal HRT (no.,%)	3 (30%)	2 (20%)	0.80

* Values presented as median with range. [1] All patients presented sinus rhythm. [2] Non-sustained tachycardia were recognized when the rate was >100 beats per minute for at least 3 consecutive beats and arrhythmia lasted <30 s. [3] SDNN—the standard deviation of N-N (normal-to-normal) interval; SDNN-I—is the mean of the standard deviations of all the NN intervals for each 5 min periods of the entire recording; SDANN—the standard deviation of the average of N-N in all 5 min periods of the entire recording; RMSSD—the square root of the mean of the sum of the squares of differences between adjacent N-N; pNN50—number of pairs of adjacent N-N differing by more than 50 ms in the entire recording divided by the total number of all N-N; HRV Index—total number of all NN intervals divided by the height of the histogram of all NN intervals measured on a discrete scale with bins of 1/128 s 23 [20]. [4] HRT values were possible to measure in only 10 obese patients before and after bariatric surgery; as proposed by International Society for Holter and Noninvasive Electrocardiology, abnormal HRT was recognized if TO value was ≥0% and/or TS value was ≤2.5 ms/RR [21].

2.3. Statistical Analysis

The tested groups were compared by either Student's *t*-test or the Mann–Whitney–Wilcoxon test, according to parameters' distribution assessed by the Shapiro–Wilk test (variables with normal distribution were presented as mean with standard deviation, not showing normal distribution as median with range values). Deletions of outliers' data were not performed. The χ2 test or McNemar's test was used to compare categorical variables (if needed, Yates's correction was applied). All tests were double-sided. Correlations were evaluated by Spearman correlation coefficients. Logistic regression analysis was carried out to explore the influence of confounding factors on cardiac autonomic function in patients with obesity. The influence of measured parameters was expressed as an odds ratio (OR) with 95% confidence interval (CI). Values of $p < 0.05$ were considered statistically significant. Analyses were performed using R, which is a free software environment for statistical computing and graphics (www.r-project.org, version 3.4.0, accessed on 1st May 2017).

3. Results

3.1. Clinical Characteristics of Study Populations

The general characteristics of the patients with obesity before and after weight loss are presented in Table 2. The median age was 36.5 years (range 18–56), and 86% of the study cohort were women. It is worth noting that after observation, the incidence of carbohydrate metabolism disorders and hypertension decreased significantly, and all laboratory tests improved—results in Table 2 and in Figure 1. During the follow-up visit, patients received previously started angiotensin converting enzyme inhibitors (in 16/32%), diuretics (in 6/12%), dihydropyridine calcium antagonists (in 5/10%) and also a statin or fibrate (in 18/36%) due to primary prevention. One patient with type 2 diabetes mellitus was taking insulin, while two patients with persistent impaired glucose tolerance were receiving metformin. None of the subjects received beta-blockers or other medications that affected heart rhythm.

Table 2. Anthropometric obesity parameters, additional diseases and parameters of carbohydrate metabolism results in patients before and after bariatric surgery.

Characteristic	Patients Before Bariatric Surgery (n = 50)	Patients After Bariatric Surgery (n = 50)	p Value
Body mass index (kg/m^2) *	43.9 (40.1–55.8)	29.7 (19.6–43.9)	<0.001
Body mass index reduction (kg/m^2) *	-	14.7 (7.2–23.9)	-
Waist circumference (cm) *	139 (127–155)	88 (67–124)	<0.001
Waist circumference reduction (cm) *	-	53 (18–74)	-
Additional diseases and parameters of carbohydrate metabolism			
Hypertension, n (%)	27 (54%)	16 (32%)	0.04
Disorders of carbohydrate metabolism (together), (n,%)	12 (24%)	3 (6%)	0.02
Type 2 diabetes mellitus, (n,%)	1 (2%)	1 (2%)	1.0
Impaired glucose tolerance, (n,%)	6 (12%)	2 (4%)	0.27
Impaired fasting glucose, (n,%)	5 (10%)	0 (0%)	0.05
Fasting glucose level (mg/dl) *	90 (76–118)	85 (64–98)	<0.001
Fasting insulin level (uIU/mL) *	13.0 (5.0–55.1)	5.0 (1.4–11.9)	<0.001
QUICKI *,[1]	0.32 (0.27–0.39)	0.38 (0.33–0.49)	<0.001
HOMA-IR *,[2]	3.1 (1.0–14.3)	1.1 (0.3–2.4)	<0.001

* Values presented as median with range. [1] QUICKI-quantitative insulin sensitivity check index. [2] HOMA-IR-homeostatic model assessment for insulin resistance.

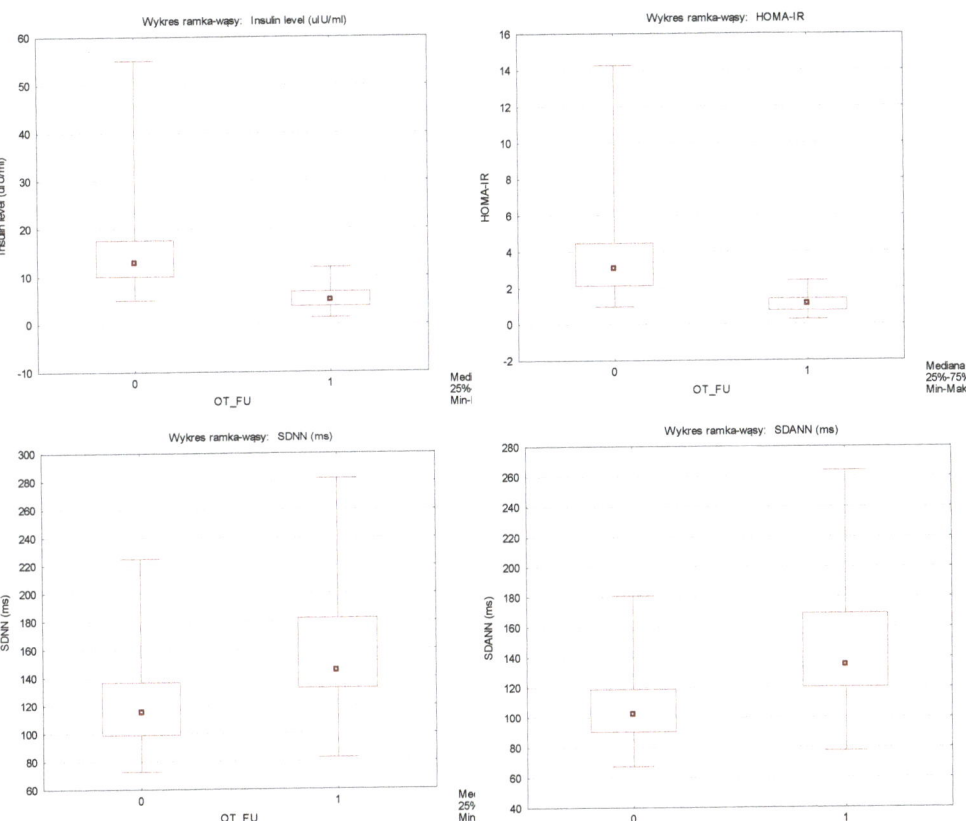

Figure 1. The values of fasting insulin level (chart **A**), homeostatic model assessment for insulin resistance HOMA-IR (chart **B**), SDNN (chart **C**) and SDANN (chart **D**) in 50 patients before and after weight loss. Charts present medians with ranges' values, while detailed results are shown in Table 2 (Y-axis: 0—patients before bariatric surgery, 0—patients after weight loss).

3.2. 24-h Holter Data

Detailed results of 24-h Holter data before and after weight loss are presented in Table 1. After observation, a significant improvement was observed in HRV indices estimating overall and long-term components, which are mainly related to the sympathetic tone (SDNN, SDANN and HRV-Index). By contrast, RMSSD and pNN50 values estimating short-term components and mainly associated with parasympathetic regulation remained unchanged. Due to rare occurrences of ventricular extrasystoles, HRT parameters were possible to count in only 10 subjects both before as well as after bariatric surgery. In the obtained results, turbulence slope (mostly triggered by a sympathetic tone) and also turbulence onset value (mostly related to transient vagal inhibition) were not significantly changed after weight loss.

Correlations were measured to estimate the association between a reduction in BMI or a reduction in WC and an increase in HRV indices. There were significant correlations between BMI reduction and increase of SDNN-I ($r = 0.281$, $p = 0.04$; Figure 2) and also nearly significant correlations for increase of SDNN ($r = 0.267$, $p = 0.05$) and SDANN ($r = 0.256$, $p = 0.07$). However, no correlations between the increase of HRV and WC reduction or HOMA-IR reduction were observed in patients after follow-up.

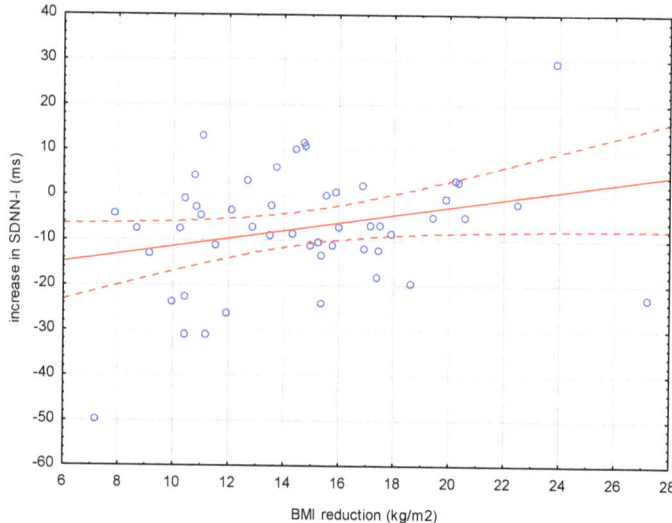

Figure 2. Correlation between the reduction in body mass index and the increase in SDNN-I value (r = 0.281, p = 0.04) in all 50 patients after follow-up period.

In addition, no significant differences in parameters of carbohydrate metabolism, HRV and HRT were observed after follow-up in patients divided according to the degree of weight reduction expressed by median of final BMI or final WC—results in Table 3. There were also no significant differences in the improvement of patients' HRV parameters according to the median follow-up period (<15 vs. ≥15 months)—detailed data are not shown.

Table 3. Comparison of indices of carbohydrate metabolism, time-domain heart rate variability and heart rate turbulence in groups divided according to the median reduction of body mass index and the median reduction of waist circumference.

Characteristic	Patients with Body Mass Index Reduction <14.7 kg/m² (n = 24)	Patients with Body mass Index Reduction ≥14.7 kg/m² (n = 26)	p value	Patients with Waist Circumference Reduction <53 cm (n = 24)	Patients with Waist Circumference Reduction ≥53 cm (n = 26)	p value
Hypertension, n (%)	10 (42%)	6 (23%)	0.23	8 (33%)	8 (31%)	1.0
Parameters of carbohydrate metabolism						
Fasting glucose level (mg/dl) *	86.6 ± 5.3	83.0 ± 6.8	0.05	85.7 ± 5.4	83.9 ± 7.0	0.33
Fasting insulin level (uIU/mL) *	5.5 ± 2.3	5.2 ± 2.4	0.69	5.7 ± 2.6	5.0 ± 2.0	0.32
QUICKI *,[1]	0.38 ± 0.03	0.39 ± 0.04	0.40	0.38 ± 0.03	0.39 ± 0.03	0.47
HOMA-IR * [1]	1.17 ± 0.51	1.09 ± 0.52	0.54	1.21 ± 0.56	1.06 ± 0.46	0.28
Time-domain heart rate variability parameters [1]						
SDNN (ms) *	156 (99–244)	138 (83–282)	0.15	143 (99–269)	143 (83–282)	0.56
SDNN-I (ms) *	54 (28–93)	44 (24–122)	0.23	49 (24–121)	44 (26–96)	0.78
SDANN (ms) *	144 (95–257)	129 (78–264)	0.25	133 (95–223)	133 (78–264)	0.36
RMSSD (ms) *	40 (19–90)	28 (16–112)	0.14	38 (16–112)	33 (18–108)	0.62
pNN50 (%) *	11.9 (1.1–37.8)	5.7 (0.4–50.8)	0.12	10.3 (0.4–50.8)	9.3 (0.8–40.9)	0.47
HRV–index *	23 (15–37)	21.8 (11–38)	0.38	27 (15–38)	29 (11–36)	0.26

Table 3. Cont.

Characteristic	Patients with Body Mass Index Reduction <14.7 kg/m² (n = 24)	Patients with Body mass Index Reduction ≥14.7 kg/m² (n = 26)	p value	Patients with Waist Circumference Reduction <53 cm (n = 24)	Patients with Waist Circumference Reduction ≥53 cm (n = 26)	p value
Heart rate turbulence parameters						
Turbulence onset (%)	−2.9 ± 3.4	−3.1 ± 2.9	0.93	−3.5 ± 2.8	-2.7 ± 3.2	0.51
Turbulence slope (ms/RR)	12.6 ± 12.9	16.2 ± 14.2	0.58	17.3 ± 13.1	12.2 ± 13.8	0.62

* Values presented as median with range. [1] For abbreviations—see Table 2.

The univariate logistic regression analysis was performed to detect potential predictors of increase of SDNN after weight loss (the main HRV parameter). This analysis revealed that only mean heart rate was significantly related to the increase in SDNN value (odds ratio 0.02, 95%CI 0.0–0.1, $p < 0.001$). Other parameters used in the univariate analysis included age, BMI reduction and WC reduction (the detailed values of the corrections applied are not presented). Due to the results of the univariate analysis, the previously planned multivariate analysis was not performed.

4. Discussion

Obesity is a multi-factorial disease, and obesity-related diseases increase the incidence of disability and mortality [1,2,22]. The main finding of our study is that the weight loss after LSG resulted in a multi-profile improvement in carbohydrate metabolism and blood pressure control, as well as overall cardiac ANS function. In addition, these health benefits were observed irrespective of degree of weight loss.

Various techniques of bariatric surgery are used for effective treatment of morbid obesity, such as Roux-en-Y gastric bypass, sleeve gastrectomy or biliopancreatic diversion with duodenal switch. In most patients, all types of bariatric surgery procedures improve metabolic status, reduce the incidence of hypertension and decrease long-term mortality [2,22]. Multiple studies and meta-analyses suggest that weight loss following bariatric surgery is associated with significant optimization of glycemia, insulin, lipids and other metabolic and hormonal changes that improve the overall metabolic profile [2,9,22]. Several hypotheses have been put forward trying to explain individually variable improvement, and one of the issues studied is the role of the ANS function in this process [13,23]. However, these mechanisms are extremely complex and still not fully understood [2,7,11,24].

Recently, one of the preferred procedures is LSG with relatively few postoperative complications. As numerous studies have shown, ANS dysfunction is often found because of morbid obesity, while weight loss improves sympathetic and parasympathetic activity and consequently decreases mean heart rate [6,10,13,25]. After analyzing the results of previous studies, we expected not only HRV and HRT recovery, but also a reduction in the incidence of hypertension and improvement in glucose homeostasis. Our study confirmed these assumptions, and we additionally showed that positive changes are present regardless of the degree of weight loss expressed by the median reduction of BMI or WC (Table 3). It has also been hypothesized that changes in the vagal-modulated neuroendocrine system have an additional effect on the beneficial effects after bariatric surgery [6,10,13,25]. Both the Roux-en-Y surgery and sleeve gastrectomy may induce metabolic improvements via different mechanisms. In a recent Greek study, both these surgical procedures resulted in comparable improvements in glucose, HOMA-IR, triglycerides and high-density lipoprotein cholesterol, while insulin levels were significantly higher in the sleeve gastrectomy group [9]. Earlier observations have suggested that LSG has more benefits in improving autonomic balance because the vagus nerve fibers are not damaged during this procedure, in contrast to the Roux-en-Y method, where induced damage to the vagus nerve innervation is similar to that of a sub-diaphragmatic trunk vagotomy [10,26,27]. However, in our study, HRV indices related to parasympathetic part did not improve after the follow-up period. Thus, our evaluation does not support the hypothesis that LSG causes significant improvements in both parts of ANS function.

Another issue concerns the relationship between anthropometric parameters and autonomic HRV indices. It seems that improvement of sympathetic parameters should be related to the decrease of WC, as abdominal obesity is just associated with hyperinsulinemia, hyperleptinemia and insulin resistance, which are considered to be contributed to the abnormal activation of the sympathetic autonomic system [28]. However, in our study, correlations between an increase of SDNN, SDNN-I and SDANN, and a reduction in BMI were revealed, but not with the reduction in waist circumference.

The results of the study by Sharma et al. suggest that sleeve gastrectomy leads to a dramatic improvement in insulin resistance as early as the first postoperative day [29]. In our study, HOMA-IR was also significantly lower after a median of 15 months of follow-up. Literature data on the association of HRV with insulin resistance parameters in patients after bariatric surgery are not consistent. As in the results of the study by Maser et al., no correlations between the increase of HRV parameters and HOMA-IR reduction were observed in our individuals after follow-up [12]. In contrast, an evaluation by Wu et al. revealed significant association between changes in HOMA-IR and increase of parasympathetic-related HRV indices 180 days after LSG [30]. Nevertheless, the Geronikolou et al. meta-analysis of 646 patients aged 34–52.5 years and BMI >50 kg/m^2 showed a positive effect of weight loss after various bariatric surgeries not only on time-domain or frequency-domain HRV parameters, but also on HOMA-IR. Interestingly, the authors concluded that gastric bypass favors insulin resistance decrease, while sleeve gastrectomy increases the vagal tone. Accordingly, in patients with severe cardiovascular involvement, a sleeve gastrectomy should be preferred to gastric bypass techniques [27]. It is worth emphasizing that studies involving many cases indicate that next to insulin resistance improvement, remission of type 2 diabetes after bariatric surgery is also possible, especially from operations with a malabsorptive component [2].

Hitherto, the assessment of HRT was infrequently performed in patients with obesity or metabolic syndrome [31,32]. In our study, the small number of people with ventricular extrasystoles suitable to calculate HRT significantly limited the statistical analysis both before and after weight loss. As far as we know, such evaluation during follow-up has not been performed in patients treated with bariatric surgery as of yet; therefore, this promising issue requires further research.

There is ample evidence that various bariatric procedures and subsequent weight loss significantly reduce the incidence of cardiovascular complications and improve the structure and function of the heart [4,15]. However, there are limited data evaluating the incidence of arrhythmias after bariatric surgery [14,15,33,34]. In the presented patients, it was surprising that numerous or severe cardiac arrhythmias were very rare, including atrial fibrillation or nocturnal bradyarrhythmia. However, our study included subjects with a median of 36.5 years, without structural heart disease and other serious comorbidities, including evident obstructive sleep apnea that might predispose to arrhythmias. In Holter monitoring, atrial tachycardia was even more common after follow-up, with the exception of atrial fibrillation. However, the prognostic value of frequent atrial tachycardia is limited, and so far, no clear association between these arrhythmias and cardiac ANS function has been demonstrated. It is noteworthy that after weight loss, short non-sustained ventricular tachycardia was also reported in two patients (both with slight left ventricular hypertrophy 10–11 mm of wall thickness recognized during at baseline visit).

One of the limitations of our study is the small number of patients enrolled, which undoubtedly influenced the obtained results, but many publications on morbid obesity are of similar size. In particular, the subgroup analysis (presented in Table 3) concerns a small number of compared patients; therefore, the differences may not be significant. An additional reason for the results obtained may be that our group was relatively young and consisted mainly of women. In addition, to eliminate the influence of various factors on examined parameters, only selected patients were included as described in the Methods section. Another possible limitation is the lack of frequency-domain (power spectral) HRV analysis. However, we are convinced that well-tried time-domain HRV and HRT analyses are sufficient for assessing ANS function.

5. Conclusions

In our study, the weight loss after LSG due to class III obesity resulted in a multi-profile improvement in carbohydrate metabolism and blood pressure control as well as overall cardiac ANS function. The improvement of HRV sympathetic-related indices were correlated with the reduction of BMI, but not with the reduction of WC. The subgroup analysis according to the degree of reduction of anthropomorphic parameters (BMI, WC) suggested that health benefits after LSG might be expected even in people with less weight loss. Serious or life-threatening cardiac arrhythmia were infrequent both before surgical treatment as well as after weight loss. However, it should be noted that patients evaluated in our study were of relatively young age and without other significant comorbidities.

Author Contributions: P.B., writing manuscript, design, conduct/data collection, analysis and supervision; Z.R., writing manuscript, design and conduct/data collection; J.D.-K., conduct/data collection; W.L., conduct/data collection and supervision; P.S., analysis; P.P., design and supervision; M.C., writing manuscript and supervision. All authors have read and agreed to the published version of the manuscript.

Funding: This research received no specific grant from any funding agency in the public, commercial, or not-for-profit sectors.

Institutional Review Board Statement: This study was conducted in accordance with the amended Declaration of Helsinki. The protocol of the study was approved by the Bioethics Committee of Medical University of Warsaw (protocol no. AKBE/108/15).

Informed Consent Statement: All patients gave their written informed consent to participate in the study.

Data Availability Statement: Not applicable.

Conflicts of Interest: The authors have no conflict of interest to declare.

References

1. Dwivedi, A.K.; Dubey, P.; Cistola, D.P.; Reddy, S.Y. Association Between Obesity and Cardiovascular Outcomes: Updated Evidence from Meta-analysis Studies. *Curr. Cardiol. Rep.* **2020**, *22*, 25. [CrossRef]
2. Keshavjee, S.H.; Schwenger, K.J.P.; Yadav, J.; Jackson, T.D.; Okrainec, A.; Allard, J.P. Factors Affecting Metabolic Outcomes Post Bariatric Surgery: Role of Adipose Tissue. *J. Clin. Med.* **2021**, *10*, 714. [CrossRef] [PubMed]
3. Straznicky, N.E.; Grima, M.T.; Eikelis, N.; Nestel, P.J.; Dawood, T.; Schlaich, M.P.; Chopra, R.; Masuo, K.; Esler, M.D.; Sari, C.I.; et al. The effects of weight loss versus weight loss maintenance on sympathetic nervous system activity and metabolic syndrome components. *J. Clin. Endocrinol. Metab.* **2011**, *96*, E503–E508. [CrossRef]
4. Aggarwal, R.; Harling, L.; Efthimiou, E.; Darzi, A.; Athanasiou, T.; Ashrafian, H. The Effects of Bariatric Surgery on Cardiac Structure and Function: A Systematic Review of Cardiac Imaging Outcomes. *Obes. Surg.* **2016**, *26*, 1030–1040. [CrossRef]
5. Azmi, S.; Ferdousi, M.; Liu, Y.; Adam, S.; Iqbal, Z.; Dhage, S.; Ponirakis, G.; Siahmansur, T.; Marshall, A.; Petropoulos, I.; et al. Bariatric surgery leads to an improvement in small nerve fibre damage in subjects with obesity. *Int. J. Obes.* **2021**, *45*, 631–638. [CrossRef] [PubMed]
6. Ibacache, P.; Carcamo, P.; Miranda, C.; Bottinelli, A.; Guzman, J.; Martinez-Rosales, E.; Artero, E.G.; Cano-Cappellacci, M. Improvements in Heart Rate Variability in Women with Obesity: Short-term Effects of Sleeve Gastrectomy. *Obes. Surg.* **2020**, *30*, 4038–4045. [CrossRef] [PubMed]
7. Gomide Braga, T.; das Gracas Coelho de Souza, M.; Maranhao, P.A.; Menezes, M.; Dellatorre-Teixeira, L.; Bouskela, E.; Le Roux, C.W.; Kraemer-Aguiar, L.G. Evaluation of Heart Rate Variability and Endothelial Function 3 Months After Bariatric Surgery. *Obes. Surg.* **2020**, *30*, 2450–2453. [CrossRef] [PubMed]
8. Ashrafian, H.; Harling, L.; Toma, T.; Athanasiou, C.; Nikiteas, N.; Efthimiou, E.; Darzi, A.; Athanasiou, T. Type 1 Diabetes Mellitus and Bariatric Surgery: A Systematic Review and Meta-Analysis. *Obes. Surg.* **2016**, *26*, 1697–1704. [CrossRef] [PubMed]
9. Magouliotis, D.E.; Tasiopoulou, V.S.; Sioka, E.; Chatedaki, C.; Zacharoulis, D. Impact of Bariatric Surgery on Metabolic and Gut Microbiota Profile: A Systematic Review and Meta-analysis. *Obes. Surg.* **2017**, *27*, 1345–1357. [CrossRef]

10. Casellini, C.M.; Parson, H.K.; Hodges, K.; Edwards, J.F.; Lieb, D.C.; Wohlgemuth, S.D.; Vinik, A.I. Bariatric Surgery Restores Cardiac and Sudomotor Autonomic C-Fiber Dysfunction towards Normal in Obese Subjects with Type 2 Diabetes. *PLoS ONE* **2016**, *11*, e0154211. [CrossRef]
11. Cornejo-Pareja, I.; Clemente-Postigo, M.; Tinahones, F.J. Metabolic and Endocrine Consequences of Bariatric Surgery. *Front Endocrinol.* **2019**, *10*, 626. [CrossRef]
12. Maser, R.E.; Lenhard, M.J.; Peters, M.B.; Irgau, I.; Wynn, G.M. Effects of surgically induced weight loss by Roux-en-Y gastric bypass on cardiovascular autonomic nerve function. *Surg. Obes. Relat. Dis.* **2013**, *9*, 221–226. [CrossRef]
13. Perugini, R.A.; Li, Y.; Rosenthal, L.; Gallagher-Dorval, K.; Kelly, J.J.; Czerniach, D.R. Reduced heart rate variability correlates with insulin resistance but not with measures of obesity in population undergoing laparoscopic Roux-en-Y gastric bypass. *Surg. Obes. Relat. Dis.* **2010**, *6*, 237–241. [CrossRef] [PubMed]
14. Clapp, B.; Amin, M.; Dodoo, C.; Harper, B.; Liggett, E.; Davis, B. New Onset Cardiac Arrhythmias after Metabolic and Bariatric Surgery. *JSLS* **2020**, *24*. [CrossRef] [PubMed]
15. Lee, G.K.; Cha, Y.M. Cardiovascular benefits of bariatric surgery. *Trends Cardiovasc. Med.* **2016**, *26*, 280–289. [CrossRef]
16. Cygankiewicz, I. Heart rate turbulence. *Prog. Cardiovasc. Dis.* **2013**, *56*, 160–171. [CrossRef] [PubMed]
17. Cygankiewicz, I.; Zareba, W. Heart rate variability. *Handb. Clin. Neurol.* **2013**, *117*, 379–393. [CrossRef]
18. Williams, S.M.; Eleftheriadou, A.; Alam, U.; Cuthbertson, D.J.; Wilding, J.P.H. Cardiac Autonomic Neuropathy in Obesity, the Metabolic Syndrome and Prediabetes: A Narrative Review. *Diabetes Ther.* **2019**, *10*, 1995–2021. [CrossRef]
19. Bienias, P.; Rymarczyk, Z.; Domieniek-Karlowicz, J.; Lisik, W.; Sobieraj, P.; Pruszczyk, P.; Ciurzynski, M. Assessment of arrhythmias and cardiac autonomic tone at a relatively young age patients with obesity class III. *Clin. Obes.* **2021**, *11*, e12424. [CrossRef]
20. Heart rate variability. Standards of measurement, physiological interpretation, and clinical use. Task Force of the European Society of Cardiology and the North American Society of Pacing and Electrophysiology. *Eur. Heart J.* **1996**, *17*, 354–381. [CrossRef]
21. Bauer, A.; Malik, M.; Schmidt, G.; Barthel, P.; Bonnemeier, H.; Cygankiewicz, I.; Guzik, P.; Lombardi, F.; Muller, A.; Oto, A.; et al. Heart rate turbulence: Standards of measurement, physiological interpretation, and clinical use: International Society for Holter and Noninvasive Electrophysiology Consensus. *J. Am. Coll. Cardiol.* **2008**, *52*, 1353–1365. [CrossRef]
22. Cardoso, L.; Rodrigues, D.; Gomes, L.; Carrilho, F. Short- and long-term mortality after bariatric surgery: A systematic review and meta-analysis. *Diabetes Obes. Metab.* **2017**, *19*, 1223–1232. [CrossRef]
23. Rossi, R.C.; Vanderlei, L.C.; Goncalves, A.C.; Vanderlei, F.M.; Bernardo, A.F.; Yamada, K.M.; da Silva, N.T.; de Abreu, L.C. Impact of obesity on autonomic modulation, heart rate and blood pressure in obese young people. *Auton. Neurosci.* **2015**, *193*, 138–141. [CrossRef]
24. Rao, R.S.; Yanagisawa, R.; Kini, S. Insulin resistance and bariatric surgery. *Obes. Rev.* **2012**, *13*, 316–328. [CrossRef] [PubMed]
25. Alam, I.; Lewis, M.J.; Lewis, K.E.; Stephens, J.W.; Baxter, J.N. Influence of bariatric surgery on indices of cardiac autonomic control. *Auton. Neurosci.* **2009**, *151*, 168–173. [CrossRef]
26. Ballsmider, L.A.; Vaughn, A.C.; David, M.; Hajnal, A.; Di Lorenzo, P.M.; Czaja, K. Sleeve gastrectomy and Roux-en-Y gastric bypass alter the gut-brain communication. *Neural Plast.* **2015**, *2015*, 601985. [CrossRef] [PubMed]
27. Geronikolou, S.A.; Albanopoulos, K.; Chrousos, G.; Cokkinos, D. Evaluating the Homeostasis Assessment Model Insulin Resistance and the Cardiac Autonomic System in Bariatric Surgery Patients: A Meta-Analysis. *Adv. Exp. Med. Biol.* **2017**, *988*, 249–259. [CrossRef] [PubMed]
28. Windham, B.G.; Fumagalli, S.; Ble, A.; Sollers, J.J.; Thayer, J.F.; Najjar, S.S.; Griswold, M.E.; Ferrucci, L. The Relationship between Heart Rate Variability and Adiposity Differs for Central and Overall Adiposity. *J. Obes.* **2012**, *2012*, 149516. [CrossRef]
29. Sharma, R.; Hassan, C.; Chaiban, J.T. Severe Insulin Resistance Improves Immediately After Sleeve Gastrectomy. *J. Investig. Med. High Impact Case Rep.* **2016**, *4*. [CrossRef]
30. Wu, J.M.; Yu, H.J.; Lai, H.S.; Yang, P.J.; Lin, M.T.; Lai, F. Improvement of heart rate variability after decreased insulin resistance after sleeve gastrectomy for morbidly obesity patients. *Surg. Obes. Relat. Dis.* **2015**, *11*, 557–563. [CrossRef]
31. Avsar, A.; Acarturk, G.; Melek, M.; Kilit, C.; Celik, A.; Onrat, E. Cardiac autonomic function evaluated by the heart rate turbulence method was not changed in obese patients without co-morbidities. *J. Korean Med. Sci.* **2007**, *22*, 629–632. [CrossRef] [PubMed]
32. Erdem, A.; Uenishi, M.; Matsumoto, K.; Kucukdurmaz, Z.; Kato, R.; Sahin, S.; Yazici, M. Cardiac autonomic function in metabolic syndrome: A comparison of ethnic Turkish and Japanese patients. *J. Interv. Card. Electrophysiol.* **2012**, *35*, 253–258. [CrossRef] [PubMed]
33. Nault, I.; Nadreau, E.; Paquet, C.; Brassard, P.; Marceau, P.; Marceau, S.; Biron, S.; Hould, F.; Lebel, S.; Richard, D.; et al. Impact of bariatric surgery–induced weight loss on heart rate variability. *Metabolism* **2007**, *56*, 1425–1430. [CrossRef]
34. Pabon, M.A.; Manocha, K.; Cheung, J.W.; Lo, J.C. Linking Arrhythmias and Adipocytes: Insights, Mechanisms, and Future Directions. *Front Physiol.* **2018**, *9*, 1752. [CrossRef] [PubMed]

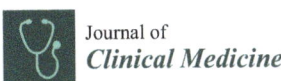

Review

Left Main Coronary Artery Disease—Current Management and Future Perspectives

Emil Julian Dąbrowski *, Marcin Kożuch and Sławomir Dobrzycki

Department of Invasive Cardiology, Medical University of Bialystok, 24A Sklodowskiej-Curie St., 15-276 Bialystok, Poland
* Correspondence: e.j.dabrowski@gmail.com

Abstract: Due to its anatomical features, patients with an obstruction of the left main coronary artery (LMCA) have an increased risk of death. For years, coronary artery bypass grafting (CABG) has been considered as a gold standard for revascularization. However, notable advancements in the field of percutaneous coronary intervention (PCI) led to its acknowledgement as an important treatment alternative, especially in patients with low and intermediate anatomical complexity. Although recent years brought several random clinical trials that investigated the safety and efficacy of the percutaneous approach in LMCA, there are still uncertainties regarding optimal revascularization strategies. In this paper, we provide a comprehensive review of state-of-the-art diagnostic and treatment methods of LMCA disease, focusing on percutaneous methods.

Keywords: left main coronary artery; percutaneous coronary intervention; coronary artery bypass grafting; coronary artery disease; coronary revascularization

1. Background

According to the latest WHO reports, in 2019 ischaemic heart disease (IHD) has strengthened its position as a leading cause of deaths since 2000, accounting for 16% of the world's total deaths. The rise was especially marked in low-, lower-middle, and upper-middle-income countries. Interestingly, although in high-income countries the number of deaths due to IHD declined, it still remained the main cause of death [1].

Since the early development of coronary artery angiography, it became evident that not all atherosclerotic lesion localizations are equally dangerous. Due to its anatomical features, patients with an obstruction of the left main coronary artery (LMCA) may be at exceptionally high risk. Depending on coronary artery dominance, LMCA supplies blood to 75–100% of the myocardium [2]. Knowing that, there is no wonder that LMCA in the past was known as 'the artery of sudden death' [3]. During the early coronarography era, clinicians reported even a 10% risk of death due to LMCA catheterization, and suggested special caution when performing angiography in patients with suspected left main coronary artery disease (LMCAD) [4]. Research available at the time reported over 50% five-year mortality among the patients who received only pharmacological treatment [5]. In the meta-analysis performed by Yusuf et al. 10-year mortality in the group of patients with LMCAD exceeded even the mortality rate of patients with the involvement of three vessels [5].

The poor prognosis of patients with LMCAD gradually improved with the development of revascularization techniques. In the 1970s, coronary artery bypass grafting (CABG) was implemented in the treatment of coronary artery disease (CAD) [6]. Surgical efficacy was proven in observational studies and early randomized clinical trials (RCT), which resulted in wide acknowledgement of this treatment as a method of choice in LMCAD [7]. The following years brought another breakthrough in the treatment of CAD. In 1978, Andreas Gruntzig published a description of five patients not suitable for CABG, including two with LMCAD, successfully treated with a novel method—percutaneous transluminal coronary angioplasty (PTCA) [8]. As he reported few severe acute complications, the initial

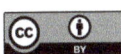

results were promising. Yet, there was still no data on its long-term complications and safety. Further research revealed that application of PTCA in LMCA was highly unfavorable, and bore a high risk of death and restenosis [9]. It led to the grounding of the CABG position as the first choice for LMCAD treatment for almost twenty years [10].

However, the development of bare-metal stents (BMS) and, finally, drug-eluting stents (DES) led to the necessity of reconsideration percutaneous coronary interventions (PCI) as the method of LMCAD treatment, at least in some subgroups [11]. In the early 2000s, multiple studies provided evidence on the effectiveness and safety of PCI in LMCA, which was eventually reflected in 2009 as the new class IIb recommendation in ACC/AHA guidelines, starting a new chapter in coronary artery revascularization [12–14]. Recent years brought several highly acclaimed multicentre RCTs and large-register analyses comparing the use of CABG and PCI in LMCAD [15–19]. Nevertheless, despite the fine quality of the aforementioned research, the long-term outcomes and prognoses of percutaneous treatment of this special disease are inconsistent.

In this article, we aim to provide a comprehensive review of state-of-the-art diagnostic and treatment techniques of left main coronary artery disease, focusing on percutaneous methods.

2. Evidence Supporting LMCA Revascularization

Decision on therapeutic strategy in ischaemic heart disease is an important issue. Current guidelines supporting significant LMCA revascularization are based on the early studies documenting the survival advantage of CABG compared to medical therapy (MT). A recent landmark ischemia trial that proved similar effects of an invasive approach compared to MT excluded individuals with significant unprotected left main coronary artery (ULMCA) stenosis [20]. Due to safety concerns, most recent studies addressing invasive and conservative strategies did not include patients with ULMCA. In fact, no RCT directly compared DES with MT in LMCAD. The meta-analysis by Shah et al. that focused on the comparison of CABG to DES to MT, revealed that an invasive approach was associated with better survival over short, intermediate, and long term [7]. To sum up, current evidence supports ULMCA revascularization over MT, however, future groundbreaking RCTs may influence physicians' approach.

The beginning of the 21st century carried rapid and notable advancements in the field of percutaneous device technology, pharmacological treatment (e.g., dual antiplatelet therapy (DAPT)), procedural techniques, and imaging. The higher risk of adverse cardiovascular events led to the abandonment of BMS in favor of more promising DES [21,22]. All the aforementioned factors have contributed to the renewed enthusiasm for the percutaneous approach in the treatment of LMCAD and resulted in registry studies and, eventually, multicentre RCTs that focused on its comparison with conventional surgical treatment.

2.1. Randomized Clinical Trials

Although early registry and nonrandomized studies suggested promising data on outcomes of percutaneous treatment, they were prone to selection bias and confounding. When the results of RCTs targeted on LMCAD treatment were finally published, they mostly suggested the comparable efficacy and safety of percutaneous and surgical treatment in terms of various endpoints [16,17,23–30]. The summary of the major studies and their findings are presented in Table 1. Recent years brought the awaited long-term follow-ups that provided new insights into differences between revascularization strategies [15,16,18,19].

Available presently, 10-year follow-up data of LE MANS (Left Main Coronary Artery Stenting), PRECOMBAT (Premier of Randomized Comparison of Bypass Surgery versus Angioplasty Using Sirolimus-Eluting Stent in Patients with Left Main Coronary Artery Disease) and SYNTAXES (SYNTAX Extended Survival) maintained the previously reported trends of comparable outcomes provided by both strategies. It is, however, noteworthy that all the above RCTs were underpowered due to either too small population or unexpectedly low event rates, thus their findings should be considered hypotheses-generating.

Table 1. Summary of random clinical trials comparing PCI with CABG in left main coronary artery disease.

	LE MANS [17]	Boudriot et al. [29]	SYNTAX-LM [27,31]	PRECOMBAT [19,25]	EXCEL [15,24]	NOBLE [16,23]
Recruitment period	2001–2004	2003–2009	2005–2007	2004–2009	2010–2014	2008–2015
Follow-up (years)	10	1	5; 10 for mortality only	10	5	5
PCI/CABG (n)	52/53	100/101	357/348	300/300	948/957	592/592
Bifurcation disease (%)	58	72	61	65	81	81
Mean LVEF (%)	54	65	N/D	61	57	60
Age (years)	61	68	65	62	66	66
IVUS (%)	Recommended	No recommendation	N/D	91	77	74
Mean SYNTAX score	N/D	23	30	25	21	22
Stents	BMS and DES (35%)	DP-SES	DP-PES	DP-SES	DP-EES	BP-BES and DP-SES (8%)
OPCAB (%)	1.9	46	N/D	64	29	16
LIMA (%)	72	99	97	94	99	96
Primary endpoint	Change in LVEF	All-cause death, MI, repeat revascularization	All-cause death, stroke, MI, repeat revascularization; 10-years all-cause death	Any-cause death, MI, stroke, TVR	Any-cause death, MI, stroke	Any-cause death, nonprocedural MI, stroke, repeat revascularization
Outcomes	Trend toward higher LVEF in PCI	PCI inferior to CABG	PCI non-inferior to CABG at 5-years; No difference in all-cause death at 10-years	PCI non-inferior to CABG	PCI non-inferior to CABG	PCI inferior to CABG

BMS—bare metal stents, BP-BES—biodegradable polymer biolimus-eluting stent, CABG—coronary artery bypass grafting, DES—drug-eluting stent, DP-EES—durable polymer everolimus-eluting stent, DP-PES—durable polymer paclitaxel-eluting stent, DP-SES—durable-polymer sirolimus-eluting stent, EXCEL—Evaluation of Xience Everolimus Eluting Stent vs. Coronary Artery Bypass Surgery for Effectiveness of Left Main Revascularization, IVUS—intravascular ultrasound, LE MANS—Left Main Stenting, LIMA—left internal mammary artery, LVEF—left ventricular ejection fraction, MI—myocardial infarction, N/D—no data, NOBLE—Nordic-Baltic-British Left Main Revascularization, OPCAB—off-pump coronary artery bypass, PCI—percutaneous coronary intervention, PRECOMBAT—Premier of Randomized Comparison of Bypass Surgery versus Angioplasty Using Sirolimus-Eluting Stent in Patients with Left Main Coronary Artery Disease, SYNTAX—Synergy Between Percutaneous Coronary Intervention With TAXUS and Cardiac Surgery, SYNTAX-LM—left main substudy of the SYNTAX, TVR—target vessel revascularization.

Only two of the RCTs focusing solely on LMCAD treatment were sufficiently powered for non-inferiority testing of prespecified major adverse cardiac and cerebrovascular events (MACCE)–EXCEL (Evaluation of Xience Everolimus Eluting Stent vs. Coronary Artery Bypass Surgery for Effectiveness of Left Main Revascularization) and NOBLE (Nordic-Baltic-British Left Main Revascularization) trials. While the highly anticipated results were expected to shed more light on the uncertainties, not only did they not break the deadlock, but also provided conflicting outcomes. Although the added value of studies is indisputable, they both have been criticized for their shortcomings and aroused various controversies. To discuss and understand the dissimilarities in outcomes, it is important to know the analogies and disparities between their design.

They have been both conducted as non-inferiority randomized trials comparing PCI with CABG in LMCAD. The EXCEL trial recruited 1,905 patients with angiographical LMCA stenosis of 70% or 50–70% stenosis with additional non-invasive or invasive testing proving hemodynamically significant lesion. Additional inclusion criterium was low or intermediate anatomical complexity (expressed as SYNTAX (Synergy between Percutaneous Coronary Intervention with TAXUS and Cardiac Surgery) score ≤ 32). Patients were randomly allocated to either PCI (n = 948) or CABG (n = 957) group. All patients received second-generation fluoropolymer-based cobalt–chromium everolimus-eluting stents (EES). The NOBLE trial consisted of 1,201 patients, 598 randomized to PCI and 603 to CABG. Inclusion criteria involved visually assessed stenosis of LMCA ≥ 50% or fractional flow reserve (FFR) ≤ 0.80. SYNTAX score was not utilized as the inclusion or exclusion criterium. Instead, patients with a complex lesion or more than three additional non-complex lesions were excluded (complex lesions were defined as chronic total occlusions, bifurcation lesions requiring two stent techniques, or lesions with calcified or tortuous vessel morphology). In the beginning, around 10% of patients were treated with first-generation sirolimus-eluting stents (SESs), and the rest received newer-generation biolimus-eluting stents (BESs). Primary composite endpoints differed between the two studies: EXCEL included all-cause death, myocardial infarction (MI), and stroke, while NOBLE predefined MACCE as all-cause death, non-procedural MI, stroke, or any repeat revascularization.

Both three-year and five-year follow-up of EXCEL presented that PCI is non-inferior to CABG in terms of primary composite endpoints. However, when analyzing individual endpoints in the five-year follow-up, it turned out that death from any cause occurred more frequently in the PCI group. On the other hand, short- and mid-term follow-up of NOBLE revealed that although PCI was inferior to CABG, all-cause mortality rates were not affected.

At a glance, contrary results of the landmark RCTs require cautious analysis. There are at least a few sources of discrepancies that could be located on the studies' timelines. At the very beginning, the assessment strategies for eligibility of patients for both revascularization techniques were different. In EXCEL there was a clear heart team (i.e., an interventional cardiologist and a cardiac surgeon) involvement in decision-making, while the multidisciplinary qualification was more ambiguous in NOBLE. It might have led to the heterogeneity of patients enrolled in the study, affecting later outcomes. Secondly, there were previously discussed differences in used device technology. According to the NOBLE authors, the average LMCA diameter is above 4 mm (average 5.7 mm), while the maximum size of used BES was 4.0 mm. Only half of the patients underwent post-dilatation with balloons larger than 4 mm, suggesting that stent underexpansion and malapposition might have contributed to the high rate of revascularizations. If we compare rates of therapy failure defined as definite stent thrombosis or symptomatic graft occlusion between two trials, there are major discrepancies. In NOBLE there were no significant differences in failure ratios between the two strategies (2% vs. 4% for PCI and CABG, respectively), while the superiority of the percutaneous method was apparent in the EXCEL trial (1.1% vs. 6.5% for PCI and CABG, respectively). Additionally, in NOBLE percutaneous treatment in patients with low SYNTAX score (<23) was unexpectedly found to be significantly inferior to surgery. Interestingly, in the PCI arm in NOBLE, there was an unexplainable high prevalence of stroke occurrence at one year, which coincides with DAPT cessation. Arguably the most important disparities concerned composite primary endpoints. EXCEL focused on the previously discussed hard endpoints, while NOBLE adopted any revascularization as well. On the one hand, the NOBLE investigators excluded periprocedural MI from MACCE, but on the other, the EXCEL researchers used the SCAI definition of MI which favored PCI [32]. As a result, NOBLE outcomes were largely driven by the inclusion of revascularization into composite endpoints, and on the other side EXCEL non-inferiority of PCI was driven by a lower incidence of periprocedural MI. Knowing the late cross-over of event curves, the longer follow-up of the studies will deliver further valuable information on both procedures' effectiveness and safety.

2.2. Meta-Analyses

The publication of numerous long-term follow-up outcomes of RCTs prompted the patient- and study-level meta-analysis. Most of them are consistent with each other, stating that PCI and CABG are similarly safe in terms of all-cause mortality, MI, and stroke, however percutaneously treated patients more frequently required repeat revascularization. The summary of selected meta-analyses is presented in Table 2.

Table 2. The summary of selected meta-analyses of RCTs comparing PCI with CABG in LMCAD.

	Palmerini et al. [33]	Head et al. [34]	Ahmad et al. [35]	Bajraktari et al. [36]	D'Ascenzo et al. [37] *	Sabatine et al. [38]
Year of publication	2017	2018	2020	2020	2021	2021
Number of analyzed RCTs	6	11	5	5	4	4
Number of patients (PCI/CABG)	4686 (2347/2339)	4478 (2233/2245)	4612 (2303/2309)	4499 (2249/2250)	4394 (2197/2197)	4394 (2197/2197)
Primary outcome	All-cause mortality	All-cause mortality	All-cause mortality	A composite of all-cause mortality, MI, or stroke	All-cause mortality	All-cause mortality
Results for primary outcome	HR = 0.99, 95% CI 0.76–1.3, p = 0.74	RR = 1.07, 95% CI 0.87–1.33, p = 0.52	RR = 1.03, 95% CI 0.82–1.30, p = 0.78	RR = 1.13, 95% CI 0.94–1.36, p = 0.19	OR = 0.93, 95% CI 0.71–1.21, p = 0.58	HR = 1.10, 95% CI 0.91–1.32, p = 0.33
Other findings	CV mortality: HR = 1.01, 95% CI 0.72–1.42, p = 0.83 MI: HR = 1.33, 95% CI 0.84–2.11, p = 0.11 Stroke: HR = 0.71, 95% CI 0.34–1.49, p = 0.31 UR: HR = 1.74, 95% CI 1.47–2.07, p < 0.001 Significant interaction for CV mortality between treatment and the SYNTAX score, p for interaction = 0.03	In diabetic patients: RR = 1.34, 95% CI 0.93–1.91, p = 0.11; In non–diabetic patients: RR = 0.94, 95% CI 0.72–1.23, p = 0.65, p for interaction = 0.13 SYNTAX score 0–22: RR = 0.91, 95% CI 0.60–1.36, p = 0.64 SYNTAX score 23–32: RR = 0.92, 95% CI 0.65–1.30, p = 0.65 SYNTAX score ≥ 33: RR = 1.39, 95% CI 0.94–2.06, p = 0.10, p for interaction = 0.38	CV mortality: RR = 1.03, 95% CI 0.79–1.34, p = 0.82 Stroke: RR = 0.74, 95% CI 0.36–1.50, p = 0.40 MI: RR = 1.22, 95% CI 0.96–1.56, p = 0.11 UR: RR = 1.73, 95% CI 1.49–2.02, p < 0.001	All-cause mortality: RR = 1.07, 95% CI 0.89–1.28, p = 0.48 CV mortality: RR 1.13, 95% CI 0.89–1.43, p = 0.31 Stroke: RR = 0.87, 95% CI 0.62–1.23, p = 0.42 MI: RR = 1.48, 95% CI 0.97–2.25, p = 0.07 UR: RR = 1.70, 95% CI 1.34–2.15, p < 0.001	MACCE (all–cause mortality, MI, stroke, repeat revascularization): OR = 0.69, 95% CI 0.60–0.79, p < 0.001 CV mortality: OR = 0.95, 95% CI 0.68–1.32, p = 0.75 Stroke: OR = 1.17, 95% CI 0.59–2.31, p = 0.66 MI: OR = 0.48, 95% CI 0.36–0.65, p < 0.001 Repeat revascularization: OR = 0.53, 95% CI 0.45–0.64, p < 0.001	CV mortality: HR = 1.07, 95% CI 0.83–1.37, p = 0.61 Stroke: HR = 0.84, 95% CI 0.59–1.21, p = 0.36 Spontaneous MI: HR = 2.35, 95% CI 1.71–3.23, p < 0.001 Repeat revascularization: HR = 1.78, 95% CI 1.51–2.10, p < 0.001 10–year all-cause death: HR = 1.10, 95% CI 0.93–1.29, p = 0.25
Interpretation	PCI and CABG showed similar mortality; interaction effect suggesting relatively lower mortality with PCI in patients with low SYNTAX score and relatively lower mortality with CABG in patients with high SYNTAX score	PCI and CABG showed similar mortality, regardless of diabetic status and SYNTAX score	PCI and CABG showed similar mortality; UR was less common after CABG	PCI and CABG showed similar mortality; UR was less common after CABG	PCI and CABG showed similar mortality; CABG reduced risk of MI, revascularization and MACCE, especially in older patients and with high SYNTAX score	PCI and CABG showed similar mortality; MI and repeat revascularization were less common after CABG

* All ORs are reported for CABG compared with PCI, CABG–coronary artery bypass grafting, CI—confidence interval, CV—cardiovascular, HR—hazard ratio, MACCE—major adverse cardiac or cerebrovascular event, OR—odds ratio, PCI–percutaneous coronary intervention, RR—risk ratio, UR—unplanned revascularization.

2.3. Special Groups

When considering the optimal strategy for LMCA revascularization, not only the severity of CAD and the possibility of achieving complete revascularization is important, as comorbidities, age, and past medical history also influence the treatment. As RCTs are prone to strict enrolment criteria, they might not appropriately reflect patients that are met in everyday practice. According to multiple reports, patients over the last years tend to be older and sicker. As a consequence, due to high surgical risk, PCI is more often a method of choice. It was well expressed by Kataruka et al. in their analysis, reporting over a two-fold increase in LMCA PCI between the years 2005 and 2017 [39]. The apparent diversity of patients and little evidence supporting management strategies in special groups may raise clinical uncertainties.

2.3.1. Diabetes Mellitus

Diabetes mellitus (DM) is one of the most challenging comorbidities associated with CAD. Patients with DM are at a higher risk of developing severe CAD, complications after revascularization, and risk of restenosis [40]. After the initial decrease of DM-related complications, such as MI, recent years have brought an alarming trend of their resurgence, mainly among younger patients [41]. Traditionally, diabetes has been a strong indication for CABG treatment, especially in patients suffering from a multivessel disease (MVD). Although there is evidence supporting CABG in such cases, the choice of optimal treatment in LMCAD is blurrier [34]. In the BMS era, there was a noticeable benefit of CABG over PCI in LMCAD with concomitant DM, but the development of DES has once again led to the need for reconsideration of optimal revascularization strategy [42]. Although no trial has solely focused on diabetic patients, there is recent evidence derived from subanalyses of the aforementioned modern RCTs and large registry studies that suggest similar outcomes of PCI compared with CABG. Head et al. in their pooled analysis of individual patient data from 11 trials, reported that five-year all-cause mortality was similar in patients treated with either method, and diabetes status did not interact with the treatment effect (p for interaction = 0.13) [34]. A more recent meta-analysis performed by Sabatine et al. supported these findings [38].

In conclusion, PCI with modern-era DES became a valuable option for diabetic patients with LMCAD. Nevertheless, CABG remains the treatment of choice for MVD involving LMCA with concomitant DM.

2.3.2. Chronic Kidney Disease

Chronic kidney disease (CKD) is a well-known condition associated not only with more diffuse CAD, but also with a poorer prognosis [43]. A recently published RCT suggested that there is no benefit of the early revascularization approach in such patients [44]. Data on LMCAD treatment with concomitant CKD is limited, but lately presented evidence mostly supports the equivalence of CABG and PCI, especially in terms of all-cause mortality rates [45–48]. Patients who obtained percutaneous treatment more often required repeat revascularization, while surgery was linked with a higher risk of stroke. However, the benefits of CABG were significant in severe CKD, which is consistent with Lee et al. findings of a patient-pooled analysis of PCI outcomes [49].

2.3.3. Left Ventricular Dysfunction

Heart failure (HF) and CAD often accompany each other, as the latter is the most common cause of left ventricular (LV) dysfunction [50]. The improved survival of patients with MI, among others, has resulted in the increasing prevalence of HF over the last years [50,51]. According to Bollano et al. the utilization of coronary angiography in patients with HF between 2000 and 2018 has increased by 5.5% per year, resulting in an increased number of revascularizations and a better long-term prognosis. Interestingly, no such increase was seen for angina pectoris and ST-elevation myocardial infarction (STEMI) [52]. The choice of revascularization method in patients with reduced left ventricular ejection fraction (LVEF) may determine their long-term survival. The STICH (Surgical Treatment for Ischemic Heart Failure) trial proved that CABG is superior to medical therapy in patients with ischemic cardiomyopathy at a ten-year follow-up [53]. On the other hand, the most recent REVIVED trial has questioned the reasonableness of PCI in patients with severe ischaemic LV dysfunction [54]. Importantly, the study included 95 patients with LMCAD. In the overall cohort and in the LMCAD subgroup, the percutaneous approach did not result in a lower incidence of death from any cause or hospitalization for heart failure when compared to medical therapy. However, there are a few concerns regarding the study design. First of all, it was an open-label trial. Secondly, lesion-significance assessment did not include intravascular imaging or physiological assessment, which may have especially influenced patients with LMCAD. Thirdly, as much as 66% of individuals in the PCI arm were asymptomatic, therefore results cannot be easily extrapolated to patients with angina. Several observational studies and meta-analyses compare invasive methods of treatment revealed better outcomes of surgery in patients with reduced LVEF and CAD [34,55–58]. When it comes to the management of patients with LMCAD, Wolff et al. reported that CABG was associated with significantly improved survival compared with PCI [57]. A recent analysis of the IRIS-MAIN (Interventional Research Incorporation Society-Left MAIN Revascularization) registry proved that PCI was inferior to CABG in terms of the primary composite outcome of death, MI, or stroke in patients with LVEF < 45% [59]. On the other hand, the results of the EXCEL trial and Bangalore et al. study showed similar results regarding primary composite endpoint and long-term survival, respectively [24,60]. Moreover, the superiority of the surgical approach was not significant in the IRIS-MAIN registry when complete revascularization was achieved. It is consistent with other studies, indicating that completeness of revascularization should be a priority in patients with reduced LVEF [57,60]. All things considered, contemporary evidence suggests that patients suffering from LMCAD and reduced LVEF may benefit best from CABG. For those ineligible for surgery, complete percutaneous revascularization may be a valuable alternative.

2.3.4. Age

With improving life expectancy, it is projected that in the United States by 2050 will be home to 18 million people aged 85 or above [61]. Age is a powerful risk factor for CAD, adverse outcomes after cardiovascular events, and complications related to invasive treatment [62]. Elderly patients undergoing cardiac surgeries may be at an especially high risk of negative outcomes. Tran et al. in their analysis revealed that frailty syndrome was remarkably more prevalent in the group of patients undergoing CABG compared with patients undergoing major noncardiac surgery (22% vs. 3%). Recent studies comparing the percutaneous approach with surgical treatment of CAD brought mixed results. The superiority of CABG was especially marked in patients with MVD, but not in LMCAD [63–65]. A substudy from the DELTA registry (Drug-Eluting stent for LefT main Artery) found no difference in the occurrence of the primary endpoint in octogenarians after CABG and PCI [66]. Recently published results of a subanalysis of the ten-year follow-up SYNTAX Extended Study which focused on elderly individuals (>70 years old) with three-vessel disease and/or LMCAD reported comparable ten-year all-cause death, life expectancy, five-year MACCE, and five-year quality of life (QOL) status irrespective of revascularization mode [67]. Moreover, there was no significant difference between the relative risks of the treatment effects in the EXCEL trial, and no interaction between age and revascularization methods for the primary outcome was found in the NOBLE trial [15,16]. Sabatine et al. in their meta-analysis found no statistically significant heterogeneity for five-year all-cause deaths in a group of patients suffering from LMCAD aged ≥65 compared with <65 years old [38]. Based on present-day evidence, providing similar effects concerning mortality and QOL, PCI is an important alternative to CABG in LMCAD treatment in the elderly. Results suggest that concomitant comorbidities, frailty syndrome, and expected QOL, rather than chronological age, might be more relevant when considering optimal revascularization strategy in this group.

2.3.5. Lesion Anatomy

When planning the optimal revascularization technique for LMCA, lesion localization and vessel anatomy must be taken into consideration. LMCA is usually divided into three segments—ostium, shaft, and distal segment (Figure 1). As atherosclerotic plaques can localize in every part, treatment strategies are different. The early RCT conducted by Boudriot et al. reported that the incidence of MACCE in the PCI arm differed dramatically regarding lesion location (1.0% in ostium/shaft and 18% in distal segment) [29]. Later, MAIN-COMPARE (Revascularization for Unprotected Left Main Coronary Artery Stenosis:

Comparison of Percutaneous Coronary Angioplasty Versus Surgical Revascularization) and DELTA registry analyses brought evidence that lesions located in the ostium and shaft treated by either revascularization method provided comparable outcomes [68,69]. Earlier, the analysis of the latter registry revealed that bifurcation compared with ostial/shaft angioplasty was associated with a higher incidence of MACCE [70]. Long-term follow-up of MAIN-COMPARE demonstrated unfavorable outcomes of PCI compared with CABG for distal LMCAD [71]. Percutaneous treatment was associated with a significantly higher risk for death and composite outcome (hazard ratio (HR): 1.78, 95% confidence interval (95% CI): 1.22–2.59; HR: 1.94, 95% CI: 1.35–2.79 for death and composite outcome, respectively). In contrast, this effect was not observed for ostial or shaft lesions. Interestingly, analysis of the EXCEL trial proved only greater rates of repeat revascularizations, with no influence on the incidence of primary composite outcome after PCI, compared with CABG in the group of patients with bifurcation disease. In the case of lesions located in the ostium/shaft, both treatment methods provided similar results in terms of primary composite outcomes and repeat revascularization rates [72]. Recent findings of a meta-analysis performed by De Filippo et al. supported the superiority of CABG in distal but not in ostial/shaft LMCAD [73]. In summary, contemporary evidence suggests that heterogeneity related to the location of atherosclerotic plaques in LMCA is an important factor that should influence the decision regarding revascularization method. For ostial/shaft lesions, both techniques provide similar prognosis and durability, whereas surgery gives better outcomes when applied to the distal LMCAD. In patients with bifurcation disease selected for percutaneous treatment, better outcomes may be achieved by preferably using the double kissing crush (DK crush) stenting technique, the appliance of intravascular imaging, and appropriate stent optimization [74,75].

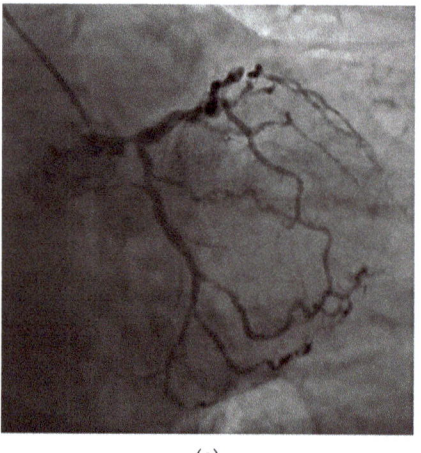
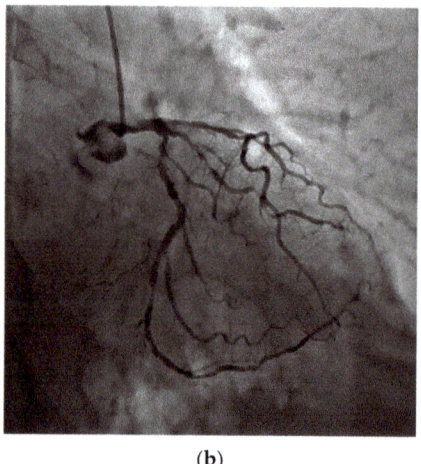

(a) (b)

Figure 1. Coronary angiograms. (**a**) Severe distal left main coronary artery (LMCA) lesion. (**b**) Disseminated coronary artery disease with shaft LMCA lesion.

3. State-of-the-Art Evaluation of LMCAD

Significant LMCA stenosis is detected in 4–6% of patients referred for coronary angiography, occasionally also in asymptomatic individuals [4]. Knowing the unfavorable prognosis of untreated LMCAD, precise evaluation of atherosclerotic plaque is essential in further management. Due to overlapping of side branches, lesion eccentricity, vessel foreshortening, and angulation, conventional coronary angiography has its limitations, especially in intermediate (40–70%) LMCA narrowing. Moreover, the significance of stenosis assessed angiographically is observer-dependent, and the reproducibility of results is low even between experienced clinicians [76,77]. To avoid misclassification of the disease, recent years brought the development of various adjunctive tools that are helpful in the decision-making process.

3.1. Intravascular Imaging

Intravascular ultrasound (IVUS) is the best-established method of intravascular imaging in LMCAD evaluation. It may provide valuable information on the plaque extent, cross-sectional characteristics of the lesion, and minimal lumen area (MLA) in LMCA and its branches (i.e., left anterior descending artery (LAD), left circumflex artery (LCx)). As it became evident that plaque burden at the MLA is an independent predictor of events, researchers strived to set an optimal threshold for determining the significance of LMCA stenosis [78,79]. Firstly, based on the analysis of 55 patients and a fractional flow reserve (FFR) of 0.75, Jasti et al. proposed a cut-off value of 5.9 mm^2 [80]. Later, the prospective multicentre LITRO study validated an MLA of 6.0 mm^2 as a safe value for LMCA revascularization deferral [81]. In a two-year follow-up period, between patients with MLA < 6.0 mm^2 who underwent revascularization and deferred patients with MLA $\geq$ 6.0 mm^2, there were no significant differences in survival and MACCE rates. Since then, the MLA of 6.0 mm^2 became a widely acknowledged cut-off value for deferring revascularization of the LMCA. Nonetheless, both of the aforementioned studies were conducted in Western populations. Park et al. in their analysis of 112 Asian individuals proposed IVUS derived MLA of 4.5 mm^2 as a cut-off value for an FFR of $\leq$0.8 [82]. A plausible explanation of these discrepancies may include ethnic differences in coronary artery dimensions. The mean MLA of patients included in the Asian study was 4.8 mm^2, while Jasti et al. reported a mean MLA of 7.65 mm^2 in their study group. Ethnic differences in LMCA anatomy were also supported by a comparative study of 99 Asian and 99 United States white patients (MLA 5.2 $\pm$ 1.8 vs. 6.2 $\pm$ 14 mm^2, respectively) [83].

Not only is IVUS a useful tool for LMCAD assessment, but also it may provide important information on stent adequate expansion and apposition. Early insights from the MAIN-COMPARE registry provided evidence on a better prognosis of patients with LMCAD who underwent PCI under the guidance of IVUS in comparison to only conventional angiography [84]. The reduction in three-year incidence of mortality was especially marked in the group of patients who received DES (4.7% vs. 16.0%, log-rank p = 0.048) and no difference was observed in the group treated with BMS (8.6% vs. 10.8%, log-rank p = 0.35). Further registry studies supported these findings [85–87]. The meta-analysis of ten studies performed by Ye et al. revealed that IVUS-guided PCI of LMCA impressively reduced the risks of all-cause death by 40% compared with angiography-guided PCI [88]. The benefit of IVUS-guidance may especially include stent optimization. It was proved in an early analysis of RCTs by Doi et al. that post-intervention minimum stent area (MSA) measured by IVUS was an important factor that could predict in-stent restenosis (ISR) after nine-months of follow-up, and the authors suggested an MSA threshold of 5.7 mm^2 for paclitaxel-eluting stents [89]. In the EXCEL trial IVUS-substudy there was a strong association between the group of patients with small final MSA (4.4–8.7 mm^2) and the occurrence of adverse events during long-term follow-up, compared with patients with the largest MSA (11.0–17.8 mm^2) [90]. The currently best-known proposed MSA cut-off values that predicted ISR are 5.0 mm^2 for LCx, 6.3 mm^2 for LAD, 7.2 mm^2 for confluence zone, and 8.2 mm^2 for LMCA [91]. However, nowadays some clinicians advocate for higher MSA thresholds, as in the DK-CRUSH VIII trial (>10 mm^2, >7 mm^2, >6 mm^2 for LMCA, LAD, and LCx, respectively) [92]. To sum up, IVUS is an important tool that can improve PCI performance, leading to fewer procedural-related complications and a better prognosis in patients with LMCAD.

Optical coherence tomography (OCT) is a newer method that can provide excellent resolution images influencing a better assessment of plaque phenotype and identification of PCI-related complications. However, due to technology that requires proper blood clearance, OCT cannot be applied to coronary artery ostia. Another drawback includes low tissue penetration which limits the utilization of this method in LMCA stenosis assessment [93]. Despite that, recent studies investigated its outcomes in PCI of LMCA in comparison with IVUS and conventional angiography, especially in bifurcation disease. In the retrospective analysis of 730 patients, OCT was found to be superior to angiography in distal LMCA stenting with no difference compared to IVUS-guidance [94]. In the LEMON trial that analyzed the feasibility, safety, and impact of OCT-guided LMCA PCI, the primary endpoint of procedural success was achieved in 86% of subjects, suggesting that OCT may be a suitable tool for PCI guidance in distal LMCA [95]. Although contemporary results are promising, further research that investigates safety, long-term outcomes in big arteries, and OCT correlation with physiological assessment is needed.

3.2. Physiological Assessment

Knowing the limited accuracy of conventional coronary angiography in the evaluation of LMCAD significance, a physiological assessment may deliver crucial information on the ischemic potential of vessel narrowing, determining further management strategy. A study conducted by Hamilos et al. proved that the FFR threshold of ≥ 0.80 for LMCA revascularization deferral is safe and clinical outcomes in such patients were similar to those who obtained surgical treatment based on the FFR values < 0.80 [96]. The data on the safety and feasibility of FFR-based deferral was later supported by various meta-analyses, RCTs, and register studies [97–100]. Moreover, decisions based on visually assessed 50% diameter stenosis (DS) may not accurately reflect the hemodynamic and functional significance of the vessel narrowing, especially in LMCA. Interestingly, an analysis of 152 patients revealed that the optimal cut-off value of DS for predicting FFR ≤ 0.80 was 43%, and multiple studies supported visual-functional mismatch in patients with LMCA lesions [96,101,102]. However, it is noteworthy that FFR interpretation in patients with bifurcation disease or downstream stenoses requires special caution, as it may cause under- or over-estimation of LMCA narrowing functional significance [103–105].

Apart from the pre-PCI assessment of LMCAD, FFR is also a useful tool in post-PCI functional optimization or jailed side branch management. According to previous studies that focused on functional significance of side branches after bifurcation crossover stenting, angiography alone tends to overestimate the functional severity of stenoses [106,107]. When it comes to LMCA, Lee et al. reported that only 16.9% of patients that underwent simple crossover stenting had FFR < 0.80 in jailed LCx, and no correlation between FFR values and angiographic percent DS was found [108]. Moreover, at five years, patients with higher FFR values had lower target lesion failure (TLF) rates, while no difference in such outcomes was found based solely on DS. It suggests insufficient angiographic accuracy in the evaluation of jailed LCx functional significance and, consequently, that in most cases complex procedures can be avoided by postinterventional FFR assessment.

Recently, instantaneous wave-free ratio (iFR) established the position of a valuable tool that provides outcomes non-inferior to FFR in CAD treatment [109–111]. However, data on its safety and long-term clinical outcomes in LMCAD assessment is currently limited. A study by Warisawa et al. indicates that iFR cutoff ≤ 0.89 for LMCA revascularization deferral is safe, and at a median follow-up of 30 months, MACCE rates were similar to patients that underwent invasive management [112]. If confirmed in further studies, iFR may become an important adenosine-free alternative to FFR in LMCAD evaluation.

4. Percutaneous Management Techniques

Evolution and pursuit of better clinical outcomes in patients with LMCAD also affected percutaneous management techniques. As mentioned before, atherosclerotic plaques localized in the distal segment of LMCA are related to a higher incidence of MACCE compared with ostial/shaft lesions. Therefore, optimal stenting technique for bifurcation disease was a subject of special interest over the last years.

Early RCTs concerning percutaneous treatment provided data on unfavorable outcomes of the two-stent technique in coronary artery bifurcations, and advocated for provisional stenting (PS) in such cases [113,114]. Contrary to them, DKCRUSH-II (Randomized

Study on Double Kissing Crush Technique Versus Provisional Stenting Technique for Coronary Artery Bifurcation Lesions) reported that the DK crush technique in selected patients was associated with lower target lesion revascularization (TLR) and target vessel revascularization (TVR) rates compared with PS [115]. The results of this study evoked scientists' interest in further research of the optimal percutaneous approach in coronary bifurcation disease, including distal LMCA. Besides RCTs that involved all-comer bifurcation lesions, two of them focused exclusively on LMCA. DKCRUSH-V trial investigated the difference in TLF between patients with LMCAD that underwent PS compared with DK crush [74]. At three years, the two-stent technique was associated with significantly better outcomes (TLF occurred in 16.9% and 8.3% of patients in the PS and DK crush groups ($p = 0.005$), respectively), and the advantage was especially marked in complex lesions. On the other hand, in the EBC MAIN (European Bifurcation Club Left Main Study) patients with true LMCA bifurcation lesions were randomly allocated to a stepwise layered provisional strategy group or systemic dual stent approach [116]. Interestingly, although none of the analyzed methods proved to be significantly superior, a single-stent approach provided numerically better outcomes in terms of primary (and most of the secondary) endpoints. As the main findings differ between studies, a closer look into procedural characteristics may clarify the source of the discrepancy. Firstly, it is noteworthy that an earlier DKCRUSH-III study which focused on differences in clinical outcome between DK crush compared with culotte in distal LMCAD proved that at three years culotte stenting was associated with significantly increased rates of MACCE and stent thrombosis (ST) [117]. Moreover, the most recent network meta-analysis comparing bifurcation techniques that included 8318 patients from 29 RCTs reported that DK crush was superior to PS and other two-stent techniques [118]. Yet, in EBC MAIN culotte was the most common, and, on the contrary, DK crush was the least common technique used in a two-stent approach (53% and 5% for culotte and DK crush, respectively). Secondly, the PS protocol differed between the two studies—in EBC MAIN kissing balloon inflation (KBI) of the side vessel after stenting was a part of the procedure, whereas in DKCRUSH-V KBI was permitted only if residual DS of the side branch was >75%, or dissection ≥ type B, or Thrombolysis In Myocardial Infarction (TIMI) flow grade < 3 was present. As the studies comparing KBI with no-KBI in a one-stent approach provide non-consistent results, this difference in protocols presumably influenced the final outcomes of the aforementioned RCTs [119]. Lastly, it is noteworthy that operators included in the DKCRUSH-V study had to be well-experienced, as it was confirmed by sending three to five cases to the trial steering committee, which to some extent might have driven favorable DK crush outcomes. The question of whether if the procedure protocols had been unified would the outcomes of both RCTs be similar is thought-provoking, and suggests that further research with the state-of-the-art approach is needed.

When it comes to the recommendations, a provisional strategy followed by a proximal optimization technique (POT) is preferred for the majority of patients, especially without a true distal LMCA lesion [120]. In case of too distal balloon positioning during POT, carina shift resulting in side branch ostium lumen reduction might occur. In such cases, as described before, FFR assessment of functional significance might be applicable. Importantly, if a suboptimal effect was achieved or complications occur, such an approach allows conversion to a two-stent technique (T-, T and protrusion (TAP) or culotte) for a better final outcome. When deciding between a one-stent and up-front two-stent strategy, the complexity of LMCA lesion should be the key-determinant. Although no universal definition of complexity has been established, developed in the DEFINITION study (Definitions and impact of complEx biFurcation lesIons on clinical outcomes after percutaNeous coronary IntervenTIOn using drug-eluting steNts) criteria are the most acknowledged [121]. Recent results of the DEFINITION II trial, including 28.8% of patients with distal LMCAD, proved that for the pre-specified coronary bifurcation lesions, the complexity criteria two-stent approach was associated with significantly better outcomes compared with PS [122]. Of note, in this study, as much as 77.8% of patients in the two-stent group were treated with the DK crush technique. Current ESC/EACTS guidelines indicate that in true bifurcation lesions of

LMCA, DK crush may be preferred over provisional T-stenting (class IIb recommendation, level of evidence B) [123]. Even though presumably superior to other methods, it should be kept in mind that DK crush is technically demanding and optimal effects may be achieved in hands of experienced operators. Selected PCI bifurcation techniques are presented in Figure 2.

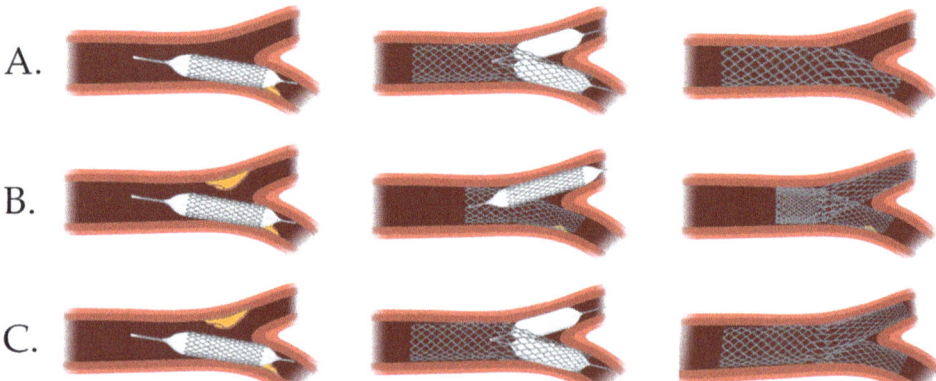

Figure 2. Selected percutaneous coronary intervention bifurcation techniques. (**A**) Provisional stenting, (**B**) culotte, (**C**) double kissing crush.

5. Current Guidelines and Future Directions

Surgical revascularization has established its position as a gold standard for LMCA revascularization, reflected in class I recommendation by European and US guidelines [123,124]. Over recent years, great progress has been made in the field of percutaneous CAD treatment, and its equivalence with CABG in selected patients was supported by gradually accumulated evidence, eventually earning a part in recommendations for LMCAD treatment. In the most recent European guidelines class of recommendation for PCI in LMCA was dependent on SYNTAX score: tertiles–I in the lowest, IIa in intermediate, or III in the highest [123]. On the other hand, last year, updated US clinical practice guidelines gave more unified class IIa recommendation for percutaneous treatment in selected patients for whom PCI can provide equivalent revascularization to that possible with CABG, without anatomical complexity stratification [124]. However, recommendations are consistent with each other when it comes to the multidisciplinary heart team involvement in the decision-making process. Such an approach can improve outcomes and minimize the risk of inappropriate use of revascularization strategies, as a marked variability in PCI-to-CABG ratios between countries was observed [125]. Surgical risk scores, such as the European System for Cardiac Operative Risk Evaluation (EuroSCORE II) and the Society of Thoracic Surgeons (STS) score, and anatomical complexity SYNTAX score may provide useful information that influences heart team discussion toward a more patient-orientated decision. If the outcomes are expected to be comparable, the preferences of the patient should be forefront. The summary of indications for PCI and CABG are presented in Figure 3.

Although great effort has been put to improve outcomes and dispel doubts concerning the optimal approach in LMCAD, not all issues have been resolved. Firstly, knowing the late cross-over of event curves, long- and very long-term follow-up of NOBLE and EXCEL are likely to deliver more information on the actual durability and effectiveness of percutaneous and surgical treatment. Secondly, more subgroup-dedicated studies that investigate optimal treatment options in specific patients are needed. Knowing the unequal clinical outcomes of various stenting techniques and the influence of adjunctive tools on PCI results, contemporary state-of-the-art percutaneous treatment comparison with CABG might start a new chapter in LMCAD revascularization.

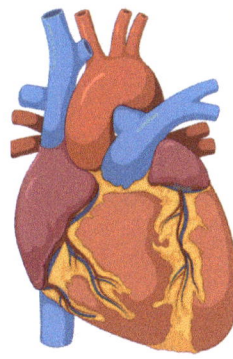
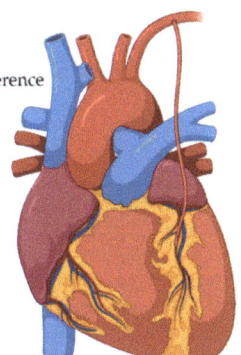

Favours PCI:
- Advanced age, comorbidities, high surgical risk, frailty
- Reduced life expectancy
- Restricted mobility
- Ostial/shaft lesion
- SYNTAX score <23
- Urgent revascularization

Favours CABG:
- Low LVEF
- Doubtful DAPT adherence or contraindications
- Diabetes and multivessel disease
- Bifurcation lesion
- SYNTAX score ≥23
- Concomitant cardiac surgery

Figure 3. Indications for percutaneous coronary intervention and coronary artery bypass grafting in left main coronary artery disease. CABG–coronary artery bypass grafting, DAPT–dual antiplatelet therapy, LVEF–left ventricular ejection fraction, PCI–percutaneous coronary intervention, SYNTAX - Synergy Between Percutaneous Coronary Intervention With TAXUS and Cardiac Surgery.

6. Conclusions

The last decades' developments and further progress in coronary revascularization methods were arguably one of the greatest steps in cardiology and changed the dramatic course of CAD. Although the declining trend in deaths due to IHD in high-income countries is caused by many factors, technical improvements and widespread access to percutaneous treatment are undoubtedly one of them. As for once-deadly LMCA stenosis, nowadays two effective treatment options are available. There is no unified algorithm for decision-making in LMCAD, but careful selection of patients and a multi-disciplinary heart team approach can provide the best management option at the time. Since the modern coronary revascularization philosophy has become patient-orientated, it is important to emphasize that PCI and CABG are not contradictory to each other but rather complementary in terms of reaching favorable outcomes in various clinical settings. Further years are expected to bring more research on LMCA treatment, but due to constant improvements in both techniques they will likely not break the deadlock and the optimal approach will remain a moving target.

Author Contributions: Conceptualization, E.J.D.; methodology, E.J.D.; writing—original draft preparation, E.J.D.; writing—review and editing, E.J.D. and M.K.; visualization, E.J.D.; supervision, M.K. and S.D. All authors have read and agreed to the published version of the manuscript.

Funding: This research received no external funding.

Institutional Review Board Statement: Not applicable.

Informed Consent Statement: Not applicable.

Data Availability Statement: Not applicable.

Conflicts of Interest: The authors declare no conflict of interest.

References

1. The Top 10 Causes of Death. Available online: https://www.who.int/news-room/fact-sheets/detail/the-top-10-causes-of-death (accessed on 22 June 2022).
2. Ramadan, R.; Boden, W.E.; Kinlay, S. Management of left main coronary artery disease. *J. Am. Heart Assoc.* **2018**, *7*, 8151. [CrossRef] [PubMed]
3. Maron, B.J.; Doerer, J.J.; Haas, T.S.; Tierney, D.M.; Mueller, F.O. Sudden Deaths in Young Competitive Athletes. *Circulation* **2009**, *119*, 1085–1092. [CrossRef] [PubMed]
4. Ragosta, M. Left main coronary artery disease: Importance, diagnosis, assessment, and management. *Curr. Probl. Cardiol.* **2015**, *40*, 93–126. [CrossRef] [PubMed]
5. Yusuf, S.; Zucker, D.; Peduzzi, P.; Fisher, L.D.; Takaro, T.; Kennedy, J.W.; Davis, K.; Killip, T.; Passamani, E.; Norris, R.; et al. Effect of coronary artery bypass graft surgery on survival: Overview of 10-year results from randomised trials by the Coronary Artery Bypass Graft Surgery Trialists Collaboration. *Lancet* **1994**, *344*, 563–570. [CrossRef]
6. Favaloro, R. Direct and Indirect Coronary Surgery. *Circulation* **1972**, *46*, 1197–1207. [CrossRef]
7. Shah, R.; Morsy, M.S.; Weiman, D.S.; Vetrovec, G.W. Meta-Analysis Comparing Coronary Artery Bypass Grafting to Drug-Eluting Stents and to Medical Therapy Alone for Left Main Coronary Artery Disease. *Am. J. Cardiol.* **2017**, *120*, 63–68. [CrossRef]
8. Grüntzig, A. Transluminal dilatation of coronary-artery stenosis. *Lancet* **1978**, *1*, 263. [CrossRef]
9. Braunwald, E. Treatment of Left Main Coronary Artery Disease. *N. Engl. J. Med.* **2016**, *375*, 2284–2285. [CrossRef]
10. Eagle, K.A.; Guyton, R.A.; Davidoff, R.; Edwards, F.H.; Ewy, G.A.; Gardner, T.J.; Hart, J.C.; Herrmann, H.C.; Hillis, L.D.; Hutter, A.; et al. ACC/AHA 2004 guideline update for coronary artery bypass graft surgery: Summary article. A report of the American College of Cardiology/American Heart Association Task Force on Practice Guidelines (Committee to Update the 1999 Guidelines for Coronary Artery Bypass Graft Surgery). *J. Am. Coll. Cardiol.* **2004**, *44*, 1146–1154. [CrossRef]
11. Kim, Y.H.; Dangas, G.D.; Solinas, E.; Aoki, J.; Parise, H.; Kimura, M.; Franklin-Bond, T.; Dasgupta, N.K.; Kirtane, A.J.; Moussa, I.; et al. Effectiveness of drug-eluting stent implantation for patients with unprotected left main coronary artery stenosis. *Am. J. Cardiol.* **2008**, *101*, 801–806. [CrossRef]
12. Seung, K.B.; Park, D.W.; Kim, Y.-H.; Lee, S.-W.; Lee, C.W.; Hong, M.-K.; Park, S.-W.; Yun, S.-C.; Gwon, H.-C.; Jeong, M.-H.; et al. Stents versus Coronary-Artery Bypass Grafting for Left Main Coronary Artery Disease. *N. Engl. J. Med.* **2008**, *358*, 1781–1792. [CrossRef] [PubMed]
13. Park, S.J.; Hong, M.K.; Lee, C.W.; Kim, J.J.; Song, J.K.; Kang, D.H.; Park, S.W.; Mintz, G.S. Elective stenting of unprotected left main coronary artery stenosis: Effect of debulking before stenting and intravascular ultrasound guidance. *J. Am. Coll. Cardiol.* **2001**, *38*, 1054–1060. [CrossRef]
14. Kushner, F.G.; Hand, M.; Smith, S.C.; King, S.B., Jr.; Anderson, J.L., 3rd; Antman, E.M.; Bailey, S.R.; Bates, E.R.; Blankenship, J.C.; Casey, D.E.; et al. 2009 Focused Updates: ACC/AHA Guidelines for the Management of Patients With ST-Elevation Myocardial Infarction (Updating the 2004 Guideline and 2007 Focused Update) and ACC/AHA/SCAI Guidelines on Percutaneous Coronary Intervention (Updating the 2005 Guideline and 2007 Focused Update): A Report of the American College of Cardiology Foundation/American Heart Association Task Force on Practice Guidelines. *J. Am. Coll. Cardiol.* **2009**, *54*, 2205–2241. [CrossRef] [PubMed]
15. Stone, G.W.; Kappetein, A.P.; Sabik, J.F.; Pocock, S.J.; Morice, M.C.; Puskas, J.; Kandzari, D.E.; Karmpaliotis, D.; Brown, W.M.; Lembo, N.J., 3rd; et al. Five-Year Outcomes after PCI or CABG for Left Main Coronary Disease. *N. Engl. J. Med.* **2019**, *381*, 1820–1830. [CrossRef] [PubMed]
16. Holm, N.R.; Mäkikallio, T.; Lindsay, M.M.; Spence, M.S.; Erglis, A.; Menown, I.; Trovik, T.; Kellerth, T.; Kalinauskas, G.; Mogensen, L.; et al. Percutaneous coronary angioplasty versus coronary artery bypass grafting in the treatment of unprotected left main stenosis: Updated 5-year outcomes from the randomised, non-inferiority NOBLE trial. *Lancet* **2020**, *395*, 191–199. [CrossRef]
17. Buszman, P.E.; Buszman, P.P.; Banasiewicz-Szkróbka, I.; Milewski, K.P.; Żurakowski, A.; Orlik, B.; Konkolewska, M.; Trela, B.; Janas, A.; Martin, J.L.; et al. Left Main Stenting in Comparison with Surgical Revascularization: 10-Year Outcomes of the (Left Main Coronary Artery Stenting) LE MANS Trial. *JACC Cardiovasc. Interv.* **2016**, *9*, 318–327. [CrossRef] [PubMed]
18. Thuijs, D.; Kappetein, A.P.; Serruys, P.W.; Mohr, F.W.; Morice, M.C.; Mack, M.J.; Holmes, D.R.; Curzen, N., Jr.; Davierwala, P.; Noack, T.; et al. Percutaneous coronary intervention versus coronary artery bypass grafting in patients with three-vessel or left main coronary artery disease: 10-year follow-up of the multicentre randomised controlled SYNTAX trial. *Lancet* **2019**, *394*, 1325–1334. [CrossRef]
19. Park, D.W.; Ahn, J.M.; Park, H.; Yun, S.C.; Kang, D.Y.; Lee, P.H.; Kim, Y.H.; Lim, D.S.; Rha, S.W.; Park, G.M.; et al. Ten-Year Outcomes After Drug-Eluting Stents Versus Coronary Artery Bypass Grafting for Left Main Coronary Disease: Extended Follow-Up of the PRECOMBAT Trial. *Circulation* **2020**, *141*, 1437–1446. [CrossRef]
20. Maron, D.J.; Hochman, J.S.; Reynolds, H.R.; Bangalore, S.; O'Brien, S.M.; Boden, W.E.; Chaitman, B.R.; Senior, R.; López-Sendón, J.; Alexander, K.P.; et al. Initial Invasive or Conservative Strategy for Stable Coronary Disease. *N. Engl. J. Med.* **2020**, *382*, 1395–1407. [CrossRef]
21. Piccolo, R.; Bonaa, K.H.; Efthimiou, O.; Varenne, O.; Baldo, A.; Urban, P.; Kaiser, C.; Remkes, W.; Räber, L.; de Belder, A.; et al. Drug-eluting or bare-metal stents for percutaneous coronary intervention: A systematic review and individual patient data meta-analysis of randomised clinical trials. *Lancet* **2019**, *393*, 2503–2510. [CrossRef]

22. Pandya, S.B.; Kim, Y.H.; Meyers, S.N.; Davidson, C.J.; Flaherty, J.D.; Park, D.W.; Mediratta, A.; Pieper, K.; Reyes, E.; Bonow, R.; et al. Drug-Eluting Stents versus Bare Metal Stents in Unprotected Left Main Coronary Artery Stenosis: A Meta-Analysis. *JACC Cardiovasc. Interv.* **2010**, *3*, 602. [CrossRef] [PubMed]
23. Mäkikallio, T.; Holm, N.R.; Lindsay, M.; Spence, M.S.; Erglis, A.; Menown, I.B.; Trovik, T.; Eskola, M.; Romppanen, H.; Kellerth, T.; et al. Percutaneous coronary angioplasty versus coronary artery bypass grafting in treatment of unprotected left main stenosis (NOBLE): A prospective, randomised, open-label, non-inferiority trial. *Lancet* **2016**, *388*, 2743–2752. [CrossRef]
24. Stone, G.W.; Sabik, J.F.; Serruys, P.W.; Simonton, C.A.; Généreux, P.; Puskas, J.; Kandzari, D.E.; Morice, M.C.; Lembo, N.; Brown, W.M.; et al. Everolimus-Eluting Stents or Bypass Surgery for Left Main Coronary Artery Disease. *N. Engl. J. Med.* **2016**, *375*, 2223–2235. [CrossRef] [PubMed]
25. Ahn, J.M.; Roh, J.H.; Kim, Y.H.; Park, D.W.; Yun, S.C.; Lee, P.H.; Chang, M.; Park, H.W.; Lee, S.W.; Lee, C.W.; et al. Randomized Trial of Stents Versus Bypass Surgery for Left Main Coronary Artery Disease: 5-Year Outcomes of the PRECOMBAT Study. *J. Am. Coll. Cardiol.* **2015**, *65*, 2198–2206. [CrossRef] [PubMed]
26. Park, S.J.; Kim, Y.H.; Park, D.W.; Yun, S.C.; Ahn, J.M.; Song, H.G.; Lee, J.Y.; Kim, W.J.; Kang, S.J.; Lee, S.W.; et al. Randomized Trial of Stents versus Bypass Surgery for Left Main Coronary Artery Disease. *N. Engl. J. Med.* **2011**, *364*, 1718–1727. [CrossRef]
27. Morice, M.C.; Serruys, P.W.; Kappetein, A.P.; Feldman, T.E.; Ståhle, E.; Colombo, A.; Mack, M.J.; Holmes, D.R.; Choi, J.W.; Ruzyllo, W.; et al. Five-Year outcomes in patients with left main disease treated with either percutaneous coronary intervention or coronary artery bypass grafting in the synergy between percutaneous coronary intervention with taxus and cardiac surgery trial. *Circulation* **2014**, *129*, 2388–2394. [CrossRef]
28. Morice, M.C.; Serruys, P.W.; Kappetein, A.P.; Feldman, T.E.; Ståhle, E.; Colombo, A.; Mack, M.J.; Holmes, D.R.; Torracca, L.; van Es, G.; et al. Outcomes in patients with de novo left main disease treated with either percutaneous coronary intervention using paclitaxel-eluting stents or coronary artery bypass graft treatment in the synergy between percutaneous coronary intervention with taxus and cardiac surgery (SYNTAX) trial. *Circulation* **2010**, *121*, 2645–2653. [CrossRef]
29. Boudriot, E.; Thiele, H.; Walther, T.; Liebetrau, C.; Boeckstegers, P.; Pohl, T.; Reichart, B.; Mudra, H.; Beier, F.; Gansera, B.; et al. Randomized Comparison of Percutaneous Coronary Intervention with Sirolimus-Eluting Stents Versus Coronary Artery Bypass Grafting in Unprotected Left Main Stem Stenosis. *J. Am. Coll. Cardiol.* **2011**, *57*, 538–545. [CrossRef]
30. Buszman, P.E.; Kiesz, S.R.; Bochenek, A.; Peszek-Przybyla, E.; Szkrobka, I.; Debinski, M.; Bialkowska, B.; Dudek, D.; Gruszka, A.; Zurakowski, A.; et al. Acute and Late Outcomes of Unprotected Left Main Stenting in Comparison with Surgical Revascularization. *J. Am. Coll. Cardiol.* **2008**, *51*, 538–545. [CrossRef]
31. Ninomiya, K.; Serruys, P.W.; Garg, S.; Gao, C.; Masuda, S.; Lunardi, M.; Lassen, J.F.; Banning, A.P.; Colombo, A.; Burzotta, F.; et al. Predicted and Observed Mortality at 10 Years in Patients with Bifurcation Lesions in the SYNTAX Trial. *JACC Cardiovasc. Interv.* **2022**, *15*, 1231–1242. [CrossRef]
32. Cho, M.S.; Ahn, J.M.; Lee, C.H.; Kang, D.Y.; Lee, J.B.; Lee, P.H.; Kang, S.J.; Lee, S.W.; Kim, Y.H.; Lee, C.W.; et al. Differential Rates and Clinical Significance of Periprocedural Myocardial Infarction After Stenting or Bypass Surgery for Multivessel Coronary Disease According to Various Definitions. *JACC Cardiovasc. Interv.* **2017**, *10*, 1498–1507. [CrossRef] [PubMed]
33. Palmerini, T.; Serruys, P.; Kappetein, A.P.; Genereux, P.; Riva, D.D.; Reggiani, L.B.; Christiansen, E.H.; Holm, N.R.; Thuesen, L.; Makikallio, T.; et al. Clinical outcomes with percutaneous coronary revascularization vs coronary artery bypass grafting surgery in patients with unprotected left main coronary artery disease: A meta-analysis of 6 randomized trials and 4686 patients. *Am. Heart J.* **2017**, *190*, 54–63. [CrossRef] [PubMed]
34. Head, S.J.; Milojevic, M.; Daemen, J.; Ahn, J.M.; Boersma, E.; Christiansen, E.H.; Domanski, M.J.; Farkouh, M.E.; Flather, M.; Fuster, V.; et al. Mortality after coronary artery bypass grafting versus percutaneous coronary intervention with stenting for coronary artery disease: A pooled analysis of individual patient data. *Lancet* **2018**, *391*, 939–948. [CrossRef]
35. Ahmad, Y.; Howard, J.P.; Arnold, A.D.; Cook, C.M.; Prasad, M.; Ali, Z.A.; Parikh, M.A.; Kosmidou, I.; Francis, D.P.; Moses, J.W.; et al. Mortality after drug-eluting stents vs. coronary artery bypass grafting for left main coronary artery disease: A meta-analysis of randomized controlled trials. *Eur. Heart J.* **2020**, *41*, 3228–3235. [CrossRef]
36. Bajraktari, G.; Zhubi-Bakija, F.; Ndrepepa, G.; Alfonso, F.; Elezi, S.; Rexhaj, Z.; Bytyçi, I.; Bajraktari, A.; Poniku, A.; Henein, M.Y. Long-Term Outcomes of Patients with Unprotected Left Main Coronary Artery Disease Treated with Percutaneous Angioplasty versus Bypass Grafting: A Meta-Analysis of Randomized Controlled Trials. *J. Clin. Med.* **2020**, *9*, 2231. [CrossRef]
37. D'Ascenzo, F.; De Filippo, O.; Elia, E.; Doronzo, M.P.; Omedè, P.; Montefusco, A.; Pennone, M.; Salizzoni, S.; Conrotto, F.; Gallone, G.; et al. Percutaneous vs. surgical revascularization for patients with unprotected left main stenosis: A meta-analysis of 5-year follow-up randomized controlled trials. *Eur. Heart J. Qual. Care Clin. Outcomes* **2021**, *7*, 476–485. [CrossRef]
38. Sabatine, M.S.; Bergmark, B.A.; Murphy, S.A.; O'Gara, P.T.; Smith, P.K.; Serruys, P.W.; Kappetein, A.P.; Park, S.J.; Park, D.W.; Christiansen, E.H.; et al. Percutaneous coronary intervention with drug-eluting stents versus coronary artery bypass grafting in left main coronary artery disease: An individual patient data meta-analysis. *Lancet* **2021**, *398*, 2247–2257. [CrossRef]
39. Kataruka, A.; Maynard, C.C.; Kearney, K.E.; Mahmoud, A.; Bell, S.; Doll, J.A.; McCabe, J.M.; Bryson, C.; Gurm, H.S.; Jneid, H.; et al. Temporal Trends in Percutaneous Coronary Intervention and Coronary Artery Bypass Grafting: Insights from the Washington Cardiac Care Outcomes Assessment Program. *J. Am. Heart Assoc.* **2020**, *9*, e015317. [CrossRef]
40. Arnold, S.V.; Bhatt, D.L.; Barsness, G.W.; Beatty, A.L.; Deedwania, P.C.; Inzucchi, S.E.; Kosiborod, M.; Leiter, L.A.; Lipska, K.J.; Newman, J.D.; et al. Clinical Management of Stable Coronary Artery Disease in Patients with Type 2 Diabetes Mellitus: A Scientific Statement from the American Heart Association. *Circulation* **2020**, *141*, e779–e806. [CrossRef]

41. Gregg, E.W.; Hora, I.; Benoit, S.R. Resurgence in Diabetes-Related Complications. *JAMA* **2019**, *321*, 1867. [CrossRef]
42. Lee, K.; Ahn, J.M.; Yoon, Y.H.; Kang, D.Y.; Park, S.Y.; Ko, E.; Park, H.; Cho, S.C.; Park, S.; Kim, T.O.; et al. Long-Term (10-Year) Outcomes of Stenting or Bypass Surgery for Left Main Coronary Artery Disease in Patients with and without Diabetes Mellitus. *J. Am. Heart Assoc.* **2020**, *9*, e015372. [CrossRef] [PubMed]
43. Tonelli, M.; Muntner, P.; Lloyd, A.; Manns, B.J.; Klarenbach, S.; Pannu, N.; James, M.T.; Hemmelgarn, B.R.; Alberta Kidney Disease Network. Risk of coronary events in people with chronic kidney disease compared with those with diabetes: A population-level cohort study. *Lancet* **2012**, *380*, 807–814. [CrossRef]
44. Bangalore, S.; Maron, D.J.; O'Brien, S.M.; Fleg, J.L.; Kretov, E.I.; Briguori, C.; Kaul, U.; Reynolds, H.R.; Mazurek, T.; Sidhu, M.S.; et al. Management of Coronary Disease in Patients with Advanced Kidney Disease. *N. Engl. J. Med.* **2020**, *382*, 1608. [CrossRef]
45. Giustino, G.; Mehran, R.; Serruys, P.W.; Sabik, J.F.; Milojevic, M., 3rd; Simonton, C.A.; Puskas, J.D.; Kandzari, D.E.; Morice, M.C.; Taggart, D.P.; et al. Left Main Revascularization with PCI or CABG in Patients with Chronic Kidney Disease: Excel Trial. *J. Am. Coll. Cardiol.* **2018**, *72*, 754–765. [CrossRef] [PubMed]
46. Gallo, M.; Blitzer, D.; Laforgia, P.L.; Doulamis, I.P.; Perrin, N.; Bortolussi, G.; Guariento, A.; Putzu, A. Percutaneous coronary intervention versus coronary artery bypass graft for left main coronary artery disease: A meta-analysis. *J. Thorac. Cardiovasc. Surg.* **2022**, *163*, 94–105.e15. [CrossRef]
47. Kim, D.W.; Om, S.Y.; Park, M.W.; Park, H.W.; Lee, P.H.; Kang, D.Y.; Ahn, J.M.; Lee, C.W.; Park, S.W.; Park, S.J.; et al. Comparative effectiveness analysis of percutaneous coronary intervention versus coronary artery bypass grafting in patients with chronic kidney disease and unprotected left main coronary artery disease. *EuroIntervention* **2020**, *16*, 27–35. [CrossRef]
48. Spinthakis, N.; Farag, M.; Gorog, D.A.; Prasad, A.; Mahmood, H.; Gue, Y.; Wellsted, D.; Nabhan, A.; Srinivasan, M. Percutaneous coronary intervention with drug-eluting stent versus coronary artery bypass grafting: A meta-analysis of patients with left main coronary artery disease. *Int. J. Cardiol.* **2017**, *249*, 101–106. [CrossRef]
49. Lee, J.M.; Kang, J.; Lee, E.; Hwang, D.; Rhee, T.M.; Park, J.; Kim, H.L.; Lee, S.E.; Han, J.K.; Yang, H.M.; et al. Chronic Kidney Disease in the Second-Generation Drug-Eluting Stent Era: Pooled Analysis of the Korean Multicenter Drug-Eluting Stent Registry. *JACC Cardiovasc. Interv.* **2016**, *9*, 2097–2109. [CrossRef]
50. Gheorghiade, M.; Sopko, G.; De Luca, L.; Velazquez, E.J.; Parker, J.D.; Binkley, P.F.; Sadowski, Z.; Golba, K.S.; Prior, D.L.; Rouleau, J.L.; et al. Navigating the Crossroads of Coronary Artery Disease and Heart Failure. *Circulation* **2006**, *114*, 1202–1213. [CrossRef]
51. Briceno, N.; Schuster, A.; Lumley, M.; Perera, D. Ischaemic cardiomyopathy: Pathophysiology, assessment and the role of revascularisation. *Heart* **2016**, *102*, 397–406. [CrossRef]
52. Bollano, E.; Redfors, B.; Rawshani, A.; Venetsanos, D.; Völz, S.; Angerås, O.; Ljungman, C.; Alfredsson, J.; Jernberg, T.; Råmunddal, T.; et al. Temporal trends in characteristics and outcome of heart failure patients with and without significant coronary artery disease. *ESC Heart Fail.* **2022**, *9*, 1812–1822. [CrossRef] [PubMed]
53. Howlett, J.G.; Stebbins, A.; Petrie, M.C.; Jhund, P.S.; Castelvecchio, S.; Cherniavsky, A.; Sueta, C.A.; Roy, A.; Piña, I.L.; Wurm, R.; et al. CABG Improves Outcomes in Patients with Ischemic Cardiomyopathy: 10-Year Follow-Up of the STICH Trial. *JACC Heart Fail.* **2019**, *7*, 878–887. [CrossRef] [PubMed]
54. Perera, D.; Clayton, T.; O'Kane, P.D.; Greenwood, J.P.; Weerackody, R.; Ryan, M.; Morgan, H.P.; Dodd, M.; Evans, R.; Canter, R.; et al. Percutaneous Revascularization for Ischemic Left Ventricular Dysfunction. *N. Engl. J. Med.* **2022**. [CrossRef] [PubMed]
55. Marui, A.; Kimura, T.; Nishiwaki, N.; Mitsudo, K.; Komiya, T.; Hanyu, M.; Shiomi, H.; Tanaka, S.; Sakata, R.; CREDO-Kyoto PCI/CABG Registry Cohort-2 Investigators. Comparison of five-year outcomes of coronary artery bypass grafting versus percutaneous coronary intervention in patients with left ventricular ejection fractions ≤50% versus >50% (from the CREDO-Kyoto PCI/CABG Registry Cohort-2). *Am. J. Cardiol.* **2014**, *114*, 988–996. [CrossRef]
56. Sun, L.Y.; Gaudino, M.; Chen, R.J.; Bader Eddeen, A.; Ruel, M. Long-term Outcomes in Patients with Severely Reduced Left Ventricular Ejection Fraction Undergoing Percutaneous Coronary Intervention vs Coronary Artery Bypass Grafting. *JAMA Cardiol.* **2020**, *5*, 631–641. [CrossRef] [PubMed]
57. Wolff, G.; Dimitroulis, D.; Andreotti, F.; Kołodziejczak, M.; Jung, C.; Scicchitano, P.; Devito, F.; Zito, A.; Occhipinti, M.; Castiglioni, B.; et al. Survival Benefits of Invasive Versus Conservative Strategies in Heart Failure in Patients with Reduced Ejection Fraction and Coronary Artery Disease: A Meta-Analysis. *Circ. Heart Fail.* **2017**, *10*, e003255. [CrossRef] [PubMed]
58. Nagendran, J.; Bozso, S.J.; Norris, C.M.; McAlister, F.A.; Appoo, J.J.; Moon, M.C.; Freed, D.H.; Nagendran, J. Coronary Artery Bypass Surgery Improves Outcomes in Patients with Diabetes and Left Ventricular Dysfunction. *J. Am. Coll. Cardiol.* **2018**, *71*, 819–827. [CrossRef]
59. Park, S.; Ahn, J.M.; Kim, T.O.; Park, H.; Kang, D.Y.; Lee, P.H.; Jeong, Y.J.; Hyun, J.; Lee, J.; Kim, J.H.; et al. Revascularization in Patients with Left Main Coronary Artery Disease and Left Ventricular Dysfunction. *J. Am. Coll. Cardiol.* **2020**, *76*, 1395–1406. [CrossRef]
60. Bangalore, S.; Guo, Y.; Samadashvili, Z.; Blecker, S.; Hannan, E.L. Revascularization in patients with multivessel coronary artery disease and severe left ventricular systolic dysfunction: Everolimus-eluting stents versus coronary artery bypass graft surgery. *Circulation* **2016**, *133*, 2132–2140. [CrossRef]
61. Schneider, E.L. Aging in the third millennium. *Science* **1999**, *283*, 796–797. [CrossRef]
62. Wenger, N.K.; Engberding, N. Acute Coronary Syndromes in the Elderly. *F1000Research* **2017**, *6*, 1791. [CrossRef]

63. Shah, A.I.; Alabaster, A.; Dontsi, M.; Rana, J.S.; Solomon, M.D.; Krishnaswami, A. Comparison of coronary revascularization strategies in older adults presenting with acute coronary syndromes. *J. Am. Geriatr. Soc.* **2022**, *70*, 2235–2245. [CrossRef] [PubMed]
64. Nicolini, F.; Contini, G.A.; Fortuna, D.; Pacini, D.; Gabbieri, D.; Vignali, L.; Campo, G.; Manari, A.; Zussa, C.; Guastaroba, P.; et al. Coronary Artery Surgery Versus Percutaneous Coronary Intervention in Octogenarians: Long-Term Results. *Ann. Thorac. Surg.* **2015**, *99*, 567–574. [CrossRef] [PubMed]
65. Zhang, Q.; Zhao, X.H.; Gu, H.F.; Xu, Z.R.; Yang, Y.M. Clinical Outcomes of Coronary Artery Bypass Grafting vs Percutaneous Coronary Intervention in Octogenarians with Coronary Artery Disease. *Can. J. Cardiol.* **2016**, *32*, 1166.e21–1166.e28. [CrossRef] [PubMed]
66. Conrotto, F.; Scacciatella, P.; D'Ascenzo, F.; Chieffo, A.; Latib, A.; Park, S.J.; Kim, Y.H.; Onuma, Y.; Capranzano, P.; Jegere, S.; et al. Long-term outcomes of percutaneous coronary interventions or coronary artery bypass grafting for left main coronary artery disease in octogenarians (from a Drug-Eluting stent for LefT main Artery registry substudy). *Am. J. Cardiol.* **2014**, *113*, 2007–2012. [CrossRef]
67. Ono, M.; Serruys, P.W.; Hara, H.; Kawashima, H.; Gao, C.; Wang, R.; Takahashi, K.; O'Leary, N.; Wykrzykowska, J.J.; Sharif, F.; et al. 10-Year Follow-Up After Revascularization in Elderly Patients with Complex Coronary Artery Disease. *J. Am. Coll. Cardiol.* **2021**, *77*, 2761–2773. [CrossRef]
68. Lee, S.W.; Kim, S.H.; Kim, S.O.; Han, S.; Kim, Y.H.; Park, D.W.; Kang, S.J.; Lee, C.W.; Park, S.W.; Park, S.J. Comparative long-term efficacy and safety of drug-eluting stent versus coronary artery bypass grafting in ostial left main coronary artery disease: Analysis of the MAIN-COMPARE registry. *Catheter Cardiovasc. Interv.* **2012**, *80*, 206–212. [CrossRef]
69. Naganuma, T.; Chieffo, A.; Meliga, E.; Capodanno, D.; Park, S.J.; Onuma, Y.; Valgimigli, M.; Jegere, S.; Makkar, R.R.; Palacios, I.F.; et al. Long-term clinical outcomes after percutaneous coronary intervention versus coronary artery bypass grafting for ostial/midshaft lesions in unprotected left main coronary artery from the DELTA registry: A multicenter registry evaluating percutaneous coronary intervention versus coronary artery bypass grafting for left main treatment. *JACC Cardiovasc. Interv.* **2014**, *7*, 354–361. [CrossRef]
70. Naganuma, T.; Chieffo, A.; Meliga, E.; Capodanno, D.; Park, S.J.; Onuma, Y.; Valgimigli, M.; Jegere, S.; Makkar, R.R.; Palacios, I.F.; et al. Long-term clinical outcomes after percutaneous coronary intervention for ostial/mid-shaft lesions versus distal bifurcation lesions in unprotected left main coronary artery: The DELTA Registry (drug-eluting stent for left main coronary artery disease): A multicenter registry evaluating percutaneous coronary intervention versus coronary artery bypass grafting for left main treatment. *JACC Cardiovasc. Interv.* **2013**, *6*, 1242–1249. [CrossRef]
71. Hyun, J.; Kim, J.H.; Jeong, Y.; Choe, K.; Lee, J.; Yang, Y.; Kim, T.O.; Park, H.; Cho, S.C.; Ko, E.; et al. Long-Term Outcomes After PCI or CABG for Left Main Coronary Artery Disease According to Lesion Location. *JACC Cardiovasc. Interv.* **2020**, *13*, 2825–2836. [CrossRef]
72. Gershlick, A.H.; Kandzari, D.E.; Banning, A.; Taggart, D.P.; Morice, M.C.; Lembo, N.J.; Brown, W.M.; Banning, A.P., 3rd; Merkely, B.; Horkay, F.; et al. Outcomes After Left Main Percutaneous Coronary Intervention Versus Coronary Artery Bypass Grafting According to Lesion Site: Results from the EXCEL Trial. *JACC Cardiovasc. Interv.* **2018**, *11*, 1224–1233. [CrossRef] [PubMed]
73. De Filippo, O.; Di Franco, A.; Boretto, P.; Bruno, F.; Cusenza, V.; Desalvo, P.; Demetres, M.; Saglietto, A.; Franchin, L.; Piroli, F.; et al. Percutaneous coronary intervention versus coronary artery surgery for left main disease according to lesion site: A meta-analysis. *J. Thorac. Cardiovasc. Surg.* **2021**. [CrossRef] [PubMed]
74. Chen, X.; Li, X.; Zhang, J.J.; Han, Y.; Kan, J.; Chen, L.; Qiu, C.; Santoso, T.; Paiboon, C.; Kwan, T.W.; et al. 3-Year Outcomes of the DKCRUSH-V Trial Comparing DK Crush with Provisional Stenting for Left Main Bifurcation Lesions. *JACC Cardiovasc. Interv.* **2019**, *12*, 1927–1937. [CrossRef] [PubMed]
75. Buccheri, S.; Franchina, G.; Romano, S.; Puglisi, S.; Venuti, G.; D'Arrigo, P.; Francaviglia, B.; Scalia, M.; Condorelli, A.; Barbanti, M.; et al. Clinical Outcomes Following Intravascular Imaging-Guided Versus Coronary Angiography-Guided Percutaneous Coronary Intervention with Stent Implantation: A Systematic Review and Bayesian Network Meta-Analysis of 31 Studies and 17,882 Patients. *JACC Cardiovasc. Interv.* **2017**, *10*, 2488–2498. [CrossRef] [PubMed]
76. Fisher, L.D.; Judkins, M.P.; Lesperance, J.; Cameron, A.; Swaye, P.; Ryan, T.; Maynard, C.; Bourassa, M.; Kennedy, J.W.; Gosselin, A.; et al. Reproducibility of coronary arteriographic reading in the coronary artery surgery study (CASS). *Cathet Cardiovasc. Diagn.* **1982**, *8*, 565–575. [CrossRef] [PubMed]
77. Lindstaedt, M.; Spiecker, M.; Perings, C.; Lawo, T.; Yazar, A.; Holland-Letz, T.; Muegge, A.; Bojara, W.; Germing, A. How good are experienced interventional cardiologists at predicting the functional significance of intermediate or equivocal left main coronary artery stenoses? *Int. J. Cardiol.* **2007**, *120*, 254–261. [CrossRef]
78. Abizaid, A.S.; Mintz, G.S.; Abizaid, A.; Mehran, R.; Lansky, A.J.; Pichard, A.D.; Satler, L.F.; Wu, H.; Kent, K.M.; Leon, M.B. One-year follow-up after intravascular ultrasound assessment of moderate left main coronary artery disease in patients with ambiguous angiograms. *J. Am. Coll. Cardiol.* **1999**, *34*, 707–715. [CrossRef]
79. Okabe, T.; Mintz, G.S.; Lee, S.Y.; Lee, B.; Roy, P.; Steinberg, D.H.; Pinto-Slottow, T.; Smith, K.A.; Xue, Z.; Satler, L.F.; et al. Five-year outcomes of moderate or ambiguous left main coronary artery disease and the intravascular ultrasound predictors of events. *J. Invasive Cardiol.* **2008**, *20*, 635–639.
80. Jasti, V.; Ivan, E.; Yalamanchili, V.; Wongpraparut, N.; Leesar, M.A. Correlations Between Fractional Flow Reserve and Intravascular Ultrasound in Patients with an Ambiguous Left Main Coronary Artery Stenosis. *Circulation* **2004**, *110*, 2831–2836. [CrossRef]

81. de la Torre Hernandez, J.M.; Hernández Hernandez, F.; Alfonso, F.; Rumoroso, J.R.; Lopez-Palop, R.; Sadaba, M.; Carrillo, P.; Rondan, J.; Lozano, I.; Nodar, J.M.R.; et al. Prospective Application of Pre-Defined Intravascular Ultrasound Criteria for Assessment of Intermediate Left Main Coronary Artery Lesions: Results from the Multicenter LITRO Study. *J. Am. Coll. Cardiol.* **2011**, *58*, 351–358. [CrossRef]
82. Rusinova, R.P.; Mintz, G.S.; Choi, S.Y.; Araki, H.; Hakim, D.; Sanidas, E.; Yakushiji, T.; Weisz, G.; Mehran, R.; Franklin-Bond, T.; et al. Intravascular ultrasound-derived minimal lumen area criteria for functionally significant left main coronary artery stenosis. *JACC Cardiovasc. Interv.* **2014**, *7*, 868–874. [CrossRef]
83. Rusinova, R.P.; Mintz, G.S.; Choi, S.Y.; Araki, H.; Hakim, D.; Sanidas, E.; Yakushiji, T.; Weisz, G.; Mehran, R.; Franklin-Bond, T.; et al. Intravascular ultrasound comparison of left main coronary artery disease between white and Asian patients. *Am. J. Cardiol.* **2013**, *111*, 979–984. [CrossRef] [PubMed]
84. Park, S.J.; Kim, Y.H.; Park, D.W.; Lee, S.W.; Kim, W.J.; Suh, J.; Yun, S.C.; Lee, C.W.; Hong, M.K.; Lee, J.H.; et al. Impact of Intravascular Ultrasound Guidance on Long-Term Mortality in Stenting for Unprotected Left Main Coronary Artery Stenosis. *Circ. Cardiovasc. Interv.* **2009**, *2*, 167–177. [CrossRef] [PubMed]
85. Claessen, B.E.; Mehran, R.; Mintz, G.S.; Weisz, G.; Leon, M.B.; Dogan, O.; de Ribamar Costa, J., Jr.; Stone, G.W.; Apostolidou, I.; Morales, A.; et al. Impact of Intravascular Ultrasound Imaging on Early and Late Clinical Outcomes Following Percutaneous Coronary Intervention with Drug-Eluting Stents. *JACC Cardiovasc. Interv.* **2011**, *4*, 974–981. [CrossRef]
86. Kinnaird, T.; Johnson, T.; Anderson, R.; Gallagher, S.; Sirker, A.; Ludman, P.; de Belder, M.; Copt, S.; Oldroyd, K.; Banning, A.; et al. Intravascular Imaging and 12-Month Mortality After Unprotected Left Main Stem PCI: An Analysis from the British Cardiovascular Intervention Society Database. *JACC Cardiovasc. Interv.* **2020**, *13*, 346–357. [CrossRef]
87. Andell, P.; Karlsson, S.; Mohammad, M.A.; Götberg, M.; James, S.; Jensen, J.; Fröbert, O.; Angerås, O.; Nilsson, J.; Omerovic, E.; et al. Intravascular Ultrasound Guidance is Associated with Better Outcome in Patients Undergoing Unprotected Left Main Coronary Artery Stenting Compared with Angiography Guidance Alone. *Circ. Cardiovasc. Interv.* **2017**, *10*, e004813. [CrossRef]
88. Ye, Y.; Yang, M.; Zhang, S.; Zeng, Y. Percutaneous coronary intervention in left main coronary artery disease with or without intravascular ultrasound: A meta-analysis. *PLoS ONE* **2017**, *12*, e0179756. [CrossRef]
89. Doi, H.; Maehara, A.; Mintz, G.S.; Yu, A.; Wang, H.; Mandinov, L.; Popma, J.J.; Ellis, S.G.; Grube, E.; Dawkins, K.D.; et al. Impact of Post-Intervention Minimal Stent Area on 9-Month Follow-Up Patency of Paclitaxel-Eluting Stents: An Integrated Intravascular Ultrasound Analysis from the TAXUS IV, V, and VI and TAXUS ATLAS Workhorse, Long Lesion, and Direct Stent Trials. *JACC Cardiovasc. Interv.* **2009**, *2*, 1269–1275. [CrossRef]
90. Maehara, A.; Mintz, G.; Serruys, P.; Kappetein, A.; Kandzari, D.; Schampaert, E.; Van Boven, A.; Horkay, F.; Ungi, I.; Mansour, S.; et al. Impact of final minimal stent area by ivus on 3-year outcome After pci of left main coronary artery Disease: The excel trial. *J. Am. Coll. Cardiol.* **2017**, *69*, 963. [CrossRef]
91. Kang, S.J.; Ahn, J.M.; Song, H.; Kim, W.J.; Lee, J.Y.; Park, D.W.; Yun, S.C.; Lee, S.W.; Kim, Y.H.; Lee, C.W.; et al. Comprehensive intravascular ultrasound assessment of stent area and its impact on restenosis and adverse cardiac events in 403 patients with unprotected left main disease. *Circ. Cardiovasc. Interv.* **2011**, *4*, 562–569. [CrossRef]
92. Ge, Z.; Kan, J.; Gao, X.F.; Kong, X.Q.; Zuo, G.F.; Ye, F.; Tian, N.L.; Lin, S.; Liu, Z.Z.; Sun, Z.Q.; et al. Comparison of intravascular ultrasound-guided with angiography-guided double kissing crush stenting for patients with complex coronary bifurcation lesions: Rationale and design of a prospective, randomized, and multicenter DKCRUSH VIII trial. *Am. Heart J.* **2021**, *234*, 101–110. [CrossRef] [PubMed]
93. Räber, L.; Mintz, G.S.; Koskinas, K.C.; Johnson, T.W.; Holm, N.R.; Onuma, Y.; Radu, M.D.; Joner, M.; Yu, B.; Jia, H.; et al. Clinical use of intracoronary imaging. Part 1: Guidance and optimization of coronary interventions. An expert consensus document of the European Association of Percutaneous Cardiovascular Interventions. *Eur. Heart J.* **2018**, *39*, 3281–3300. [CrossRef] [PubMed]
94. Cortese, B.; de la Torre Hernandez, J.M.; Lanocha, M.; Ielasi, A.; Giannini, F.; Campo, G.; D'Ascenzo, F.; Latini, R.A.; Krestianinov, O.; Alfonso, F.; et al. Optical coherence tomography, intravascular ultrasound or angiography guidance for distal left main coronary stenting. The ROCK cohort II study. *Catheter. Cardiovasc. Interv.* **2022**, *99*, 664–673. [CrossRef]
95. Amabile, N.; Rangé, G.; Souteyrand, G.; Godin, M.; Boussaada, M.M.; Meneveau, N.; Cayla, G.; Casassus, F.; Lefèvre, T.; Hakim, R.; et al. Optical coherence tomography to guide percutaneous coronary intervention of the left main coronary artery: The LEMON study. *EuroIntervention* **2021**, *17*, E124–E131. [CrossRef] [PubMed]
96. Hamilos, M.; Muller, O.; Cuisset, T.; Ntalianis, A.; Chlouverakis, G.; Sarno, G.; Nelis, O.; Bartunek, J.; Vanderheyden, M.; Wyffels, E.; et al. Long-Term Clinical Outcome After Fractional Flow Reserve–Guided Treatment in Patients with Angiographically Equivocal Left Main Coronary Artery Stenosis. *Circulation* **2009**, *120*, 1505–1512. [CrossRef] [PubMed]
97. Kuramitsu, S.; Matsuo, H.; Shinozaki, T.; Horie, K.; Takashima, H.; Terai, H.; Kikuta, Y.; Ishihara, T.; Saigusa, T.; Sakamoto, T.; et al. Two-Year Outcomes after Deferral of Revascularization Based on Fractional Flow Reserve: The J-CONFIRM Registry. *Circ. Cardiovasc. Interv.* **2020**, *12*, 8355. [CrossRef]
98. Pijls, N.H.; Fearon, W.F.; Tonino, P.A.; Siebert, U.; Ikeno, F.; Bornschein, B.; van't Veer, M.; Klauss, V.; Manoharan, G.; Engstrøm, T.; et al. Fractional Flow Reserve Versus Angiography for Guiding Percutaneous Coronary Intervention in Patients with Multi-vessel Coronary Artery Disease: 2-Year Follow-Up of the FAME (Fractional Flow Reserve Versus Angiography for Multivessel Evaluation) Study. *J. Am. Coll. Cardiol.* **2010**, *56*, 177–184. [CrossRef]

99. Zimmermann, F.M.; Ferrara, A.; Johnson, N.P.; van Nunen, L.X.; Escaned, J.; Albertsson, P.; Erbel, R.; Legrand, V.; Gwon, H.C.; Remkes, W.S.; et al. Deferral vs. performance of percutaneous coronary intervention of functionally non-significant coronary stenosis: 15-year follow-up of the DEFER trial. *Eur. Heart J.* **2015**, *36*, 3182–3188. [CrossRef]
100. Cerrato, E.; Echavarria-Pinto, M.; D'Ascenzo, F.; Gonzalo, N.; Quadri, G.; Quirós, A.; de la Torre Hernández, J.M.; Tomassini, F.; Barbero, U.; Nombela-Franco, L.; et al. Safety of intermediate left main stenosis revascularization deferral based on fractional flow reserve and intravascular ultrasound: A systematic review and meta-regression including 908 deferred left main stenosis from 12 studies. *Int. J. Cardiol.* **2018**, *271*, 42–48. [CrossRef]
101. Toth, G.; Hamilos, M.; Pyxaras, S.; Mangiacapra, F.; Nelis, O.; De Vroey, F.; Di Serafino, L.; Muller, O.; Van Mieghem, C.; Wyffels, E.; et al. Evolving concepts of angiogram: Fractional flow reserve discordances in 4000 coronary stenoses. *Eur. Heart J.* **2014**, *35*, 2831–2838. [CrossRef]
102. Park, S.J.; Kang, S.J.; Ahn, J.M.; Shim, E.B.; Kim, Y.T.; Yun, S.C.; Song, H.; Lee, J.Y.; Kim, W.J.; Park, D.W.; et al. Visual-Functional Mismatch Between Coronary Angiography and Fractional Flow Reserve. *JACC Cardiovasc. Interv.* **2012**, *5*, 1029–1036. [CrossRef] [PubMed]
103. Yong, A.S.; Daniels, D.; De Bruyne, B.; Kim, H.S.; Ikeno, F.; Lyons, J.; Pijls, N.H.; Fearon, W.F. Fractional flow reserve assessment of left main stenosis in the presence of downstream coronary stenoses. *Circ. Cardiovasc. Interv.* **2013**, *6*, 161–165. [CrossRef] [PubMed]
104. Fearon, W.F.; Yong, A.S.; Lenders, G.; Toth, G.G.; Dao, C.; Daniels, D.V.; Pijls, N.; De Bruyne, B. The impact of downstream coronary stenosis on fractional flow reserve assessment of intermediate left main coronary artery disease: Human validation. *JACC Cardiovasc. Interv.* **2015**, *8*, 398–403. [CrossRef] [PubMed]
105. Modi, B.N.; van de Hoef, T.P.; Piek, J.J.; Perera, D. Physiological assessment of left main coronary artery disease. *EuroIntervention* **2017**, *13*, 820–827. [CrossRef]
106. Koo, B.K.; Kang, H.J.; Youn, T.J.; Chae, I.H.; Choi, D.J.; Kim, H.S.; Sohn, D.W.; Oh, B.H.; Lee, M.M.; Park, Y.B.; et al. Physiologic Assessment of Jailed Side Branch Lesions Using Fractional Flow Reserve. *J. Am. Coll. Cardiol.* **2005**, *46*, 633–637. [CrossRef]
107. Ahn, J.M.; Lee, J.Y.; Kang, S.J.; Kim, Y.H.; Song, H.G.; Oh, J.H.; Park, J.S.; Kim, W.J.; Lee, S.W.; Lee, C.W.; et al. Functional Assessment of Jailed Side Branches in Coronary Bifurcation Lesions Using Fractional Flow Reserve. *JACC Cardiovasc. Interv.* **2012**, *5*, 155–161. [CrossRef]
108. Lee, C.H.; Choi, S.W.; Hwang, J.; Kim, I.C.; Cho, Y.K.; Park, H.S.; Yoon, H.J.; Kim, H.; Han, S.; Kim, J.Y.; et al. 5-Year Outcomes According to FFR of Left Circumflex Coronary Artery After Left Main Crossover Stenting. *JACC Cardiovasc. Interv.* **2019**, *12*, 847–855. [CrossRef]
109. Davies, J.E.; Sen, S.; Dehbi, H.M.; Al-Lamee, R.; Petraco, R.; Nijjer, S.S.; Bhindi, R.; Lehman, S.J.; Walters, D.; Sapontis, J.; et al. Use of the Instantaneous Wave-free Ratio or Fractional Flow Reserve in PCI. *N. Engl. J. Med.* **2017**, *376*, 1824–1834. [CrossRef]
110. Götberg, M.; Christiansen, E.H.; Gudmundsdottir, I.J.; Sandhall, L.; Danielewicz, M.; Jakobsen, L.; Olsson, S.E.; Öhagen, P.; Olsson, H.; Omerovic, E.; et al. Instantaneous Wave-free Ratio versus Fractional Flow Reserve to Guide PCI. *N. Engl. J. Med.* **2017**, *376*, 1813–1823. [CrossRef]
111. Götberg, M.; Berntorp, K.; Rylance, R.; Christiansen, E.H.; Yndigegn, T.; Gudmundsdottir, I.J.; Koul, S.; Sandhall, L.; Danielewicz, M.; Jakobsen, L.; et al. 5-Year Outcomes of PCI Guided by Measurement of Instantaneous Wave-Free Ratio Versus Fractional Flow Reserve. *J. Am. Coll. Cardiol.* **2022**, *79*, 965–974. [CrossRef]
112. Warisawa, T.; Cook, C.M.; Rajkumar, C.; Howard, J.P.; Seligman, H.; Ahmad, Y.; El Hajj, S.; Doi, S.; Nakajima, A.; Nakayama, M.; et al. Safety of Revascularization Deferral of Left Main Stenosis Based on Instantaneous Wave-Free Ratio Evaluation. *JACC Cardiovasc. Interv.* **2020**, *13*, 1655–1664. [CrossRef]
113. Maeng, M.; Holm, N.R.; Erglis, A.; Kumsars, I.; Niemelä, M.; Kervinen, K.; Jensen, J.S.; Galløe, A.; Steigen, T.K.; Wiseth, R.; et al. Long-term results after simple versus complex stenting of coronary artery bifurcation lesions: Nordic Bifurcation Study 5-year follow-up results. *J. Am. Coll. Cardiol.* **2013**, *62*, 30–34. [CrossRef] [PubMed]
114. Hildick-Smith, D.; de Belder, A.J.; Cooter, N.; Curzen, N.P.; Clayton, T.C.; Oldroyd, K.G.; Bennett, L.; Holmberg, S.; Cotton, J.M.; Glennon, P.E.; et al. Randomized Trial of Simple Versus Complex Drug-Eluting Stenting for Bifurcation Lesions. *Circulation* **2010**, *121*, 1235–1243. [CrossRef]
115. Chen, S.L.; Santoso, T.; Zhang, J.J.; Ye, F.; Xu, Y.W.; Fu, Q.; Kan, J.; Paiboon, C.; Zhou, Y.; Ding, S.Q.; et al. A Randomized Clinical Study Comparing Double Kissing Crush with Provisional Stenting for Treatment of Coronary Bifurcation Lesions: Results From the DKCRUSH-II (Double Kissing Crush versus Provisional Stenting Technique for Treatment of Coronary Bifurcation Lesions) Trial. *J. Am. Coll. Cardiol.* **2011**, *57*, 914–920. [CrossRef] [PubMed]
116. Hildick-Smith, D.; Egred, M.; Banning, A.; Brunel, P.; Ferenc, M.; Hovasse, T.; Wlodarczak, A.; Pan, M.; Schmitz, T.; Silvestri, M.; et al. The European bifurcation club Left Main Coronary Stent study: A randomized comparison of stepwise provisional vs. systematic dual stenting strategies (EBC MAIN). *Eur. Heart J.* **2021**, *42*, 3829–3839. [CrossRef]
117. Chen, S.L.; Xu, B.; Han, Y.L.; Sheiban, I.; Zhang, J.J.; Ye, F.; Kwan, T.W.; Paiboon, C.; Zhou, Y.J.; Lv, S.Z.; et al. Clinical Outcome After DK Crush Versus Culotte Stenting of Distal Left Main Bifurcation Lesions: The 3-Year Follow-Up Results of the DKCRUSH-III Study. *JACC Cardiovasc. Interv.* **2015**, *8*, 1335–1342. [CrossRef]
118. Park, D.Y.; An, S.; Jolly, N.; Attanasio, S.; Yadav, N.; Rao, S.; Vij, A. Systematic Review and Network Meta-Analysis Comparing Bifurcation Techniques for Percutaneous Coronary Intervention. *J. Am. Heart Assoc.* **2022**, *11*, e025394. [CrossRef]

119. Zhong, M.; Tang, B.; Zhao, Q.; Cheng, J.; Jin, Q.; Fu, S. Should kissing balloon inflation after main vessel stenting be routine in the one-stent approach? A systematic review and meta-analysis of randomized trials. *PLoS ONE* **2018**, *13*, e0197580. [CrossRef]
120. Burzotta, F.; Lassen, J.F.; Lefèvre, T.; Banning, A.P.; Chatzizisis, Y.S.; Johnson, T.W.; Ferenc, M.; Rathore, S.; Albiero, R.; Pan, M.; et al. Percutaneous coronary intervention for bifurcation coronary lesions: The 15th consensus document from the European Bifurcation Club. *EuroIntervention* **2021**, *16*, 1307–1317. [CrossRef]
121. Chen, S.L.; Sheiban, I.; Xu, B.; Jepson, N.; Paiboon, C.; Zhang, J.J.; Ye, F.; Sansoto, T.; Kwan, T.W.; Lee, M.; et al. Impact of the Complexity of Bifurcation Lesions Treated with Drug-Eluting Stents: The DEFINITION Study (Definitions and impact of complEx biFurcation lesIons on clinical outcomes after percutaNeous coronary IntervenTIOn using drug-eluting steNts). *JACC Cardiovasc. Interv.* **2014**, *7*, 1266–1276. [CrossRef]
122. Zhang, J.J.; Ye, F.; Xu, K.; Kan, J.; Tao, L.; Santoso, T.; Munawar, M.; Tresukosol, D.; Li, L.; Sheiban, I.; et al. Multicentre, randomized comparison of two-stent and provisional stenting techniques in patients with complex coronary bifurcation lesions: The Definition II trial. *Eur. Heart J.* **2020**, *41*, 2523–2536. [CrossRef] [PubMed]
123. Neumann, F.J.; Sousa-Uva, M.; Ahlsson, A.; Alfonso, F.; Banning, A.P.; Benedetto, U.; Byrne, R.A.; Collet, J.P.; Falk, V.; Head, S.J.; et al. 2018 ESC/EACTS Guidelines on myocardial revascularization. *Eur. Heart J.* **2019**, *40*, 87–165. [CrossRef] [PubMed]
124. Lawton, J.S.; Tamis-Holland, J.E.; Bangalore, S.; Bates, E.R.; Beckie, T.M.; Bischoff, J.M.; Bittl, J.A.; Cohen, M.G.; DiMaio, J.M.; Don, C.W.; et al. 2021 ACC/AHA/SCAI Guideline for Coronary Artery Revascularization: A Report of the American College of Cardiology/American Heart Association Joint Committee on Clinical Practice Guidelines. *J. Am. Coll. Cardiol.* **2022**, *79*, e21–e129. [CrossRef]
125. Head, S.J.; Kaul, S.; Mack, M.J.; Serruys, P.W.; Taggart, D.P.; Holmes, D.R.; Leon, M.B., Jr.; Marco, J.; Bogers, A.J.; Kappetein, A.P.; et al. The rationale for Heart Team decision-making for patients with stable, complex coronary artery disease. *Eur. Heart J.* **2013**, *34*, 2510–2518. [CrossRef]

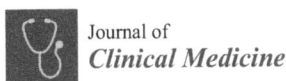

Review

An Up-to-Date Article Regarding Particularities of Drug Treatment in Patients with Chronic Heart Failure

Valentina Buda [1,2,†], Andreea Prelipcean [1,†], Dragos Cozma [3,4,*], Dana Emilia Man [3,4], Simona Negres [5], Alexandra Scurtu [1,2], Maria Suciu [1,2], Minodora Andor [3], Corina Danciu [1,2], Simina Crisan [3,4], Cristina Adriana Dehelean [1,2], Lucian Petrescu [3,4] and Ciprian Rachieru [3,6]

1. Faculty of Pharmacy, "Victor Babes" University of Medicine and Pharmacy, Eftimie Murgu Square, No. 2, 300041 Timisoara, Romania; buda.valentina@umft.ro (V.B.); andreea.preli@yahoo.com (A.P.); alexandra.scurtu@umft.ro (A.S.); suciu.maria@umft.ro (M.S.); corina.danciu@umft.ro (C.D.); cadehelean@umft.ro (C.A.D.)
2. Research Center for Pharmaco-Toxicological Evaluation, "Victor Babes" University of Medicine and Pharmacy, Eftimie Murgu Square, No. 2, 300041 Timisoara, Romania
3. Faculty of Medicine, "Victor Babes" University of Medicine and Pharmacy, Eftimie Murgu Square, No. 2, 300041 Timisoara, Romania; man.dana@umft.ro (D.E.M.); andor.minodora@umft.ro (M.A.); simina.crisan@umft.ro (S.C.); petrescu_lucian@yahoo.com (L.P.); ciprian.rachieru@umft.ro (C.R.)
4. Institute of Cardiovascular Diseases Timisoara, 13A Gheorghe Adam Street, 300310 Timisoara, Romania
5. Faculty of Pharmacy, "Carol Davila" University of Medicine and Pharmacy, Traian Vuia 6, 020956 Bucharest, Romania; simona_negres@yahoo.com
6. Center for Advanced Research in Cardiovascular Pathology and Hemostasis, "Victor Babes" University of Medicine and Pharmacy, Eftimie Murgu Square, No. 2, 300041 Timisoara, Romania

* Correspondence: dragos.cozma@umft.ro
† These authors contributed equally to this work.

Abstract: Since the prevalence of heart failure (HF) increases with age, HF is now one of the most common reasons for the hospitalization of elderly people. Although the treatment strategies and overall outcomes of HF patients have improved over time, hospitalization and mortality rates remain elevated, especially in developed countries where populations are aging. Therefore, this paper is intended to be a valuable multidisciplinary source of information for both doctors (cardiologists and general physicians) and pharmacists in order to decrease the morbidity and mortality of heart failure patients. We address several aspects regarding pharmacological treatment (including new approaches in HF treatment strategies [sacubitril/valsartan combination and sodium glucose co-transporter-2 inhibitors]), as well as the particularities of patients (age-induced changes and sex differences) and treatment (pharmacokinetic and pharmacodynamic changes in drugs; cardiorenal syndrome). The article also highlights several drugs and food supplements that may worsen the prognosis of HF patients and discusses some potential drug–drug interactions, their consequences and recommendations for health care providers, as well as the risks of adverse drug reactions and treatment discontinuation, as an interdisciplinary approach to treatment is essential for HF patients.

Keywords: heart failure; treatment strategies; new pharmacological approaches; age-induced changes; sex-related differences; pharmacokinetics; pharmacodynamics; discontinuation of treatment; food supplements; drug interactions

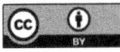

1. Introduction

Heart failure is defined by the European Society of Cardiology Guidelines as a clinical syndrome derived from structural and/or functional cardiac abnormalities [1]. This syndrome is characterized by common symptoms (such as fatigue, breathlessness, or ankle swelling) and typical signs (such as peripheral edema, elevated jugular venous pressure, or pulmonary crackles), all leading to reduced cardiac output and/or high intracardiac pressure (at rest or during stress periods) [2]. Thus, heart failure (HF) can be defined as the inability of the heart to ensure optimal blood flow, which is necessary for the organs to maintain the metabolic and functional processes of all organs. Currently, several HF definitions are available, which differ in the function of the setting (from the medical literature to medical practice, including the current guidelines) [3]. Moreover, several classification frameworks also exist, which aim to properly characterize different subsets of HF (from NYHA classification to EF categories or HF etiology) [3].

Drug therapy is a well-established strategy in treating heart failure (HF) and there are guidelines that cover most of the long-standing and recent research, although specific situations cannot be extensively analyzed [2].

HF affects a wide range of patients and thus occurs in several forms that are widely based on the assessment of left ventricular (LV) ejection fraction (EF): heart failure with preserved ejection fraction (HFpEF), with mildly reduced ejection fraction (HFmrEF), and with reduced ejection fraction (HFrEF) [4]. HFpEF is considered in patients with normal LVEF (commonly considered to be $\geq$50%, with symptoms and signs, elevated levels of natriuretic peptides and 1 additional criterion of relevant structural heart disease/diastolic dysfunction at least) [3]. The HFrEF designation is typically applied to patients presenting with less than 40% EF. Patients with LVEF between 40 and 49% represent a gray area, nowadays referred to as HFmrEF [5].

The diagnosis of HFpEF is relatively demanding, as patients usually have a normal LV, with a certain degree of wall hypertrophy and/or increased left atrial (LA) volume. Diagnosis requires proof of increased LV filling pressure or impaired LV filling, which explains the terminology of diastolic HF/dysfunction. However, diastolic dysfunction is also found in most HFrEF and HFmrEF patients (previously referred to as systolic HF) [2].

It seems that the prevalence of HF significantly varies with age, starting from approximately 1–2% among adults and increasing strikingly to more than 10% in people older than 70 years, and is more common in men than in women [2,6]. Since HF incidence and prevalence increase with age, HF is nowadays one of the most common reasons for hospitalization of elderly people [7]. Although treatment strategies and overall outcomes of HF patients have improved over time, hospitalization and mortality rates still remain elevated, especially in developed countries where the population is aging, which represents an economic burden for healthcare budgets [7].

Except for the pathology itself, HF is also associated with co-morbidities such as prior stroke or myocardial infarction, atrial fibrillation, diabetes mellitus, chronic lung disease, osteoarthritis, thyroid disease, dementia, depression, and chronic renal/hepatic failure, and all of these pathologies require additional treatment strategies [8].

Moreover, several aspects, such as changes in the mechanisms (neuroendocrine, inflammatory, immunological, or metabolic) involved in the physiopathogenesis of HF [7], the presence of co-morbidities, the use of polypharmacy in HF patients, and altered pharmacokinetics and pharmacodynamics of drugs in elderly people [9,10], require a patient-centered approach in order to avoid inappropriate medical prescriptions, drug interactions, exacerbation of adverse drug effects [11], and low adherence to pharmacological treatment, with altered prognosis of HF patients being a major consequence [12–14].

Moreover, because the worldwide population is aging and the number of people $\geq$80 years old will triple by 2050, it is extremely important to decrease the prevalence and incidence of cardiovascular pathologies in order to decrease multi-morbidity and health care costs [15].

Herein, we discuss the main important aspects regarding pharmacological approaches, treatment strategies, and the particularities of patients and treatment that should absolutely be taken into account in order to improve treatment outcomes for HF patients.

2. General Considerations Regarding HF Treatment

The pharmacological treatment of HF is oriented towards the following: long-term management of the pathology and improvement in survival (e.g., ACEIs (angiotensin-converting enzyme inhibitors), ARBs (angiotensin receptor blockers), beta-blockers, MRA (mineralocorticoid receptor antagonists), ARNI (angiotensin receptor-neprilysin inhibitors), SGLT2 (sodium-glucose cotransporter-2) inhibitors and ivabradine, an I_f channel blocker, highly selective for sinoatrial node pacemaker current) and symptom relief medication (e.g., administration of diuretics, nitrates or digoxin). Except for loop diuretics and digoxin, all of these options for treatment have been shown to improve symptoms, reduce hospitalization rates and/or prolong survival, in large randomized controlled trials [16,17].

Drug selection for HF depends on the type of HF and on the personal characteristics of the patients, the most important goals being as already mentioned: to reduce mortality, to improve clinical status and functional capacity and to prevent hospitalization [16,17].

2.1. Mechanisms of Action of the Classical Therapy in Chronic HF Patients

Later, we summarize the mechanisms of actions and the benefits of the main classes of drugs/pharmaceutical substances used in the treatment of HF.

Beta-blockers bind to β adrenergic receptors ($β_1$-receptors located in the heart and kidneys; $β_2$-receptors located in the vessels, lungs, gastrointestinal tract, liver, uterus, and skeletal muscle; $β_3$-receptors located in the adipocytes). By binding to $β_1$-receptors, they block the deleterious actions of catecholamines: noradrenaline and adrenaline [18]. As a result, the heart rate and the contractility decrease and thus, the cardiac output and blood pressure will also decrease. As the heart rate will decrease, this will allow a longer time for diastolic filling, without typically reducing the stroke volume. Moreover, certain beta-blockers (cardioselective ones) will also reduce rennin secretion (via the blockade of $β_1$ receptors in the juxtaglomerular apparatus), thus decreasing the severity of angiotensin II-induced vasoconstriction and aldosterone-induced volume expansion [19]. They are classified into noncardioselective beta-blockers (e.g., propranolol, carvedilol, and labetalol) and cardioselective beta-blockers ($β_1$-selective, e.g., atenolol, metoprolol, bisoprolol and nebivolol). Certain beta-blockers are associated with vasodilating properties (nebivolol improves nitric oxide release, whereas carvedilol and labetalol block the $α_1$-receptor). The vasodilating properties are beneficial because they decrease the peripheral vascular resistance, thus improving stroke volume, left ventricular function and therefore, cardiac output [18].

ACEIs selectively inhibit the angiotensin-converting enzyme leading to decreased angiotensin II production and, therefore, limit its negative effects, such as vasoconstriction, antidiuretic hormones, and aldosterone secretion. Moreover, ACEIs will increase the levels of the potent vasoactive peptide bradykinin, an endogenous vasodilator. Thus, ACEIs will induce vasodilatation, decreasing the total peripheral resistance (both arterial and venous) and blood pressure. In this way, they decrease the left ventricular afterload, thus increasing cardiac output and decreasing filling pressures (both left and right), which will improve pulmonary and systemic venous congestion [20].

ARBs work on the same angiotensin pathway, the difference being the fact that they bind to AT1 receptors located on the vascular smooth muscle, as well as in other tissues (e.g., heart) and thus, they block the damaging actions of angiotensin II. They induce less vasoconstriction and antidiuretic hormone and aldosterone secretion and lower blood pressure. Therefore, as well as ACEIs, they prevent damage to the vasculature, heart and kidneys [20].

As in some cases, the ACEIs or ARBs do not suppress the excessive formation of aldosterone sufficiently, patients with moderate to severe heart failure can also benefit from aldosterone antagonists. MRAs work by competitively blocking the binding of aldosterone to the mineralocorticoid receptor, thus decreasing the reabsorption of sodium and water, as well as decreasing the excretion of potassium, leading to cardioprotective effects [21].

Loop diuretics act by inhibiting the luminal sodium-potassium chloride cotransporter located in the thick ascending limb of the loop of Henle, where approximately 20–30% of the filtration of sodium occurs. Therefore, compared with other diuretics, loop diuretics reduce the reabsorption of a much greater proportion of sodium, leading to the excretion of it, alongside water. This will decrease the plasma volume, cardiac workload, and oxygen demand, thereby relieving the signs and symptoms of volume excess. They are currently used to relieve symptoms associated with pulmonary congestion and peripheral edema in HF patients [22].

If the patient is intolerant to ACEIs/ARBs/ARNIs, other vasodilators can be used, such as isosorbide dinitrate or hydralazine. Isosorbide dinitrate acts by releasing nitric oxide into the vascular smooth muscle cell, which activates guanylyl cyclase (an enzyme that catalyzes the formation of cyclic guanosine monophosphate-cGMP from guanosine triphosphate–GTP). Therefore, the increased intracellular cGMP will activate a series of reactions, which will decrease the intracellular calcium and thus, the contractility of vascular smooth muscle, leading to smooth muscle relaxation and vasodilatation. Hydralazine also acts on the vascular smooth muscle, with multiple effects such as the stimulation of nitric oxide release from the vascular endothelium (with cGMP production and low-intracellular calcium concentration), opening of potassium channels and inhibition of calcium release from the sarcoplasmic reticulum, thus inducing smooth muscle relaxation and subsequent vasodilatation [23].

Digoxin increases cardiac muscle cells' contractility by inhibiting $Na^+/K^+/ATPaze$ pump in the cardiac muscle, a pump responsible for moving sodium ions out of the cells and bringing potassium ions into the cells. When sodium concentrations in the cardiac cell increases, another electrolyte mover known as the sodium-calcium exchanger pushes the excess of the sodium ions out, while bringing additional calcium ions in. Therefore, the intracellular calcium increases, which will later increase the force of contraction and thus the cardiac output. Cardiac output increases followed by a decrease in ventricular filling pressures. Moreover, it inhibits the atrio-ventricular node, by stimulating the parasympathetic nervous system. Therefore, it diminishes the electrical conduction in the AV node and thus the heart rate. However, it has not been shown to reduce mortality [24].

Ivabradine acts by blocking the I_f current channel, responsible for the cardiac peacemaker, which regulates the heart rate. In this way, it prolongs the diastolic time and decreases the heart rate without affecting myocardial contraction/relaxation or ventricular repolarization [25].

2.2. New Approaches in HF Pharmacological Treatment

As several pharmacological classes of drugs have emerged in recent years with proven long-term benefits, in the following, we describe some of the most important aspects, as they are currently underused.

2.2.1. Sacubitril/Valsartan

The combination of sacubitril and valsartan is the first from the class of angiotensin receptor–neprilysin inhibitors (ARNI). Agents in this new therapeutic class (sacubitril/valsartan) act at the level of RAAS and the neutral endopeptidase system. Sacubitril acts by inhibiting neprilysin and slowing down the degradation of natriuretic peptides, bradykinin, adrenomedullin, and other peptides [26]. It is indicated in chronic symptomatic heart failure with reduced ejection fraction [27].

Sacubitril/valsartan also improves symptom severity and heart functionality in patients with HFpEF, reducing the serum levels of the biomarker NT-pro BNP (and increasing BNP), an indicator of heart failure severity, and improves quality of life after 24 weeks [28].

One of the largest HF trials ever performed (PARADIGM-HF trial) compared enalapril with sacubitril/valsartan. In this trial, 8442 patients with HFrEF with FEVS $\leq$ 40% were enrolled and randomly received enalapril or sacubitril/valsartan twice daily. The trial was stopped early after 27 months because sacubitril/valsartan met the pre-specified stopping endpoint for an overwhelming benefit. All of the outcomes showed a 20% lower event rate in favor of sacubitril/valsartan; even the death rate from any cause was 16% lower in the group receiving sacubitril/valsartan [29]. ARNIs have been associated with improvements in diastolic function, left ventricular function, quality of life and decrease in ventricular arrythmias [30,31].

In the PROVE-HF and EVALUATE-HF trials, sacubitril/valsartan showed efficacy in improving the structural and functional changes that occur during heart failure. It improves cardiac remodeling and decreases the biomarker NT-pro BNP, so the drug reverses the damage to the heart in HFrEF patients [32].

Sacubitril/valsartan is recommended to replace ACE inhibitors when HFrEF patients are still symptomatic after optimal therapy. When initiating therapy with sacubitril/valsartan, there are some safety issues, including symptomatic hypotension, angioedema, and risk of hyperkalemia, so monitoring blood pressure levels, kidney function, and kalemia is extremely important [27,33]. Although the new combination was approved for the market starting from 2015, it is currently still underused, despite its proven benefits [34].

Figure 1 presents the mechanism of action of sacubitril/valsartan association and its consequences [27–34].

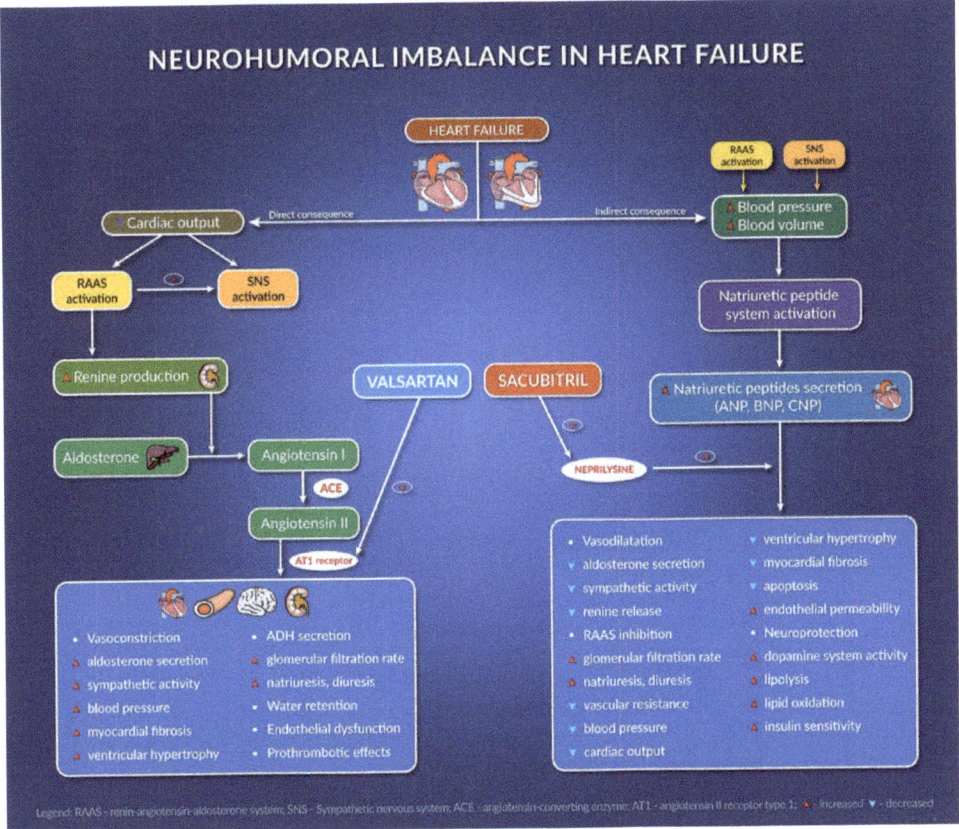

Figure 1. Neurohumoral imbalance in heart failure.

2.2.2. Sodium Glucose Co-Transporter-2 Inhibitors

It is known that patients with type 2 diabetes mellitus (T2DM) are prone to developing cardiovascular events and heart failure, which can lead to high rates of hospitalization and premature mortality [35].

A new class of antidiabetics, sodium glucose co-transporter-2 (SGLT2) inhibitors, has also been found to have beneficial effects in patients with cardiac diseases [36,37]. The compounds in this class are represented by empagliflozin, dapagliflozin, canagliflozin, and ertugliflozin [38]. They act by inhibiting glucose transport in the proximal tube of the kidney, resulting in glucosuria and, as a result, lower blood glucose levels [35].

Aside from the direct mechanism of action on glucose control, other indirect mechanisms are taken into account regarding possible cardiovascular benefits [39].

In Figure 2, we summarize the possible mechanisms involved, their actions, and their effect on the heart [39,40].

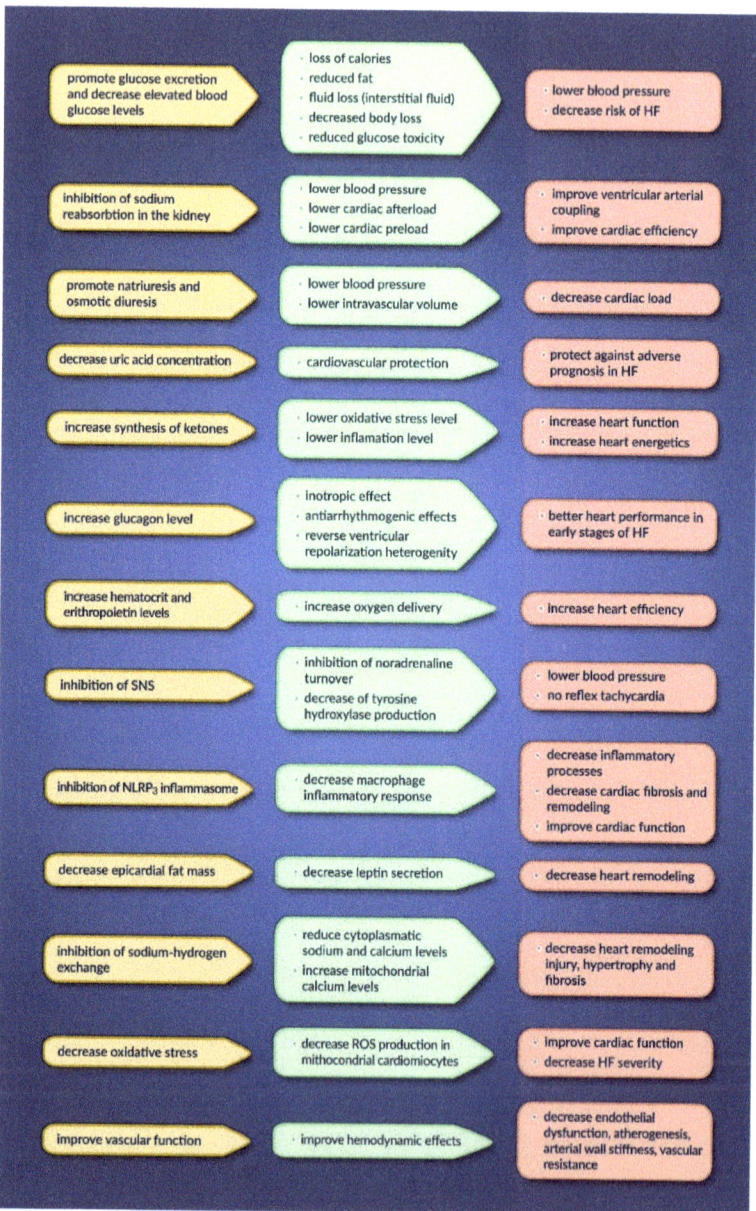

Figure 2. Mechanisms, actions and effects of SGLT2 inhibitors on the heart.

The main trials reporting the benefits of SGLT2 inhibitors in HF patients with reduced EF, more precisely of dapagliflozin and empagliflozin, are as follows: DAPA-HF [41], DEFINE-HF [42] and EMPEROR-reduced [43].

The DAPA-HF trial evaluated the long-term effects of dapagliflozin on the incidence of cardiovascular death or HF hospitalization, regardless of the presence of diabetes. It was a phase 3 randomized placebo-controlled study, enrolling 4744 patients suffering from chronic HFrEF (NYHA class II-IV, LVEF $\leq$ 40% in addition to the recommended HF therapy, NT-proBNP high and eGFR $\geq$ 30 mL/min/1.73 m^2) and having a median period of 18 months. The obtained results were as follows: a reduction in all-cause mortality and HF symptom aggravation, and the improvement in physical condition and overall quality of life. Their excellent benefits were seen very soon after starting the treatment with dapagliflozin. Regarding the incidence of adverse effects, they were attributed to volume depletion, renal dysfunction or hypoglycemia, but they did not differ between the studied groups [41].

The DEFINE-HF trial assessed the effect of dapagliflozin on the symptoms and biomarker plasmatic concentration of HFrEF patients (NYHA class II-III, LVEF $\leq$ 40%, eGFR $\geq$ 30 mL/min/1.73 m^2 and with elevated natriuretic peptides). In total, 263 patients were included (taking either dapagliflozin 10 mg/once, daily, or a placebo, for a period of 12 weeks, in addition to the recommended HF therapy). Dapagliflozin induced an improvement in the patients' health conditions or in their natriuretic peptides' plasmatic concentrations [42].

The EMPEROR-reduced clinical trial evaluated the outcome of empagliflozin in patients with chronic HFrEF (NYHA class II-IV, LVEF $\leq$ 40%, eGFR $\geq$ 20 mL/min/1.73 m^2). It was a double-blind clinical trial involving 3730 patients who received either empagliflozin (10 mg/once daily) or a placebo, in addition to the recommended HF therapy, for a median period of 18 months. Cardiovascular death and hospitalization rates (due to the worsening of HF) were reduced by empagliflozin, regardless of the presence of diabetes mellitus. The annual decline in the renal filtration rate was reduced, as well as the severity of renal complications. Non-complicated fungal infections of the genital tract were reported more often in patients taking empagliflozin [43].

Therefore, both substances are included as recommend treatments for HFrEF patients by the American and European guidelines [1,17].

The EMPEROR-preserved study assessed the effects of empagliflozin in patients with chronic HFpEF (NYHA class II-IV, LVEF $\geq$ 40%, eGFR $\geq$ 20 mL/min/1.73 m^2). In total, 5988 patients were included, who were randomized 1:1 and received either empagliflozin (10 mg/once daily) or a placebo, in addition to their classical HF therapy. Over a period of 26.2 months, the primary outcome was obtained (decreased risk of hospitalization in HF patients, regardless of the presence/absence of diabetes). Beneficial effects were also seen in eGFR, without considering the renal outcomes by themselves. It is important to note the fact that the most used medicines for HFrEF have not shown benefits in patients with HFpEF; therefore, empagliflozin is superior in improving HF outcomes even in patients with HFpEF, which are symptomatic and stable [44,45].

In Table 1, we summarize the indications, contra-indications and cautions worth considering for ARNI and SGLT2 inhibitors [17].

Table 1. The indications, contra-indications and cautions for ARNI and SGLT2 inhibitors.

	ARNI	SGLT2 Inhibitors
Indications	· HFrEF ($\leq$40%) · NYHA class II-IV · Alternative of ACEI/ARB	· HFrEF ($\leq$40%) ± diabetes mellitus · NYHA class II-IV
Contra-indications	- hypersensitivity to the active substances - history of angioedema - severe hepatic impairment - $\leq$36 h of the last ACEI dose	- hypersensitivity to the active substance - type I diabetes - dialysis - eGFR < 30 mL/min/1.73 m^2 (dapagliflozin) - eGFR < 20 mL/min/1.73 m^2 (empagliflozin)

Table 1. Cont.

	ARNI	SGLT2 Inhibitors
Cautions	◊ severe renal impairment (starting dose: 24/26 mg × 2/day) ◊ moderate hepatic impairment (starting dose: 24/26 mg × 2/day) ◊ SBP < 100 mmHg ◊ volume depletion ◊ renal artery stenosis ◊ pregnancy/lactation	◊ high risk of genital infections (especially mycotic) and urinary infections ◊ hypovolemia ◊ ketoacidosis ◊ acute renal impairment ◊ necrotizing fasciitis of the perineum (Fournier gangrene) ◊ bladder cancer ◊ pregnancy

3. Treatment Strategies in HF Patients

For the treatment of heart failure with preserved ejection fraction or with mildly reduced ejection fraction (LVEF $\geq$ 50% or LVEF between 40 and 49), the guidelines recommend the prescription of diuretics, as first line therapy [1]. The other drugs (ACEI or ARB, beta-blockers or MRA) may be considered as a second alternative [1].

The treatment strategy also focuses on treating co-morbidities such as: hypertension, atrial fibrillation, cardiac ischemic disease, pulmonary hypertension, diabetes mellitus, chronic kidney disease, COPD (chronic obstructive pulmonary disease), anemia and obesity. The optimal management of co-morbidities has been shown to improve symptoms and to improve the patient's quality of life [2].

In the case of congestion, diuretics will be very effective and will improve the symptomatology. There is proof that nebivolol, candesartan, digoxin and spironolactone might reduce hospitalization for patients with HFpEF in sinus rhythm [46]. Moreover, besides empagliflozin, none of other drugs consistently met their primary endpoint in the clinical trials that were performed, and none reduced mortality and morbidity [44,45].

For patients in atrial fibrillation, the prescription of an anticoagulant is very important for reducing thrombo-embolic events [47]. For the control of heart rate, the use of digoxin, beta-blockers or verapamil/diltiazem is recommended, targeting an optimal rate control between 60 and 100 bpm [48].

Amiodarone and non-dihydropyridine calcium-channel blockers (CCB) are able to reduce heart rate, but due to their adverse effects profile, they should be replaced, if possible. In the case of a fast ventricular rate and symptoms, it might be appropriate to consider AV node ablation, and if there are indications for ICD (implantable cardioverter-defibrillator), AV node ablation with the implantation of CRT-D (cardiac resynchronization therapy–defibrillator) might be preferred. The rhythm control strategy has not been shown to be superior to the rate control strategy. Urgent cardioversion is indicated if atrial fibrillation is life threatening [49].

Regarding HFrEF treatment, the evidence base for drug treatment in HF is for HFrEF. Either an ACEI/ARB/ARNI or a beta-blocker should be started (sometimes also ACEI/ARB/ARNI and beta-blocker at the same time), with doses up-titrated to the maximum tolerated/targeted dose every 2 weeks. ACEI, beta-blockers and MRA proved to improve survival and are recommended for the treatment of every patient with HFrEF. The new ARNI (sacubitril/valsartan) has been shown to be superior to ACEI in reducing the risk of death and hospitalization. Thus, ARNI is recommended to replace ACEI in cases of HFrEF patients if they are symptomatic despite optimal therapy [26].

In the case of decompensated patients, beta-blockers should not be initiated or if already initiated but patients develop worsening of HF symptoms (e.g., fatigue, dyspnea, dizziness or erectile dysfunction) caution should be applied regarding their prescription. Moreover, in the case of frailty or other complications (e.g., marginal hemodynamics), a longer period of time may be required for dose up-titration [17].

ARNI can be prescribed as an alternative to ACEI/ARB intolerance (e.g., angioedema) or in the absence of hypotension, electrolyte or renal imbalance. It is recommended to avoid the association of an ARNI with an ACEI and if previously administered ACEI, to ensure a 36 h washout period before the initiation of an ARNI, due to the high risk of angioedema [50]. This delay is not required when switching from ARB to ARNI. When up-titrating ARNI/ACEI/ARB (every 2 weeks or more), the monitoring of the potassium level, renal function and blood pressure is required. Lower loop diuretic doses may be necessary for the optimal titration of ARNI/ACEI/ARB and caution regarding the potassium concentration is required, as well as the dietary restriction of/supplementation with potassium, as the kaliuretic effect of loop diuretics might no longer be present [17].

If the patients have LVEF $\leq$ 35%, the guidelines recommend the use of MRAs to reduce mortality and hospitalization. MRAs (e.g., spironolactone or eplerenone) are added in patients with symptomatic chronic HFrEF, as a triple therapy (ACEI/ARB/ARNI + beta-blockers + MRA), in the absence of contra-indications. It is essential to achieve the targeted dose of other drugs before initiating the treatment with an aldosterone antagonist and to monitor the potassium levels and renal function under the treatment [17].

SGLT2 inhibitors can also be added, as part of the quadruple therapy (ACEI/ARB/ARNI + beta-blocker + MRA + SGLT2 inhibitor), in the absence of contra-indications. There is no need to achieve targeted doses of other drugs before adding SGLT2 inhibitors, although the loop diuretic dose might require adjustments based on the close monitoring of symptoms and weight [17].

Isosorbide dinitrate/Hydralazine could be prescribed especially for African American patients once the targeted dose of ACEI/ARB/ARNI + beta-blockers + MRA has been achieved [17].

The I_f channel inhibitor ivabradine is recommended in patients with symptomatic HFrEF or LVEF $\leq$ 35%, in sinus rhythm and heart rate $\geq$ 70 bpm, and in patients that have been hospitalized for HF in the last year, despite receiving beta-blockers at the maximum tolerated dose, ACEI and an MRA. The titration of the dose should be performed every 2 weeks in order to decrease the heart rate. In the case of patients $\geq$ 75 years old or in those with a history of conduction defects, the recommended initial dose is 2.5 mg twice daily, administered with meals [17].

4. Particularities of Patients

4.1. Age-Induced Changes

4.1.1. Cardiovascular Structure and Function

A reduction in the response after beta adrenergic stimulation was observed (due to impaired coupling of G-protein receptors to adenyl cyclase and a decrease in adenyl cyclase concentration), which damages the capacity of the aging heart to increase cAMP as a response to the stimulation of beta receptors [7,51]. Thus, age-related cardiovascular changes are associated with a reduction in chronotropic and inotropic responses, which decline with age (peak contractility and heart rate decline almost linearly with age) [52].

The filling of left ventricular diastole is impaired by the aging process, as it is a process that depends on energy and active myocardial relaxation. Altered calcium release by the cardiomyocytes, with resulting prolonged contractile period of the heart, was also observed in elderly people [7,53].

The high deposits of collagen, amyloid, and lipofuscin in the interstitial space and myocyte hypertrophy seen in older people increase cardiac stiffness and decrease cardiac compliance, altering cardiac filling, especially in critical situations [7,54–56].

The increased vascular (arterial) stiffness (due to collagen deposition and cross-linking in the vascular media and to fragmentation of arterial elastin), together with impaired endothelium-dependent vasorelaxation (a consequence of vascular inflammation and altered endothelial nitric oxide synthesis) observed in aging lead to a higher afterload and a predisposition to systolic hypertension in the elderly [57,58].

Inadequate mitochondrial synthesis of adenosine triphosphate in response to stress will lead to altered energy release, thus altered cellular reactions, such as gene expression, chromatin remodeling, intra/extra-cellular signaling, ion homeostasis, muscle contraction, protein and hormone synthesis and secretion, and neurotransmitter release and reuptake [59].

4.1.2. Other Organs

Age-associated modifications in the glomerular filtration rate and electrolyte imbalances [60,61] often seen in the elderly (due to dehydration, diuretic use, etc.) can raise the risk of HF decompensation and exacerbate the risk of drug side effects, with dangerous consequences, especially if the patient also has chronic kidney disease [62].

The aging of the respiratory system can lead to decreased compliance in pulmonary function. Moreover, the presence of chronic lung disease or sleep-related breathing disorders can increase the risk of pulmonary hypertension, exacerbate the sensation of dyspnea, and decrease biventricular filling [7,63,64].

The aging of the autonomic nervous system is characterized by sympathetic hyperreactivity and increased plasma concentrations of catecholamines, but a reduced sympathetic response is observed due to the diminished response of catecholamine receptors. Thus, tachycardia is felt less in elderly than middle-aged adults [65].

4.2. Sex Differences in HF

Regarding sex differences in heart failure, it seems that a large percentage of women tend to develop HRpEF, with the etiology of HF being either hypertension, diastolic dysfunction, or valvular pathology, whereas men tend to develop HFrEF or HFmrEF (HF with mid-range ejection fraction), with the etiology usually being an ischemic condition [66]. Moreover, it seems that women with HF are usually older and present with increased EF and more frequent symptoms linked to HF. Although they tend to also have multiple comorbidities compared to men, a meta-analysis showed that they have a better prognostic rate regarding hospitalization and mortality risk, regardless of EF [67].

The cardioprotection found in women seems to be due to the secretion of 17β-estradiol, an estrogen with a very clear established role in counteracting ischemic, hypertrophic, apoptotic, and cytotoxic impulses related to the heart [66,68,69].

Animal studies have shown that the cardiomyocytes of female models had a higher rate of survival after they were exposed to oxidative stress, which led to cell death, with the explanation relying on the fact that highly expressed estrogen receptor alpha (ER-α) can mediate the inhibition of pro-apoptotic pathways and the activation of the Akt signaling pathway [66,70].

Other differences regarding plasma B-type natriuretic peptide (BNP) levels, left ventricular mass index, left ventricular ejection fraction, and peak oxygen consumption between the sexes were also noted, suggesting that men are more susceptible to HF development than women [66,71,72].

Concerning treatment, it seems that although angiotensin-converting enzyme (ACE) inhibitors decrease the morbidity and mortality rates in both men and women, their effect seems to be more pronounced in men [73]. On the contrary, angiotensin II receptor blockers (ARBs) seem to have a higher mortality reduction rate in women than in men, although no difference was observed between the two classes of drugs (ACE inhibitors and ARBs) in terms of reduced mortality rates [74]. All of these aspects could be due to the action of estrogen on the receptor expression of angiotensin II by the ACE2 gene, located on chromosome X, and to the higher incidence of coughing and thus higher rate of discontinuation of ACE inhibitors in women [75].

No sex-related differences were observed in terms of treatment outcomes in patients under treatment with beta blockers or mineralocorticoid receptor antagonist [66].

Differences between the sexes were also noted in the case of digoxin treatment; women with a digoxin plasma concentration of 1.2–2.0 ng/mL had a higher mortality rate than men, although plasma levels of 0.5–0.9 ng/mL in men were associated with reduced mortality, but not any effect in women [76].

5. Particularities of Treatment

5.1. Pharmacokinetic Considerations and Their Consequences in HF Patients

Reduced blood flow to the gastrointestinal tract causes decreased absorption of drugs [77]. In the case of medicines with low permeability into the intestinal tissue, edema in the intestinal mucosa may affect their transport into the intestine [13,78].

Intestinal wall dysfunction secondary to hypoperfusion can, over time, induce chronic enteral inflammation and malnutrition. On the other hand, increased intestinal permeability in patients with HF can stimulate the transfer of drugs from the gastrointestinal tract to the portal blood [13].

Decreased blood perfusion in the central and peripheral organs results in an irregular tissue distribution of drugs [79]. Differences in the body's water load can also affect the distribution of drugs [80,81].

Plasma protein binding may also be affected, especially after a myocardial infarction (production of α1-glycoproteins in the liver increases tissue necrosis and inflammatory reactions in the myocardium) or in patients with cachexia [82].

Reduced hepatic and renal blood flow induces an altered metabolism and elimination of administered drugs and their metabolites. In addition to an irregular distribution of drugs in the liver (a consequence of poor hepatic blood infusion), hepatic congestion and/or hypoxia (as a major consequence) and hepatocellular lesions may occur, manifested by hepatocytolysis (and thus increased liver transaminases) and disorders affecting enzymatic activity [83,84].

Since the concentration of active substances at the site of action cannot yet be directly determined, plasma concentration is often measured as a surrogate marker of the drug effect, depending on the concentration of active substances at the site of action [80].

Practically, changes in pharmacokinetics have been only observed in patients with renal and/or hepatic complications [13,84,85].

Increased action of the following drugs was observed after oral administration in patients with decompensated HF: captopril, enalapril, perindopril, carvedilol, felodipine, candesartan, furosemide, milrinone, and enoximone [13,84,85].

Since most studies to date (clinical trials) have not included patients with decompensated HF or major renal or hepatic problems (which involve more severe changes in PK and PD), the pharmacokinetic and pharmacodynamic parameters are currently under-studied in patients with HF. Thus, we recommend paying more attention to monitoring the efficacy and safety of drugs used in HF. Furthermore, the progressive titration of drugs should be implemented and the benefit/risk ratio should be periodically evaluated [13,84,85].

5.2. Pharmadynamic Considerations

The pharmacodynamics of drugs, as well as their tolerability, may also be affected by several neuronal and endocrinological compensatory mechanisms in HF, including the activation of the renin-angiotensin (RAA) and sympathetic system. Moreover, nodal activity and baroreceptor sensitivity are affected, and peripheral vascular resistance is increased; these are aspects that could cause an altered response to administered drugs [13,84,85].

The activation of the sympathetic nervous system can alter the perfusion of the viscera, especially the splenic organs (liver, gastrointestinal tract, kidneys), to maintain the perfusion of vital organs (brain and heart), resulting in hypoperfusion in the liver and kidneys. Furthermore, increased central pressure in patients with right HF causes hepatic congestion and dilation of the central vein in the hepatic acini, inducing hepatocellular ischemia and necrosis, and reducing the activity of microsomal enzymes [13,84–86].

Therefore, it is advisable to consider all changes that might occur in heart failure patients (Figure 3) [13,84–86].

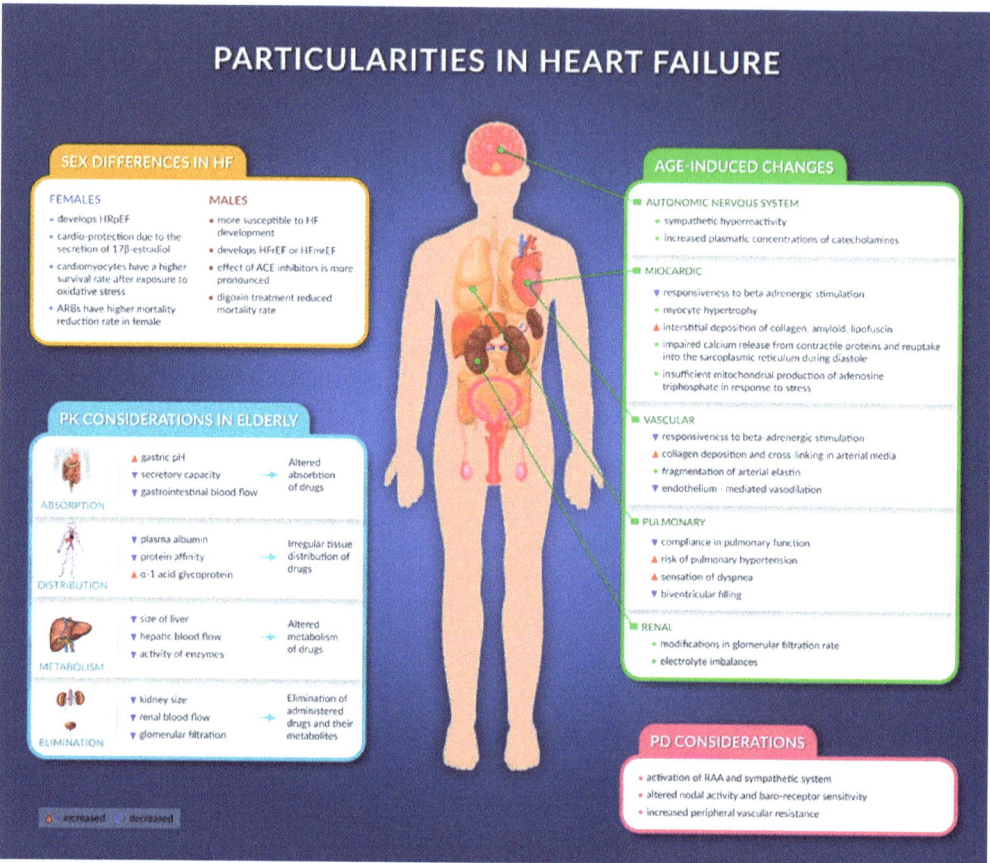

Figure 3. Particularities in heart failure.

5.3. HF Treatment in Patients with Cardiorenal Syndrome

It is well known that the acute/chronic dysfunction of one organ could induce the acute/chronic dysfunction of the other organ [87], therefore, cardiorenal syndrome has been defined as a spectrum of diseases involving the heart and the kidneys. This syndrome implies a "hemodynamic cross-talk" between the injured heart and the kidneys' responses and vice versa [87,88]. Several mechanisms underline this cardiorenal syndrome, such as the hemodynamic interactions between the heart and kidneys in HF patients; cytokine production; the impact of atherosclerotic disease on both organs; biochemical perturbations due to the installation of chronic kidney disease; and the structural changes that appear in the heart, which are due to kidney disease progression [87,89].

In summary, the drop in cardiac output induces the activation of the sympathetic nervous system which will increase the stroke volume and the heart rate, as a compensatory mechanism. Sympathetic nervous system activation will also stimulate the release of renin from the kidneys, with the consequence of RAAS activation. Moreover, the drop in cardiac output will also induce a decreased perfusion of the kidneys, leading to kidney injuries (the beginning of cardiorenal syndrome). A reduced perfusion in the kidneys will stimulate renin release, RAAS activation and thus sodium and water retention (due to aldosterone secretion and antidiuretic hormone release), which will later increase the mean arterial pressure and the preload and decrease the cardiac output. RAAS activation will also cause vasoconstriction, which will contribute to reduced renal perfusion [87,89,90].

Moreover, chronic kidney disease (CKD) can lead to cardiovascular dysfunction, as a low glomerular filtration rate activates RAAS, which will lead, in time, to cardiac remodeling and left ventricular hypertrophy. CKD also implies a reduction in erythropoietin production over time, leading to anemia, which will increase the risk of ischemic events in the heart. Moreover, CKD induces a decrease in vitamin D production and parathormone stimulation, leading to an increase in calcium and phosphate levels and thus, increased risk of coronary and vessel calcification, augmenting the high risk of ischemic events [91]. Electrolyte imbalances are also observed in CKD patients, more precisely, hyperkalemia, which can increase the risk of cardiovascular complications [87].

Therefore, the management of cardiorenal syndrome is challenging and must be directed towards the specific pathophysiologic mechanism involved. The volume overload can be either addressed by prescribing diuretics (usually loop diuretics, as they are the most potent diuretics e.g., furosemide, torsemide and bumetanide) or using ultrafiltration methods. The addition of a thiazide diuretic to a loop diuretic may be preferred in the case of diuretic resistance, as an initial approach to restore euvolemia [87,89]. Regarding HF treatment in patients with renal disease, the renal function and potassium level should be checked within 1–2 weeks of the initiation or up-titration of an ACEI/ARB/ARN. Regarding aldosterone antagonists (MRA), in patients with preserved renal function or mild to moderate impairment, potassium levels and renal function should be checked within 2–3 days after the initiation of the therapy, followed by a check after 7 days of treatment, and at least monthly for the first 3 months and then, every 3 months [17].

In patients with severe renal impairment (eGFR < 30 mL/min/1.73 m^2), the ARBs/ACEIs are considered safe. The starting dose of ARNI (Sacubitril/Valsartan) should be reduced to 24/26 mg, twice a day, in patients with severe renal impairment. The dose of ARNI might also need to be reduced in the case of hypotension or hyperkalemia. MRAs are contraindicated in patients with severe renal impairment, creatinine > 2.5 mg/dL in men, creatinine > 2 mg/dL in women or potassium > 5.0 mEq/L. As for SGLT2 inhibitors, there is currently no evidence regarding dose adjustments in patients with eGFR < 30 mL/min/1.73 m^2 for dapagliflozin and eGFR < 20 mL/min/1.73 m^2 for empagliflozin [17]. As a general rule, a decrease in eGFR of more than 30% or the apparition of hyperkalemia should alert the clinician to adjust (decrease) the doses of HF drugs [17].

5.4. HF Treatment in Pregnancy and Lactation

During pregnancy, the increased physiological requirements are partially fulfilled through changes in the physiology of the cardiovascular system, which has to adapt to the extra metabolic demands of the fetus and of the other organ systems. Therefore, the augmentation of the size and activity of the uterus, as well as the increase in blood flow in the choriodecidual space, represents extra work for the cardiovascular system. Moreover, during pregnancy, the skin and kidneys have an increased perfusion which allows them to disperse heat and retain sodium and water [92,93].

Symptoms of HF are more likely to appear in the second trimester as a consequence of an increased cardiac output and of intravascular volume (during pregnancy, the plasma volume increases by 40% and the cardiac output by 30–50%) [94]. Therefore, the therapeutical management of HF during pregnancy will be adapted to the clinical setting and the severity of the pathology. For cases in which the oral administration of drugs is sufficient, diuretics, betablockers, hydralazine or nitrates can be recommended. Usually, diuretics represent the first line treatment for pregnant HF women due to the increased preload associated with pregnancy (therefore, reducing preload will diminish the left side filling pressure and the pulmonary capillary pressure, and thus, it will allow the resorption of the pulmonary interstitial fluid). Currently, there is no evidence that diuretics are directly responsible for fetal growth restrictions. Betablockers decrease the heart rate and allow a greater filling during diastole. Beta-1-selective blockers (for example metoprolol succinate or bisoprolol) are preferred and better tolerated [1,92].

Regarding the management of HF before pregnancy, ACEIs, ARBs, ARNI, MRA and SGLT2 inhibitors, as well as ivabradine should all be avoided and stopped prior to conception due to an increased risk of fetal harm. It is recommended that the pregnancy be planned and closely monitored by a multidisciplinary team of specialists in order to avoid HF decompensation and fetal harm (induced by either the pathology or the treatment) [1].

Hydralazine, methyldopa, or oral nitrates can also be recommended during pregnancy [1].

In patients with atrial fibrillation, low-molecular-weight heparins are the first choice of anticoagulant treatment (NOAC should be avoided due to insufficient data regarding their safety) [1].

Concerning the breastfeeding period in HF women, it is important to know that the mother's treatment prevail over breastfeeding compatibility, and that the benefits of breastfeeding are important for both the mother and child [95,96]. Enalapril is among the preferred options of ACEIs (as it has the most assuring safety data) and can be used from birth. [95]. As a second option, among the ARBs, losartan can be a good choice, due to its extensive first-pass metabolism and thus low systemic concentration, but breastfeeding should be performed with caution [95]. From the betablockers, metoprolol succinate or propranolol are the preferred choices (favorable PK profile and assuring data). Additionally, carvedilol or bisoprolol can be seen as a second option of treatment. Sacubitril/valsartan association should be avoided due to lack of data regarding their use during pregnancy, as well as SGLT2 inhibitors. Moreover, there is good evidence for digoxin, hydralazine and spironolactone use during breastfeeding period. The monitorization of babies exposed to either betablockers or ACEIs is recommended for hypotension (especially in neonates), lethargy, drowsiness, bradycardia, poor feeding, or weight gain [95].

6. Drugs and Food Supplements That Can Aggravate HF

The treatment of HF patients is very complex and includes not only lifestyle changes but also multiple pharmacological therapies, as well as the presence of co-morbidities and individual pharmacological strategies; this leads to polypharmacy in HF patients, generating increased iatrogenic risks [97,98].

In Appendix A we summarize the main/most used drugs and food supplements that can worsen the prognosis of heart failure patients; thus, it is recommended to avoid them by this category of patients [99–170].

7. Potential Drug–Drug Interactions in HF Patients

Several studies have shown a strong association between the number of drugs taken by HF patients (usually more than five) and the occurrence of potential drug–drug interactions, leading to the conclusion that the incidence of drug–drug interactions in HF patients is extremely high [97,171,172].

The coordinated efforts of a multidisciplinary team of healthcare providers also involving a clinical pharmacist could reduce the medication-related problems and improve the efficacy, tolerability, and safety of the pharmacological strategies implemented by physicians [171,173,174].

Appendix B summarizes the main important drug–drug interactions that should be considered in HF patients, their consequences, and some recommendations regarding their management [174–185].

8. Adverse Drug Reactions in HF Patients

Adverse drug reactions (ADRs) have been estimated to account for approximatively 10–20% of hospital admissions in geriatric units [186]. Moreover, an observational study performed in 1996 highlighted that the iatrogenic problems accounted for nearly 7% of HF admissions and were associated with higher mortality and prolonged hospital stays compared with those of non-iatrogenic causes [187,188]. Thus, the decompensation of HF patients due to iatrogenic conditions is a well-known and documented problem, which leads to increased morbidity and mortality rates. Therefore, good management of all prescribed drugs is mandatory for HF patients.

It seems that there are also sex-related differences between men and women regarding ADRs. Although women are underrepresented in all phases of clinical trials and little is known about this aspect, several meta-analyses concluded that women are more susceptible (1.5–1.7×) to developing ADRs than men and are also at higher risk of hospitalization due to the severity of ADRs [189,190].

As women usually present HFpEF with additional risk factors (co-morbidities and advanced age) compared with other types of HF, there seems to be a high incidence of polypharmacy, as they tend to take more drugs than men (including over-the-counter drugs and food supplements); thus, they have an increased risk of iatrogenic events (due to ADRs and drug interactions) and low adherence to treatment. Other explanations may underline this problem of high iatrogenic risk. Sex differences in the pharmacokinetics and pharmacodynamics of administered drugs (regarding distribution volume, hepatic/renal clearance, sex hormones, alterations in drug target expression and signal transduction pathways, immunological conditions, etc.) predispose women to a higher probability of overdosing than men [190–194]. Drug-induced ventricular arrhythmia (torsade de pointes) is more often encountered in women, as women have longer QTc intervals, probably due to the sex hormone modulation of Ca^{2+} and K^+ channels implicated in ventricular repolarization [190,195]. Differences in prescribing habits for men and women compared with the recommended guidelines is another reason supporting the high incidence of ADRs in women, as well as the overall poor quality of life observed in women HF patients [189,190].

All of the aforementioned sex-related differences in female patients predispose women to a higher probability of drug-induced complications such as bleeding problems (e.g., under antithrombotics), electrolyte abnormalities (e.g., under diuretics), cough and increased creatinine (under treatment with ACE inhibitors), myopathy (under statin treatment), hepatotoxicity, skin diseases, etc. [190,196,197].

Thus, it is important to adjust the drug dosage as a function of total body weight/size or glomerular filtration rate and titrate it to the required clinical effect, especially in those with a narrow therapeutic index, in order to avoid the incidence of ADRs [189,190].

9. Discontinuation of Drugs in HF Patients

Several articles also discuss the negative outcomes of HF patients after discontinuing chronic HF treatment [2,187,198–200].

It was observed that RAAS (renin-angiotensin-aldosterone system) inhibitors provide the most beneficial outcomes in terms of mortality reduction in patients with HFrEF, although renal function is affected at baseline [201]. The cessation of these drugs in patients with HFrEF was associated with increased mortality and re-hospitalization admissions after 1 month, 3 months, and 1 year, which led to the conclusion that RAAS inhibitors should not be discontinued in patients with moderate to several renal dysfunction if the benefits outweigh the risks [202].

Regarding beta blocker discontinuation, although they are associated with a risk of negative inotropic effects and hypotension, ESC has recommended not to disrupt beta blocker treatment unless severe hypotension is present, due to the risk of rebound effects (such as rebound tachycardia, aggravation of angina pectoris, risk of ventricular arrhythmia) and the correlation with increased mortality and readmissions rates after cessation of treatment [2,199,203]. Several trials highlighted that continuous administration of beta blockers in patients with decompensated HF reduced the mortality and readmission rates [203–205].

10. Conclusions

In order to reduce exacerbations, hospital readmission rates, morbidity, and mortality and to improve the overall quality of life, an interdisciplinary approach to treatment strategies is mandatory for HF patients. The treatment strategy must be individualized for each

HF patient, periodically monitored and reviewed by the healthcare team. Moreover, patient education, including topics such as dietary counseling, healthy lifestyle habits, regular exercise in a tolerable amount, alcohol and smoking cessation; moreover, understanding the alarming signs and symptoms of HF decompensation (shortness of breath, fatigue, ankle swelling, sudden weight modification) is another extremely important action that needs to be urgently implemented by societies with aging populations.

Author Contributions: Conceptualization, V.B., A.P., D.C., S.N. and L.P.; methodology, V.B., A.P., C.R. and C.D.; resources, D.E.M., M.S., M.A., C.D. and S.C.; data curation, L.P., S.C. and S.N.; writing—original draft preparation, V.B., A.P., A.S., D.E.M., D.C. and C.R.; writing—review and editing, M.A., M.S., L.P. and C.A.D. All authors have read and agreed to the published version of the manuscript.

Funding: This research received no external funding.

Conflicts of Interest: The authors declare no conflict of interest.

Appendix A

Table A1. Drugs and food supplements that can worsen HF prognosis.

Drugs [99]	Possible Mechanism Involved	Results	References
NSAIDs	Inhibition of cyclooxygenase enzyme Inhibition of renal prostaglandin synthesis	Sodium and water retention Higher systemic vascular resistance Reduction in renal perfusion, glomerular filtration rate, sodium excretion	[100–106]
Alpha-1 blockers (e.g., doxazosin)	Beta-1 receptor stimulation Stimulation of renin and aldosterone release Chronic alfa1 antagonism Stimulation of heart fibrosis factor galectin-3 expression	Edema Tachyphylaxis Cardiomyocyte apoptosis Myocardial hypertrophy	[107]
Calcium channel blockers (e.g., verapamil, diltiazem)	Negative inotrope Calcium channel blockade	Cardiac depression Atrioventricular conduction block	[103,106]
Moxonidine (centrally acting α-adrenergic drug)	Possible sympathetic withdrawal	Myocardial depression Hypotension Rebound norepinephrine increase	[108]
Class I antiarrhythmic (e.g., flecainide, disopyramide)	Negative inotrope Pro-arrhythmic stimulation	Myocardial infarction Premature ventricular beats Myocardial depressant effects	[106,109]
Class III antiarrhythmic (e.g., sotalol)	Beta inhibition Pro-arrhythmic stimulation Potassium channel blockade	Bradycardia Prolonged QT interval Torsades de pointes T-wave abnormalities	[109–111]
Inhibitors of dipeptidyl peptidase 4 (e.g., sitagliptin, saxagliptin)	Dipeptidyl peptidase 4 enzyme interference Direct interaction in myocytes Calcium channel interference Interference in substance P degradation Sympathetic nervous system stimulation	Myocardial infarction Stroke	[103,112–115]
Thiazolidinediones (e.g., rosiglitazone, pioglitazone)	Possible calcium channel blockade Interference with mitochondrial respiration or oxidative stress	Sodium and water retention Peripheral edema Myocardial infarction Stroke Transient ischemic attacks	[106,115–117]

Table A1. Cont.

Drugs [99]	Possible Mechanism Involved	Results	References
Itraconazole	Negative inotropic effect Mitochondrial dysfunction Inhibition of 11 beta-hydroxysteroid dehydrogenase 2 Cytochrome P450 inhibition	Peripheral edema Hypertension Prolonged QT interval Cardiac depression Excess mineralocorticoid Myofibroblast damage	[118–120]
Amphotericin B	Unknown	Cardiotoxicity Dilated cardiomyopathy	[121]
Carbamazepine(overdose)	Negative inotropic and chronotropic effects Depression of phase 2 repolarization Direct toxic effect on myocardial fibers Anticholinergic action Increased automaticity of ectopic pacemakers Sodium channel blockade	Left ventricular dysfunction Suppressed sinus nodal activity Atrioventricular conduction disturbances Hypotension	[122–124]
Pregabalin	Alterations in cardiac renin angiotensin system (RAS) L-type calcium channel blockade	Peripheral edema Decreased calcium influx in cardiomyocytes Left ventricular deterioration	[125–127]
Tricyclic antidepressants	Negative inotrope Pro-arrhythmic stimulation Norepinephrine and serotonin reuptake blockade Sodium channel blockade Suppression of potassium channels in myocytes Vasoconstriction of cerebral arteries	Arrhythmias Impaired heart conduction Prolonged intraventricular conduction Prolonged QT interval Hemorrhagic stroke Ischemic stroke	[128,129]
Citalopram	Inhibition of depolarizing current mediated by L-type calcium channels Antagonistic effects on myocardial potassium channels	Prolonged QT interval Episodes of torsades de pointes Arrhythmias	[130,131]
Pergolide, cabergoline, pramipexole	Potent agonists at cardiac myocyte 5-HT2B serotonin receptors Induction of fibroblast activation	Valvular damage Cardiac valvular regurgitation Pulmonary arterial hypertension Peripheral edema	[132–134]
Clozapine	Calcium channel blockade Ig-E mediated hypersensitivity Reduced left ventricular function	Myocarditis Cardiomyopathy Prolonged QT interval Elevated troponin	[135–138]
Lithium	Altered acetylcholinesterase activity Direct myofibril degeneration Induction of oxidative stress Interference with calcium ion influx	Cardiac fibrosis Cardiomyocyte apoptosis Rhythm disturbances Edema, ascites Complete heart block and first-degree AV block	[139–143]
β2 adrenergic agonists (e.g., salbutamol)	Decreased β-receptor responsiveness Small positive inotropic and chronotropic effects Activation of Gs/cAMP/PKA Inhibition of Gi/PDE	Arrhythmias Prolonged QT interval	[144,145]

Table A1. Cont.

Drugs [99]	Possible Mechanism Involved	Results	References
Tumor necrosis factor-α (TNF-α) inhibitors	Cytokine mediation Sympathetic excitation Inflammation and renin-angiotensin system upregulation	Peripheral inflammation Cardiac dysfunction	[146–148]
Topical beta-blockers (e.g., timolol)	Hemodynamic effects due to beta blockade	Arrhythmias Myocardial ischemia Hypotension Pulmonary edema	[99]
Food supplements [149]	Possible mechanism involved	Results	Reference
Aconitum spp. (Monkshood)	Alkaloids block potassium channels	Ventricular fibrillation Bradycardia Hypotension	[150]
Aesculus hippocastanum L. (Horse chestnut)	Antiplatelet effect	Increased risk of bleeding when associated with anticoagulant drugs	[151]
Allium sativum L. (Garlic)	Inhibition of platelet aggregation (dose-dependent)	Increased risk of bleeding when associated with anti-thrombotic drugs	[152]
Aloe barbadensis Mill. (Aloe vera)	Laxative effect	Risk of hypokalemia with increased toxicity of cardiotonic glycosides or antiarrhythmia drugs	[153]
Angelica sinensis (Oliv.) Diels (Angelica)	Antiplatelet and anticoagulant effect	Increased anticoagulant effect	[154]
Cassia senna L. (Senna)	Laxative effect	Risk of hypokalemia with increased toxicity of digitalis or antiarrhythmia drugs	[153]
Citrus paradisi Macfad. (Grapefruit)	Inhibition of CYP3A4 enzyme	Increased effects (therapeutic or toxic) of co-administered drugs (e.g., calcium channel blockers, antiarrhythmia drugs) Inefficacy of pro-drugs metabolized by CYP3A4	[155,156]
Cratageus spp. (Hawthorn)	Increases digitalis toxicity (incompletely elucidated)	Risk of digitalis intoxication if co-administered	[157,158]
Ephedra sinica Stapf (Chinese ephera)	Alkaloids stimulate adrenergic receptors Indirect agonist stimulation and noradrenaline release	Tachycardia Hypertension Arrythmias Heart attack Stroke	[159]
Ginkgo biloba L. (Ginkgo)	Antiplatelet effect	Increased risk of bleeding when co-administered with antithrombotic drugs	[160,161]
Glycyrrhiza glabra L. (Licorice)	Hypokalemia Reduced sodium and water excretion	Increased toxicity of digitalis or antiarrhythmic drugs Decreased effect of diuretics	[153]
Harpagophytum procumbens Burch. (Devil's claw)	Inhibition of CYP1A2 and CYP2D6	Increased effects of diuretics, antihypertensives, statins, and anticoagulants	[162,163]

Table A1. *Cont.*

Food supplements [149]	Possible mechanism involved	Results	Reference
Hypericum perforatum L. (St. John's Wort)	Induction of CYP3A4 isoenzyme activity	Decreases plasma levels of co-administered drugs metabolized by this enzyme	[164–166]
Leonurus cardiaca L. (Motherwort)	Antiplatelet effect	Increased risk of bleeding when co-administered with antithrombotic drugs	[152]
Oenothera biennis L. (Evening primrose)	Inhibition of platelet activating factor	Increased risk of bleeding when co-administered with antithrombotic drugs	[167,168]
Panax ginseng C.A. Meyer (Asian ginseng)	Decreased prothrombin time	Decreased warfarin effect and increased risk of thrombo-embolic events	[152]
Stephania tetrandra S. Moore	Calcium channel blockade	Cardiac depression	[169]
Zingiber officinale Roscoe (Ginger)	Thromboxane synthase inhibition Prostacyclin agonist	Increased risk of bleeding when co-administered with antithrombotic drugs Increased effects of antihypertensive drugs	[170]

Appendix B

Table A2. Drug-drug interactions in HF.

Main Drug for HF	Co-Administered Drugs	Consequences	Recommendations
ACE inhibitors	ARBs/aliskiren (angiotensin II receptor blockers)	Increased risk of impaired renal function, acute renal failure, hyperkalemia, hypotension, syncope and falls, thus increased risk of fractures in the elderly	Avoid association
	Sacubitril	High risk of angioedema	Avoid association
	NSAIDs (nonsteroidal anti-inflammatory drugs)	Risk of acute renal failure due to decreased glomerular filtration rate (decreased synthesis of renal vasodilating prostaglandins), especially if patient is elderly, dehydrated, or under diuretic treatment	If possible, avoid association If association is needed, proper hydration is recommended, monitoring of renal function, administering the lowest therapeutic NSAID dose and for the shortest period of time
	Spironolactone, amiloride, triamterene	High risk of hyperkalemia, especially in patients with chronic renal failure	Evaluate renal function before beginning of treatment (determine creatinine clearance), administer in therapeutically effective minimum doses and periodically check potassium
	Allopurinol	Higher risk of hypersensitivity reactions (Steven-Johnson syndrome)	If associated, ensure clinical supervision and adjust dose [177]
	Gliptins	Increased risk of angioedema through decreased DPPIV by gliptin	Avoid association If associated, ensure clinical supervision and adjust dose

Table A2. Cont.

Main Drug for HF	Co-Administered Drugs	Consequences	Recommendations
	Insulin	High risk of hypoglycemia	Monitor blood glucose and adjust insulin dosage
	Hypoglycemic sulfonamides	Hypoglycemic risk through improved glucose tolerance and decreased hypoglycemic sulfonamide dose requirements	Monitor blood glucose and adjust dosage of hypoglycemic sulfonamides
	Racecadotril	High risk of allergic side effects (angioneurotic edema)	Avoid association If associated, ensure clinical supervision and adjust dose
	Lithium	Increased lithium plasma concentration through decreased elimination	Avoiding association If associated, ensure clinical supervision and adjust lithium dose
ARBs	ACE inhibitors NSAIDs Spironolactone Lithium	Same as for ACE inhibitors	
Sacubitril/valsartan	Statins	Increased effects of statins	Adjust statin dose [178]
	Sildenafil	Additional blood pressure reduction	Use caution when associated and adjust dose of sildenafil [179]
Beta blockers (carvedilol, bisoprolol, metoprolol, nebivolol)	Amiodarone	Cardiac conduction disorders, bradycardia, atrioventricular block	Preferably avoid association, or adapt drug dosages and conduct patient monitoring (ECG, heart rate)
	Verapamil Diltiazem	Cardiac depression, HF decompensation, AV block	Preferably avoid association
	Antidiabetic drugs	Risk of masking signs of hypoglycemia (palpitations, tachycardia, tremor of extremities)	Preferably avoid association or closely monitor dosage of antidiabetic drugs
	Digitalis	Automatic disorders (bradycardia, sinus arrest), AV block	Preferably avoid association or adjust dosages
	NSAIDs	Decreased antihypertensive effect due to inhibition of renal vasodilating prostaglandin synthesis by NSAIDs	Preferably avoid association or adjust dosages
	Mexiletine	Negative inotropic effect Automation disorders Risk of cardiac decompensation	Preferably avoid association
	Central antihypertensives	Decreased central sympathetic tone and vasodilating effect of central blood-lowering drugs	Preferably avoid association
	Imipramine antidepressants (e.g., amitriptyline)	Intensification of vasodilating effect and risk of orthostatic hypotension	Avoid association or adapt beta blocker dosage
	Neuroleptics	Vasodilator effect Risk of orthostatic hypotension	Monitor blood pressure and adapt dosages if needed

Table A2. Cont.

Main Drug for HF	Co-Administered Drugs	Consequences	Recommendations
	Anticholinesterases	Excessive bradycardia	Avoid association or monitor heart rate with adjustment of beta blocker dosage
Diuretics	NSAIDs	Decreased diuretic effect and risk of kidney failure	Avoid association if possible
	Carbamazepine	Increased risk of hyponatremia	Hydrate patient and correct electrolyte imbalances
	Lithium	Decreased renal elimination of lithium with high risk of accumulation	Avoid association if possible or adapt lithium dosage
SGLT2 inhibitors Dapagliflozin Empagliflozin	Thiazide diuretics/loop diuretics	Increased diuretic effect	Adjust dosage Monitor the blood pressure. Hydrate patients and monitor the electrolyte balance
Nitrates	Sildenafil	Increased risk of hypotension, blood pressure collapse	Avoid association or adjust dosage
	Heparins	Increased excretion of heparins	Adjust dosage
Digoxin	Amiodarone Propafenone Quinidine Clarithromycin Hypokalemic diuretics	Digoxin toxicity	Avoid association or adjust dosage
	Carbamazepine Dronedarone	Decreased plasma concentration of digoxin Cardiac deprivation Increased digoxinemia	Therapeutic supervision Therapeutic supervision (clinical and ECG) Reduce digoxin dosage by half
Amiodarone	Verapamil/ Diltiazem	Cardiac deprivation with high risk of bradycardia and atrioventricular block	Avoid intravenous administration, use ECG surveillance when administered orally
	Levofloxacin/ moxifloxacin	Ventricular rhythm disorders (risk of torsades des pointes)	Therapeutic supervision (clinical and ECG)
	Statins	Increased effects of statins	Adjust statin dose (maximum 20 mg/day for simvastatin)
Ivabradine	Verapamil/ diltiazem	Increased ivabradine plasma concentration with increased risk of side effects Marked bradycardia	Avoid association
	Azithromycin	Ventricular rhythm disorders (risk of torsades des pointes)	Therapeutic supervision (clinical and ECG)
AVK	Amiodarone	Increased AVK effects Hemorrhagic risk	INR (International Normalized Ratio) control Adjust dosage (up to 4 weeks after stopping amiodarone treatment)

Table A2. Cont.

Main Drug for HF	Co-Administered Drugs	Consequences	Recommendations
	Allopurinol	Increased hemorrhagic risk	INR surveillance and adjust AVK dosage up to 8 days after stopping allopurinol treatment [180]
	Cefamandole/ cefazolin/ ceftriaxone	Increased AVK plasma concentration with high hemorrhagic risk	INR surveillance and adjust AVK dosage
	Fluoroquinolones	Increased AVK plasma concentration with high hemorrhagic risk	INR surveillance and adjust AVK dosage
	Fenofibrate	Increased AVK plasma concentration with high hemorrhagic risk	INR surveillance and adjust AVK dosage
	Paracetamol	Increased AVK plasma concentration with high hemorrhagic risk when given paracetamol in high dosage (>4 g/day), >4 days	INR surveillance and adjust AVK and paracetamol dosage
	Thiamazole (methimazole)	Increased risk of bleeding due to hypoprothrombinemia caused by methimazole	If possible, avoid association or conduct INR surveillance and adjust AVK dosage [181]
	NSAIDs	Increased AVK plasmatic concentration with high hemorrhagic risk	If possible, avoid association or conduct INR surveillance and adjust AVK dosage
NOAC (New Oral Anticoagulants)	Rifampicin	Decreased NOAC efficacy and increased thromboembolic risk	Clinical supervision Adjust NOAC dose up to 8 days after stopping rifampicin treatment [180]
	Itraconazole/ ketoconazole/ voriconazole	Increased NOAC plasma concentration and efficacy with high risk of bleeding	Clinical surveillance and adjust dose of NOAC
	Carbamazepine/ levetiracetam/ phenobarbital/ valproic acid	Decreased NOAC efficacy and increased thromboembolic risk	Clinical supervision and adjust NOAC dose
Dabigatran	Amiodarone	High plasma concentration of dabigatran and increased risk of bleeding	Clinical supervision and adjust dabigatran dose (maximum 150 mg/day) [182]
	Dronedarone	High plasma concentration of dabigatran (also rivaroxaban) with increased risk of bleeding	Clinical supervision and adjust dabigatran/rivaroxaban dose
	Quinidine	High plasma concentration of dabigatran with increased risk of bleeding	Avoid association If associated, clinical supervision and adjust dabigatran dose
	Fluconazole/ itraconazole/ ketoconazole	High plasma concentration of dabigatran with increased risk of bleeding	Avoid association If associated, clinical supervision and adjust dabigatran dose

Table A2. *Cont.*

Main Drug for HF	Co-Administered Drugs	Consequences	Recommendations
Apixaban	Diltiazem	Increased plasma concentration of apixaban with increased risk of bleeding [182,183]	Clinical supervision and adjust apixaban dose
	Clarithromycin/ Erythromycin	High plasma concentration of apixaban/rivaroxaban with increased risk of bleeding	Clinical supervision and adjust apixaban/rivaroxaban dose
	Fluconazole	High plasma concentration of apixaban/rivaroxaban with increased risk of bleeding	Avoid association If associated, clinical supervision and adjust apixaban dose
Antiplatelet agents	NSAIDs	Increased risk of bleeding (especially gastro-intestinal)	Avoid association If associated, clinical supervision and adjust dose
	Heparins/ oral anticoagulants	Increased risk of bleeding	Avoid association If associated, clinical supervision and adjust dose
	Selective serotonin reuptake inhibitors (SSRIs)	Increased risk of bleeding	Avoid association If associated, clinical supervision and adjust dose
	Antidepressants with mixed adrenergic–serotoninergic mechanism	Increased risk of bleeding	Avoid association If associated, clinical supervision and adjust dose
	Pentoxifylline	Increased risk of bleeding	Clinical supervision and dose adjustments
Clopidogrel	Proton pump inhibitors (PPIs)	High thromboembolic risk	Avoid association [184]
	Repaglinide	Increased plasma concentration of oral antidiabetic with intensified side effects	Adjust repaglinide dose
Ticagrelor	Dabigatran	High plasma concentration of dabigatran and increased risk of bleeding	Avoid association If associated, clinical supervision and adjust dabigatran dose
	Diltiazem/ verapamil	High plasma concentration of ticagrelor and increased risk of bleeding	Avoid association If associated, clinical supervision and adjust ticagrelor dose
	Atorvastatin	Increased plasma concentration of statin	Adjust statin dosage (maximum 40 mg/day) [178,185]

References

1. McDonagh, T.A.; Metra, M.; Adamo, M.; Gardner, R.S.; Baumbach, A.; Böhm, M.; Burri, H.; Butler, J.; Čelutkienė, J.; Chioncel, O.; et al. 2021 ESC Guidelines for the diagnosis and treatment of acute and chronic heart failure. *Eur. Heart J.* **2021**, *42*, 3599–3726. [CrossRef] [PubMed]
2. Ponikowski, P.; Voors, A.A.; Anker, S.D.; Bueno, H.; Cleland, J.G.; Coats, A.J.; Falk, V.; González-Juanatey, J.R.; Harjola, V.P.; Jankowska, E.A.; et al. 2016 ESC Guidelines for the diagnosis and treatment of acute and chronic heart failure: The Task Force for the diagnosis and treatment of acute and chronic heart failure of the European Society of Cardiology (ESC). Developed with the special contribution of the Heart Failure Association (HFA) of the ESC. *Eur. J. Heart Fail.* **2016**, *18*, 891–975. [CrossRef]

3. Bozkurt, B.; Coats, A.J.S.; Tsutsui, H.; Abdelhamid, C.M.; Adamopoulos, S.; Albert, N.; Anker, S.D.; Atherton, J.; Böhm, M.; Butler, J.; et al. Universal definition and classification of heart failure: A report of the Heart Failure Society of America, Heart Failure Association of the European Society of Cardiology, Japanese Heart Failure Society and Writing Committee of the Universal Definition of Heart Failure: Endorsed by the Canadian Heart Failure Society, Heart Failure Association of India, Cardiac Society of Australia and New Zealand, and Chinese Heart Failure Association. *Eur. J. Heart Fail.* **2021**, *23*, 352–380. [CrossRef]
4. Andronic, A.A.; Mihaila, S.; Cinteza, M. Heart Failure with Mid-Range Ejection Fraction—A New Category of Heart Failure or Still a Gray Zone. *Maedica* **2016**, *11*, 320–324. [PubMed]
5. Delepaul, B.; Robin, G.; Delmas, C.; Moine, T.; Blanc, A.; Fournier, P.; Roger-Rollé, A.; Domain, G.; Delon, C.; Uzan, C.; et al. Who are patients classified within the new terminology of heart failure from the 2016 ESC guidelines? *ESC Heart Fail.* **2017**, *4*, 99–104. [CrossRef]
6. Mosterd, A.; Hoes, A.W. Clinical epidemiology of heart failure. *Heart* **2007**, *93*, 1137–1146. [CrossRef] [PubMed]
7. Dharmarajan, K.; Rich, M.W. Epidemiology, Pathophysiology, and Prognosis of Heart Failure in Older Adults. *Heart Fail. Clin.* **2017**, *13*, 417–426. [CrossRef]
8. Snipelisky, D.; Chaudhry, S.P.; Stewart, G.C. The Many Faces of Heart Failure. *Card. Electrophysiol. Clin.* **2019**, *11*, 11–20. [CrossRef]
9. Crooks, J.; O'Malley, K.; Stevenson, I.H. Pharmacokinetics in the elderly. *Clin. Pharmacokinet.* **1976**, *1*, 280–296. [CrossRef] [PubMed]
10. Turnheim, K. When drug therapy gets old: Pharmacokinetics and pharmacodynamics in the elderly. *Exp. Gerontol.* **2003**, *38*, 843–853. [CrossRef] [PubMed]
11. Salwe, K.J.; Kalyansundaram, D.; Bahurupi, Y. A Study on Polypharmacy and Potential Drug-Drug Interactions among Elderly Patients Admitted in Department of Medicine of a Tertiary Care Hospital in Puducherry. *J. Clin. Diagn. Res.* **2016**, *10*, FC06. [CrossRef] [PubMed]
12. Mastromarino, V.; Casenghi, M.; Testa, M.; Gabriele, E.; Coluccia, R.; Rubattu, S.; Volpe, M. Polypharmacy in heart failure patients. *Curr. Heart Fail. Rep.* **2014**, *11*, 212–219. [CrossRef] [PubMed]
13. Lainscak, M.; Vitale, C.; Seferovic, P.; Spoletini, I.; Cvan Trobec, K.; Rosano, G.M. Pharmacokinetics and pharmacodynamics of cardiovascular drugs in chronic heart failure. *Int. J. Cardiol.* **2016**, *224*, 191–198. [CrossRef] [PubMed]
14. Lainscak, M.; Vitale, C. Biological and chronological age in heart failure: Role of immunosenescence. *J. Cardiovasc. Med.* **2016**, *17*, 857–859. [CrossRef]
15. United Nations. Population Ageing. 2015. Available online: WPA2015_Report.pdf(un.org) (accessed on 25 January 2022).
16. Yancy, C.W.; Jessup, M.; Bozkurt, B.; Butler, J.; Casey, D.E., Jr.; Drazner, M.H.; Fonarow, G.C.; Geraci, S.A.; Horwich, T.; Januzzi, J.L.; et al. 2013 ACCF/AHA guideline for the management of heart failure: A report of the American College of Cardiology Foundation/American Heart Association Task Force on Practice Guidelines. *J. Am. Coll. Cardiol.* **2013**, *62*, e147–e239. [CrossRef]
17. Writing Committee; Maddox, T.M.; Januzzi, J.L., Jr.; Allen, L.A.; Breathett, K.; Butler, J.; Davis, L.L.; Fonarow, G.C.; Ibrahim, N.E.; Lindenfeld, J.; et al. 2021 Update to the 2017 ACC Expert Consensus Decision Pathway for Optimization of Heart Failure Treatment: Answers to 10 Pivotal Issues About Heart Failure with Reduced Ejection Fraction: A Report of the American College of Cardiology Solution Set Oversight Committee. *J. Am. Coll. Cardiol.* **2021**, *77*, 772–810. [CrossRef]
18. Oliver, E.; Mayor, F., Jr.; D'Ocon, P. Beta-blockers: Historical Perspective and Mechanisms of Action. *Rev. Española Cardiol.* **2019**, *72*, 853–862, (In English and Spanish). [CrossRef]
19. Bie, P.; Mølstrøm, S.; Wamberg, S. Normotensive sodium loading in conscious dogs: Regulation of renin secretion during beta-receptor blockade. *Am. J. Physiol.-Regul. Integr. Comp. Physiol.* **2009**, *296*, R428–R435. [CrossRef]
20. Sayer, G.; Bhat, G. The renin-angiotensin-aldosterone system and heart failure. *Cardiol. Clin.* **2014**, *32*, 21–32. [CrossRef]
21. Bruno, N.; Sinagra, G.; Paolillo, S.; Bonomi, A.; Corrà, U.; Piepoli, M.; Veglia, F.; Salvioni, E.; Lagioia, R.; Metra, M.; et al. Mineralocorticoid receptor antagonists for heart failure: A real-life observational study. *ESC Heart Fail.* **2018**, *5*, 267–274. [CrossRef]
22. Casu, G.; Merella, P. Diuretic Therapy in Heart Failure-Current Approaches. *Eur. Cardiol.* **2015**, *10*, 42–47. [CrossRef] [PubMed]
23. Levine, T.B. Role of vasodilators in the treatment of congestive heart failure. *Am. J. Cardiol.* **1985**, *55*, 32A–35A. [CrossRef]
24. David, M.N.V.; Shetty, M. Digoxin Toxicity. In *StatPearls [Internet]*; StatPearls Publishing: Treasure Island, FL, USA, 2021. Available online: https://www.ncbi.nlm.nih.gov/books/NBK556025/ (accessed on 25 January 2022).
25. Reed, M.; Kerndt, C.C.; Nicolas, D. Ivabradine. In *StatPearls [Internet]*; StatPearls Publishing: Treasure Island, FL, USA, 2021. Available online: https://www.ncbi.nlm.nih.gov/books/NBK507783/ (accessed on 25 January 2022).
26. Yancy, C.; Jessup, M.; Butler, J.; Butler, J.; Casey, D.E., Jr.; Colvin, M.M.; Drazner, M.H.; Filippatos, G.S.; Fonarow, G.C.; Givertz, M.M.; et al. 2017 ACC/AHA/HFSA Focused Update of the 2013 ACCF/AHA Guideline for the Management of Heart Failure: A Report of the American College of Cardiology/American Heart Association Task Force on Clinical Practice Guidelines and the Heart Failure Society of America. *Circulation* **2017**, *136*, e137–e161. [CrossRef] [PubMed]
27. Sauer, A.J.; Cole, R.; Jensen, B.C.; Pal, J.; Sharma, N.; Yehya, A.; Vader, J. Practical guidance on the use of sacubitril/valsartan for heart failure. *Heart Fail. Rev.* **2019**, *24*, 167–176. [CrossRef]
28. Chandra, A.; Lewis, E.; Claggertt, B.; Desai, A.S.; Packer, M.; Zile, M.R.; Swedberg, K.; Rouleau, J.L.; Shi, V.C.; Lefkowitz, M.P.; et al. The Effects of Sacubitril/Valsartan on Physical and Social Activity Limitations in Heart Failure Patients: The PARADIGM-HF Trial. *JAMA Cardiol.* **2018**, *3*, 498–505. [CrossRef]
29. Velazquez, E.; Morrow, D.; DeVore, A.; Duffy, C.I.; Ambrosy, A.P.; McCague, K.; Rocha, R.; Braunwald, E.; PIONEER-HF Investigators. Angiotensin-Neprilysin Inhibition in Acute Decompensated Heart Failure. *N. Engl. J. Med.* **2019**, *380*, 539–548. [CrossRef]

30. Myhre, P.L.; Vaduganathan, M.; Claggett, B.; Packer, M.; Desai, A.S.; Rouleau, J.L.; Zile, M.R.; Swedberg, K.; Lefkowitz, M.; Shi, V.; et al. B-type natriuretic peptide during treatment with sacubitril/valsartan: The PARADIGM-HF trial. *J. Am. Coll. Cardiol.* **2019**, *73*, 1264–1272. [CrossRef]
31. Lewis, E.F.; Claggett, B.L.; McMurray, J.J.V.; Packer, M.; Lefkowitz, M.P.; Rouleau, J.L.; Liu, J.; Shi, V.C.; Zile, M.R.; Desai, A.S.; et al. Health-related quality of life outcomes in PARADIGM-HF. *Circ. Heart Fail.* **2017**, *10*, e003430. [CrossRef]
32. Seferovic, P.; Ponikowski, P.; Anker, S.; Bauersachs, J.; Chioncel, O.; Cleland, J.G.F.; de Boer, R.A.; Drexel, H.; Ben Gal, T.; Hill, L.; et al. Clinical practice update on heart failure 2019: Pharmacotherapy, procedures, devices and patient management. An expert consensus meeting report of The Heart Failure Association of the European Society of Cardiology. *Eur. J. Heart Fail.* **2019**, *21*, 1169–1186. [CrossRef]
33. Gillette, M.; Bozkurt, B. Ins and Outs: Perspectives of Inpatient Prescribing for Sacubitril/Valsartan. *Ann. Pharmacother.* **2020**, *55*, 805–813. [CrossRef]
34. Byrne, D.; Fahey, T.; Moriarty, F. Efficacy and safety of sacubitril/valsartan in the treatment of heart failure: Protocol for a systematic review incorporating unpublished clinical study reports. *HRB Open Res.* **2020**, *3*, 5. [CrossRef]
35. Scheen, A.J. Sodium-glucose cotransporter type 2 inhibitors for the treatment of type 2 diabetes mellitus. *Nat. Rev. Endocrinol.* **2020**, *16*, 556–577. [CrossRef]
36. Al Hamed, F.A.; Elewa, H. Potential Therapeutic Effects of Sodium Glucose-linked Cotransporter 2 Inhibitors in Stroke. *Clin. Ther.* **2020**, *42*, e242–e249. [CrossRef] [PubMed]
37. Ling, A.W.; Chan, C.C.; Chen, S.W.; Kao, Y.W.; Huang, C.Y.; Chan, Y.H.; Chu, P.H. The risk of new-onset atrial fibrillation in patients with type 2 diabetes mellitus treated with sodium glucose cotransporter 2 inhibitors versus dipeptidyl peptidase-4 inhibitors. *Cardiovasc. Diabetol.* **2020**, *19*, 188. [CrossRef] [PubMed]
38. Lee, H.C.; Shiou, Y.L.; Jhuo, S.J.; Chang, C.Y.; Liu, P.L.; Jhuang, W.J.; Dai, Z.K.; Chen, W.Y.; Chen, Y.F.; Lee, A.S. The sodium-glucose co-transporter 2 inhibitor empagliflozin attenuates cardiac fibrosis and improves ventricular hemodynamics in hypertensive heart failure rats. *Cardiovasc. Diabetol.* **2019**, *18*, 45. [CrossRef] [PubMed]
39. GrubićRotkvić, P.; CigrovskiBerković, M.; Bulj, N.; Rotkvić, L. Minireview: Are SGLT2 inhibitors heart savers in diabetes? *Heart Fail. Rev.* **2020**, *25*, 899–905. [CrossRef] [PubMed]
40. Lopaschuk, G.D.; Verma, S. Mechanisms of Cardiovascular Benefits of Sodium Glucose Co-Transporter 2 (SGLT2) Inhibitors: A State-of-the-Art Review. *JACC Basic Transl. Sci.* **2020**, *5*, 632–644. [CrossRef]
41. McMurray, J.J.V.; Solomon, S.D.; Inzucchi, S.E.; Køber, L.; Kosiborod, M.N.; Martinez, F.A.; Ponikowski, P.; Sabatine, M.S.; Anand, I.S.; Bělohlávek, J.; et al. Dapagliflozin in Patients with Heart Failure and Reduced Ejection Fraction. *N. Engl. J. Med.* **2019**, *381*, 1995–2008. [CrossRef]
42. Nassif, M.E.; Windsor, S.L.; Tang, F.; Khariton, Y.; Husain, M.; Inzucchi, S.E.; McGuire, D.K.; Pitt, B.; Scirica, B.M.; Austin, B.; et al. Dapagliflozin Effects on Biomarkers, Symptoms, and Functional Status in Patients with Heart Failure with Reduced Ejection Fraction: The DEFINE-HF Trial. *Circulation* **2019**, *140*, 1463–1476. [CrossRef]
43. Packer, M.; Anker, S.D.; Butler, J.; Filippatos, G.; Pocock, S.J.; Carson, P.; Januzzi, J.; Verma, S.; Tsutsui, H.; Brueckmann, M.; et al. EMPEROR-Reduced Trial Investigators. Cardiovascular and Renal Outcomes with Empagliflozin in Heart Failure. *N. Engl. J. Med.* **2020**, *383*, 1413–1424. [CrossRef]
44. Anker, S.D.; Butler, J.; Filippatos, G.; Shahzeb Khan, M.; Ferreira, J.P.; Bocchi, E.; Böhm, M.; Brunner-La Rocca, H.P.; Choi, D.J.; EMPEROR-Preserved Trial Committees and Investigators; et al. Baseline characteristics of patients with heart failure with preserved ejection fraction in the EMPEROR-Preserved trial. *Eur. J. Heart Fail.* **2020**, *22*, 2383–2392. [CrossRef] [PubMed]
45. Packer, M.; Butler, J.; Zannad, F.; Filippatos, G.; Ferreira, J.P.; Pocock, S.J.; Carson, P.; Anand, I.; Doehner, W.; Haass, M.; et al. Effect of Empagliflozin on Worsening Heart Failure Events in Patients with Heart Failure and Preserved Ejection Fraction: EMPEROR-Preserved Trial. *Circulation* **2021**, *144*, 1284–1294. [CrossRef] [PubMed]
46. Gazewood, J.D.; Turner, P.L. Heart failure with preserved ejection fraction: Diagnosis and management. *Am. Fam. Physician* **2017**, *96*, 582–588.
47. Mulder, B.A.; Schnabel, R.B.; Rienstra, M. Predicting the future in patients with atrial fibrillation: Who develops heart failure? *Eur. J. Heart Fail.* **2013**, *15*, 366–367. [CrossRef] [PubMed]
48. Ouyang, A.J.; Lv, Y.N.; Zhong, H.L.; Wen, J.H.; Wei, X.H.; Peng, H.W.; Zhou, J.; Liu, L.L. Meta-analysis of digoxin use and risk of mortality in patients with atrial fibrillation. *Am. J. Cardiol.* **2015**, *115*, 901–906. [CrossRef] [PubMed]
49. Van Gelder, I.C.; Haegeli, L.M.; Brandes, A.; Heidbuchel, H.; Aliot, E.; Kautzner, J.; Szumowski, L.; Mont, L.; Morgan, J.; Willems, S.; et al. Rationale and current perspective for early rhythm control therapy in atrial fibrillation. *Europace* **2011**, *13*, 1517–1525. [CrossRef] [PubMed]
50. Packer, M.; Califf, R.M.; Konstam, M.A.; Krum, H.; McMurray, J.J.; Rouleau, J.L.; Swedberg, K. Comparison of omapatrilat and enalapril in patients with chronic heart failure: The Omapatrilat Versus Enalapril Randomized Trial of Utility in Reducing Events (OVERTURE). *Circulation* **2002**, *106*, 920–926. [CrossRef] [PubMed]
51. Fleg, J.L.; Strait, J. Age-associated changes in cardiovascular structure and function: A fertile milieu for future disease. *Heart Fail. Rev.* **2012**, *17*, 545–554. [CrossRef]
52. Lakatta, E.G. Diminished beta-adrenergic modulation of cardiovascular function in advanced age. *Cardiol. Clin.* **1986**, *4*, 185–200. [CrossRef]

53. Loffredo, F.S.; Nikolova, A.P.; Pancoast, J.R.; Lee, R.T. Heart failure with preserved ejection fraction: Molecular pathways of the aging myocardium. *Circ. Res.* **2014**, *115*, 97–107. [CrossRef]
54. Olivetti, G.; Melissari, M.; Capasso, J.M.; Anversa, P. Cardiomyopathy of the aging human heart. Myocyte loss and reactive cellular hypertrophy. *Circ. Res.* **1991**, *68*, 1560–1568. [CrossRef] [PubMed]
55. Burgess, M.L.; McCrea, J.C.; Hedrick, H.L. Age-associated changes in cardiac matrix and integrins. *Mech. Ageing Dev.* **2001**, *122*, 1739–1756. [CrossRef]
56. Eghbali, M.; Eghbali, M.; Robinson, T.F.; Seifter, S.; Blumenfeld, O.O. Collagen accumulation in heart ventricles as a function of growth and aging. *Cardiovasc. Res.* **1989**, *23*, 723–729. [CrossRef] [PubMed]
57. Lakatta, E.G.; Levy, D. Arterial and cardiac aging: Major shareholders in cardiovascular disease enterprises: Part I: Aging arteries: A "set up" for vascular disease. *Circulation* **2003**, *107*, 139–146. [CrossRef]
58. Lakatta, E.G.; Levy, D. Arterial and cardiac aging: Major shareholders in cardiovascular disease enterprises: Part II: The aging heart in health: Links to heart disease. *Circulation* **2003**, *107*, 346–354. [CrossRef]
59. Picard, M.; McEwen, B.S. Psychological Stress and Mitochondria: A Conceptual Framework. *Psychosom. Med.* **2018**, *80*, 126–140. [CrossRef]
60. Liamis, G.; Milionis, H.J.; Elisaf, M. A review of drug-induced hypernatraemia. *NDT Plus* **2009**, *2*, 339–346. [CrossRef]
61. Miller, M. Fluid and electrolyte homeostasis in the elderly: Physiological changes of ageing and clinical consequences. *Baillière's Clin. Endocrinol. Metab.* **1997**, *11*, 367–387. [CrossRef]
62. Peeters, L.E.J.; Kester, M.P.; Feyz, L.; Van Den Bemt, P.M.L.A.; Koch, B.C.P.; Van Gelder, T.; Versmissen, J. Pharmacokinetic and pharmacodynamic considerations in the treatment of the elderly patient with hypertension. *Expert Opin. Drug Metab. Toxicol.* **2019**, *15*, 287–297. [CrossRef]
63. Barr, R.G.; Bluemke, D.A.; Ahmed, F.S.; Carr, J.J.; Enright, P.L.; Hoffman, E.A.; Jiang, R.; Kawut, S.M.; Kronmal, R.A.; Lima, J.A.; et al. Percent emphysema, airflow obstruction, and impaired left ventricular filling. *N. Engl. J. Med.* **2010**, *362*, 217–227. [CrossRef]
64. Petrescu, C.; Schlink, U.; Richter, M.; Suciu, O.; Ionovici, R.; Herbarth, O. Risk assessment of the respiratory health effects due to air pollution and meteorological factors in a population from Drobeta Turnu Severin, Romania. In Proceedings of the 17th European Symposium on Computer Aided Process Engineering, Cluj, Romania, 27–30 May 2007; Volume 24, pp. 1205–1210.
65. Monfredi, O.; Lakatta, E.G. Complexities in cardiovascular rhythmicity: Perspectives on circadian normality, ageing and disease. *Cardiovasc. Res.* **2019**, *115*, 1576–1595. [CrossRef] [PubMed]
66. Savarese, G.; D'Amario, D. Sex Differences in Heart Failure. *Adv. Exp. Med. Biol.* **2018**, *1065*, 529–544. [CrossRef] [PubMed]
67. Aimo, A.; Vergaro, G.; Barison, A.; Maffei, S.; Borrelli, C.; Morrone, D.; Cameli, M.; Palazzuoli, A.; Ambrosio, G.; Coiro, S.; et al. Sex-related differences in chronic heart failure. *Int. J. Cardiol.* **2018**, *255*, 145–151. [CrossRef] [PubMed]
68. Luo, T.; Kim, J.K. The Role of Estrogen and Estrogen Receptors on Cardiomyocytes: An Overview. *Can. J. Cardiol.* **2016**, *32*, 1017–1025. [CrossRef] [PubMed]
69. Bouma, W.; Noma, M.; Kanemoto, S.; Matsubara, M.; Leshnower, B.G.; Hinmon, R.; Gorman, J.H., 3rd; Gorman, R.C. Sex-related resistance to myocardial ischemia-reperfusion injury is associated with high constitutive ARC expression. *Am. J. Physiol. Heart Circ. Physiol.* **2010**, *298*, H1510–H1517. [CrossRef]
70. Jia, M.; Dahlman-Wright, K.; Gustafsson, J.Å. Estrogen receptor alpha and beta in health and disease. *Best Pract. Res. Clin. Endocrinol. Metab.* **2015**, *29*, 557–568. [CrossRef]
71. Tasevska-Dinevska, G.; Kennedy, L.M.; Cline-Iwarson, A.; Cline, C.; Erhardt, L.; Willenheimer, R. Gender differences in variables related to B-natriuretic peptide, left ventricular ejection fraction and mass, and peak oxygen consumption, in patients with heart failure. *Int. J. Cardiol.* **2011**, *149*, 364–371. [CrossRef]
72. Elmariah, S.; Goldberg, L.R.; Allen, M.T.; Kao, A. Effects of gender on peak oxygen consumption and the timing of cardiac transplantation. *J. Am. Coll. Cardiol.* **2006**, *47*, 2237–2242. [CrossRef]
73. vanDeursen, V.M.; Urso, R.; Laroche, C.; Damman, K.; Dahlström, U.; Tavazzi, L.; Maggioni, A.P.; Voors, A.A. Co-morbidities in patients with heart failure: An analysis of the European Heart Failure Pilot Survey. *Eur. J. Heart Fail.* **2014**, *16*, 103–111. [CrossRef]
74. Hudson, M.; Rahme, E.; Behlouli, H.; Sheppard, R.; Pilote, L. Sex differences in the effectiveness of angiotensin receptor blockers and angiotensin converting enzyme inhibitors in patients with congestive heart failure—A population study. *Eur. J. Heart Fail.* **2007**, *9*, 602–609. [CrossRef]
75. Ghali, J.K.; Lindenfeld, J. Sex differences in response to chronic heart failure therapies. *Expert Rev. Cardiovasc. Ther.* **2008**, *6*, 555–565. [CrossRef]
76. Adams, K.F., Jr.; Patterson, J.H.; Gattis, W.A.; O'Connor, C.M.; Lee, C.R.; Schwartz, T.A.; Gheorghiade, M. Relationship of serum digoxin concentration to mortality and morbidity in women in the digitalis investigation group trial: A retrospective analysis. *J. Am. Coll. Cardiol.* **2005**, *46*, 497–504. [CrossRef] [PubMed]
77. Valentova, M.; von Haehling, S. An overview of recent developments in the treatment of heart failure: Update from the ESC Congress 2013. *Expert Opin. Investig. Drugs* **2014**, *23*, 573–578. [CrossRef] [PubMed]
78. Arutyunov, G.P.; Kostyukevich, O.I.; Serov, R.A.; Rylova, N.V.; Bylova, N.A. Collagen accumulation and dysfunctional mucosal barrier of the small intestine in patients with chronic heart failure. *Int. J. Cardiol.* **2008**, *125*, 240–245. [CrossRef] [PubMed]

79. Sandek, A.; Bauditz, J.; Swidsinski, A.; Buhner, S.; Weber-Eibel, J.; von Haehling, S.; Schroedl, W.; Karhausen, T.; Doehner, W.; Rauchhaus, M.; et al. Altered intestinal function in patients with chronic heart failure. *J. Am. Coll. Cardiol.* **2007**, *50*, 1561–1569. [CrossRef]
80. Schwartz, J.B. The current state of knowledge on age, sex, and their interactions on clinical pharmacology. *Clin. Pharmacol. Ther.* **2007**, *82*, 87–96. [CrossRef] [PubMed]
81. Sica, D.A.; Wood, M.; Hess, M. Gender and its effect in cardiovascular pharmacotherapeutics: Recent considerations. *Congest. Heart Fail.* **2005**, *11*, 163–166. [CrossRef] [PubMed]
82. Ogawa, R.; Stachnik, J.M.; Echizen, H. Clinical pharmacokinetics of drugs in patients with heart failure: An update (part 1, drugs administered intravenously). *Clin. Pharmacokinet.* **2013**, *52*, 169–185. [CrossRef]
83. Valentová, M.; von Haehling, S.; Doehner, W.; Murín, J.; Anker, S.D.; Sandek, A. Liver dysfunction and its nutritional implications in heart failure. *Nutrition* **2013**, *29*, 370–378. [CrossRef]
84. Ogawa, R.; Stachnik, J.M.; Echizen, H. Clinical pharmacokinetics of drugs in patients with heart failure: An update (part 2, drugs administered orally). *Clin. Pharmacokinet.* **2014**, *53*, 1083–1114. [CrossRef]
85. Mangoni, A.A.; Jarmuzewska, E.A. The influence of heart failure on the pharmacokinetics of cardiovascular and non-cardiovascular drugs: A critical appraisal of the evidence. *Br. J. Clin. Pharmacol.* **2019**, *85*, 20–36. [CrossRef] [PubMed]
86. Bader, F.; Atallah, B.; Brennan, L.F.; Rimawi, R.H.; Khalil, M.E. Heart failure in the elderly: Ten peculiar management considerations. *Heart Fail. Rev.* **2017**, *22*, 219–228. [CrossRef] [PubMed]
87. Rangaswami, J.; Bhalla, V.; Blair, J.E.A.; Chang, T.I.; Costa, S.; Lentine, K.L.; Lerma, E.V.; Mezue, K.; Molitch, M.; Mullens, W.; et al. Cardiorenal Syndrome: Classification, Pathophysiology, Diagnosis, and Treatment Strategies: A Scientific Statement From the American Heart Association. *Circulation* **2019**, *139*, e840–e878. [CrossRef] [PubMed]
88. Rangaswami, J.; Mathew, R.O. Pathophysiological Mechanisms in Cardiorenal Syndrome. *Adv. Chronic. Kidney Dis.* **2018**, *25*, 400–407. [CrossRef]
89. Kousa, O.; Mullane, R.; Aboeata, A. Cardiorenal Syndrome. In *StatPearls [Internet]*; StatPearls Publishing: Treasure Island, FL, USA, 2021. Available online: https://www.ncbi.nlm.nih.gov/books/NBK542305/ (accessed on 25 January 2022).
90. Damman, K.; Testani, J.M. The kidney in heart failure: An update. *Eur. Heart J.* **2015**, *36*, 1437–1444. [CrossRef]
91. Ronco, C.; Chionh, C.Y.; Haapio, M.; Anavekar, N.S.; House, A.; Bellomo, R. The cardiorenal syndrome. *Blood Purif.* **2009**, *27*, 114–126. [CrossRef]
92. Anthony, J.; Sliwa, K. Decompensated Heart Failure in Pregnancy. *Card Fail. Rev.* **2016**, *2*, 20–26. [CrossRef]
93. Stergiopoulos, K.; Lima, F.V.; Butler, J. Heart Failure in Pregnancy: A Problem Hiding in Plain Sight. *J. Am. Heart Assoc.* **2019**, *8*, e012905. [CrossRef]
94. Dorn, G.W., 2nd. The fuzzy logic of physiological cardiac hypertrophy. *Hypertension* **2007**, *49*, 962–970. [CrossRef]
95. Kearney, L.; Wright, P.; Fhadil, S.; Thomas, M. Postpartum Cardiomyopathy and Considerations for Breastfeeding. *Card. Fail. Rev.* **2018**, *4*, 112–118. [CrossRef]
96. Tschiderer, L.; Seekircher, L.; Kunutsor, S.K.; Peters, S.A.E.; O'Keeffe, L.M.; Willeit, P. Breastfeeding Is Associated with a Reduced Maternal Cardiovascular Risk: Systematic Review and Meta-Analysis Involving Data from 8 Studies and 1 192 700 Parous Women. *J. Am. Heart Assoc.* **2022**, *11*, e022746. [CrossRef] [PubMed]
97. Von Lueder, T.G.; Atar, D. Comorbidities and polypharmacy. *Heart Fail. Clin.* **2014**, *10*, 367–372. [CrossRef] [PubMed]
98. Brockhattingen, K.K.; Anru, P.L.; Masud, T.; Petrovic, M.; Ryg, J. Association between number of medications and mortality in geriatric inpatients: A Danish nationwide register-based cohort study. *Eur. Geriatr. Med.* **2020**, *11*, 1063–1071. [CrossRef] [PubMed]
99. Page, R.L., 2nd; O'Bryant, C.L.; Cheng, D.; Dow, T.J.; Ky, B.; Stein, C.M.; Spencer, A.P.; Trupp, R.J.; Lindenfeld, J.; American Heart Association Clinical Pharmacology and Heart Failure and Transplantation Committees of the Council on Clinical Cardiology; et al. Drugs That May Cause or Exacerbate Heart Failure: A Scientific Statement from the American Heart Association. *Circulation* **2016**, *134*, e32–e69. [CrossRef] [PubMed]
100. Sunaga, T.; Yokoyama, A.; Nakamura, S.; Miyamoto, N.; Watanabe, S.; Tsujiuchi, M.; Nagumo, S.; Nogi, A.; Maezawa, H.; Mizukami, T.; et al. Association of Potentially Inappropriate Medications with All-Cause Mortality in the Elderly Acute Decompensated Heart Failure Patients: Importance of Nonsteroidal Anti-Inflammatory Drug Prescription. *Cardiol. Res.* **2020**, *11*, 239–246. [CrossRef] [PubMed]
101. Jödicke, A.M.; Burden, A.M.; Zellweger, U.; Tomka, I.T.; Neuer, T.; Roos, M.; Kullak-Ublick, G.A.; Curkovic, I.; Egbring, M. Medication as a risk factor for hospitalization due to heart failure and shock: A series of case-crossover studies in Swiss claims data. *Eur. J. Clin. Pharmacol.* **2020**, *76*, 979–989. [CrossRef] [PubMed]
102. Huerta, C.; Varas-Lorenzo, C.; Castellsague, J.; García Rodríguez, L.A. Non-steroidal anti-inflammatory drugs and risk of first hospital admission for heart failure in the general population. *Heart* **2006**, *92*, 1610–1615. [CrossRef]
103. Silva Almodóvar, A.; Nahata, M.C. Potentially Harmful Medication Use among Medicare Patients with Heart Failure. *Am. J. Cardiovasc. Drugs* **2020**, *20*, 603–610. [CrossRef]
104. Arfè, A.; Scotti, L.; Varas-Lorenzo, C.; Zambon, A.; Kollhorst, B.; Schink, T.; Garbe, E.; Herings, R.; Straatman, H.; Schade, R.; et al. Safety of Non-steroidal Anti-inflammatory Drugs (SOS) Project Consortium. Non-steroidal anti-inflammatory drugs and risk of heart failure in four European countries: Nested case-control study. *BMJ* **2016**, *354*, i4857. [CrossRef]

105. Alvarez, P.A.; Putney, D.; Ogunti, R.; Puppala, M.; Ganduglia, C.; Torre-Amione, G.; Schutt, R.; Wong, S.T.C.; Estep, J.D. Prevalence of in-hospital nonsteroidal antiinflammatory drug exposure in patients with a primary diagnosis of heart failure. *Cardiovasc. Ther.* **2017**, *35*, e12256. [CrossRef] [PubMed]
106. Alvarez, P.A.; Gao, Y.; Girotra, S.; Mentias, A.; Briasoulis, A.; Vaughan Sarrazin, M.S. Potentially harmful drug prescription in elderly patients with heart failure with reduced ejection fraction. *ESC Heart Fail.* **2020**, *7*, 1862–1871. [CrossRef] [PubMed]
107. Qian, X.; Li, M.; Wagner, M.B.; Chen, G.; Song, X. Doxazosin Stimulates Galectin-3 Expression and Collagen Synthesis in HL-1 Cardiomyocytes Independent of Protein Kinase C Pathway. *Front. Pharmacol.* **2016**, *7*, 495. [CrossRef] [PubMed]
108. Edwards, L.P.; Brown-Bryan, T.A.; McLean, L.; Ernsberger, P. Pharmacological properties of the central antihypertensive agent, moxonidine. *Cardiovasc. Ther.* **2012**, *30*, 199–208. [CrossRef] [PubMed]
109. Valembois, L.; Audureau, E.; Takeda, A.; Jarzebowski, W.; Belmin, J.; Lafuente-Lafuente, C. Antiarrhythmics for maintaining sinus rhythm after cardioversion of atrial fibrillation. *Cochrane Database Syst. Rev.* **2019**, *9*, CD005049. [CrossRef]
110. Frommeyer, G.; Milberg, P.; Witte, P.; Stypmann, J.; Koopmann, M.; Lücke, M.; Osada, N.; Breithardt, G.; Fehr, M.; Eckardt, L. A new mechanism preventing proarrhythmia in chronic heart failure: Rapid phase-III repolarization explains the low proarrhythmic potential of amiodarone in contrast to sotalol in a model of pacing-induced heart failure. *Eur. J. Heart Fail.* **2011**, *13*, 1060–1069. [CrossRef]
111. Finks, S.W.; Rogers, K.C.; Manguso, A.H. Assessment of sotalol prescribing in a community hospital: Opportunities for clinical pharmacist involvement. *Int. J. Pharm. Pract.* **2011**, *19*, 281–286. [CrossRef]
112. Kongwatcharapong, J.; Dilokthornsakul, P.; Nathisuwan, S.; Phrommintikul, A.; Chaiyakunapruk, N. Effect of dipeptidyl peptidase-4 inhibitors on heart failure: A meta-analysis of randomized clinical trials. *Int. J. Cardiol.* **2016**, *211*, 88–95. [CrossRef]
113. Savarese, G.; Schrage, B.; Cosentino, F.; Lund, L.H.; Rosano, G.M.C.; Seferovic, P.; Butler, J. Non-insulin antihyperglycaemic drugs and heart failure: An overview of current evidence from randomized controlled trials. *ESC Heart Fail.* **2020**, *7*, 3438–3451. [CrossRef]
114. Patel, K.V.; Sarraju, A.; Neeland, I.J.; McGuire, D.K. Cardiovascular Effects of Dipeptidyl Peptidase-4 Inhibitors and Glucagon-Like Peptide-1 Receptor Agonists: A Review for the General Cardiologist. *Curr. Cardiol. Rep.* **2020**, *22*, 105. [CrossRef]
115. Nassif, M.E.; Kosiborod, M. A Review of Cardiovascular Outcomes Trials of Glucose-Lowering Therapies and Their Effects on Heart Failure Outcomes. *Am. J. Cardiol.* **2019**, *124* (Suppl. S1), S12–S19. [CrossRef]
116. Hantson, P. Mechanisms of toxic cardiomyopathy. *Clin. Toxicol.* **2019**, *57*, 1–9. [CrossRef] [PubMed]
117. Wallach, J.D.; Wang, K.; Zhang, A.D.; Cheng, D.; Grossetta Nardini, H.K.; Lin, H.; Bracken, M.B.; Desai, M.; Krumholz, H.M.; Ross, J.S. Updating insights into rosiglitazone and cardiovascular risk through shared data: Individual patient and summary level meta-analyses. *BMJ* **2020**, *368*, l7078. [CrossRef] [PubMed]
118. Teaford, H.R.; Abu Saleh, O.M.; Villarraga, H.R.; Enzler, M.J.; Rivera, C.G. The Many Faces of Itraconazole Cardiac Toxicity. *Mayo Clin. Proc. Innov. Qual. Outcomes* **2020**, *4*, 588–594. [CrossRef] [PubMed]
119. Abraham, A.O.; Panda, P.K. Itraconazole Induced Congestive Heart Failure, A Case Study. *Curr. Drug Saf.* **2018**, *13*, 59–61. [CrossRef] [PubMed]
120. Paul, V.; Rawal, H. Cardiotoxicity with Itraconazole. *BMJ Case Rep.* **2017**, *2017*, bcr2017219376. [CrossRef]
121. Soares, J.R.; Nunes, M.C.; Leite, A.F.; Falqueto, E.B.; Lacerda, B.E.; Ferrari, T.C. Reversible dilated cardiomyopathy associated with amphotericin B therapy. *J. Clin. Pharm. Ther.* **2015**, *40*, 333–335. [CrossRef]
122. Mégarbane, B.; Leprince, P.; Deye, N.; Guerrier, G.; Résière, D.; Bloch, V.; Baud, F.J. Extracorporeal life support in a case of acute carbamazepine poisoning with life-threatening refractory myocardial failure. *Intensive Care Med.* **2006**, *32*, 1409–1413. [CrossRef]
123. Faisy, C.; Guerot, E.; Diehl, J.L.; Rezgui, N.; Labrousse, J. Carbamazepine-associated severe left ventricular dysfunction. *J. Toxicol. Clin. Toxicol.* **2000**, *38*, 339–342. [CrossRef]
124. Takamiya, M.; Aoki, Y.; Niitsu, H.; Saigusa, K. A case of carbamazepine overdose with focal myocarditis. *Leg. Med.* **2006**, *8*, 243–247. [CrossRef]
125. Lund, M.; Poulsen, G.; Pasternak, B.; Worm Andersson, N.; Melbye, M.; Svanström, H. Use of Pregabalin and Worsening Heart Failure: A Nationwide Cohort Study. *Drug Saf.* **2020**, *43*, 1035–1044. [CrossRef]
126. Awwad, Z.M.; El-Ganainy, S.O.; ElMallah, A.I.; Khedr, S.M.; Khattab, M.M.; El-Khatib, A.S. Assessment of Pregabalin-Induced Cardiotoxicity in Rats: Mechanistic Role of Angiotensin 1-7. *Cardiovasc. Toxicol.* **2020**, *20*, 301–311. [CrossRef] [PubMed]
127. Ho, J.M.; Tricco, A.C.; Perrier, L.; Chen, M.; Juurlink, D.N.; Straus, S.E. Risk of heart failure and edema associated with the use of pregabalin: A systematic review. *Syst. Rev.* **2013**, *2*, 25. [CrossRef] [PubMed]
128. Nezafati, M.H.; Vojdanparast, M.; Nezafati, P. Antidepressants and cardiovascular adverse events: A narrative review. *ARYA Atheroscler.* **2015**, *11*, 295–304. [PubMed]
129. Biffi, A.; Rea, F.; Scotti, L.; Lucenteforte, E.; Vannacci, A.; Lombardi, N.; Chinellato, A.; Onder, G.; Vitale, C.; Cascini, S.; et al. Antidepressants and the Risk of Cardiovascular Events in Elderly Affected by Cardiovascular Disease: A Real-Life Investigation From Italy. *J. Clin. Psychopharmacol* **2020**, *40*, 112–121. [CrossRef]
130. Deshmukh, A.; Ulveling, K.; Alla, V.; Abuissa, H.; Airey, K. Prolonged QTc interval and torsades de pointes induced by citalopram. *Tex. Heart Inst. J.* **2012**, *39*, 68–70.
131. Assimon, M.M.; Brookhart, M.A.; Flythe, J.E. Comparative Cardiac Safety of Selective Serotonin Reuptake Inhibitors among Individuals Receiving Maintenance Hemodialysis. *J. Am. Soc. Nephrol.* **2019**, *30*, 611–623. [CrossRef]

132. Tran, T.; Brophy, J.M.; Suissa, S.; Renoux, C. Risks of Cardiac Valve Regurgitation and Heart Failure Associated with Ergot- and Non-Ergot-Derived Dopamine Agonist Use in Patients with Parkinson's Disease: A Systematic Review of Observational Studies. *CNS Drugs* **2015**, *29*, 985–998. [CrossRef]
133. Montastruc, F.; Moulis, F.; Araujo, M.; Chebane, L.; Rascol, O.; Montastruc, J.L. Ergot and non-ergot dopamine agonists and heart failure in patients with Parkinson's disease. *Eur. J. Clin. Pharmacol.* **2017**, *73*, 99–103. [CrossRef]
134. Renoux, C.; Dell'Aniello, S.; Brophy, J.M.; Suissa, S. Dopamine agonist use and the risk of heart failure. *Pharmacoepidemiol. Drug Saf.* **2012**, *21*, 34–41. [CrossRef]
135. Patuszynski, D.; Applegate, P.M. Suspected Clozapine-Induced Cardiomyopathy and Heart Failure with Reduced Ejection Fraction. *Fed. Pract.* **2017**, *34*, 20–22.
136. Whiskey, E.; Yuen, S.; Khosla, E.; Piper, S.; O'Flynn, D.; Taylor, D. Resolution without discontinuation: Heart failure during clozapine treatment. *Ther. Adv. Psychopharmacol.* **2020**, *10*, 2045125320924786. [CrossRef]
137. Garg, A.; Bath, A.S.; Kalavakunta, J.K. Non-ischemic Cardiomyopathy: A Rare Adverse Effect of Clozapine. *Cureus* **2020**, *12*, e7901. [CrossRef] [PubMed]
138. Chow, V.; Yeoh, T.; Ng, A.C.; Pasqualon, T.; Scott, E.; Plater, J.; Whitwell, B.; Hanzek, D.; Chung, T.; Thomas, L.; et al. Asymptomatic left ventricular dysfunction with long-term clozapine treatment for schizophrenia: A multicentre cross-sectional cohort study. *Open Heart* **2014**, *1*, e000030. [CrossRef] [PubMed]
139. Salimi, A.; Gholamifar, E.; Naserzadeh, P.; Hosseini, M.J.; Pourahmad, J. Toxicity of lithium on isolated heart mitochondria and cardiomyocyte: A justification for its cardiotoxic adverse effect. *J. Biochem. Mol. Toxicol.* **2017**, *31*, e21836. [CrossRef] [PubMed]
140. Mezni, A.; Aoua, H.; Khazri, O.; Limam, F.; Aouani, E. Lithium induced oxidative damage and inflammation in the rat's heart: Protective effect of grape seed and skin extract. *Biomed. Pharmacother.* **2017**, *95*, 1103–1111. [CrossRef]
141. Asim, K.; Selman, Y.; Suleyman, Y.; Ozgur, K.; Ozlem, B.; Gokhan, E. Heart Attack in the Course of Lithium Overdose. *Iran. Red Crescent Med. J.* **2016**, *18*, e21731. [CrossRef]
142. Acharya, S.; Siddiqui, A.H.; Anwar, S.; Habib, S.; Anwar, S. Lithium-induced Cardiotoxicity: A Rare Clinical Entity. *Cureus* **2020**, *12*, e7286, Erratum in *Cureus* **2020**, *12*, c33. [CrossRef]
143. Ataallah, B.; Al-Zakhari, R.; Sharma, A.; Tofano, M.; Haggerty, G. A Rare but Reversible Cause of Lithium-Induced Bradycardia. *Cureus* **2020**, *12*, e8600. [CrossRef]
144. Wang, Y.; Yuan, J.; Qian, Z.; Zhang, X.; Chen, Y.; Hou, X.; Zou, J. β2 adrenergic receptor activation governs cardiac repolarization and arrhythmogenesis in a guinea pig model of heart failure. *Sci. Rep.* **2015**, *5*, 7681. [CrossRef]
145. Say, B.; Degirmencioglu, H.; Kutman, H.; Uras, N.; Dilmen, U. Supraventricular tachycardia after nebulized salbutamol therapy in a neonate: Case report. *Arch. Argent. Pediatr.* **2015**, *113*, e98–e100, (In English and Spanish). [CrossRef]
146. Yu, Y.; Wei, S.G.; Weiss, R.M.; Felder, R.B. TNF-α receptor 1 knockdown in the subfornical organ ameliorates sympathetic excitation and cardiac hemodynamics in heart failure rats. *Am. J. Physiol. Heart Circ. Physiol.* **2017**, *313*, H744–H756. [CrossRef] [PubMed]
147. Yu, Y.; Cao, Y.; Bell, B.; Chen, X.; Weiss, R.M.; Felder, R.B.; Wei, S.G. Brain TACE (Tumor Necrosis Factor-α-Converting Enzyme) Contributes to Sympathetic Excitation in Heart Failure Rats. *Hypertension* **2019**, *74*, 63–72. [CrossRef] [PubMed]
148. Schumacher, S.M.; Naga Prasad, S.V. Tumor Necrosis Factor-α in Heart Failure: An Updated Review. *Curr. Cardiol. Rep.* **2018**, *20*, 117. [CrossRef] [PubMed]
149. Suroowan, S.; Mahomoodally, F. Common phyto-remedies used against cardiovascular diseases and their potential to induce adverse events in cardiovascular patients. *Clin. Phytoscience* **2015**, *1*, 1. [CrossRef]
150. Kim, E.J.Y.; Chen, Y.; Huang, J.Q.; Li, K.M.; Razmovski-Naumovski, V.; Poon, J.; Li, K.M.; Razmovski-Naumovski, V.; Poon, J.; Chan, K.; et al. Evidence-based toxicity evaluation and scheduling of Chinese herbal medicines. *J. Ethnopharmacol.* **2013**, *146*, 40–61. [CrossRef]
151. Alternative Medicine Review. *Aesculus hippocacastanum*. **2009**, *14*, 278–283.
152. Tachjian, A.; Maria, V.; Jahangir, A. Use of herbal products and potential interactions in patients with cardiovascular diseases. *J. Am. Coll. Cardiol.* **2010**, *55*, 515–525. [CrossRef]
153. World Health Organization. Aloe. Folium Sennae, Fructus Sennae. Radix Glycyrrhizae. WHO Monograph on Selected Medicinal Plants—Volume 1. ISBN: 9241545178. Available online: http://apps.who.int/medicinedocs/en/d/Js2200e/5.html (accessed on 25 January 2022)ISBN 9241545178.
154. World Health Organization. Radix Angelicae Sinensis. WHO Monograph on Selected Medicinal Plants—Volume 2. Available online: http://apps.who.int/medicinedocs/en/d/Js4927e/5.html (accessed on 25 January 2022).
155. Agosti, S.; Casalino, L.; Bertero, G.; Barsotti, A.; Brunelli, C.; Morelloni, S. A dangerous fruit juice. *Am. J. Emerg. Med.* **2012**, *30*, 248.e5–248.e8. [CrossRef]
156. Papandreou, D.; Phily, A. An updated mini review on grapefruit: Interactions with drugs, obesity and cardiovascular Risk factors. *Food Nutr. Sci.* **2014**, *5*, 376–381. [CrossRef]
157. Tassell, M.; Kingston, R.; Gilroy, D.; Lehane, M.; Furey, A. Hawthorn (*Crataegus* spp.) in the treatment of cardiovascular disease. *Pharmacogn. Rev.* **2010**, *4*, 32.
158. Pittler, M.H.; Schmidt, K.; Ernst, E. Hawthorn extract for treating chronic heart failure: Meta-analysis of randomized trials. *Am. J. Med.* **2003**, *114*, 665–674. [CrossRef]

159. Chen, W.L.; Tsai, T.H.; Yang, C.C.H.; Kuo, T.B.J. Effects of ephedra on autonomic nervous modulation in healthy young adults. *J. Ethnopharmacol.* **2010**, *130*, 563–568. [CrossRef] [PubMed]
160. Koch, E. Inhibition of platelet activating factor (PAF)-induced aggregation of human thrombocytes by ginkgolides: Considerations on possible bleeding complications after oral intake of Ginkgo biloba extracts. *Phytomed* **2005**, *12*, 10–16. [CrossRef] [PubMed]
161. Bone, K.M. Potential interaction of *Ginkgo biloba* leaf with antiplatelet or anticoagulant drugs: What is the evidence? *Mol. Nutr. Food Res.* **2008**, *52*, 764–771. [CrossRef]
162. Pengelly, A. Harpagophytum procumbens. *Altern. Med. Rev.* **2008**, *13*, 248–252.
163. Calitz, C.; Steenekamp, J.H.; Steyn, J.D.; Gouws, C.; Viljoen, J.M.; Hamman, J.H. Impact of traditional African medicine on drug metabolism and transport. *Expert Opin. Drug Metab. Toxicol.* **2014**, *10*, 991–1003. [CrossRef]
164. Johne, A.; Brockmoller, J.; Bauer, S.; Maurer, A.; Langheinrich, M.; Roots, I. Pharmacokinetic interaction of digoxin with an herbal extract from St John's wort (*Hypericum perforatum*). *Clin. Pharmacol. Ther.* **1999**, *66*, 338–345. [CrossRef]
165. Yue, Q.Y.; Bergquist, C.; Gerden, B. Safety of St John's wort (*Hypericum perforatum*). *Lancet* **2002**, *355*, 576–577. [CrossRef]
166. Henderson, L.; Yue, Q.Y.; Bergquist, C.; Gerden, B.; Arlett, P. St John's wort (*Hypericum perforatum*): Drug interactions and clinical outcomes. *Br. J. Clin. Pharmacol.* **2002**, *54*, 349–356. [CrossRef]
167. World Health Organization. Oleum OenotheraeBiennis. WHO Monograph on Selected Medicinal Plants—Volume 2. Available online: http://apps.who.int/medicinedocs/en/d/Js4927e/22.html (accessed on 25 January 2022).
168. Fecker, R.; Buda, V.; Alexa, E.; Avram, S.; Pavel, I.Z.; Muntean, D.; Cocan, I.; Watz, C.; Minda, D.; Dehelean, C.A.; et al. Phytochemical and biological screening of *Oenothera biennis* L. Hydroalcoholic extract. *Biomolecules* **2020**, *10*, 818. [CrossRef]
169. Frishman, W.H.; Beravol, P.; Carosella, C. Alternative and complementary medicine for preventing and treating cardiovascular disease. *Dis. Mon.* **2009**, *55*, 121–192. [CrossRef] [PubMed]
170. World Health Organization. RhizomaZingiberis. WHO Monograph on Selected Medicinal Plants–Volume 1. Available online: http://apps.who.int/medicinedocs/en/d/Js2200e/30.html (accessed on 25 January 2022).
171. Georgiev, K.D.; Hvarchanova, N.; Georgieva, M.; Kanazirev, B. The role of the clinical pharmacist in the prevention of potential drug interactions in geriatric heart failure patients. *Int. J. Clin. Pharm.* **2019**, *41*, 1555–1561. [CrossRef] [PubMed]
172. Bhagat, A.A.; Greene, S.J.; Vaduganathan, M.; Fonarow, G.C.; Butler, J. Initiation, Continuation, Switching, and Withdrawal of Heart Failure Medical Therapies During Hospitalization. *JACC Heart Fail.* **2019**, *7*, 1–12. [CrossRef] [PubMed]
173. Anderson, S.L.; Marrs, J.C. A Review of the Role of the Pharmacist in Heart Failure Transition of Care. *Adv. Ther.* **2018**, *35*, 311–323. [CrossRef]
174. Investigators of the MAGIC-PHARM Study; Khazaka, M.; Laverdière, J.; Li, C.C.; Correal, F.; Mallet, L.; Poitras, M.; Nguyen, P.V. Medication appropriateness on an acute geriatric care unit: The impact of the removal of a clinical pharmacist. *Age Ageing* **2020**, *50*, afaa175. [CrossRef]
175. Association Nationale Des Enseignants de Pharmacie Clinique; Limat, S.; Dupuis, A.; Fagnoni, P.; Deamore, B.; Fernandez, C.; Aulagner, G.; Cazin, J.L. *Pharmacie Clinique et Therapeutique*; Elsevier: Amsterdam, The Netherlands, 2018; ISBN 9782294750779.
176. Preston, C.L. *Stockley's Drug Interactions*, 12th ed.; Pharmaceutical Press: London, UK, 2019; ISBN 978-0-85-711347-4.
177. Sica, D.A. Angiotensin-converting enzyme inhibitors side effects—Physiologic and non-physiologic considerations. *J. Clin. Hypertens* **2004**, *6*, 410–416. [CrossRef]
178. Wiggins, B.S.; Saseen, J.J.; Page, R.L., 2nd; Reed, B.N.; Sneed, K.; Kostis, J.B.; Lanfear, D.; Virani, S.; Morris, P.B.; American Heart Association Clinical Pharmacology Committee of the Council on Clinical Cardiology; et al. Recommendations for Management of Clinically Significant Drug-Drug Interactions With Statins and Select Agents Used in Patients With Cardiovascular Disease: A Scientific Statement From the American Heart Association. *Circulation* **2016**, *134*, e468–e495. [CrossRef]
179. Hsiao, H.L.; Langenickel, T.H.; Petruck, J.; Kode, K.; Ayalasomayajula, S.; Schuehly, U.; Greeley, M.; Pal, P.; Zhou, W.; Prescott, M.F.; et al. Evaluation of Pharmacokinetic and Pharmacodynamic Drug-Drug Interaction of Sacubitril/Valsartan (LCZ696) and Sildenafil in Patients with Mild-to-Moderate Hypertension. *Clin. Pharmacol. Ther.* **2018**, *103*, 468–476. [CrossRef]
180. Referentiel National des Interactions Medicamenteuses—ANSM. Thesaurus des Interactions Medicamenteuses 2019. Available online: https://ansm.sante.fr/var/ansm_site/storage/original/application/0002510e4ab3a9c13793a1fdc0d4c955.pdf (accessed on 25 January 2022).
181. Singh, G.; Correa, R. Methimazole. StatPearls [Internet]. 2020. Available online: https://www.ncbi.nlm.nih.gov/books/NBK545223/ (accessed on 25 January 2022).
182. Steffel, J.; Verhamme, P.; Potpara, T.S.; Albaladejo, P.; Antz, M.; Desteghe, L.; Haeusler, K.G.; Oldgren, J.; Reinecke, H.; Roldan-Schilling, V.; et al. The 2018 European Heart Rhythm Association Practical Guide on the use of non-vitamin K antagonist oral anticoagulants in patients with atrial fibrillation. *Eur. Heart J.* **2018**, *39*, 1330–1393. [CrossRef]
183. Frost, C.E.; Byon, W.; Song, Y.; Wang, J.; Schuster, A.E.; Boyd, R.A.; Zhang, D.; Yu, Z.; Dias, C.; Shenker, A.; et al. Effect of ketoconazole and diltiazem on the pharmacokinetics of apixaban, an oral direct factor Xa inhibitor. *Br. J. Clin. Pharmacol.* **2015**, *79*, 838–846. [CrossRef]
184. Bundhun, P.K.; Teeluck, A.R.; Bhurtu, A.; Huang, W.Q. Is the concomitant use of clopidogrel and Proton Pump Inhibitors still associated with increased adverse cardiovascular outcomes following coronary angioplasty? A systematic review and meta-analysis of recently published studies (2012–2016). *BMC Cardiovasc. Disord.* **2017**, *17*, 3. [CrossRef] [PubMed]

185. Kariyanna, P.T.; Haseeb, S.; Chowdhury, Y.S.; Jayarangaiah, A.; Maryniak, A.; Mo, G.; Hegde, S.; Marmur, J.D.; McFarlane, I.M. Ticagrelor and Statin Interaction Induces Rhabdomyolysis and Acute Renal Failure: Case reports and Scoping Review. *Am. J. Med. Case Rep.* **2019**, *7*, 337–341. [CrossRef] [PubMed]
186. Oscanoa, T.J.; Lizaraso, F.; Carvajal, A. Hospital admissions due to adverse drug reactions in the elderly. A meta-analysis. *Eur. J. Clin. Pharmacol.* **2017**, *73*, 759–770. [CrossRef] [PubMed]
187. Tran, P.; Banerjee, P. Iatrogenic Decompensated Heart Failure. *Curr. Heart Fail. Rep.* **2020**, *17*, 21–27. [CrossRef] [PubMed]
188. Rich, M.W.; Shah, A.S.; Vinson, J.M.; Freedland, K.E.; Kuru, T.; Sperry, J.C. Iatrogenic congestive heart failure in older adults: Clinical course and prognosis. *J. Am. Geriatr. Soc.* **1996**, *44*, 638–643. [CrossRef]
189. Bots, S.H.; Groepenhoff, F.; Eikendal, A.L.M.; Tannenbaum, C.; Rochon, P.A.; Regitz-Zagrosek, V.; Miller, V.M.; Day, D.; Asselbergs, F.W.; den Ruijter, H.M. Adverse Drug Reactions to Guideline-Recommended Heart Failure Drugs in Women: A Systematic Review of the Literature. *JACC Heart Fail.* **2019**, *7*, 258–266. [CrossRef]
190. Tamargo, J.; Rosano, G.; Walther, T.; Duarte, J.; Niessner, A.; Kaski, J.C.; Ceconi, C.; Drexel, H.; Kjeldsen, K.; Savarese, G.; et al. Gender differences in the effects of cardiovascular drugs. *Eur. Heart J. Cardiovasc. Pharmacother.* **2017**, *3*, 163–182. [CrossRef]
191. Soldin, O.P.; Chung, S.; Mattison, D.R. Sex differences in drug disposition. *J. Biomed. Biotechnol.* **2011**, *2011*, 187103. [CrossRef]
192. Soldin, O.P.; Mattison, D.R. Sex differences in pharmacokinetics and pharmacodynamics. *Clin. Pharmacokinet.* **2009**, *48*, 143–158. [CrossRef]
193. Drici, M.D.; Clement, N. Is gender a risk factor for adverse drug reactions? The example of drug-induced long QT syndrome. *Drug Saf.* **2001**, *24*, 575–585. [CrossRef]
194. Yap, Y.G.; Camm, A.J. Drug induced QT prolongation and torsades de pointes. *Heart* **2003**, *89*, 1363–1372. [CrossRef] [PubMed]
195. Pratt, C.M.; Camm, A.J.; Cooper, W.; Friedman, P.L.; MacNeil, D.J.; Moulton, K.M.; Pitt, B.; Schwartz, P.J.; Veltri, E.P.; Waldo, A.L.; et al. Mortality in the Survival WithORal D-Sotalol (SWORD) trial: Why did patients die? *Am. J. Cardiol.* **1998**, *81*, 869–876. [CrossRef]
196. Jochmann, N.; Stangl, K.; Garbe, E.; Baumann, G.; Stangl, V. Female-specific aspects in the pharmacotherapy of chronic cardiovascular diseases. *Eur. Heart J.* **2005**, *26*, 1585–1595. [CrossRef] [PubMed]
197. Capodanno, D.; Angiolillo, D.J. Impact of race and gender on antithrombotic therapy. *Thromb. Haemost.* **2012**, *104*, 471–484. [CrossRef]
198. Gilstrap, L.G.; Fonarow, G.C.; Desai, A.S.; Fonarow, G.C.; Butler, J. Initiation, Continuation, or Withdrawal of Angiotensin-Converting Enzyme Inhibitors/Angiotensin Receptor Blockers and Outcomes in Patients Hospitalized with Heart Failure with Reduced Ejection Fraction. *J. Am. Heart Assoc.* **2017**, *6*, e004675. [CrossRef] [PubMed]
199. O'Brien, E.T. Beta-blockade withdrawal. *Lancet* **1975**, *2*, 819. [CrossRef]
200. Miller, R.R.; Olson, H.G.; Amsterdam, E.A.; Mason, D.T. Propranolol-withdrawal rebound phenomenon. Exacerbation of coronary events after abrupt cessation of antianginal therapy. *N. Engl. J. Med.* **1975**, *293*, 416–418. [CrossRef]
201. Clark, H.; Krum, H.; Hopper, I. Worsening renal function during renin-angiotensin-aldosterone system inhibitor initiation and long-term outcomes in patients with left ventricular systolic dysfunction. *Eur. J. Heart Fail.* **2014**, *16*, 41–48. [CrossRef]
202. Clark, A.L.; Kalra, P.R.; Petrie, M.C.; Mark, P.B.; Tomlinson, L.A.; Tomson, C.R. Change in renal function associated with drug treatment in heart failure: National guidance. *Heart* **2019**, *105*, 904–910. [CrossRef]
203. Jondeau, G.; Neuder, Y.; Eicher, J.C.; Jourdain, P.; Fauveau, E.; Galinier, M.; Jegou, A.; Bauer, F.; Trochu, J.N.; Bouzamondo, A.; et al. B-CONVINCED: Beta-blocker CONtinuationVs. INterruption in patients with Congestive heart failure hospitalizED for a decompensation episode. *Eur. Heart J.* **2009**, *30*, 2186–2192. [CrossRef]
204. Fonarow, G.C.; Abraham, W.T.; Albert, N.M.; Stough, W.G.; Gheorghiade, M.; Greenberg, B.H.; O'Connor, C.M.; Nunez, E.; Yancy, C.W.; Young, J.B. A smoker's paradox in patients hospitalized for heart failure: Findings from OPTIMIZE-HF. *Eur. Heart J.* **2008**, *29*, 1983–1991. [CrossRef] [PubMed]
205. Halliday, B.P.; Wassall, R.; Lota, A.S.; Khalique, Z.; Gregson, J.; Newsome, S.; Jackson, R.; Rahneva, T.; Wage, R.; Smith, G.; et al. Withdrawal of pharmacological treatment for heart failure in patients with recovered dilated cardiomyopathy (TRED-HF): An open-label, pilot, randomized trial. *Lancet* **2019**, *393*, 61–73. [CrossRef]

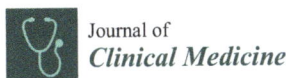

Review

Adaptive Servo-Ventilation as a Novel Therapeutic Strategy for Chronic Heart Failure

Teruhiko Imamura [1,*], Nikhil Narang [2] and Koichiro Kinugawa [1]

1. Second Department of Internal Medicine, University of Toyama, 2630 Sugitani, Toyama 930-0194, Japan; kinugawa-tky@umin.ac.jp
2. Advocate Christ Medical Center, Oak Lawn, IL 60453, USA; nikhil.narang@gmail.com
* Correspondence: teimamu@med.u-toyama.ac.jp; Tel.: +81-76-434-2281; Fax: +81-76-434-5026

Abstract: The introduction of new therapeutics for patients with chronic heart failure, including sacubitril/valsartan, sodium-glucose cotransporter 2 inhibitors, and ivabradine, in addition to beta-blockers, angiotensin converting enzyme inhibitors, and mineralocorticoid receptor antagonists, lends an opportunity for significant clinical risk reduction compared to what was available just one decade ago. Further clinical options are needed, however, for patients with residual clinical congestion refractory to these therapies. Adaptive servo-ventilation is a novel therapeutic option to address significant clinical volume in cases resistant to medical therapy. The aggregate benefit of these additional therapeutic strategies in addition to foundational medical therapy may be a promising option in the selected candidates who do not achieve acceptable clinical and quality-of-life improvements with oral medical therapy alone. Now is the era to reconsider the implication of an adaptive servo-ventilation-therapy-incorporated medical therapeutic strategy for patients with congestive heart failure.

Keywords: heart failure; hemodynamics; congestion

1. Introduction

Several novel therapies have been introduced over the last decade that both improve quality of life and reduce mortality in patients with chronic heart failure, including sacubitril/valsartan (ARNI), sodium-glucose cotransporter 2 (SGLT2) inhibitor, and ivabradine [1]. Up-titration of neurohormonal agents including beta-blockers and mineralocorticoid receptor antagonists to maximal doses in addition to these new therapies is essential to achieve the best clinical benefit [2]. The additional risk reduction for heart failure hospitalization or death with contemporary four-tier guideline-directed medical therapy (ARNI, beta-blocker, mineralocorticoid inhibitor, and SGLT2i) compared to angiotensin-converting enzyme inhibitors and beta-blockers alone is >50%. The guidelines of the Japanese Circulation Society recently published a focused update to emphasize the importance of these life-saving therapies, with a clear recommendation of urgency to rapidly up-titrate these therapies to doses specified in respective landmark clinical trials [3].

In addition to the survival benefit, improvement in patient-reported outcomes including functional status and quality of life is also of paramount importance [4]. Much of this is related to the treatment of congestion. Although these new medical therapies significantly reduce the burden of congestions, some patients suffer from residual volume overload that considerably reduces functional capacity. Furthermore, adequate decongestion at index discharge following heart failure hospitalization is unsurprisingly strongly associated with clinical outcomes [5]. Loop diuretics are conventional tools to treat pulmonary and systemic congestion [6]. Tolvaptan, vasopressin type-2 receptor antagonist, is a potent natriuretic agent that has been utilized for a decade [7]. Tolvaptan as a diuretic therapy improves pulmonary/systemic congestion while not worsening renal function [8]. The cost of this medication in addition to lack of evidence when combined with contemporary heart

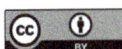

failure therapies are limiting factors to justify the widespread implementation of tolvaptan. There remains a gap in care for patients with residual congestion, for which nonmedical therapeutic strategies should be considered.

Adaptive servo-ventilation (ASV; AutoSet-CS; ResMed, Sydney, Australia) is a noninvasive, positive pressure ventilation tool that reduces work of breathing, suppresses sympathetic nervous system activation, and improves pulmonary/systemic congestion via decreasing cardiac preload and afterload in patients with congestive heart failure, if appropriately utilized at least for 4 h during the night (Figure 1) [9]. Importantly, this occurs irrespective of the existence of sleep-disordered breathing [10]. Although large-scale randomized control trials of ASV in patients with chronic heart failure did not demonstrate a mortality benefit [11], ASV is still being utilized with success in some scenarios to improve patient symptomology [12].

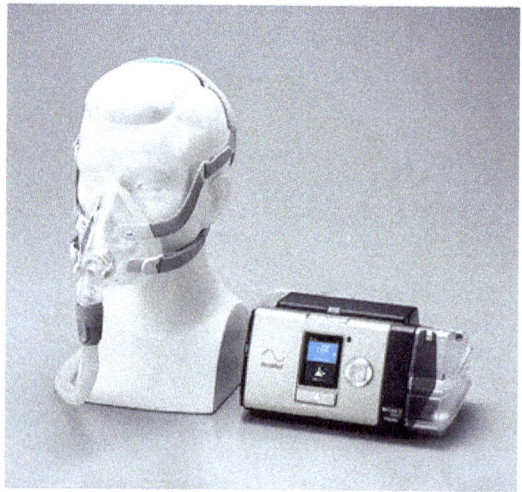

Figure 1. Adaptive servo-ventilation device set.

We believe that ASV therapy can be an effective strategy in managing persistent pulmonary/systemic congestion refractory to medical treatment [13], and should be reconsidered as part of the therapeutic armamentarium in patients with chronic heart failure, even in the era when novel medical agents have been introduced, if appropriately utilized as discussed in this review.

2. Management of Congestion in the Current Era

Adequate control of congestion is a critically important goal in chronic heart failure management to both reduce mortality and morbidity and improve patients' symptomology and quality of life [14]. Furthermore, residual pulmonary congestion misdiagnosed by clinical assessment at index discharge is associated with worse clinical outcomes [5].

Sacubitril/valsartan was the first of the new medical therapies in patients with chronic heart failure shown to reduce mortality and morbidity compared to the enalapril arm in the PARADIGM-HF trial [15]. However, the secondary analysis demonstrated reduced efficacy of sacubitril/valsartan in patients with multiple signs of congestion based on clinical exam [16]. SGLT2 inhibitors have pleiotropic benefits with no single direct mechanism to explain the substantial clinical benefit in patients with heart failure and reduced ejection fraction. Furthermore, there is a longitudinal benefit in patients with chronic kidney disease with and without heart failure, which is unique among the current heart failure-specific therapies [17]. However, the renoprotective effect of SGLT2 inhibitors was less expected in patients with insufficient cardiac unloading, indicated as higher plasma B-type natriuretic peptide levels [18]. The additive effects of these novel medical therapies may potentiate clinical benefit with alternative therapies such as ASV, whereas this benefit was not realized in prior clinical trials before the debut of both ARNI and SGLT2 inhibitor therapy.

In the acute phase of decompensated heart failure, early de novo administration of beta-blocker therapy is generally contraindicated given the risk of worsening cardiac output due to negative inotropic effects in the presence of pulmonary congestion [19]. This may be a time point when ASV can be utilized to more immediately alleviate congestion and thus shorten the period to initiation of foundational medical therapy [20].

3. Adjustment of Adaptive Servo-Ventilation Therapy

The indications, pressure settings, and timing of termination need to be identified during ASV therapy. For successful ASV therapy and avoidance of congestion, the baseline existence of pulmonary congestion is necessary to be confirmed [13]. Inappropriate ASV therapy for those without pulmonary/systemic congestion would rather decrease cardiac output, deteriorate hemodynamics, and increase cardiovascular mortality and morbidity.

Recently, remote dielectric sensing (ReDS^{TM}, Sensible Medical Innovations Ltd., Netanya, Israel) system, which is a noninvasive electromagnetic-based technology to quantify lung fluid volume, has been introduced in the clinical setting (Figure 2) [21]. Prior work has demonstrated the correlation between ReDS value and lung fluid level measured by high-resolution computed tomography [22,23]. The ReDS system is a promising tool to accurately assess for pulmonary congestion and may be an appropriate precursor modality to screen for patients that may benefit from early ASV therapy when decompensated heart failure is suspected.

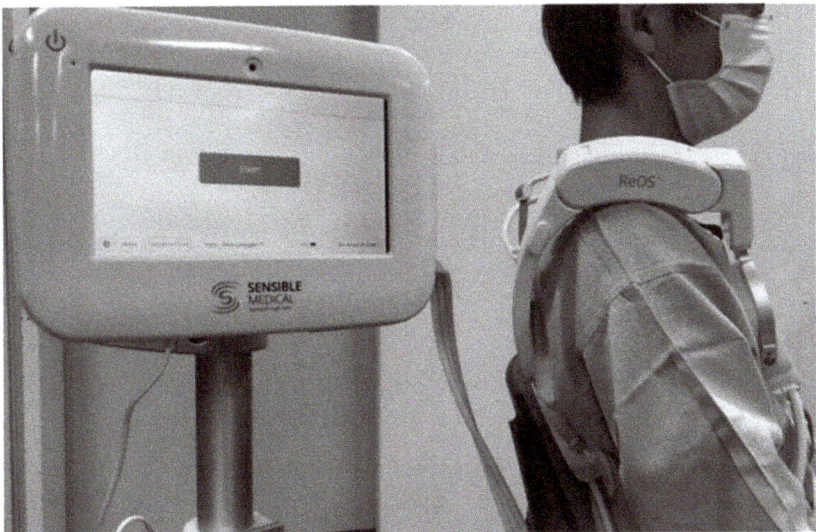

Figure 2. A monitor and a sensor of the remote dielectric sensing system.

Another novel tool in the care of heart failure patients is the AESCULON mini^{TM} (Osypka Medical, Berlin, Germany), which noninvasively estimates cardiac output (Figure 3) [24]. With ASV therapy, inappropriately high pressure settings may rather lower cardiac output during the ASV therapy [12]. We thus propose a pressure ramp test, during which cardiac output is measured at each pressure setting to optimize end-expiratory pressure to accompany maximum cardiac output (Figure 3) [25]. ReDS values might also be measured during the pressure ramp test to assess lung fluid levels at each pressure setting [26].

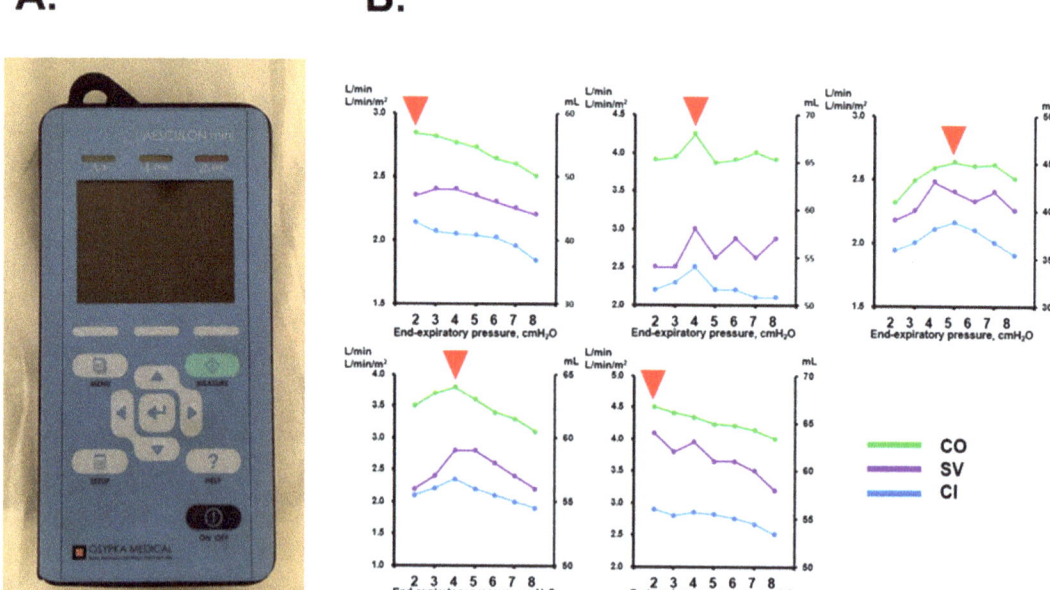

Figure 3. ASESCULON mini device (**A**) and examples of pressure ramp test (**B**) [25]. Red arrow heads indicate end-expiratory pressures with maximum cardiac output. CO, cardiac output; SV, stroke volume; CI, cardiac index.

Continuation of ASV after improvement in clinical congestion is not encouraged and may explain the lack of superior clinical benefit in the SAVIOR-C randomized control trial [10]. However, optimal methodologies for clinicians deciding the appropriate timing to terminate ASV therapy remain unestablished. Monitoring of daily congestion through utilization of the ReDS system, in addition to congestion-related biomarkers including adrenomedullin, should allow the clinicians to accurately tailor the use of ASV. When ReDS value trends to decrease, we should consider terminating the ASV therapy to avoid hemodynamic deterioration.

4. Renoprotection

A cardiorenal syndrome is an additional clinical syndrome within heart failure presentations which is independently associated with worse clinical outcomes [27]. Unoptimized chronic heart failure can lead to renal congestion, decreased renal perfusion and further downstream activation of inflammatory and maladaptive neurohormonal pathways. Renal impairment worsens volume overload, subsequentially increasing cardiovascular preload and afterload.

Up-titration of loop diuretics is one option to manage volume overload triggered by progressive chronic kidney disease. However, high-dose diuretics are associated with inappropriate stimulation of the renin–angiotensin system, and may further worsen renal function [4]. Angiotensin-converting enzyme inhibitor, ARNIs, and mineralocorticoid receptor antagonist may increase serum creatinine and potassium levels particularly in elderly patients with chronic kidney disease [28,29].

ASV therapy might be a promising alternative to manage congestion while maintaining renal function. We recently demonstrated that ASV therapy maintained renal function by comparison with the pre-ASV treatment period (i.e., pretreatment versus on-treatment) [30]. Underlying mechanisms should be multifactorial. Improvement of cardiac output following the initiation of ASV supports would enhance renal perfusion and ameliorate renal ischemia.

Suppression of sympathetic nerve activity by respiratory stabilization would dilate the renal artery and maintain renal perfusion, as well as prevent the progression of renal tissue apoptosis and fibrosis. Of note, those who achieved a reduction in diuretics dosage had greater long-term renal function preservation. Thus, ASV therapy might have a direct and indirect protective effect on kidney function.

Other therapies may also have the potential to preserve kidney function. Tolvaptan, a vasopressin type-2 receptor antagonist, may have a neutral impact on renal function as opposed to conventional loop diuretics. Tolvaptan has potent aquaretic properties and may decrease the dosage needed of typical loop diuretics, though in some countries this presents a cost challenge [8]. SGLT2 inhibitors, in addition to being associated with significant clinical benefits in patients with chronic heart failure, have also been shown to have considerable renoprotective effects in a large-scale randomized control trial [17]. One of the proposed mechanisms is the regulation of tubularglomerular feedback. Although further studies are needed, sacubitril/valsartan might also slow the worsening of renal function through an improvement in ventricular function and lowering the volume and pressure burden experienced by kidneys [31]. Although categorized as a mineralocorticoid receptor antagonist, the newly introduced esaxerenone might reduce proteinuria and better preserve renal function [32]. Another nonsteroidal, selective mineralocorticoid receptor antagonist, finerenone, may also suppress progression of chronic kidney disease and prevent cardiovascular events [33]. The combination of these heart failure therapies with ASV may be a promising strategy to manage cardiorenal syndrome.

5. Conclusions

In the current era with a new regimen of available medical therapies for heart failure, a combination of ASV and medical therapy may be a promising option for patients with considerable congestion and impaired renal function.

Author Contributions: Conceptualization, T.I.; methodology, T.I.; software, T.I.; validation, K.K.; formal analysis, T.I.; investigation, T.I.; resources, K.K.; data curation, T.I.; writing—original draft preparation, T.I.; writing—review and editing, N.N.; visualization, T.I.; supervision, K.K.; project administration, T.I.; funding acquisition, K.K. All authors have read and agreed to the published version of the manuscript.

Funding: This research received no external funding.

Informed Consent Statement: Informed consent was obtained from the volunteer.

Data Availability Statement: Data are available on appropriate requests.

Conflicts of Interest: The authors declare no conflict of interest.

References

1. Crespo-Leiro, M.G.; Metra, M.; Lund, L.H.; Milicic, D.; Costanzo, M.R.; Filippatos, G.; Gustafsson, F.; Tsui, S.; Barge-Caballero, E.; De Jonge, N.; et al. Advanced heart failure: A position statement of the Heart Failure Association of the European Society of Cardiology. *Eur. J. Heart Fail.* **2018**, *20*, 1505–1535. [CrossRef]
2. Vaduganathan, M.; Claggett, B.L.; Jhund, P.S.; Cunningham, J.W.; Pedro Ferreira, J.; Zannad, F.; Packer, M.; Fonarow, G.C.; McMurray, J.J.V.; Solomon, S.D. Estimating lifetime benefits of comprehensive disease-modifying pharmacological therapies in patients with heart failure with reduced ejection fraction: A comparative analysis of three randomised controlled trials. *Lancet* **2020**, *396*, 121–128. [CrossRef]
3. Tsutsui, H.; Ide, T.; Ito, H.; Kihara, Y.; Kinugawa, K.; Kinugawa, S.; Makaya, M.; Murohara, T.; Node, K.; Saito, Y.; et al. JCS/JHFS 2021 Guideline Focused Update on Diagnosis and Treatment of Acute and Chronic Heart Failure. *Circ. J. Off. J. Jpn. Circ. Soc.* **2021**, *85*, 2252–2291. [CrossRef]
4. Mullens, W.; Damman, K.; Harjola, V.P.; Mebazaa, A.; Brunner-La Rocca, H.P.; Martens, P.; Testani, J.M.; Tang, W.H.W.; Orso, F.; Rossignol, P.; et al. The use of diuretics in heart failure with congestion—A position statement from the Heart Failure Association of the European Society of Cardiology. *Eur. J. Heart Fail.* **2019**, *21*, 137–155. [CrossRef]
5. Rivas-Lasarte, M.; Maestro, A.; Fernandez-Martinez, J.; Lopez-Lopez, L.; Sole-Gonzalez, E.; Vives-Borras, M.; Montero, S.; Mesado, N.; Pirla, M.J.; Mirabet, S.; et al. Prevalence and prognostic impact of subclinical pulmonary congestion at discharge in patients with acute heart failure. *ESC Heart Fail.* **2020**, *7*, 2621–2628. [CrossRef] [PubMed]

6. Jentzer, J.C.; DeWald, T.A.; Hernandez, A.F. Combination of loop diuretics with thiazide-type diuretics in heart failure. *J. Am. Coll. Cardiol.* **2010**, *56*, 1527–1534. [CrossRef] [PubMed]
7. Plosker, G.L. Tolvaptan. *Drugs* **2010**, *70*, 443–454. [CrossRef]
8. Imamura, T.; Kinugawa, K. Update of acute and long-term tolvaptan therapy. *J. Cardiol.* **2019**, *73*, 102–107. [CrossRef]
9. Momomura, S. Treatment of Cheyne-Stokes respiration-central sleep apnea in patients with heart failure. *J. Cardiol.* **2012**, *59*, 110–116. [CrossRef]
10. Momomura, S.; Seino, Y.; Kihara, Y.; Adachi, H.; Yasumura, Y.; Yokoyama, H.; Wada, H.; Ise, T.; Tanaka, K.; SAVIOR-C investigators. Adaptive servo-ventilation therapy for patients with chronic heart failure in a confirmatory, multicenter, randomized, controlled study. *Circ. J. Off. J. Jpn. Circ. Soc.* **2015**, *79*, 981–990. [CrossRef]
11. Cowie, M.R.; Woehrle, H.; Wegscheider, K.; Angermann, C.; d'Ortho, M.P.; Erdmann, E.; Levy, P.; Simonds, A.K.; Somers, V.K.; Zannad, F.; et al. Adaptive Servo-Ventilation for Central Sleep Apnea in Systolic Heart Failure. *N. Engl. J. Med.* **2015**, *373*, 1095–1105. [CrossRef] [PubMed]
12. Cowie, M.R.; Wegscheider, K.; Teschler, H. Adaptive Servo-Ventilation for Central Sleep Apnea in Heart Failure. *N. Engl. J. Med.* **2016**, *374*, 687–688. [CrossRef]
13. Imamura, T.; Kinugawa, K. What is the Optimal Strategy for Adaptive Servo-Ventilation Therapy? *Int. Heart J.* **2018**, *59*, 683–688. [CrossRef] [PubMed]
14. Boorsma, E.M.; Ter Maaten, J.M.; Damman, K.; Dinh, W.; Gustafsson, F.; Goldsmith, S.; Burkhoff, D.; Zannad, F.; Udelson, J.E.; Voors, A.A. Congestion in heart failure: A contemporary look at physiology, diagnosis and treatment. *Nat. Rev. Cardiol.* **2020**, *17*, 641–655. [CrossRef] [PubMed]
15. McMurray, J.J.; Packer, M.; Desai, A.S.; Gong, J.; Lefkowitz, M.P.; Rizkala, A.R.; Rouleau, J.L.; Shi, V.C.; Solomon, S.D.; Swedberg, K.; et al. Angiotensin-neprilysin inhibition versus enalapril in heart failure. *N. Engl. J. Med.* **2014**, *371*, 993–1004. [CrossRef]
16. Selvaraj, S.; Claggett, B.; Pozzi, A.; McMurray, J.J.V.; Jhund, P.S.; Packer, M.; Desai, A.S.; Lewis, E.F.; Vaduganathan, M.; Lefkowitz, M.P.; et al. Prognostic Implications of Congestion on Physical Examination Among Contemporary Patients With Heart Failure and Reduced Ejection Fraction: PARADIGM-HF. *Circulation* **2019**, *140*, 1369–1379. [CrossRef]
17. Heerspink, H.J.L.; Stefansson, B.V.; Correa-Rotter, R.; Chertow, G.M.; Greene, T.; Hou, F.F.; Mann, J.F.E.; McMurray, J.J.V.; Lindberg, M.; Rossing, P.; et al. Dapagliflozin in Patients with Chronic Kidney Disease. *N. Engl. J. Med.* **2020**, *383*, 1436–1446. [CrossRef]
18. Nakagaito, M.; Imamura, T.; Joho, S.; Ushijima, R.; Nakamura, M.; Kinugawa, K. Renoprotective effects of sodium glucose cotransporter 2 inhibitors in type 2 diabetes patients with decompensated heart failure. *BMC Cardiovasc. Disord.* **2021**, *21*, 347. [CrossRef]
19. Lee, H.Y.; Baek, S.H. Optimal Use of Beta-Blockers for Congestive Heart Failure. *Circ. J. Off. J. Jpn. Circ. Soc.* **2016**, *80*, 565–571. [CrossRef]
20. Nakano, S.; Kasai, T.; Tanno, J.; Sugi, K.; Sekine, Y.; Muramatsu, T.; Senbonmatsu, T.; Nishimura, S. The effect of adaptive servo-ventilation on dyspnoea, haemodynamic parameters and plasma catecholamine concentrations in acute cardiogenic pulmonary oedema. *Eur. Heart J. Acute Cardiovasc. Care* **2015**, *4*, 305–315. [CrossRef]
21. Amir, O.; Rappaport, D.; Zafrir, B.; Abraham, W.T. A novel approach to monitoring pulmonary congestion in heart failure: Initial animal and clinical experiences using remote dielectric sensing technology. *Congest. Heart Fail.* **2013**, *19*, 149–155. [CrossRef]
22. Amir, O.; Azzam, Z.S.; Gaspar, T.; Faranesh-Abboud, S.; Andria, N.; Burkhoff, D.; Abbo, A.; Abraham, W.T. Validation of remote dielectric sensing (ReDS) technology for quantification of lung fluid status: Comparison to high resolution chest computed tomography in patients with and without acute heart failure. *Int. J. Cardiol.* **2016**, *221*, 841–846. [CrossRef] [PubMed]
23. Imamura, T.; Gonoi, W.; Hori, M.; Ueno, Y.; Narang, N.; Onoda, H.; Tanaka, S.; Nakamura, M.; Kataoka, N.; Ushijima, R.; et al. Validation of Noninvasive Remote Dielectric Sensing System to Quantify Lung Fluid Levels. *J. Clin. Med.* **2021**, *11*, 164. [CrossRef]
24. Nakayama, A.; Iwama, K.; Makise, N.; Domoto, Y.; Ishida, J.; Morita, H.; Komuro, I. Use of a Non-invasive Cardiac Output Measurement in a Patient with Low-output Dilated Cardiomyopathy. *Intern. Med.* **2020**, *59*, 1525–1530. [CrossRef] [PubMed]
25. Hori, M.; Imamura, T.; Narang, N.; Kinugawa, K. Pressure ramp testing for optimization of end-expiratory pressure settings in adaptive servo-ventilation therapy. *Circ. Rep.* **2022**, *4*, 17–24. [CrossRef]
26. Hori, M.; Imamura, T.; Oshima, A.; Onoda, H.; Kinugawa, K. Novel ramp test to optimize pressure setting of adaptive servo-ventilation using non-invasive lung fluid level quantification. *Am. J. Case Rep.* **2022**; *in press*.
27. Schefold, J.C.; Filippatos, G.; Hasenfuss, G.; Anker, S.D.; von Haehling, S. Heart failure and kidney dysfunction: Epidemiology, mechanisms and management. *Nat. Rev. Nephrol.* **2016**, *12*, 610–623. [CrossRef] [PubMed]
28. Vardeny, O.; Claggett, B.; Anand, I.; Rossignol, P.; Desai, A.S.; Zannad, F.; Pitt, B.; Solomon, S.D.; Randomized Aldactone Evaluation Study (RALES) Investigators. Incidence, predictors, and outcomes related to hypo- and hyperkalemia in patients with severe heart failure treated with a mineralocorticoid receptor antagonist. *Circ. Heart Fail.* **2014**, *7*, 573–579. [CrossRef]
29. Rossignol, P.; Dobre, D.; McMurray, J.J.; Swedberg, K.; Krum, H.; van Veldhuisen, D.J.; Shi, H.; Messig, M.; Vincent, J.; Girerd, N.; et al. Incidence, determinants, and prognostic significance of hyperkalemia and worsening renal function in patients with heart failure receiving the mineralocorticoid receptor antagonist eplerenone or placebo in addition to optimal medical therapy: Results from the Eplerenone in Mild Patients Hospitalization and Survival Study in Heart Failure (EMPHASIS-HF). *Circ. Heart Fail.* **2014**, *7*, 51–58. [CrossRef] [PubMed]
30. Imamura, T.; Hori, M.; Narang, N.; Kinugawa, K. Association Between Adaptive Servo-Ventilation Therapy and Renal Function. *Int. Heart J.* **2021**, *62*, 1052–1056. [CrossRef]

31. Spannella, F.; Giulietti, F.; Filipponi, A.; Sarzani, R. Effect of sacubitril/valsartan on renal function: A systematic review and meta-analysis of randomized controlled trials. *ESC Heart Fail.* **2020**, *7*, 3487–3496. [CrossRef] [PubMed]
32. Oshima, A.; Imamura, T.; Narang, N.; Kinugawa, K. Renoprotective Effect of the Mineralocorticoid Receptor Antagonist Esaxerenone. *Circ. Rep.* **2021**, *3*, 333–337. [CrossRef] [PubMed]
33. Bakris, G.L.; Agarwal, R.; Anker, S.D.; Pitt, B.; Ruilope, L.M.; Rossing, P.; Kolkhof, P.; Nowack, C.; Schloemer, P.; Joseph, A.; et al. Effect of Finerenone on Chronic Kidney Disease Outcomes in Type 2 Diabetes. *N. Engl. J. Med.* **2020**, *383*, 2219–2229. [CrossRef] [PubMed]

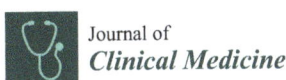

Review

A Systematic Review of the Efficacy and Safety of Direct Oral Anticoagulants in Atrial Fibrillation Patients with Diabetes Using a Risk Index

Domenico Acanfora [1,*], Marco Matteo Ciccone [2], Valentina Carlomagno [1], Pietro Scicchitano [2,3], Chiara Acanfora [1,4], Alessandro Santo Bortone [5], Massimo Uguccioni [6] and Gerardo Casucci [1,*]

1. Unit of Internal Medicine, San Francesco Hospital, Viale Europa 21, 82037 Telese Terme, Italy; vale.carlomagno@gmail.com (V.C.); acanforachiara@gmail.com (C.A.)
2. Section of Cardiovascular Diseases, Department of Emergency and Organ Transplantation, School of Medicine, University of Bari, Piazza Umberto I, 1, 70121 Bari, Italy; marcomatteo.ciccone@uniba.it (M.M.C.); piero.sc@hotmail.it (P.S.)
3. Cardiology Unit, Hospital "F. Perinei", Strada Statale 96 per Gravina in Puglia, 70022 Altamura, Italy
4. Department of Biotechnological and Applied Clinical Sciences, University of L'Aquila, 67100 L'Aquila, Italy
5. Division of Cardiac Surgery, Department of Emergency and Organ Transplantation, University of Bari, 70121 Bari, Italy; alessandro.bortone@gmail.com
6. Cardiology Unit, San Camillo Hospital, 00152 Rome, Italy; muguccioni@hotmail.com
* Correspondence: domenico.acanfora29@gmail.com (D.A.); segr.dott.gerardocasucci@virgilio.it (G.C.); Tel.: +39-0824-9747-26 (G.C.)

Citation: Acanfora, D.; Ciccone, M.M.; Carlomagno, V.; Scicchitano, P.; Acanfora, C.; Bortone, A.S.; Uguccioni, M.; Casucci, G. A Systematic Review of the Efficacy and Safety of Direct Oral Anticoagulants in Atrial Fibrillation Patients with Diabetes Using a Risk Index. *J. Clin. Med.* **2021**, *10*, 2924. https://doi.org/10.3390/jcm10132924

Academic Editors: Michał Ciurzyński and Justyna Domienik-Karłowicz

Received: 31 May 2021
Accepted: 26 June 2021
Published: 29 June 2021

Publisher's Note: MDPI stays neutral with regard to jurisdictional claims in published maps and institutional affiliations.

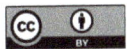

Copyright: © 2021 by the authors. Licensee MDPI, Basel, Switzerland. This article is an open access article distributed under the terms and conditions of the Creative Commons Attribution (CC BY) license (https://creativecommons.org/licenses/by/4.0/).

Abstract: Diabetes mellitus (DM) represents an independent risk factor for chronic AF and is associated with unfavorable outcomes. We aimed to evaluate the efficacy and safety of direct oral anticoagulants (DOACs) in patients with atrial fibrillation (AF), with and without diabetes mellitus (DM), using a new risk index (RI) defined as: $RI = \frac{\text{Rate of Events}}{\text{Rate of Patients at Risk}}$. In particular, an RI lower than 1 suggests a favorable treatment effect. We searched MEDLINE, MEDLINE In-Process, EMBASE, PubMed, and the Cochrane Central Register of Controlled Trials. The risk index (RI) was calculated in terms of efficacy (rate of stroke/systemic embolism (stroke SEE)/rate of patients with and without DM; rate of cardiovascular death/rate of patients with and without DM) and safety (rate of major bleeding/rate of patients with and without DM) outcomes. AF patients with DM (n = 22,057) and 49,596 without DM were considered from pivotal trials. DM doubles the risk index for stroke/SEE, major bleeding (MB), and cardiovascular (CV) death. The RI for stroke/SEE, MB, and CV death was comparable in patients treated with warfarin or DOACs. The lowest RI was in DM patients treated with Rivaroxaban (stroke/SEE, RI = 0.08; CV death, RI = 0.13). The RIs for bleeding were higher in DM patients treated with Dabigatran (RI110 = 0.32; RI150 = 0.40). Our study is the first to use RI to homogenize the efficacy and safety data reported in the DOACs pivotal studies against warfarin in patients with and without DM. Anticoagulation therapy is effective and safe in DM patients. DOACs appear to have a better efficacy and safety profile than warfarin. The use of DOACs is a reasonable alternative to vitamin-K antagonists in AF patients with DM. The RI can be a reasonable tool to help clinicians choose between DOACs or warfarin in the peculiar set of AF patients with DM.

Keywords: atrial fibrillation; DOACs; diabetes mellitus; risk index

1. Introduction

Atrial fibrillation (AF) is the most common arrhythmia worldwide. The prevalence of AF is expected to increase 2.5-fold in the next 50 years due to the growing mean age of the population [1]. Diabetes can be considered a pandemic too [2,3]. Diabetes mellitus (DM) represents an independent risk factor for chronic AF [4]. The development of AF is likely to be multifactorial and the mechanism is elusive, while evidence is emerging on the correlation between AF and DM [4]. DM and AF certainly share common risk factors, including hypertension, dyslipidemia, atherosclerosis, and obesity. Population-based studies suggested that DM is an independent risk factor for atrial fibrillation [5]. In patients with hypertension, DM did not act as an independent predictor for new onset AF in a post-hoc analysis from ALLHAT [6]. Nevertheless, a retrospective analysis of the VALUE study showed that hypertensive patients with new onset DM had a significantly higher event rate of new onset AF compared to patients without DM, even after adjusting for body mass index [7]. On the other hand, DM is one of the most common concomitant diseases in patients with AF [8]. Indeed, DM and AF are both predictors for stroke and mortality [9].

DM itself is associated with increased thrombin production and consequently may increase thromboembolic risk [10,11]. Anticoagulation therapy is mandatory in DM patients with AF. The use of VKA in these patients is to be implemented with caution. Hyperglycemia induces an increase in glycated albumin in DM patients. Glycated albumin has a reduced binding affinity for warfarin, resulting in a higher free fraction of the anticoagulant [12]. Consequently, there is a greater variability of the INR in AF patients with an increased risk of Stroke/SEE and MB [13].

Prevention of thromboembolic events was improved with the use of direct oral anticoagulants (DOACs) (Dabigatran, Rivaroxaban, Apixaban, and Edoxaban), which overcame the limitations of therapeutic standard of dose-adjusted vitamin K antagonists (VKAs) [14–18]. These drugs were approved based on the results from their respective dose-adjusted phase III, warfarin-controlled, randomized controlled trials (RCTs) [14–17].

The proportion of patients with DM enrolled in the four trials was 23% in the Randomized Evaluation of Long-Term Anticoagulant Therapy (RE-LY) study, 40% in the Rivaroxaban Once-daily oral direct factor Xa inhibition Compared with vitamin K antagonism for prevention of stroke and Embolism Trial in Atrial Fibrillation (ROCKET-AF) study, 25% in the Apixaban for Reduction in Stroke and Other Thromboembolic Events in Atrial Fibrillation (ARISTOTLE) study, and 36% in the Effective Anticoagulation With Factor Xa Next Generation in Atrial Fibrillation (ENGAGE-AF TIMI 48) study [14–17].

This systematic review aimed at evaluating the efficacy and safety of DOACs versus warfarin in patients with AF, with and without DM, by applying the risk index (RI) proposed by Uguccioni et al. [19,20].

2. Methods

We performed an extensive literature search to identify studies reporting stroke and systemic embolism, major bleeding, and cardiovascular (CV) death in patients with AF, randomized to VKA or DOAC, with and without DM. The search was performed in MEDLINE, MEDLINE In-Process, and Other Non-Indexed Citations, EMBASE, PubMed, and the Cochrane Central Register of Controlled Trials through the Ovid interface to identify English-language clinical articles published from 2002 (first marketed DOAC) to February 2020 related to phase III RCTs of dabigatran, rivaroxaban, apixaban, or edoxaban versus warfarin for the prevention of thrombotic events in AF patients. Keywords used were: "atrial fibrillation", "warfarin", "oral thrombin inhibitor", "oral factor Xa inhibitor", "dabigatran", "rivaroxaban", "apixaban", "edoxaban", and "diabetes".

We also established regular alerts and complemented the electronic search strategy with a direct, manual reference review.

Systematic reviews, which included RCTs that evaluated stroke/systemic embolic events (SEE), major bleeding, and/or cardiovascular (CV) death and evaluated DOACs and VKAs were eligible for inclusion. PICOS (patients, intervention, comparator, outcomes, and study design) criteria for inclusion and exclusion of network meta-analyses (NMAs) are described in Table 1.

Table 1. PICOS criteria for inclusion and exclusion of systematic review.

	Inclusion Criteria	Exclusion Criteria
Population	Patients with NVAF receiving any of the treatments below. All studies in the SLR must include $\geq$ 90% patients with NVAF. SLRs including studies with < 90% patients with NVAF must report data separately for the NVAF studies	Not a population of interest (ie, non-NVAF patients) Studies of patients receiving ablation, cardioversion, or left-atrial appendage closure
Intervention/comparator	DOACs (apixaban, dabigatran, rivaroxaban, edoxaban) and warfarin studies need to have compared 1 or more DOACs and/or warfarin	Studies not reporting outcomes for population of interest
Outcome	Clinical outcomes: • Stroke/systemic embolism • Major bleeding (ISTH or modified ISTH). • Cardiovascular death • Patients with and without diabetes mellitus Doses included: Apixaban: 5 or 2.5 mg [a] Rivaroxaban: 20 or 15 mg Dabigatran: 150 or 110 mg Edoxaban: 30 or 60 mg	SLRs/NMAs of observational studies, nonsystematic reviews, primary research trials, primary observational studies, case reports, case series, narrative reviews Letters to the editor, guidelines, meeting abstracts In vitro pharmacodynamic or pharmacokinetic studies only, animal studies, genetic studies only
Study design	SLR of randomized controlled trials	

PICOS, patients, intervention, comparator, outcomes, study design; DOAC, direct oral anticoagulant; ISTH, International Society on Thrombosis and Hemostasis; $CHADS_2$ = (congestive heart failure, hypertension, age $\geq$ 75 years), diabetes mellitus, stroke (double weight)); NMA, network meta-analysis; NVAF, nonvalvular atrial fibrillation; SLR, systematic literature review. [a] Any network meta-analysis comparison of apixaban 2.5 mg only with another DOAC was not included.

The search results were compared and the duplicates eliminated. An initial screening of the studies was performed on the basis of titles and abstracts, and then the full texts were reviewed by five. Five reviewers (D.A., P.S., C.A., V.C., and G.C.) independently performed the revision, while discrepancies were solved by a consensus, involving two additional authors (M.U., M.M.C.).

Data were derived from four pivotal trials (Figure 1). Details of the search strategy according to PRISMA-P were described in all of the tables in the supplementary materials section.

The RI was computed in terms of efficacy (rate of stroke-systemic embolism/rate of patients with and without diabetes) and safety (rate of major bleeding/rate of patients with and without diabetes; rate of cardiovascular death/rate of patients with and without diabetes) of DOACs and VKAs.

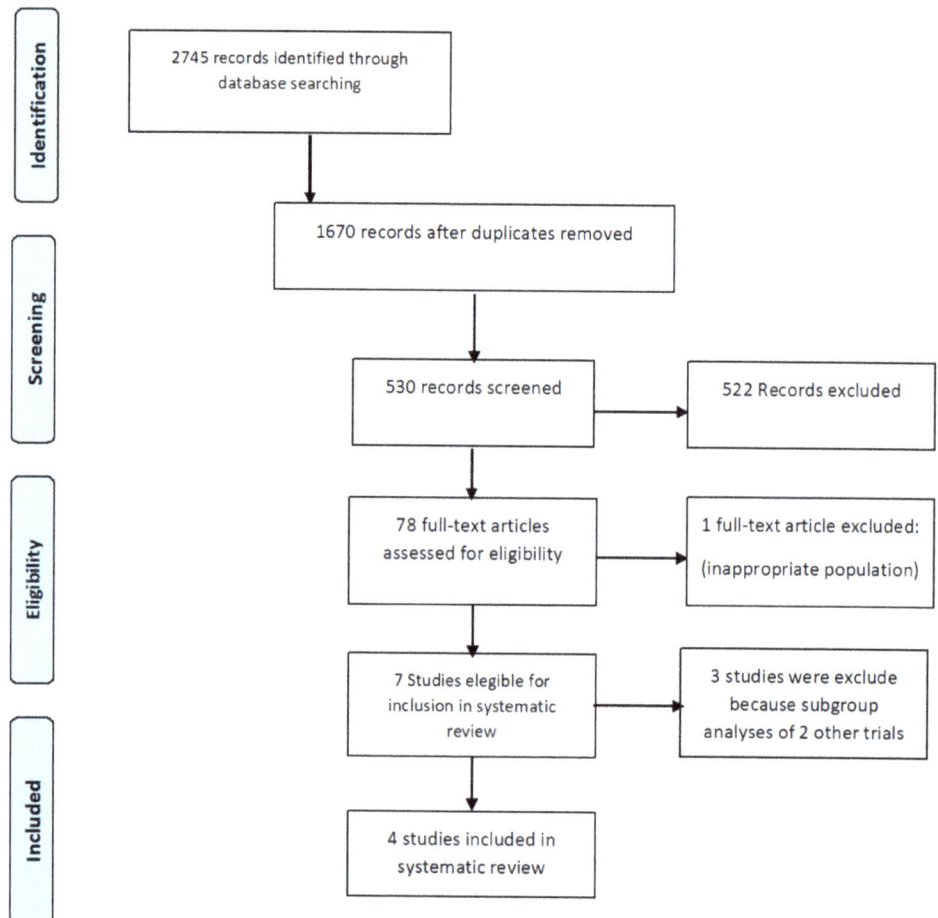

Figure 1. Preferred Reporting Items for Systematic Reviews and Meta-Analyses (PRISMA-P) flow diagram: search and selection process.

3. Statistical Analysis

No statistical analyses were conducted; according to the authors, indirect, comparative meta-analyses among DOACs are a hypothesis generator that cannot provide definitive answers.

Furthermore, the RI does not allow the comparisons of rates among non-homogeneous studies.

4. Main Results

The main characteristics of the four RCTs involving DOACs are summarized in Table 2. About 22,057 patients with AF and DM and 49,596 AF patients without DM were finally included. The results of our systematic review are summarized in Table 3. The percentages of patients with DM ranged from 23.3% to 39.9%. The highest number of patients with DM was in the patient population treated with Rivaroxaban (40.3%).

Table 2. Main characteristics of the four DOACs pivotal trials.

	ROCKET AF Rivaroxaban	ARISTOTLE Apixaban	RE-LY Dabigatran	ENGAGE Edoxaban
Effect	Anti-Xa	Anti-Xa	Anti-IIa	Anti-Xa
Dose	20/15 mg QD	5/2.5 mg BID	150/110 mg BID	60/30 mg QD
Mean $CHADS_2$ score	3.5	2.1	2.1	2.8
Target INR (Warfarin arm)	2–3	2–3	2–3	2–3
TTR (%)	58	62	64	68
Asia Pacific Region N (%)	2109 (14.8%)	2916 (16%)	3854 (21%)	3383 (16%)
Median Follow-up duration	1.9 y	1.8 y	2 y	2.8 y

ROCKET-AF = Rivaroxaban Once-daily oral direct factor Xa inhibition Compared with vitamin K antagonism for prevention of stroke and Embolism Trial in Atrial Fibrillation [17]; ARISTOTLE = Apixaban for Reduction in Stroke and Other Thromboembolic Events in Atrial Fibrillation [16]; RE-LY = Randomized Evaluation of Long-Term Anticoagulant Therapy [14]; ENGAGE-AF TIMI 48 = Effective Anticoagulation With Factor Xa Next Generation in Atrial Fibrillation [15]; Xa = Factor X activated; IIa = Thrombin; QD = Quaque die; BID = Bis in die; $CHADS_2$ = Congestive Heart Failure, Hypertension, Age, Diabetes, Stroke; INR = International Normalized Ratio; TTR = Time to Range; N = Number; y = year.

Table 3. Patients with and without diabetes in the pivotal trials.

RCTs	Pts on DOACs (N)	Diabetes N (%)	No Diabetes N (%)	Pts on Warfarin (N)	Diabetes N (%)	No Diabetes N (%)
ROCKET AF	7131	2878 (40.3%)	4253 (59.7%)	7133	2817 (39.5%)	4316 (60.5%)
ARISTOTLE	9120	2284 (25.0%)	6836 (75%)	9087	2263 (24.9%)	6818 (75.1%)
RE-LY $_{110\ mg}$	6015	1409 (23.4%)	4606 (66.6%)	6022	1410 (23.4%)	4612 (66.6%)
RE-LY $_{150\ mg}$	6076	1402 (23.1%)	4674 (63.9%)	6022	1410 (23.4%)	4612 (66.6%)
ENGAGE $_{30\ mg}$	7034	2544 (36.2%)	4490 (63.8%)	7036	2521 (35.8%)	4515 (64.2%)
ENGAGE $_{60\ mg}$	7035	2529 (35.9%)	4476 (64.1%)	7036	2521 (35.8%)	4515 (64.2%)

RCTs = randomized controlled trials; DOACs = non-VKA antagonist drugs; Pts = Patients; N = Number; ROCKET-AF = Rivaroxaban Once-daily oral direct factor Xa inhibition Compared with vitamin K antagonism for prevention of stroke and Embolism Trial in Atrial Fibrillation [17]; ARISTOTLE = Apixaban for Reduction in Stroke and Other Thromboembolic Events in Atrial Fibrillation [16]; RE-LY = Randomized Evaluation of Long-Term Anticoagulant Therapy [14]; ENGAGE-AF TIMI 48 = Effective Anticoagulation With Factor Xa Next Generation in Atrial Fibrillation [15].

Table 4 summarized data regarding the rate of stroke/SEE, major bleeding, and CV death related to warfarin, Dabigatran 110 mg and 150 mg BID, Rivaroxaban 20 mg QD, Apixaban 5 mg BID, and Edoxaban high and low dose (60–30 mg) QD.

The RIs for stroke/SEE and CV death were similar between patients treated with DOACs and patients treated with warfarin (Figures 2 and 3, Table 5), except for Edoxaban 30 mg QD, which showed a higher RI than warfarin for stroke/SEE. Indeed, Rivaroxaban QD had the lowest RI values in terms of both stroke/SEE and CV death (Figures 2 and 3, Table 5). Nevertheless, no data about CV death were reported for Edoxaban low doses, as none of the patients on Edoxaban low dose were included in the pivotal RCT (Table 5).

Table 4. Stroke/systemic embolism, major bleeding, and cardiovascular death in patients with and without diabetes in the pivotal trials.

RCTs	Diabetes					
	Stroke o SEE (N)%		MB (N)%		CV Death N (%)	
	DOACs	Warfarin	DOACs	Warfarin	DOACs	Warfarin
ROCKET AF	95 (3.3%)	114 (4.0%)	165 (5.7%)	169 (6.0%)	152 (5.3%)	192 (6.8%)
ARISTOTLE	57 (2.5%)	75 (3.3%)	112 (4.9%)	114 (5.0%)	79 (3.5%)	88 (3.9%)
RE-LY $_{110}$	49 (3.5%)	64 (4.5%)	106 (7.5%)	114 (8.0%)	91 (6.5%)	109 (7.7%)
RE-LY $_{150}$	40 (2.9%)		129 (9.2%)		95 (6.8%)	
ENGAGE $_{30 mg}$	135 (5.3%)	107 (4.2%)	123 (4.9%)	278 (11%)	NA	NA
ENGAGE $_{60 mg}$	102 (4.0%)		219 (8.6%)		209 (8.1%)	219 (8.6%)
	No Diabetes					
RCTs	Stroke o SEE (N)%		MB (N)%		CV Death N (%)	
ROCKET AF	174 (4.0%)	192 (4.4%)	230 (5.4%)	217(5.0%)	223 (5.2%)	209 (4.8%)
ARISTOTLE	155 (2.3%)	190 (2.8%)	215 (3.2%)	348 (5.1%)	229 (3.4%)	256 (3.7%)
RE-LY $_{110}$	134 (2.9%)	138 (2.9%)	236 (5.1%)	307 (6.6%)	198 (4.3%)	208 (4.5%)
RE-LY $_{150}$	94 (2.0%)		271 (5.8%)		179 (3.8%)	
ENGAGE $_{30 mg}$	NA	NA	NA	NA	NA	NA
ENGAGE $_{60 mg}$	207 (4.6%)	248 (5.4%)	335 (7.5%)	417 (9.2%)	331 (7.4%)	406 (8.9%)

RCTs = randomized controlled trials; DOAC = non-VKA antagonist drugs; N = Number; SEE = systemic embolism; MB = major bleeding; CV = cardiovascular death; ROCKET-AF = Rivaroxaban Once-daily oral direct factor Xa inhibition Compared with vitamin K antagonism for prevention of stroke and Embolism Trial in Atrial Fibrillation [17]; ARISTOTLE = Apixaban for Reduction in Stroke and Other Thromboembolic Events in Atrial Fibrillation [16]; RE-LY = Randomized Evaluation of Long-Term Anticoagulant Therapy [14]; ENGAGE-AF TIMI 48 = Effective Anticoagulation With Factor Xa Next Generation in Atrial Fibrillation [15].

Table 5. Risk index of stroke/systemic embolism, major bleeding, and cardiovascular death in patients with and without diabetes in the pivotal trials.

RCTs	Diabetes					
	Stroke o SEE		MB		CV Death	
	DOACs	Warfarin	DOACs	Warfarin	DOACs	Warfarin
ROCKET AF	0.08	0.10	0.14	0.15	0.13	0.17
ARISTOTLE	0.10	0.13	0.19	0.20	0.14	0.15
RE-LY $_{110}$	0.14	0.19	0.32	0.34	0.27	0.33
RE-LY $_{150}$	0.12		0.40		0.29	
ENGAGE $_{30 mg}$	0.15	0.12	0.13	0.30	NA	NA
ENGAGE $_{60 mg}$	0.11		0.23		0.22	0.24
	No Diabetes					
RCTs	Stroke o SEE		MB		CV Death	
ROCKET AF	0.06	0.07	0.09	0.08	0.08	0.08
ARISTOTLE	0.03	0.03	0.04	0.06	0.04	0.04
RE-LY $_{110}$	0.04	0.04	0.07	0.09	0.06	0.06
RE-LY $_{150}$	0.03		0.09		0.06	
ENGAGE $_{30 mg}$	NA	NA	NA	NA	NA	NA
ENGAGE $_{60 mg}$	0.07	0.08	0.11	0.14	0.11	0.13

RCTs = randomized controlled trials; N = Number; SEE = systemic embolism; MB = major bleeding; CV = cardiovascular death; DOAC = non-VKA antagonist drugs; ROCKET-AF = Rivaroxaban Once-daily oral direct factor Xa inhibition Compared with vitamin K antagonism for prevention of stroke and Embolism Trial in Atrial Fibrillation [17]; ARISTOTLE = Apixaban for Reduction in Stroke and Other Thromboembolic Events in Atrial Fibrillation [16]; RE-LY = Randomized Evaluation of Long-Term Anticoagulant Therapy [14]; ENGAGE-AF TIMI 48 = Effective Anticoagulation With Factor Xa Next Generation in Atrial Fibrillation [15].

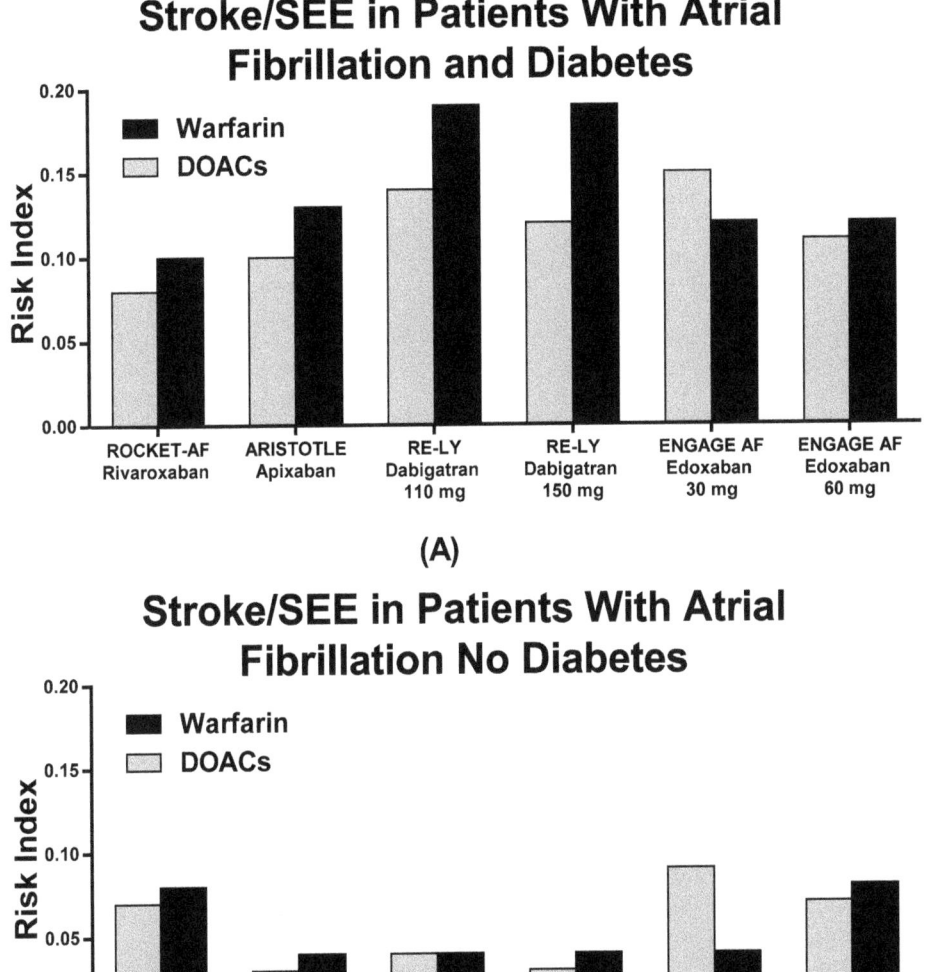

Figure 2. Risk index of stroke/systemic embolism in patients with (**A**) and without (**B**) diabetes in the pivotal trials.

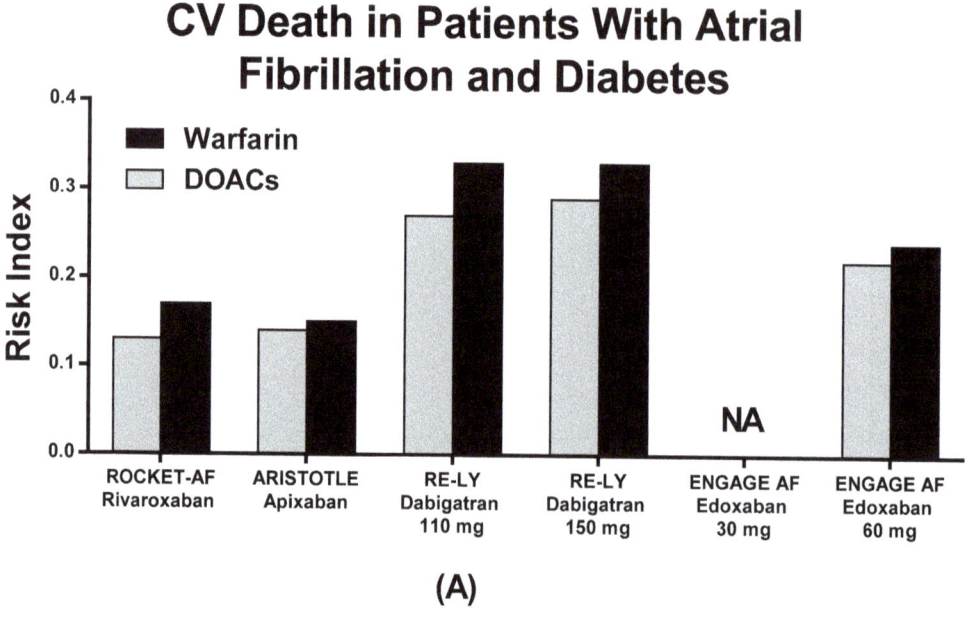

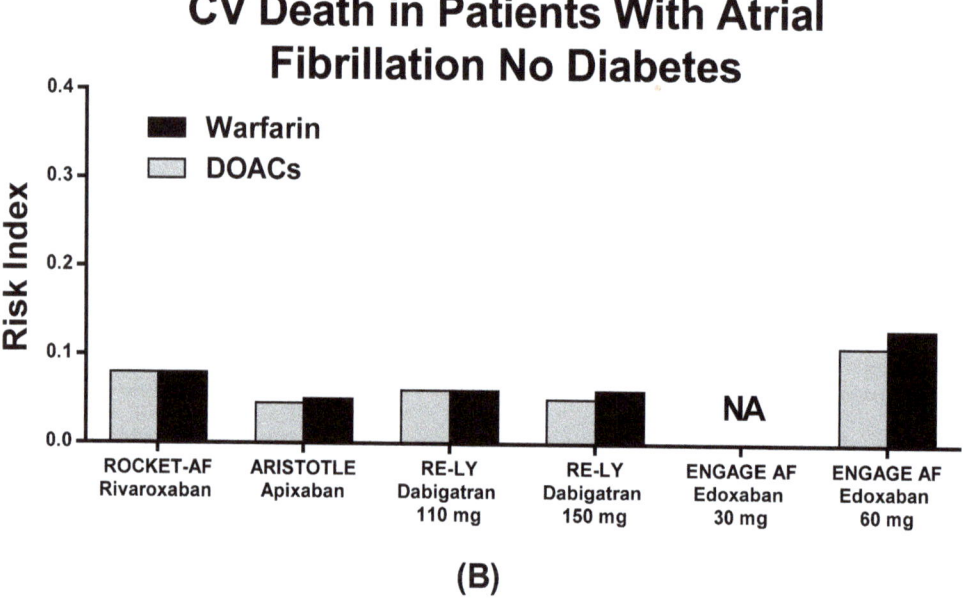

Figure 3. Risk index of CV Death in patients with (**A**) and without (**B**) diabetes in the pivotal trials.

The RIs for major bleedings are shown in Table 5 and Figure 4. Dabigatran 150 mg BID showed a higher risk for bleeding compared to warfarin, while other DOACs showed substantially equal RIs in comparison with warfarin (Table 5 and Figure 4). No DM patients with AF as compared to DM patients without AF showed lower RIs (Table 5, Figures 2–4).

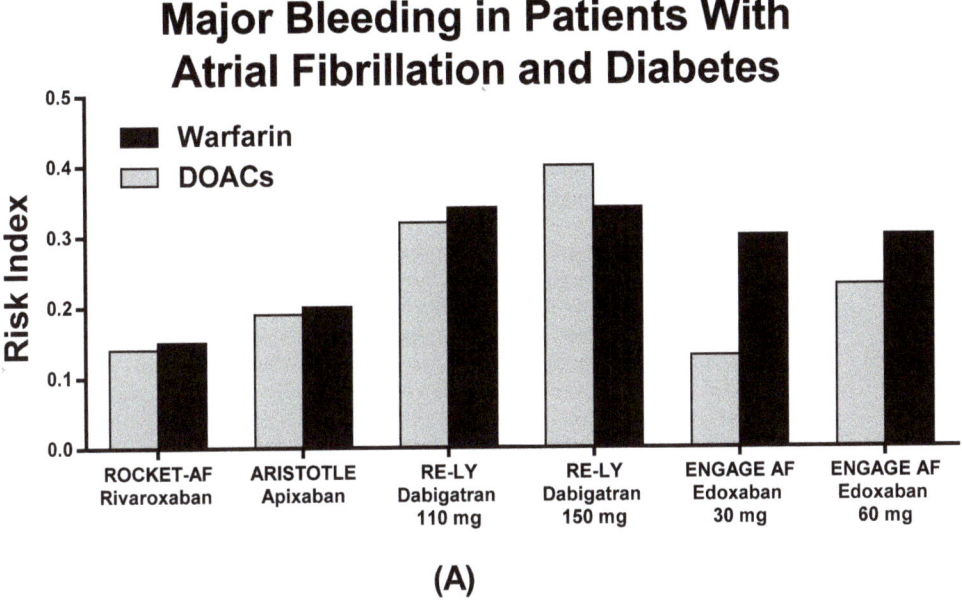

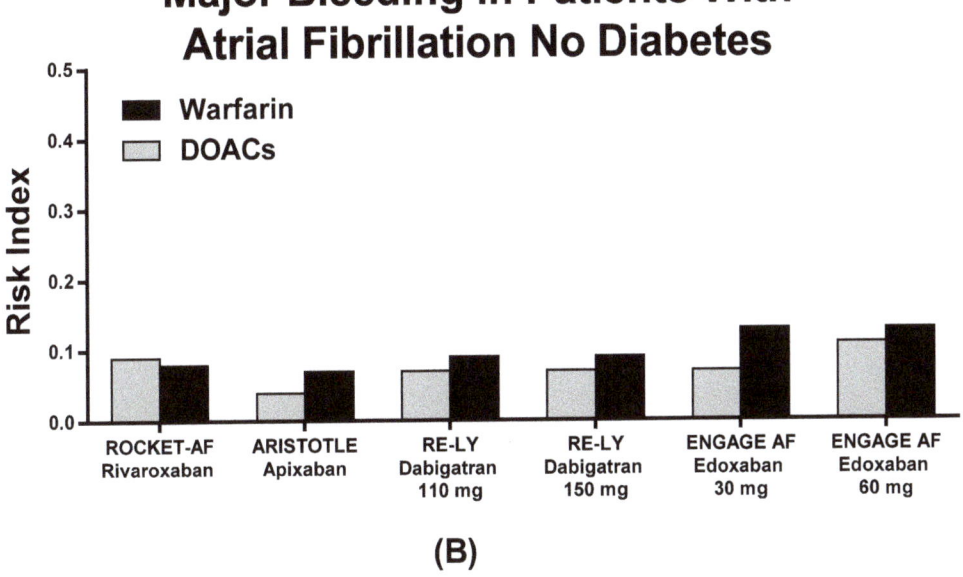

Figure 4. Risk index of Major Bleeding in patients with (**A**) and without (**B**) diabetes in the pivotal trials.

5. Discussion

Diabetes mellitus per se increases the risk of systemic stroke/embolism or cardiovascular death in patients with atrial fibrillation [21]. Therefore, anticoagulant therapy is mandatory in these patients [22]. Choosing the correct anticoagulant therapy in patients with AF is a challenge, especially in patients at higher risk such as DM patients. DM and AF are two sides of the same coin due to the tight correlation between these two pathological conditions [4]. The frequency of NVAF increases by 40% in patients with Type 2 diabetes, while thromboembolic risk is 79% higher compared to non-diabetic patients [14,22–24]. Indeed, both conditions can potentiate their negative effects on systemic tissue and organs: for example, they can both promote kidney failure [25,26]. In such a setting, choosing the correct anticoagulation remains challenging as these drugs may also promote systemic alterations. Warfarin, the traditional anticoagulant used to prevent thromboembolism, can also be dangerous due to a supposed negative influence on kidneys and systemic vessels by promoting arterial calcification and decreasing renal function [27]. Indeed, DOACs seemed to be safer and more efficacious [27], especially when dealing with Type 2 diabetic patient [22–24].

Using RI as suggested by Uguccioni et al. could help reduce heterogeneity enrolled in RCTs and provide a better approach for the selection of the correct anticoagulant based on the different patient characteristics [19,20]. In particular, an RI lower than 1 suggests a favorable treatment effect. The lower the RI value, the better the performance of the drug within the specific context [19,20]. This is the first report that evaluates the risk for stroke/SEE, CV death, and major bleeding in patients with AF with and without DM by means of RI.

In our study, both DOACs and warfarin appear to be effective in preventing stroke and systemic embolism, with lower rates of CV death and major bleeding. The RI of each drug is lower than one, although some differences should be outlined. In particular, Dabigatran 150 mg BID might increase major bleeding risk as compared to warfarin, while the risk for stroke/SEE seems higher with Edoxaban 30 mg QD as compared to warfarin in DM patients. These data are the most contradictory in the panel of RIs comparisons as all of the other drugs and dosages revealed protective and efficient effects on patients' outcomes as compared to warfarin (Figures 2 and 4). By considering the absolute measurements, Rivaroxaban QD demonstrated the lowest RI value in terms of stroke/SEE outcomes, while Edoxaban 30 mg QD showed the lowest RI in terms of major bleeding outcomes, although no data are reported on pivotal Edoxaban Low Dose RCT with regard to CV death in patients with and without DM.

The literature offers evidence about the DOACs performances in AF patients in terms of efficacy and safety, but the reproducibility of the data and indirect comparisons among drugs may interfere with the correct choice of anticoagulants [28]. A meta-analysis by Ruff et al. involving the 71,683 patients with AF from registration RCTs showed a significant reduction in the incidence of stroke and SEE (relative risk (RR) 0.81, confidence interval (CI) 95% 0.73–0.91; $p < 0.0001$) in patients with DOACs versus warfarin, as well as all-cause mortality (RR 0.90, CI 95% 0.85–0.95; $p = 0.0003$) and intracranial hemorrhages (RR 0.48, 95% CI 0.39–0:59; $p < 0.0001$), despite the increase in gastrointestinal bleeding (RR 1.25, 95% CI 1.01–1.55; $p = 0.04$) [18].

6. Study Limitations

Unfortunately, a number of methodological discrepancies, including study design, different selection of the populations, and different definitions of outcomes among the four phase-III RCTs, reduce the generalization of results and the comparisons among drugs [14–17]. The selection of DM patients among RCTs populations aimed at evaluating a uniform subset of individuals.

Registration studies differ in terms of thromboembolic risk of the enrolled populations, age, heart failure, and active cancer. Active cancer is a high thromboembolic risk condition, and DAOCs appear to be an effective and safe therapeutic option in these patients [29]. The highest rate of DM patients was in Rocket-AF (40%) while ARISTOTLE had 25% and RE-LY had 23%.

The incidence of major bleeding was similar in AF patients with DM treated with Rivaroxaban or warfarin, while increasing when Dabigatran 110 mg, Dabigatran 150 mg, or warfarin were adopted. This difference might be associated with patients' risk profiles, as well as other factors that may influence the pharmacokinetics and pharmacodynamics (co-morbidities, advanced age, HF, diabetes, hepatic or renal insufficiency). RCTs did not provide routine information about blood glucose levels and HbA_{1c}, while patients with creatinine clearance < 30 mL/min were excluded. Therefore, patients with severe diabetic nephropathy, who are at even higher risk for cardiovascular complications, were excluded from RCTs. In these RCTs, no interactions were found between diabetic status and clinical efficacy of DOACs versus warfarin. Interestingly, the superiority of Apixaban over warfarin in terms of safety was lost when patients with AF and DM were considered (p = 0.003 for interaction) [30]. Moreover, a study-level meta-analysis in patients with DM and AF demonstrated a significant reduction in stroke and systemic embolism event rates (−20%) in patients treated with DOACs as compared to warfarin, as well as vascular mortality (−17%) and intracranial bleeding (−43%), while no influence was observed in terms of incidence of major bleeding [23].

We did not conduct any statistical analyses; indirect, comparative meta-analyses among DOACs are hypothesis generators and cannot provide definitive answers.

Conversely, it has been shown that published RCT data can be affected by the insertion of controversial data. In addition, they could invalidate the medical literature, alter the results of meta-analyses, and consequently compromise future research, political decisions, and above all patient care [31].

7. Conclusions

To our knowledge, no data are available about direct comparisons between DOACs in patients with DM. The choice of DOAC in patients with DM is not supported by specific evidence, but it should be guided by general principles, taking into account age and comorbidities (hypertension, coronary artery disease, heart failure, kidney disease, obesity, and dyslipidemia).

Diabetic patients show a doubled RI compared to non-diabetic patients. Data from the systematic evaluation of the four phase-III RCTs with DOACs in patients with AF and DM showed that Rivaroxaban had the lowest RI with regard to MB, CV death, and stroke/SEE. The use of DOACs is a reasonable alternative to VKAs in the management of patients with AF and DM. The risk index is a useful additional tool to help clinicians to choose DOACs or warfarin in a particular category of AF patients.

Supplementary Materials: The following are available online at https://www.mdpi.com/2077-0383/10/13/2924/s1, File S1: The search strategy according to PRISMA-P.

Author Contributions: D.A., M.M.C., C.A., V.C., G.C., A.S.B., M.U., and P.S. devised and designed the study, collected and interpreted the data, drafted the article and critically reviewed its content, and approved the final version for publication. All authors have read and agreed to the published version of the manuscript.

Funding: The authors received no financial support for the research, authorship, and/or publication of this article.

Data Availability Statement: Data are available on request by contacting the corresponding author.

Conflicts of Interest: The authors declare that there is no conflict of interests. None of the authors have any financial or other relations that could lead to a conflict of interest.

References

1. Go, A.S.; Hylek, E.M.; Phillips, K.A.; Chang, Y.; Henault, L.E.; Selby, J.V.; Singer, D.E. Prevalence of diagnosed atrial fibrillation in adults: National implications for rhythm management and stroke prevention: The AnTicoagulation and Risk Factors in Atrial Fibrillation (ATRIA) Study. *JAMA* **2001**, *285*, 2370–2375. [CrossRef]
2. GBD 2016 Disease and Injury Incidence and Prevalence Collaborators. Global, regional, and national incidence, preva-lence, and years lived with disability for 328 diseases and injuries for 195 countries, 1990–2016: A systematic analysis for the Global Burden of Disease Study 2016. *Lancet* **2017**, *390*, 1211–1259.
3. GBD 2016 Causes of Death Collaborators. Global, regional, and national age-sex specific mortality for 264 causes of death, 1980–2016: A systematic analysis for the Global Burden of Disease Study 2016. *Lancet* **2017**, *390*, 1151–1210. [CrossRef]
4. Bell, D.S.H.; Goncalves, E. Atrial fibrillation and type 2 diabetes: Prevalence, etiology, pathophysiology and effect of an-ti-diabetic therapies. *Diabetes Obes. Metab.* **2019**, *21*, 210–217. [CrossRef] [PubMed]

5. Benjamin, E.J.; Levy, D.; Vaziri, S.M.; D'Agostino, R.B.; Belanger, A.J.; Wolf, P.A. Independent risk factors for atrial fibrillation in a population-based cohort. The Framingham Heart Study. *JAMA* **1994**, *271*, 840–844. [CrossRef] [PubMed]
6. Haywood, L.J.; Ford, C.E.; Crow, R.S.; Davis, B.R.; Massie, B.M.; Einhorn, P.T.; Williard, A. Atrial Fibrillation at Baseline and During Follow-Up in ALLHAT (Antihypertensive and Lipid-Lowering Treatment to Prevent Heart Attack Trial). *J. Am. Coll. Cardiol.* **2009**, *54*, 2023–2031. [CrossRef]
7. Aksnes, T.A.; Schmieder, R.E.; Kjeldsen, S.E.; Ghani, S.; Hua, T.A.; Julius, S. Impact of new-onset diabetes mellitus on development of atrial fibrillation and heart failure in high-risk hypertension (from the VALUE Trial). *Am. J. Cardiol.* **2008**, *101*, 634–638. [CrossRef] [PubMed]
8. Murphy, N.F.; Simpson, C.; Jhund, P.; Stewart, S.; Kirkpatrick, M.; Chalmers, J.; Macintyre, K.; McMurray, J.J.V. A national survey of the prevalence, incidence, primary care burden and treatment of atrial fibrillation in Scotland. *Heart* **2007**, *93*, 606–612. [CrossRef] [PubMed]
9. Chung, M.K.; Eckhardt, L.L.; Chen, L.Y.; Ahmed, H.M.; Gopinathannair, R.; Joglar, J.A.; Noseworthy, P.A.; Pack, Q.R.; Sanders, P.; Trulock, K.M. Lifestyle and Risk Factor Modification for Reduction of Atrial Fibrillation: A Scientific Statement From the American Heart Association. *Circulation* **2020**, *141*, e750–e772. [CrossRef] [PubMed]
10. Ceriello, A.; Giacomello, R.; Stel, G.; Motz, E.; Taboga, C.; Tonutti, L.; Pirisi, M.; Falleti, E.; Bartoli, E. Hyperglycemia-induced thrombin formation in diabetes. The possible role of oxidative stress. *Diabetes* **1995**, *44*, 924–928. [CrossRef] [PubMed]
11. Lee, S.; Ay, C.; Kopp, C.W.; Panzer, S.; Gremmel, T. Impaired glucose metabolism is associated with increased thrombin generation potential in patients undergoing angioplasty and stenting. *Cardiovasc. Diabetol.* **2018**, *17*, 131. [CrossRef] [PubMed]
12. Baraka-Vidot, J.; Guerin-Dubourg, A.; Bourdon, E.; Rondeau, P. Impaired drug-binding capacities of in vitro and in vivo glycated albumin. *Biochimie* **2012**, *94*, 1960–1967. [CrossRef] [PubMed]
13. Nelson, W.W.; Desai, S.; Damaraju, C.V.; Lu, L.; Fields, L.E.; Wildgoose, P.; Schein, J.R. International normalized ratio stability in warfarin-experienced patients with nonvalvular atrial fbrillation. *Am. J. Cardiovasc. Drugs* **2015**, *15*, 205–211. [CrossRef] [PubMed]
14. Connolly, S.J.; Ezekowitz, M.D.; Yusuf, S.; Eikelboom, J.; Oldgren, J.; Parekh, A.; Pogue, J.; Reilly, P.A.; Themeles, E.; Varrone, J.; et al. Dabigatran versus Warfarin in Patients with Atrial Fibrillation. *N. Engl. J. Med.* **2009**, *361*, 1139–1151. [CrossRef] [PubMed]
15. Giugliano, R.P.; Ruff, C.T.; Braunwald, E.; Murphy, A.; Wiviott, S.D.; Halperin, J.L.; Waldo, A.L.; Ezekowitz, M.D.; Weitz, J.I.; Špinar, J.; et al. Edoxaban versus Warfarin in Patients with Atrial Fibrillation. *N. Engl. J. Med.* **2013**, *369*, 2093–2104. [CrossRef] [PubMed]
16. Granger, C.B.; Alexander, J.H.; McMurray, J.J.V.; Lopes, R.D.; Hylek, E.M.; Hanna, M.; Al-Khalidi, H.R.; Ansell, J.; Atar, D.; Avezum, A.; et al. Apixaban versus warfarin in patients with atrial fibrillation. *N. Engl. J. Med.* **2011**, *365*, 981–992. [CrossRef] [PubMed]
17. Patel, M.R.; Mahaffey, K.W.; Garg, J.; Pan, G.; Singer, D.E.; Hacke, W.; Breithardt, G.; Halperin, J.L.; Hankey, G.J.; Piccini, J.P.; et al. Rivaroxaban versus warfarin in nonvalvular atrial fibrillation. *N. Engl. J. Med.* **2011**, *365*, 883–891. [CrossRef] [PubMed]
18. Ruff, C.T.; Giugliano, R.P.; Braunwald, E.; Hoffman, E.B.; Deenadayalu, N.; Ezekowitz, M.D.; Camm, A.J.; Weitz, J.I.; Lewis, B.S.; Parkhomenko, A.; et al. Comparison of the efficacy and safety of new oral anticoagulants with warfarin in patients with atrial fibrillation: A meta-analysis of randomised trials. *Lancet* **2014**, *383*, 955–962. [CrossRef]
19. Acanfora, D.; Ciccone, M.M.; Scicchitano, P.; Ricci, G.; Acanfora, C.; Uguccioni, M.; Casucci, G. Efficacy and Safety of Direct Oral Anticoagulants in Patients With Atrial Fibrillation and High Thromboembolic Risk. A Systematic Review. *Front. Pharmacol.* **2019**, *10*, 1048. [CrossRef] [PubMed]
20. Uguccioni, M.; Terranova, A.; Di Lullo, L. Valutazione delle reazioni avverse agli anticoagulanti orali diretti registrate nella Rete Nazionale di Farmacovigilanza mediante uno specifico indice di rischio. *Ital. Cardiol.* **2018**, *19*, 3–11.
21. Du, X.; Ninomiya, T.; De Galan, B.; Abadir, E.; Chalmers, J.; Pillai, A.; Woodward, M.; Cooper, M.; Harrap, S.; Hamet, P.; et al. Risks of cardiovascular events and effects of routine blood pressure lowering among patients with type 2 diabetes and atrial fibrillation: Results of the ADVANCE study. *Eur. Hear. J.* **2009**, *30*, 1128–1135. [CrossRef]
22. Patti, G.; Cavallari, I.; Andreotti, F.; Calabrò, P.; Cirillo, P.; Denas, G.; Galli, M.; Golia, E.; Maddaloni, E.; Marcucci, R.; et al. Prevention of atherothrombotic events in patients with diabetes mellitus: From antithrombotic therapies to new-generation glucose-lowering drugs. *Nat. Rev. Cardiol.* **2019**, *16*, 113–130. [CrossRef] [PubMed]
23. Patti, G.; Di Gioia, G.; Cavallari, I.; Nenna, A. Safety and efficacy of nonvitamin K antagonist oral anticoagulants versus warfarin in diabetic patients with atrial fibrillation: A study-level meta-analysis of phase III randomized trials. *Diabetes Metab. Res. Rev.* **2017**, *33*, e2876. [CrossRef] [PubMed]
24. Stroke Risk in Atrial Fibrillation Working Group. Independent predictors of stroke in patients with atrial fibrillation: A systematic review. *Neurology* **2007**, *69*, 546–554. [CrossRef] [PubMed]
25. Braunwald, E. Diabetes, heart failure, and renal dysfunction: The vicious circles. *Prog. Cardiovasc. Dis.* **2019**, *62*, 298–302. [CrossRef] [PubMed]
26. Hu, L.; Xiong, Q.; Chen, Z.; Fu, L.; Hu, J.; Chen, Q.; Tu, W.; Xu, C.; Xu, G.; Li, J.; et al. Factors Associated with a Large Decline in Renal Function or Progression to Renal Insufficiency in Hospitalized Atrial Fibrillation Patients with Early-Stage CKD. *Int. Hear. J.* **2020**, *61*, 239–248. [CrossRef] [PubMed]
27. Yao, X.; Tangri, N.; Gersh, B.J.; Sangaralingham, L.R.; Shah, N.D.; Nath, K.A.; Noseworthy, P.A. Renal Outcomes in Anticoagulated Patients With Atrial Fibrillation. *J. Am. Coll. Cardiol.* **2017**, *70*, 2621–2632. [CrossRef] [PubMed]

28. Acanfora, D.; Casucci, G.; Ciccone, M.M.; Scicchitano, P.; Montefusco, G.; Lanzillo, A.; Acanfora, C.; Lanzillo, B. Direct Oral Anti-coagulants, Bleeding Risk in Patients with Atrial Fibrillation, CHADS2 $\geq$ 3 or HAS-BLED $\geq$ 3. *Cardiovasc. Pharm.* **2018**, *240*, 2–4.
29. Pacholczak-Madej, R.; Bazan-Socha, S.; Zaręba, L.; Undas, A.; Dropiński, J. Direct oral anticoagulants in the prevention of stroke in breast cancer patients with atrial fibrillation during adjuvant endocrine therapy: A cohort study. *Int. J. Cardiol.* **2021**, *324*, 78–83. [CrossRef] [PubMed]
30. Zadok, O.I.B.; Eisen, A. Use of non-vitamin K oral anticoagulants in people with atrial fibrillation and diabetes mellitus. *Diabetes Med.* **2018**, *35*, 548–556. [CrossRef] [PubMed]
31. Garmendia, C.A.; Nassar Gorra, L.; Rodriguez, A.L.; Trepka, M.J.; Veledar, E.; Madhivanan, P. Evaluation of the inclusion of studies identified by the FDA as having falsified data in the results of meta-analyses: The example of the apixaban trials. *JAMA Int. Med.* **2019**, *179*, 582–584. [CrossRef] [PubMed]

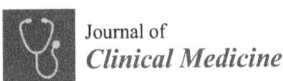

Review

Pleiotropic Effects of Acetylsalicylic Acid after Coronary Artery Bypass Grafting—Beyond Platelet Inhibition

Dominika Siwik [1,†], Magdalena Gajewska [1,†], Katarzyna Karoń [1], Kinga Pluta [1], Mateusz Wondołkowski [2], Radosław Wilimski [2], Łukasz Szarpak [3,4], Krzysztof J. Filipiak [1] and Aleksandra Gąsecka [1,*]

1. 1st Chair and Department of Cardiology, Medical University of Warsaw, Banacha 1a, 02-097 Warsaw, Poland; dominika.siwik@gmail.com (D.S.); gmgajewska@gmail.com (M.G.); katarzkar@gmail.com (K.K.); plutakinga.01@gmail.com (K.P.); krzysztof.filipiak@wum.edu.pl (K.J.F.)
2. Department of Cardiac Surgery, Medical University of Warsaw, 02-097 Warsaw, Poland; mateusz.wondolkowski@gmail.com (M.W.); rwilimski@gmail.com (R.W.)
3. Bialystok Oncology Center, 15-027 Bialystok, Poland; lukasz.szarpak@gmail.com
4. Maria Sklodowska-Curie Medical Academy in Warsaw, 00-001 Warsaw, Poland
* Correspondence: aleksandra.gasecka@wum.edu.pl
† D.S. and M.G. contributed equally to the manuscript and share the first authorship.

Abstract: Acetylsalicylic acid (ASA) is one of the most frequently used medications worldwide. Yet, the main indications for ASA are the atherosclerosis-based cardiovascular diseases, including coronary artery disease (CAD). Despite the increasing number of percutaneous procedures to treat CAD, coronary artery bypass grafting (CABG) remains the treatment of choice in patients with multivessel CAD and intermediate or high anatomical lesion complexity. Taking into account that CABG is a potent activator of inflammation, ASA is an important part in the postoperative therapy, not only due to ASA antiplatelet action, but also as an anti-inflammatory agent. Additional benefits of ASA after CABG include anticancerogenic, hypotensive, antiproliferative, anti-osteoporotic, and neuroprotective effects, which are especially important in patients after CABG, prone to hypertension, graft occlusion, atherosclerosis progression, and cognitive impairment. Here, we discuss the pleiotropic effects of ASA after CABG and provide insights into the mechanisms underlying the benefits of treatment with ASA, beyond platelet inhibition. Since some of ASA pleiotropic effects seem to increase the risk of bleeding, it could be considered a starting point to investigate whether the increase of the intensity of the treatment with ASA after CABG is beneficial for the CABG group of patients.

Keywords: acetylsalicylic acid; ASA; CABG; coronary artery bypass grafting; Alzheimer's disease; hypertension; osteoporosis; cancer; inflammation; atherosclerosis

Citation: Siwik, D.; Gajewska, M.; Karoń, K.; Pluta, K.; Wondołkowski, M.; Wilimski, R.; Szarpak, Ł.; Filipiak, K.J.; Gąsecka, A. Pleiotropic Effects of Acetylsalicylic Acid after Coronary Artery Bypass Grafting—Beyond Platelet Inhibition. *J. Clin. Med.* 2021, 10, 2317. https://doi.org/10.3390/jcm10112317

Academic Editor: Michał Ciurzyński

Received: 23 April 2021
Accepted: 22 May 2021
Published: 26 May 2021

Publisher's Note: MDPI stays neutral with regard to jurisdictional claims in published maps and institutional affiliations.

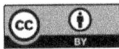

Copyright: © 2021 by the authors. Licensee MDPI, Basel, Switzerland. This article is an open access article distributed under the terms and conditions of the Creative Commons Attribution (CC BY) license (https://creativecommons.org/licenses/by/4.0/).

1. Introduction

Acetylsalicylic acid (ASA), commonly known as aspirin, is one of the most renowned drugs of all times. It was firstly introduced into clinical practice in 1899. Its centuries-long fame remains vivid thanks to its antipyretic, analgesic, and anti-inflammatory effects. Yet, the ubiquitous ASA is generally indicated in the secondary prevention of major cardiovascular and neurovascular events. However, more and more studies indicate the pleiotropy of this well-known anti-inflammatory agent.

ASA in a standard dose of 75–160 mg once daily is commonly used for secondary prevention of thromboembolic events after coronary artery bypass grafting (CABG) [1]. CABG is the treatment of choice in patients with stable multivessel coronary artery disease (CAD) or left main CAD with intermediate or high anatomical complexity of CAD [2]. During CABG, an artery or vein from the patient's body is used to create a bypass for the coronary artery around the significant atherosclerotic lesions. The goal of CABG is to provide adequate blood flow to the ischemic myocardium and thus restore its viability and function [3].

Patients after CABG procedure may benefit from ASA not only due to its antiplatelet activity, but also due to other features, including anti-inflammatory, anticancerogenic, hypotensive, antithrombotic, anti-osteoporotic, and neuroprotective effects.

Taking into account that CABG is a potent activator of inflammation, ASA is an important part in postoperative therapy not only as an antiplatelet action, but also as an anti-inflammatory agent [4,5]. Furthermore, since CAD and some types of cancer have common risk factors—including diabetes, obesity, and smoking—the use of ASA as a complementary therapy in cancer patients might limit the side effects from chemotherapeutics [6–8]. Moreover, ASA seems to have a hypotensive effect, especially when administered in the evening with statins, which indicates the benefits of the combined therapy after CABG. ASA therapy also prevents excessive and dysfunctional vascular smooth muscle cell proliferation (VSMCs), thereby decreasing the risk of late graft failure and further atherosclerosis progression [9]. Furthermore, ASA may increase bone marrow density (BMD) and reduce the potential fracture risk after CABG, thus facilitating rehabilitation. Finally, the neuroprotective features of ASA might be especially beneficial in elderly patients after CABG, who are susceptible to cognitive impairment and dementia [10].

CABG can be performed with (on-pump) or without cardiopulmonary bypass application (off-pump). On- and off-pump CABG have a different effect on inflammatory response and platelet homeostasis [11,12]. Off-pump CABG affects platelet function less than the on-pump CABG and is associated with higher rate of high on-ASA platelet reactivity after the operation [13].

Though well-recognized for its beneficial effects, ASA is also associated with several serious complications, with increased risk of bleeding being the most important one. In 2018 Tsoi et al. compared clinical outcomes of 204,170 ASA users and 408,339 non-users and observed significantly higher incidence of gastrointestinal bleeding in long-term aspirin users (4.64% vs. 2.74%) [14]. A meta-analysis of 35 randomized controlled trials showed a 55% increased risk for a major gastrointestinal bleeding due to ASA administration in daily doses of 75 to 325 mg [15]. The risk of bleeding associated with ASA has been established to be dose-related and further elevated by combining it with other antiplatelet agents or gastrotoxic drugs such as corticosteroids [16].

ASA has been examined several times as a potential drug for primary prevention of cardiovascular diseases and most of the studies concluded that ASA offered little to no benefit for primary prevention, while it increased the risk of major bleeding [17]. Recently, a randomized controlled trial of healthy participants aged ≥70, who were randomly assigned to receive 100 mg of ASA or placebo, confirmed no significant difference in the risk of cardiovascular disease, but markedly higher risk of major hemorrhage was significantly higher in the ASA group, than in placebo group (8.6 events per 1000 vs. 6.2 events per 1000 person-years, respectively) [18].

The threat of bleeding is the most important concern when it comes to the use of ASA in cardiac surgery. Several randomized controlled trials conducted in the 1980s and 1990s showed a rise in transfusion, re-exploration, and chest tube drainage in patients treated with preoperative ASA [19–22]. However, the results of more recent studies do not entirely confirm the previous findings. A 2015 study examined the effect of preoperative ASA administration in patients undergoing CABG, valve or combined CABG/valve surgery [23]. Preoperative ASA was associated with an increased incidence of red blood cell transfusion. On the contrary, a 2005 retrospective cohort study showed lower postoperative mortality rate among patients who received preoperative aspirin without significant increases in hemorrhage and transfusion [24].

In this review, we report data on the studies regarding off-pump CABG procedures [13]. We discuss the plethora of the underestimated applications of ASA, which might underlie its possible additional benefits in patients after CABG, who are a unique group of multimorbid patients. The accompanying diseases in this patient group include arterial hypertension (84%), hypercholesterolemia (47%), type 2 diabetes mellitus (32%), lower limb atherosclerosis (28%), chronic kidney disease (9%), and chronic obstructive pulmonary disease (9%) [13]. In addition, these elderly patients are more prone to post-operative wound healing disturbances and bleeding complications, and are at high risk of age-associated disease including osteoporosis, cancer, and cognitive impairment [25,26]. Based on ASA pleiotropic effects, we suggest that it could be considered to study the intensification of the postoperative treatment with ASA after CABG, by increasing either the frequency of ASA administration (e.g., 75–81 mg twice daily) or by increasing a single dose (e.g., 150–162 mg once daily).

The possible targets for ASA pleiotropic effects in patients after CABG are shown in Figure 1. The summary of ASA pleiotropic effects discussed in this review are summarized in Figure 2.

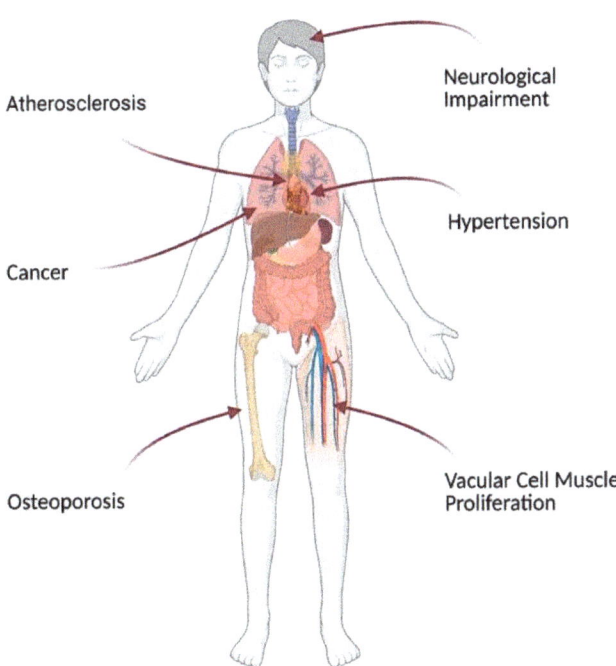

Figure 1. Possible targets for pleiotropic effects of acetylsalicylic acid in patients after coronary artery bypass grafting Figure created with BioRender.com.

2. Mechanism of Action

ASA belongs to the non-salicylate nonsteroidal anti-inflammatory drugs (NSAIDs), which mechanism of action is based on cyclooxygenase (COX) inhibition. COX plays the main role in the conversion of arachidonic acid, which is released from membrane phospholipids, into prostaglandin H2 (PGH2) [27]. PGH2 has two active sites: one for peroxidase and one for COX. The latter is the binding site for ASA and NSAIDs. Eventually, COX by binding to the COX site of PGH2 leads to transformation into various prostaglandins (PGI2, PGE2, PGF2, PGD2) and thromboxane A2. By inhibiting COX, ASA reduces the inflammatory response and inhibits platelet function. The antiplatelet effect of ASA, in turn, results from inhibition of TXA2 production, which is formed in platelets from arachidonate by the aspirin-dependent COX pathway [28]. Since platelets are anucleated bone marrow fragments, unable to produce the COX-1 protein, the effect of ASA lasts for the lifetime of a platelet, around 10 days [29]. At least two different isoenzymes are the targets of ASA: COX-1 and COX-2. COX-1 is constitutively expressed on most cells, especially platelets and gastric mucosal cells. By stimulating prostaglandin production, COX-1 takes maintains homeostasis, for example activates platelets when required and protects the gastric mucosa.

Conversely, COX-2 is periodically produced by the inflammatory cells in response to cytokine and growth factor stimulation. ASA irreversibly blocks both COX isoenzymes, but it has a stronger effect on COX-1, in comparison to COX-2. The dose-dependence of the ASA effect is crucial to understand its mode of action. Low doses of ASA (75–81 mg per day) inhibit COX-1, providing an antithrombotic effect. Intermediate doses (650 mg to 4 g per day) target both COX-1 and COX-2, exerting analgesic and antipyretic effects by impeding prostaglandin production. Finally, high doses (4–8 g per day) have anti-inflammatory effects [27].

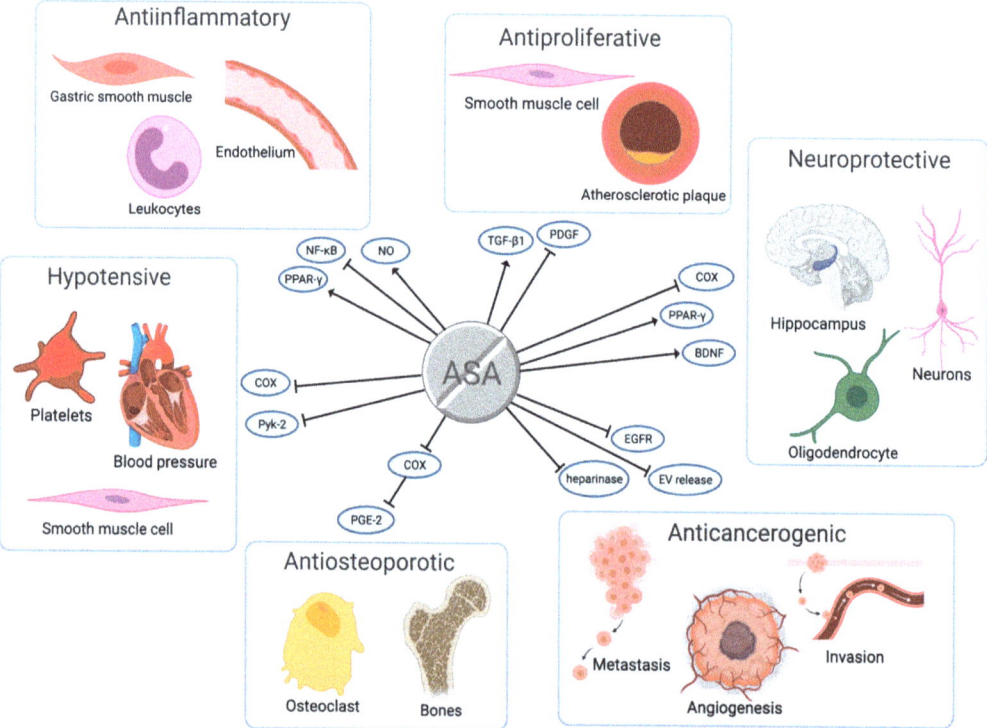

Figure 2. Pleiotropic effects of acetylsalicylic acid (ASA) discussed in this review. For details regarding the mechanisms, please see the main text. BDNF—brain-derived neurotrophic factor; COX—cyclooxygenase; EGFR—epidermal growth factor receptor; EV—extracellular vesicles; NF-κB—nuclear factor kappa-light-chain-enhancer of activated B cells; NO—nitric oxide; PDGF—platelet-derived growth factor; PGE-2—prostaglandin E-2; PPARγ—peroxisome proliferator-activated receptor gamma; Pyk-2—proline-rich tyrosine kinase 2; TGF-β1- transforming growth factor β1. Figure created with BioRender.com.

3. Anti-Inflammatory Effect

ASA activity is primarily associated with dose-dependent COX-1 and COX-2 inhibition. The most common ones are (i) inhibition of nuclear factor kappa-light-chain-enhancer of activated B cells (NF-κB) pathway; (ii) endothelial nitric oxide (NO) release; and (iii) acting as a peroxisome proliferator-activated receptor gamma (PPARγ) agonist (Figure 2). Since these pathways were mostly investigated in vitro and in animal models and not always associated with myocardial ischemia, the results should be interpreted with caution, as they may not be directly applicable to patients undergoing CABG.

ASA improved alveolar bone defects healing in rats by impeding lipopolysaccharides (LPS)-induced macrophages via the inhibition of NF-κB pathway [30]. Moreover, ASA treatment improved the inflammatory response in cerebral infarction in mice thanks to downregulation of both TLR4 (toll-like receptor 4) and NF-κB expression, which led to endoplasmic reticulum (ER) stress inhibition [31]. Another promising target point for ASA is preeclampsia, which is known to depend on oxidative stress and inflammation via activation of NF-kB. By decreasing the translocation of NF-kB, low doses of ASA are used in preeclampsia prevention and treatment [32,33]. Also, ASA inhibits the growth and the metastasis of osteosarcoma through the NF-κB pathway [34].

Another alternative anti-inflammatory pathway of ASA is stimulation of direct endothelial NO release, independent of COX suppression, but presumably associated with endothelial nitric oxide synthase activation [35]. The NO-dependent effects of ASA include vasoprotection, gastric smooth muscle relaxation, and improvement of endothelial function, and they are directly associated with the reduction of cardiovascular risk. Moreover, ASA by indirectly activating alternate compensatory pathway including mainly heme oxygenase-1 and NO reduces the frequency of gastric injury. This gastric pathway works protectively, in contrast to the well-known ASA-dependent increased risk of disturbing gastrointestinal mucosal integrity [35,36].

The third possible pathway responsible for the anti-inflammatory effects of ASA is acting as a PPARγ agonist with subsequent downregulation of the WNT/β-catenin pathway. Upregulated WNT/β-catenin pathway participates in tumor growth, whereas PPARγ reduces inflammation, oxidative stress, cell proliferation, and invasion. NSAIDs such as ASA seem to work opposite on the two above mentioned pathways: downregulating WNT/β-catenin pathway and being a PPARγ agonist.

CABG is considered to be a trigger for the 'cytokine storm' phenomenon, which manifests in the increased concentrations of cytokines (e.g., interleukin 6 (IL-6), IL-8, tumor necrosis factor alpha) [37]. Taking into account that CABG is a potent activator of inflammation, ASA could be an important part in the postoperative therapy as an anti-inflammatory agent [4,5]. However, to achieve the ASA anti-inflammatory effect, it would be necessary to substantially increase the daily dose to at least 4 g per day.

4. Anticancerogenic Effect

There is increasing data demonstrating the role of ASA both in prevention and treatment in many cancer types. Cancer cells not only upregulate platelet production, but also generate extracellular vesicles (EVs) which stimulate platelet and leukocyte activation, leading to phosphatidylserine and tissue factor exposure on platelets and leukocytes and overall prothrombotic state in cancer patients [38].

The mechanisms of anticarcinogenic activity of ASA include: (i) inhibition of EV release; (ii) inhibition of the enzymatic activity of heparinase; and (iii) inhibition of epidermal growth factor receptor (EGFR) expression (Figure 2).

EVs are nanosized particles which are key players in intercellular communications [39] and have gathered a lot of attention as potential biomarkers of cancer development and progression [40,41]. For example, increased concentration of cancer-derived EVs was found in patients with many cancer types, including breast cancer [42], prostate cancer [43], or lung cancer [44]. Concurrently, ASA administration decreases both plasma concentrations of EVs and their procoagulant properties [45], suggesting that modulation of EV concentration and composition might be one of the mechanisms underlying ASA pleiotropic effects [46].

Heparanase is an extracellular matrix enzyme responsible for polymeric heparan sulphate degradation at the cell surface and in the extracellular matrix, which may be another key point for ASA application. By changing the constitution of extracellular matrix, heparanase promotes (i) cancer metastasis by assisting cancer cell migration and invasion and (ii) angiogenesis by releasing heparin-binding cytokines including hepatocyte growth factor (HGF), vascular endothelial growth factor (VEGF), and basic fibroblast growth factor (bFGF). By inhibiting heparanase activity, ASA was found to delay cancer progress (metastasis, angiogenesis) both in vitro and in vivo [47].

EGFR is a receptor commonly linked to epithelial malignancies [48]. It is upregulated in tumor microenvironment, resulting in tumor growth, invasion and metastasis [48]. ASA inhibits EGFR signaling, therefore exerting anticancerogenic effect in various cancer types. For example, ASA was shown to normalize EGFR expression and inhibit EGFR signaling both in human colorectal cancer (CRC) cells and ovarian cancer cells in vitro [32]. Consequently, ASA has gained a lot of attention as probably the most promising chemopreventive medication of CRC. Consequently, the United States Preventive Services Task Force recommended the use of low-dose ASA for the prevention of CRC in patients with specific cardiovascular profiles (aged 50–69 years with a 10% or greater 10-year cardiovascular risk, who are not at increased risk for bleeding, have a life expectancy of at least 10 years and are willing to take ASA for at least 10 years) [49]. Hence, ASA has become a part of the CRC prevention strategy [8].

In addition, ASA was shown to have a synergic effect with temozolomide, bevacizumab, and sunitinib in the glioblastoma therapy. The combined therapy of ASA and chemotherapeutics could improve the glioblastoma treatment efficacy [50]. Finally, a meta-analysis of four cohort studies and seven case-control studies including 653,828 participants with 12,637 incident cases showed that the increased dose of ASA (per two prescriptions per week increment) was related to a 5% relative risk reduction of head and neck cancers, compared to no prior use.

Since CAD and cancer are two prominent causes of death worldwide, the coexistence of both diseases is frequent. The prevalence of CAD in patients with different cancer types ranges from 43% in patients with lung cancer to 17% in patients with breast cancer [51]. Moreover, from the clinical experience the number of elderly patients undergoing CABG increases. Since age is a risk factor of cancer development, the above-mentioned group suffers often from both CAD and cancer simultaneously. Hence, a therapy which targets both disorders simultaneously seems promising. Taking into account that CAD and some cancer types have common risk factors including diabetes, obesity and smoking, the use of ASA as a complementary therapy in cancer patients might both prevent and/or delay cancer development, and limit the side effects of chemotherapeutics [6–8]. Thus, some experts have suggested to incorporate ASA in primary cancer prevention due to the reduction of cancer incidence and mortality after 3–5 years treatment with ASA [52].

5. Hypotensive Effect

ASA hypotensive effect has been the subject of many studies, and the majority of studies agreed on three outcomes: (i) low-dose ASA treatment is associated with a stronger decrease in blood pressure, compared to high-dose; (ii) evening ASA administration decreases blood pressure more effective than morning administration; and (iii) combination of ASA and statin reduces cardiovascular risk (Figure 2).

First, low-dose ASA treatment is associated with stronger decrease in blood pressure, in comparison to high-dose [53]. The underlying mechanism is based on the inhibition of COX-2 by high-dose ASA, but not by low-dose ASA. High-dose ASA leads to reduction of renal blood flow, glomerular filtration rate, sodium, and water excretion [53], which are the reasons for against using high doses of ASA in clinical practice. Another mechanism which seems to play a role in ASA hypotensive effect is a COX-independent pathway which revolves around proline-rich tyrosine kinase 2 (Pyk2). Pyk2 is a key player in RhoA/Rho activation, which is necessary for the vascular smooth muscle constriction. RhoA/rho is dysregulated in hypertension. Through the inhibition of the Pyk2-associated pathway in vascular smooth muscle cells, ASA and other salicylates may lower the blood pressure. This phenomenon is unique for ASA doses of higher concentrations than those required to inhibit COX [53].

Second, low doses of ASA may increase the efficacy of both antiplatelet and antihypertensive therapy, if administered in the evening. ASA administration in the evening increases its antiplatelet effect due to the release of young platelets from the bone marrow in the morning. The mechanism of ASA hypotensive effect, in turn, is possibly related to the increase in the nocturnal angiotensin II-dependent NO production [54]. Moreover, a greater decrease in blood pressure was noted in non-dipper patients who became dippers while taking ASA in the evening. The observed hypotensive effect in non-dippers is of great importance, because non-dippers are at higher risk of cardiovascular events.

Third, the combined therapy of ASA and statins is beneficial for cardiovascular risk reduction. The addition of ASA to statin therapy resulted in the decrease of SBP and DBP, in comparison to the control group treated with placebo [55,56]. Furthermore, the flow-mediated vasodilatation of brachial artery increased with aspirin-statin therapy, compared to placebo. However, it is inconclusive whether this effect was truly a result of the combined aspirin-statin therapy, or just the well-established impact of statins on endothelial functions [55].

About 24% of patients after CABG admitted for in-hospital cardiac rehabilitation presented with maximum systolic pressure of 200 mmHg and diastolic of 110 mmHg, caused most often by stress and withdrawal of antihypertensive medications used preoperatively [57]. The majority of patients have arterial hypertension prior to CABG, as it is a well-established risk factor for CAD development [58]. The most presumed mechanism underlying the development of CAD in hypertensive patients is the increase in pulsatile aortic wall stress, which enhances degradation of elastin, leading to arterial stiffness [59]. Arterial stiffness is strongly associated with vascular calcification, which is a major pathology underlying CAD development [60]. The synergy of action between ASA and statins demonstrates the complementary benefits of the combined therapy after CABG.

Altogether, ASA seems to have a hypotensive effect, especially when administered with statins. However, since the majority of previous studies were conducted in healthy volunteers or mildly hypertensive patients who were not treated with anti-hypertensive drugs before, there are yet no firm conclusions on the hypotensive effect of ASA and more studies are needed to clarify it [54].

6. Antiproliferative Effect

It has been established that ASA exerts antiproliferative effect on VSMCs in patients after CABG [61]. So far, several mechanisms underlying this specific effect of ASA have been discovered. They are mainly related to (i) transforming growth factor β1 (TGF-β1) and (ii) platelet-derived growth factor (PDGF) (Figure 2).

Primarily, ASA increases the secretion of TGF-β1. TGF-β1 directly inhibits VSMCs proliferation by inducing G0/G1 phase cell cycle arrest [62]. Additionally, TGF-β1 reduces the production of matrix metalloelastase (MMP-12) in macrophages [63]. MMP-12 is one of metalloproteinases—enzymes associated with instability and rupture of atherosclerotic plaque. By increasing TGF-β1 secretion, ASA therapy might promote atherosclerotic plaque stability.

Second, ASA suppresses PDGF release from thrombocytes [64]. PDGF is one of the most important growth factors for VSMCs. Its excessive expression contributes to the development of atherosclerosis or organ fibrosis, but also to the late graft occlusion and late restenosis in patients after CABG [65,66].

One in vitro study evaluated the effect of ASA on PDGF-treated VSMCs and on retinoblastoma protein hyperphosphorylation, which is known to regulate cell cycle progression. This study found that ASA arrests the cell cycle also at the G1/S phase. Therefore, the high-dose of ASA treatment may be beneficial in treatment of vascular proliferative disorders [67].

The main factors which determine graft failure after CABG include endothelial damage, thrombosis and VSMCs proliferation. VSMC proliferation is associated with atherosclerotic plaque formation and neointimal hyperplasia, which lead to graft stenosis and finally to (mainly late) graft occlusion [9]. ASA therapy seems to prevent excessive and dysfunctional VSMC proliferation, therefore decreasing the risk of late graft failure and further suppressing atherosclerosis progression [9].

7. Influence on Bone Mineral Density

Osteoporosis is a metabolic bone disease that mainly affects elderly, postmenopausal women. It is associated with low bone mineral density (BMD) which can be measured by dual-energy X-ray absorptiometry scan. Osteoporosis leads to pathologic fractures of the hip, spine, and wrist and is a significant cause of disability and mortality among elderly patients. Osteoporosis develops due to the imbalance between bone formation and resorption, with the latter being predominant. It has been established that ASA affects bone remodeling. PGE2 stimulates the proliferation of osteoclast precursors and their differentiation and transformation to mature osteoclasts [68]. Furthermore, PGE2 stimulates bone resorption and may contribute to increased bone loss [69]. By inhibiting COX-2 activity, ASA reduces PGE2 production. Furthermore, ASA promotes the survival of bone marrow mesenchymal stem cells [70], the progenitors of osteoblasts. In this manner, ASA supports bone formation and decreases bone resorption.

Prolonged ASA intake was associated with higher total hip and lumbar BMD in women [71–73] and men [71,72,74] and with lower fracture risk in observational studies [72]. For example, ASA users between the age of 70–79 were found to have higher BMD, compared with non-users [71]. In a multicenter study which included 7786 women aged ≥65 years, the hip and lumbar BMD was higher in patients who used ASA for more than a year, compared to non-users [73]. However, more studies should be conducted to confirm these findings, as the heretofore conducted studies had methodological differences including different study groups, different ASA dosages, and questionable patient compliance [75].

Patients undergoing CABG are more likely to develop osteoporosis due to several risk factors, such as elderly age or immobilization after surgery. A study comprising 26 patients revealed considerable, progressive bone mineral density decrease during the first year after CABG [76]. Despite the small sample size, this study implies that patients undergoing CABG may be at higher risk of osteoporosis. Fragility and osteoporotic fractures significantly worsen the quality of life, diminish physical activity and may disturb rehabilitation after CABG. Hence, ASA therapy, even in low doses (<150 mg) may bring additional benefits of BMD increase and reduced fracture risk.

8. Neuroprotective Effect

Thanks to its potential neuroprotective effect, ASA found its place in the neuropsychiatric field in the treatment of Alzheimer's disease, schizophrenia, bipolar disease, and depression. The precise mechanism underlying ASA neuroprotective effect has not been well established yet. However, studies show few promising possibilities related to (i) PPARα, (ii) brain-derived neurotrophic factor (BDNF), (iii) COX-1 and COX-2, and (iv) glutamate excitotoxicity (Figure 2).

ASA binding to PPARα was found to up-regulate the hippocampal plasticity [77]. Moreover, ASA was found to enhance expression of BDNF messenger RNA in the neurons of the hippocampus in mice. BDNF is a neurotrophin promoting cell survival and synaptic plasticity which plays a key role in pathogenesis of different neurodegenerative diseases, such as Alzheimer's disease [78]. Accordingly, low-dose ASA was observed to improve spatial learning and memory in animal model of Alzheimer's disease [77].

Another pathway underlying ASA neuroprotective function may involve COX-2 modification and COX-1 irreversible inhibition, which leads to suppression of inflammatory reaction [79]. As schizophrenia has an inflammatory background, ASA is recommended also in the treatment of the first episode of schizophrenia [80]. However, in schizophrenia, high doses of ASA are needed because of difficulties to cross the blood brain barrier [79].

ASA anti-inflammatory activity appears to improve symptoms of mood disorders, such as depression or bipolar relapse [81]. Another animal study demonstrated ASA positive impact on oligodendrocyte precursor cell (OPCs) proliferation and differentiation after white matter lesion, using low and high doses of ASA, respectively [82]. It was shown that low doses of ASA (25 mg/kg) increase the amount of OPCs, while relatively high doses of ASA (100–200 mg/kg) elevate the number of oligodendrocytes and improve myelin thickness after white matter lesions [82]. Thus, both doses seemed to have neuroprotective effects.

A case report described a woman with electroencephalogram abnormalities in the left temporal-occipital area reversed and symptoms relieved after low-dose ASA therapy alone. A potential mechanism underlying the neuroprotective abilities of ASA seems to be related to its activity against glutamate excitotoxicity. However, this hypothesis is based on case reports and more research should be carried out to prove a direct link between ASA and neurotransmitter dysfunction [83].

CABG is a procedure performed in the elderly patients who are known to be at higher risk of atherosclerotic vascular changes. Moreover, atherosclerosis is an established risk factor of Alzheimer's disease. In addition, especially elderly patients who underwent CABG are susceptible to cognitive impairment and dementia [10]. Therefore, the neuroprotective features of ASA related to BDNF, PPARα, and glutamate excitotoxicity may complement the standard therapy for patients suffering from both cognitive impairment/dementia and atherosclerosis. Altogether, the framework of ASA as a neuroprotective agent is broad, but furthermore, more specific research is essential to draw firm conclusions.

9. COVID-19 and ASA

In the times of global pandemic, the application of various drugs in the treatment and prophylaxis of COVID-19 and the following complications is an important research topic. Accumulating data prove the relationship between COVID-19 and thrombosis [84]. The clinical and autopsy studies indicate that the risks of microvascular thrombosis, venous thromboembolism, and ischemic stroke are higher in COVID-19 patients [85,86]. Also, it was found that platelets have high affinity receptors for SARS-CoV-2, suggesting that platelets may participate in the development of COVID-19 [85]. Thus, the application of antiplatelet drugs in the prophylaxis and treatment of COVID-19 and related complications might be a viable treatment strategy. Currently, the clinical data regarding the efficacy of ASA to improve outcomes in COVID-19 patients remains ambiguous. CAD patients treated with ASA (75–150 mg per day) prior to COVID-19-related hospitalization have comparable in-hospital mortality as patients not receiving ASA (21.2% vs. 22.1%) [87]. On the other hand, when comparing in-hospital ASA intake to no antiplatelet therapy, a decrease in the rate of in-hospital death in the ASA group was found [88]. In addition, ASA in-hospital administration was associated with lower need of mechanical ventilation, in comparison to the non-ASA group [89]. Altogether, more studies are needed to obtain reliable conclusions regarding the effect of ASA use in the prophylaxis and treatment of COVID-19 and related complications.

10. Conclusions and Future Directions

In spite of ASA's long medical history, novel possible applications for ASA therapy still arise. Recent data demonstrates a variety of new targets for ASA beyond platelet inhibition, including cancer, hypertension, vascular cell muscle proliferation, osteoporosis, and neurological impairment. Many of these disorders have a higher prevalence in patients undergoing CABG, demonstrating the potential benefits of ASA beyond platelet inhibition. The pathophysiological mechanisms underlying these disorders after CABG include peripheral and central atherosclerosis, thrombosis, hypertension, and risk of fractures. They are often based on chronic inflammatory state associated with such pathways as WNT/β-catenin, NF-κB, PPARα, PPARγ, and different growth factors (e.g., BDNF, TGF-β1) which are affected by ASA. Some of the proposed mechanisms remain innovative and not evident yet, as they were observed in vitro and in animal models only. Many of the above-described mechanisms were not confirmed in the CABG patients and thus, they should be interpreted with caution. The risks of adverse effects of ASA (e.g., bleeding) should be taken into account, especially when the higher dose therapy of ASA is considered.

Considering ASA pleiotropic effect, a hypothesis arises that the intensification of ASA therapy might improve outcomes after CABG. The American Heart Association guidelines recommend the use of 81–325 mg ASA daily to reduce the risk of graft occlusion and adverse cardiac events [1]. One meta-analysis implied that the intermediate ASA dose (300–325 mg) may decrease the rate of reduce graft occlusion, compared to the low dose (75–160 mg) regimes within the first year after CABG [90]. There is a need for further clinical studies to establish whether the intermediate dose is superior to low dose in patients after CABG, taking into account both the graft patency and other beneficial effects; including hypotensive or neuroprotective effects, as well as adverse effects such as the risk of bleeding, gastric complaints, and reduction of glomerular filtration rate.

It is important to mention another antiplatelet drug with pleiotropic effects—ticagrelor, which could be combined with ASA to maximize the treatment benefits [91]. In the Dual Ticagrelor Plus Aspirin Antiplatelet Strategy After Coronary Artery Bypass Grafting (DACAB) study, 500 patients were randomized to receive ticagrelor (90 mg twice daily) + ASA (100 mg once daily), ticagrelor (90 mg twice daily), or ASA (100 mg once daily) within 24 h post-CABG. Although the combination of ticagrelor and ASA was superior to aspirin alone in maintaining the saphenous vein graft patency for up to 1 year after elective CABG, there were no differences between ticagrelor and ASA. Although the rate of cardiovascular events and bleeding events was low, the combination of ticagrelor and ASA numerically decreased the risk of the major cardiovascular events after CABG (cardiovascular death, myocardial infarction, stroke), but also increased the risk of bleeding (CABG-related, non-CABG-related, and major bleeding events) [92], compared to ASA. The main results of DACAB study are presented in Figure 3. Altogether, the combinations of ticagrelor and ASA might improve graft patency after CABG, but further studies are needed to assess the bleeding risk.

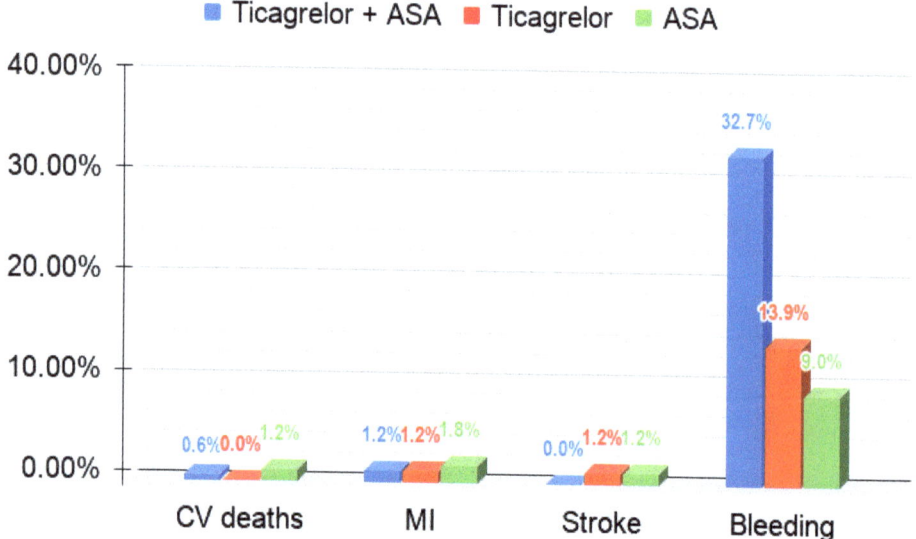

Figure 3. Postoperative complications after CABG with different treatment regimens. CV deaths—cardiovascular deaths; MI—myocardial infarction.

In another population—patients undergoing transcatheter aortic valve implantation (TAVI), those treated with ASA monotherapy for 3 months after TAVI has lower incidence of a composite end-point of bleeding and thrombotic events at 1 year, compared to ASA and clopidogrel [93]. Hence, ASA monotherapy seems to be associated with decreased bleeding risk, compared to dual antiplatelet therapy. It could be hypothesized that increasing the ASA dose might also be associated with reduced rate major cardiovascular events. However, in absence if evidence-based data, this hypothesis remains a speculation.

Until now, only a few studies have compared the bleeding risk with different ASA doses. For example, a review of 39 studies conducted in the field of gastroenterology proved that the risk for upper gastrointestinal bleeding was comparable, regardless of the ASA dose and treatment duration [94]. Hence, it is crucial to investigate whether higher doses of ASA indeed significantly increase the bleeding risk, and if so, whether it is higher than the bleeding risk during dual antiplatelet therapy.

Altogether, individualization of the postoperative dose of ASA after CABG based on the patients' individual risk of graft occlusion and bleeding is worth consideration. At least in some patients, the possible benefits of ASA pleiotropism might outweigh the risk of bleeding. However, these groups of patients still remain to be identified. Moreover, although the results of pre-clinical studies are very promising, the evidence-based data from randomized controlled trials are lacking. Further research is required to confirm the pleiotropic effects of ASA in the clinical setting.

Author Contributions: Conceptualization, D.S., M.G., A.G. and K.K.; Methodology, D.S., M.G., A.G. and K.K.; Literature investigation D.S., M.G., A.G., K.K., K.P., M.W. and Ł.S.; Resources, D.S., M.G., A.G., R.W., K.J.F. and Ł.S.; Writing—original draft preparation, D.S. and M.G.; Writing—review and editing, D.S., M.G., K.K., A.G., M.W., R.W., K.J.F., K.P., Ł.S.; Visualization, all authors; supervision, A.G., R.W., K.J.F.; Funding acquisition, A.G. and K.J.F. All authors have read and agreed to the published version of the manuscript.

Funding: This research received no external funding.

Conflicts of Interest: The authors declare no conflict of interest.

References

1. Ruel, M.; Kulik, A. Secondary prevention after coronary artery bypass graft surgery: Presentation of a scientific statement. *Can. J. Cardiol.* **2014**, *30*, S237. [CrossRef]
2. Developed with the special contribution of the European Association for Percutaneous Cardiovascular Interventions (EAPCI); Wijns, W.; Kolh, P.; Danchin, N.; Di Mario, C.; Falk, V.; Folliguet, T.; Garg, S.; Huber, K.; James, S.; et al. Guidelines on myocardial revascularization: The Task Force on Myocardial Revascularization of the European Society of Cardiology (ESC) and the European Association for Cardio-Thoracic Surgery (EACTS). *Eur. Heart J.* **2010**, *31*, 2501–2555.
3. Bachar, B.J.; Manna, B. Coronary Artery Bypass Graft. In *StatPearls*; StatPearls Publishing: Treasure Island, FL, USA, 2021.
4. Pamukcu, B.; Lip, G.Y.; Shantsila, E. The nuclear factor—Kappa B pathway in atherosclerosis: A potential therapeutic target for atherothrombotic vascular disease. *Thromb. Res.* **2011**, *128*, 117–123. [CrossRef] [PubMed]
5. Boucher, P.; Matz, R.L.; Terrand, J. Atherosclerosis: Gone with the Wnt? *Atherosclerosis* **2020**, *301*, 15–22. [CrossRef] [PubMed]
6. Pinto, C.A.; Marcella, S.; August, D.A.; Holland, B.; Kostis, J.B.; Demissie, K. Cardiopulmonary bypass has a modest association with cancer progression: A retrospective cohort study. *BMC Cancer* **2013**, *13*, 519. [CrossRef] [PubMed]
7. Malakar, A.K.; Choudhury, D.; Halder, B.; Paul, P.; Uddin, A.; Chakraborty, S. A review on coronary artery disease, its risk factors, and therapeutics. *J. Cell. Physiol.* **2019**, *234*, 16812–16823. [CrossRef] [PubMed]
8. Thrumurthy, S.G.; Thrumurthy, S.S.D.; Gilbert, C.E.; Ross, P.; Haji, A. Colorectal adenocarcinoma: Risks, prevention and diagnosis. *BMJ* **2016**, *354*, i3590. [CrossRef] [PubMed]
9. Gaudino, M.; Antoniades, C.; Benedetto, U.; Deb, S.; Di Franco, A.; Di Giammarco, G.; Fremes, S.; Glineur, D.; Grau, J.; He, G.-W.; et al. Mechanisms, Consequences, and Prevention of Coronary Graft Failure. *Circulation* **2017**, *136*, 1749–1764. [CrossRef]
10. Royter, V.; MBornstein, N.; Russell, D. Coronary artery bypass grafting (CABG) and cognitive decline: A review. *J. Neurol. Sci.* **2005**, *229–230*, 65–67. [CrossRef]
11. Jongman, R.M.; Zijlstra, J.G.; Kok, W.F.; van Harten, A.E.; Mariani, M.A.; Moser, J.; Struys, M.M.R.F.; Absalom, A.; Molema, G.; Scheeren, T.; et al. Off-Pump CABG Surgery Reduces Systemic Inflammation Compared with On-Pump Surgery but Does Not Change Systemic Endothelial Responses. *Shock* **2014**, *42*, 121–128. [CrossRef]
12. Rimmelé, T.; Venkataraman, R.; Madden, N.J.; Elder, M.M.; Wei, L.M.; Pellegrini, R.V.; Kellum, J.A. Comparison of inflammatory response during on-pump and off-pump coro-nary artery bypass surgery. *Int. J. Artif. Organ.* **2010**, *33*, 131–138. [CrossRef]
13. Wilimski, R.; Huczek, Z.; Kondracka, A.; Zborowska, H.; Wondołkowski, M.; Wancerz, A.; Puchta, D.; Ciechowska, W.; Hendzel, P.; Cichoń, R. Reaktywność płytek krwi we wczesnym okresie po pomostowaniu tętnic wieńcowych bez użycia krążenia pozaustrojowego u pacjentów stosujących małą dawkę kwasu acetylosalicylowego. *Folia Cardiol.* **2018**, *13*, 407–415. [CrossRef]
14. Tsoi, K.K.F.; Chan, F.C.H.; Hirai, H.W.; Sung, J.J.Y. Risk of gastrointestinal bleeding and benefit from colorectal cancer reduction from long-term use of low-dose aspirin: A retrospective study of 612 509 patients. *J. Gastroenterol. Hepatol.* **2018**, *33*, 1728–1736. [CrossRef]

15. Lanas, A.; Wu, P.; Medin, J.; Mills, E.J. Low Doses of Acetylsalicylic Acid Increase Risk of Gastrointestinal Bleeding in a Meta-Analysis. *Clin. Gastroenterol. Hepatol.* **2011**, *9*, 762–768. [CrossRef] [PubMed]
16. García Rodríguez, L.A.; Lin, K.J.; Hernández-Díaz, S.; Johansson, S. Risk of upper gastrointestinal bleeding with low-dose acetylsal-icylic acid alone and in combination with clopidogrel and other medications. *Circulation* **2011**, *123*, 1108–1115. [CrossRef]
17. Truong, C. Update on acetylsalicylic acid for primary prevention of cardiovascular disease: Not initiating is not the same thing as discontinuing. *Can. Fam. Physician* **2019**, *65*, 481–482. [PubMed]
18. McNeil, J.J.; Wolfe, R.; Woods, R.L.; Tonkin, A.M.; Donnan, G.A.; Nelson, M.R.; Reid, C.M.; Lockery, J.E.; Kirpach, B.; Storey, E.; et al. Effect of Aspirin on Cardiovascular Events and Bleeding in the Healthy Elderly. *N. Engl. J. Med.* **2018**, *379*, 1509–1518. [CrossRef]
19. Goldman, S.; Copeland, J.; Moritz, T.; Henderson, W.; Zadina, K.; Ovitt, T.; Kern, K.B.; Sethi, G.; Sharma, G.V.; Khuri, S. Starting aspirin therapy after operation. Effects on early graft patency. Department of Veterans Affairs Cooperative Study Group. *Circulation* **1991**, *84*, 520–526. [CrossRef] [PubMed]
20. Sethi, G.K.; Copeland, J.G.; Goldman, S.; Moritz, T.; Zadina, K.; Henderson, W.G. Implications of preoperative administration of aspi-rin in patients undergoing coronary artery bypass grafting. Department of Veterans Affairs Cooperative Study on Antiplatelet Therapy. *J. Am. Coll. Cardiol.* **1990**, *15*, 15–20. [CrossRef]
21. Ferraris, V.A.; Ferraris, S.P.; Lough, F.C.; Berry, W.R. Preoperative Aspirin Ingestion Increases Operative Blood Loss after Coronary Artery Bypass Grafting. *Ann. Thorac. Surg.* **1988**, *45*, 71–74. [CrossRef]
22. Kallis, P.; Tooze, J.A.; Talbot, S.; Cowans, D.; Bevan, D.H.; Treasure, T. Pre-operative aspirin decreases platelet aggregation and in-creases post-operative blood loss—A prospective, randomised, placebo controlled, double-blind clinical trial in 100 patients with chronic stable angina. *Eur. J. Cardiothorac. Surg.* **1994**, *8*, 404–409. [CrossRef]
23. Goldhammer, J.E.; Marhefka, G.D.; Daskalakis, C.; Berguson, M.W.; Bowen, J.E.; Diehl, J.T.; Sun, J. The Effect of Aspirin on Bleeding and Transfusion in Contemporary Cardiac Surgery. *PLoS ONE* **2015**, *10*, e0134670. [CrossRef]
24. Bybee, K.A.; Powell, B.D.; Valeti, U.; Rosales, A.G.; Kopecky, S.L.; Mullany, C.; Wright, R.S. Preoperative Aspirin Therapy Is Associated with Improved Postoperative Outcomes in Patients Undergoing Coronary Artery Bypass Grafting. *Circulation* **2005**, *112* (Suppl. 9), I-286–I-292.
25. Varma, P.K.; Kundan, S.; Ananthanarayanan, C.; Panicker, V.T.; Pillai, V.V.; Sarma, P.S.; Karunakaran, J. Demographic profile, clinical characteristics and outcomes of patients undergoing coronary artery bypass grafting—Retrospective analysis of 4024 patients. *Indian J. Thorac. Cardiovasc. Surg.* **2014**, *30*, 272–277. [CrossRef]
26. Olufajo, O.A.; Wilson, A.; Zeineddin, A.; Williams, M.; Aziz, S. Coronary Artery Bypass Grafting Among Older Adults: Patterns, Outcomes, and Trends. *J. Surg. Res.* **2021**, *258*, 345–351. [CrossRef] [PubMed]
27. Abramson, S.B.; Howard, R. Aspirin: Mechanism of Action, Major Toxicities, and Use in Rheumatic Diseases. UptoDate, Waltham (MA). Published Online 2012. Available online: https://www.uptodate.com/contents/aspirin-mechanism-of-action-major-toxicities-and-use-in-rheumatic-diseases (accessed on 30 January 2012).
28. Abrams, C.S. Platelet Biology. UptoDate. Published 2017. Available online: https://www.uptodate.com/contents/platelet-biology (accessed on 22 November 2020).
29. Altman, R.; Luciardi, H.L.; Muntaner, J.; Herrera, R.N. The antithrombotic profile of aspirin. Aspirin resistance, or simply failure? *Thromb. J.* **2004**, *2*, 1. [CrossRef] [PubMed]
30. Liu, Y.; Fang, S.; Li, X.; Feng, J.; Du, J.; Guo, L.; Su, Y.; Zhou, J.; Ding, G.; Bai, Y.; et al. Aspirin inhibits LPS-induced macrophage activation via the NF-κB pathway. *Sci. Rep.* **2017**, *7*, 11549. [CrossRef]
31. Wang, X.; Shen, B.; Sun, D.; Cui, X. Aspirin ameliorates cerebral infarction through regulation of TLR4/NF-κB-mediated endo-plasmic reticulum stress in mouse model. *Mol. Med. Rep.* **2018**, *17*, 479–487.
32. Vaughan, J.E.; Walsh, S.W. Activation of NF-κB in placentas of women with preeclampsia. *Hypertens. Pregnancy* **2012**, *31*, 243–251. [CrossRef]
33. Gil-Villa, A.M.; Alvarez, A.M.; Velásquez-Berrío, M.; Rojas-López, M.; Cadavid, J.A.P. Role of aspirin-triggered lipoxin A4, aspirin, and salicylic acid in the modulation of the oxidative and inflammatory responses induced by plasma from women with pre-eclampsia. *Am. J. Reprod. Immunol.* **2020**, *83*, e13207. [CrossRef]
34. Liao, D.; Zhong, L.; Duan, T.; Zhang, R.H.; Wang, X. Aspirin Suppresses the Growth and Metastasis of Osteosarcoma through the NF-κB Pathway. *Clin. Cancer Res.* **2015**. Available online: https://clincancerres.aacrjournals.org/content/21/23/5349.short (accessed on 14 February 2021). [CrossRef]
35. Taubert, D.; Berkels, R.; Grosser, N.; Schröder, H.; Gründemann, D.; Schömig, E. Aspirin induces nitric oxide release from vascular endothelium: A novel mechanism of action. *Br. J. Pharmacol.* **2004**, *143*, 159–165. [CrossRef] [PubMed]
36. Schröder, H. Nitric oxide and aspirin: A new mediator for an old drug. *Am. J. Ther.* **2009**, *16*, 17–23. [CrossRef] [PubMed]
37. Strüber, M.; Cremer, J.T.; Gohrbandt, B.; Hagl, C.; Jankowski, M.; Völker, B.; Rückoldt, H.; Martin, M.; Haverich, A. Human cytokine responses to coronary artery bypass grafting with and without cardiopulmonary bypass. *Ann. Thorac. Surg.* **1999**, *68*, 1330–1335. [CrossRef]
38. Plantureux, L.; Mège, D.; Crescence, L.; Dignat-George, F.; Dubois, C.; Panicot-Dubois, L. Impacts of Cancer on Platelet Production, Activation and Education and Mechanisms of Cancer-Associated Thrombosis. *Cancers* **2018**, *10*, 441. [CrossRef] [PubMed]
39. Gasecka, A.; Nieuwland, R.; Siljander, P.R.-M. Platelet-Derived Extracellular Vesicles. *Platelets* **2019**, *2019*, 401–416. [CrossRef]

40. Scholl, J.N.; Dias, C.K.; Muller, L.; Battastini, A.M.O.; Figueiró, F. Extracellular vesicles in cancer progression: Are they part of the problem or part of the solution? *Nanomedicine* **2020**, *15*, 2625–2641. [CrossRef]
41. Hu, T.; Wolfram, J.; Srivastava, S. Extracellular Vesicles in Cancer Detection: Hopes and Hypes. *Trends Cancer* **2021**, *7*, 122–133. [CrossRef] [PubMed]
42. Green, T.M.; Alpaugh, M.L.; Barsky, S.H.; Rappa, G.; Lorico, A. Breast Cancer-Derived Extracellular Vesicles: Characterization and Contribution to the Metastatic Phenotype. *BioMed Res. Int.* **2015**, *2015*, 634865. [CrossRef]
43. Park, Y.H.; Shin, H.W.; Jung, A.R.; Kwon, O.S.; Choi, Y.-J.; Park, J.; Lee, J.Y. Author Correction: Prostate-specific extracellular vesicles as a novel biomarker in human prostate cancer. *Sci. Rep.* **2019**, *9*, 6051. [CrossRef] [PubMed]
44. Choi, B.H.; Quan, Y.H.; Rho, J.; Hong, S.; Park, Y.; Choi, Y.; Park, J.-H.; Yong, H.S.; Han, K.N.; Choi, Y.H.; et al. Levels of Extracellular Vesicles in Pulmonary and Peripheral Blood Correlate with Stages of Lung Cancer Patients. *World J. Surg.* **2020**, *44*, 3522–3529. [CrossRef]
45. Goetzl, E.J.; Goetzl, L.; Karliner, J.S.; Tang, N.; Pulliam, L. Human plasma platelet-derived exosomes: Effects of aspirin. *FASEB J.* **2016**, *30*, 2058–2063. [CrossRef] [PubMed]
46. Connor, D.E.; Ly, K.; Aslam, A.; Boland, J.; Low, J.; Jarvis, S.; Muller, D.W.; Joseph, J.E. Effects of antiplatelet therapy on platelet extracellular vesicle release and procoagulant activity in health and in cardiovascular disease. *Platelets* **2016**, *27*, 805–811. [CrossRef] [PubMed]
47. Dai, X.; Yan, J.; Fu, X.; Pan, Q.; Sun, D.; Xu, Y.; Wang, J.; Nie, L.; Tong, L.; Shen, A.; et al. Aspirin Inhibits Cancer Metastasis and Angiogenesis via Targeting Heparanase. *Clin. Cancer Res.* **2017**, *23*, 6267–6278. [CrossRef]
48. Sasaki, T.; Hiroki, K.; Yamashita, Y. The Role of Epidermal Growth Factor Receptor in Cancer Metastasis and Microenviroment. *BioMed Res. Int.* **2013**, *2013*, 546318. [CrossRef] [PubMed]
49. Drew, D.A.; Cao, Y.; Chan, A.T. Aspirin and colorectal cancer: The promise of precision chemoprevention. *Nat. Rev. Cancer* **2016**, *16*, 173–186. [CrossRef] [PubMed]
50. Navone, S.E.; Guarnaccia, L.; Cordiglieri, C.; Crisà, F.M.; Caroli, M.; Locatelli, M.; Schisano, L.; Rampini, P.; Miozzo, M.; Verde, N.; et al. Aspirin Affects Tumor Angiogenesis and Sensitizes Human Glioblastoma Endo-thelial Cells to Temozolomide, Bevacizumab, and Sunitinib, Impairing Vascular Endothelial Growth Factor-Related Signaling. *World Neurosurg.* **2018**, *120*, e380–e391. [CrossRef] [PubMed]
51. Al-Kindi, S.G.; Oliveira, G.H. Prevalence of Preexisting Cardiovascular Disease in Patients with Different Types of Cancer: The Unmet Need for Onco-Cardiology. *Mayo Clin. Proc.* **2016**, *91*, 81–83. [CrossRef] [PubMed]
52. Brotons, C.; Benamouzig, R.; Filipiak, K.J.; Limmroth, V.; Borghi, C. A Systematic Review of Aspirin in Primary Prevention: Is It Time for a New Approach? *Am. J. Cardiovasc. Drugs* **2015**, *15*, 113–133. [CrossRef]
53. Costa, A.C.; Reina-Couto, M.; Albino-Teixeira, A.; Sousa, T. Aspirin and blood pressure: Effects when used alone or in combination with antihypertensive drugs. *Rev. Port. Cardiol. (Engl. Ed.)* **2017**, *36*, 551–567. [CrossRef]
54. Ruíz-Arzalluz, M.V.; Fernández, M.C.G.; Burgos-Alonso, N.; Vinyoles, E.; Blanco, R.S.V.; Grandes, G. Protocol for assessing the hypotensive effect of evening admin-istration of acetylsalicylic acid: Study protocol for a randomized, cross-over controlled trial. *Trials* **2013**, *14*, 236. [CrossRef] [PubMed]
55. Magen, E.; Viskoper, J.R.; Mishal, J.; Priluk, R.; London, D.; Yosefy, C. Effects of low-dose aspirin on blood pressure and endothelial function of treated hypertensive hypercholesterolaemic subjects. *J. Hum. Hypertens.* **2005**, *19*, 667–673. [CrossRef] [PubMed]
56. Lafeber, M.; Spiering, W.; van der Graaf, Y.; Nathoe, H.; Bots, M.L.; Grobbee, D.E.; Visseren, F.L. The combined use of aspirin, a statin, and blood pressure–lowering agents (polypill components) and the risk of vascular morbidity and mortality in patients with coronary artery disease. *Am. Hear. J.* **2013**, *166*, 282–289. [CrossRef] [PubMed]
57. Burazor, I.; Lazovic, M.; Sprioski, D.; Andjic, M.; Moraca, M. PP.01.04: High blood pressure after coronary artery bypass surgery in patients referred to in-house cardiac rehabilitation. Single center experience. *J. Hypertens.* **2015**, *33*, e130. [CrossRef]
58. Weber, T.; Lang, I.; Zweiker, R.; Zweiker, R.; Horn, S.; Wenzel, R.R.; Watschinger, B.; Slany, J.; Eber, B.; Roithinger, F.X.; et al. Hypertension and coronary artery disease: Epidemiology, physiology, effects of treatment, and recommendations: A joint scientific statement from the Austrian Society of Cardiology and the Austrian Society of Hy-pertension. *Wiener Klinische Wochenschrift* **2016**, *128*, 467–479. [CrossRef] [PubMed]
59. Mitchell, G.F. Arterial stiffness and hypertension: Chicken or egg? *Hypertension* **2014**, *64*, 210–214. [CrossRef] [PubMed]
60. Cecelja, M.; Chowienczyk, P. Role of arterial stiffness in cardiovascular disease. *JRSM Cardiovasc. Dis.* **2012**, *1*, 1–10. [CrossRef]
61. Redondo, S.; Ruiz, E.; Gordillo-Moscoso, A.; Navarro-Dorado, J.; Ramajo, M.; Carnero, M.; Reguillo, F.; Rodriguez, E.; Tejerina, T. Role of TGF-β1 and MAP Kinases in the Antiproliferative Effect of Aspirin in Human Vascular Smooth Muscle Cells. *PLoS ONE* **2010**, *5*, e9800. [CrossRef]
62. Redondo, S.; Santos-Gallego, C.G.; Ganado, P.; García, M.; Rico, L.; Del Rio, M.; Tejerina, T. Acetylsalicylic Acid Inhibits Cell Proliferation by Involving Transforming Growth Factor-β. *Circulation* **2003**, *107*, 626–629. [CrossRef]
63. Feinberg, M.W.; Jain, M.K.; Werner, F.; Sibinga, N.E.S. Transforming growth factor-β1 inhibits cytokine-mediated induction of hu-man metalloelastase in macrophages. *J. Biol.* **2000**, *275*, 25766–25773.
64. Vissinger, H.; Husted, S.E.; Kristensen, S.D.; Nielsen, H.K. Platelet-Derived Growth Factor Release and Antiplatelet Treatment with Low-Dose Acetylsalicylic Acid. *Angiology* **1993**, *44*, 633–638. [CrossRef]
65. Jawien, A.; Bowen-Pope, D.F.; Lindner, V.; Schwartz, S.M.; Clowes, A.W. Platelet-derived growth factor promotes smooth muscle migration and intimal thickening in a rat model of balloon angioplasty. *J. Clin. Investig.* **1992**, *89*, 507–511. [CrossRef] [PubMed]

66. Kappert, K.; Paulsson, J.; Sparwel, J.; Leppänen, O.; Hellberg, C.; Östman, A.; Micke, P. Dynamic changes in the expression of DEP-1 and other PDGF receptor-antagonizing PTPs during onset and termination of neointima formation. *FASEB J.* **2006**, *21*, 523–534. [CrossRef] [PubMed]
67. Marra Diego, E.; Simoncini, T.; Liao, J.K. Inhibition of Vascular Smooth Muscle Cell Proliferation by Sodium Salicy-late Mediated by Upregulation of p21Waf1 and p27Kip1. *Circulation* **2000**, *102*, 2124–2130. [CrossRef]
68. Blackwell, K.A.; Raisz, L.G.; Pilbeam, C.C. Prostaglandins in bone: Bad cop, good cop? *Trends Endocrinol. Metab.* **2010**, *21*, 294–301. [CrossRef] [PubMed]
69. Raisz, L.G. Potential impact of selective cyclooxygenase-2 inhibitors on bone metabolism in health and disease. *Am. J. Med.* **2001**, *110*, 43–45. [CrossRef]
70. Yamaza, T.; Miura, Y.; Bi, Y.; Liu, Y.; Akiyama, K.; Sonoyama, W.; Patel, V.; Gutkind, S.; Young, M.; Gronthos, S.; et al. Pharmacologic Stem Cell Based Intervention as a New Approach to Osteoporosis Treatment in Rodents. *PLoS ONE* **2008**, *3*, e2615. [CrossRef] [PubMed]
71. Carbone, L.D.; Tylavsky, F.A.; Cauley, J.A.; Harris, T.B.; Lang, T.F.; Bauer, U.C.; Barrow, K.D.; Kritchevsky, S.B. Association Between Bone Mineral Density and the Use of Nonsteroidal Anti-Inflammatory Drugs and Aspirin: Impact of Cyclooxygenase Selectivity. *J. Bone Miner. Res.* **2003**, *18*, 1795–1802. [CrossRef] [PubMed]
72. Barker, A.L.; Soh, S.-E.; Sanders, K.M.; Pasco, J.; Khosla, S.; Ebeling, P.R.; Ward, S.A.; Peeters, G.; Talevski, J.; Cumming, R.G.; et al. Aspirin and fracture risk: A systematic review and exploratory meta-analysis of obser-vational studies. *BMJ Open* **2020**, *10*, e026876. [CrossRef]
73. Bauer, D.C.; Orwoll, E.S.; Fox, K.M.; Vogt, T.M.; Lane, N.E.; Hochberg, M.C.; Stone, K.; Nevitt, M.C. Aspirin and NSAID use in older women: Effect on bone mineral density and fracture risk. *J. Bone Miner. Res.* **2009**, *11*, 29–35. [CrossRef]
74. Bleicher, K.; Cumming, R.G.; Naganathan, V.; Seibel, M.J.; Sambrook, P.N.; Blyth, F.M.; Le Couteur, D.G.; Handelsman, D.J.; Creasey, H.M.; Waite, L.M. Lifestyle factors, medications, and disease influence bone mineral density in older men: Findings from the CHAMP study. *Osteoporos. Int.* **2010**, *22*, 2421–2437. [CrossRef]
75. Vestergaard, P.; Steinberg, T.H.; Schwarz, P.; Jørgensen, N.R. Use of the oral platelet inhibitors dipyridamole and acetylsalicylic acid is associated with increased risk of fracture. *Int. J. Cardiol.* **2012**, *160*, 36–40. [CrossRef] [PubMed]
76. Miller, L.E.; Pierson, L.M.; Pierson, M.E.; Kiebzak, G.M.; Ramp, W.K.; Herbert, W.G.; Cook, J.W. Changes in Bone Mineral and Body Composition Following Coronary Artery Bypass Grafting in Men. *Am. J. Cardiol.* **2007**, *99*, 585–587. [CrossRef] [PubMed]
77. Patel, D.; Roy, A.; Kundu, M.; Jana, M.; Luan, C.-H.; Gonzalez, F.J.; Pahan, K. Aspirin binds to PPARα to stimulate hippocampal plasticity and protect memory. *Proc. Natl. Acad. Sci. USA* **2018**, *115*, E7408–E7417. [CrossRef]
78. Gasecka, A.; Siwik, D.; Gajewska, M.; Jaguszewski, M.J.; Mazurek, T.; Filipiak, K.J.; Postuła, M.; Eyileten, C. Early Biomarkers of Neurodegenerative and Neurovascular Disorders in Diabetes. *J. Clin. Med.* **2020**, *9*, 2807. [CrossRef]
79. Çakici, N.; Van Beveren, N.J.M.; Judge-Hundal, G.; Koola, M.M.; Sommer, I.E.C. An update on the efficacy of anti-inflammatory agents for patients with schizophrenia: A meta-analysis. *Psychol. Med.* **2019**, *49*, 2307–2319. [CrossRef] [PubMed]
80. Müller, N. Inflammation in Schizophrenia: Pathogenetic Aspects and Therapeutic Considerations. *Schizophr. Bull.* **2018**, *44*, 973–982. [CrossRef] [PubMed]
81. Ng, Q.X.; Ramamoorthy, K.; Loke, W.; Lee, M.W.L.; Yeo, W.S.; Lim, D.Y.; Sivalingam, V. Clinical Role of Aspirin in Mood Disorders: A Systematic Review. *Brain Sci.* **2019**, *9*, 296. [CrossRef] [PubMed]
82. Chen, J.; Zuo, S.; Wang, J.; Huang, J.; Zhang, X.; Liu, Y.; Zhang, Y.; Zhao, J.; Han, J.; Xiong, L.; et al. Aspirin promotes oligodendrocyte precursor cell proliferation and differentiation after white matter lesion. *Front. Aging Neurosci.* **2014**, *6*, 7. [CrossRef] [PubMed]
83. Persegani, C.; Russo, P.; Lugaresi, E.; Nicolini, M.; Torlini, M. Neuroprotective effects of low-doses of aspirin. *Hum. Psychopharmacol.* **2001**, *16*, 193–194. [CrossRef]
84. Gąsecka, A.; Borovac, J.A.; Guerreiro, R.A.; Giustozzi, M.; Parker, W.; Caldeira, D.; Chiva-Blanch, G. Thrombotic Complications in Patients with COVID-19: Pathophysiological Mech-anisms, Diagnosis, and Treatment. *Cardiovasc. Drugs Ther.* **2021**, *35*, 215–229. [CrossRef] [PubMed]
85. Sahai, A.; Bhandari, R.; Koupenova, M.; Freedman, J.; Godwin, M.; McIntyre, T.; Chung, M.; Iskandar, J.; Kamran, H.; Aggarwal, A.; et al. SARS-CoV-2 Receptors are Expressed on Human Platelets and the Effect of Aspirin on Clinical Outcomes in COVID-19 Patients. *Res. Sq.* **2020**. [CrossRef]
86. Gąsecka, A.; Filipiak, K.J.; Jaguszewski, M.J. Impaired microcirculation function in COVID-19 and implications for potential ther-apies. *Cardiol. J.* **2020**, *27*, 485–488. [PubMed]
87. Yuan, S.; Chen, P.; Li, H.; Chen, C.; Wang, F.; Wang, D.W. Mortality and pre-hospitalization use of low-dose aspirin in COVID-19 patients with coronary artery disease. *J. Cell Mol. Med.* **2021**, *25*, 1263–1273. [CrossRef]
88. Meizlish, M.L.; Goshua, G.; Liu, Y.; Fine, R.; Amin, K.; Chang, E.; DeFilippo, N.; Keating, C.; Liu, Y.; Mankbadi, M.; et al. Intermediate-dose anticoagulation, aspirin, and in-hospital mortality in COVID-19: A propensity score-matched analysis. *medRxiv* **2021**, *96*, 471–479. [CrossRef]
89. Chow, J.H.; Khanna, A.K.; Kethireddy, S.; Yamane, D.; Levine, A.; Jackson, A.M.; McCurdy, M.T.; Tabatabai, A.; Kumar, G.; Park, P.; et al. Aspirin Use is Associated with Decreased Mechanical Ventilation, Intensive Care Unit Admission, and In-Hospital Mortality in Hospitalized Patients with Coronavirus Disease 2019. *Anesthesia Analg.* **2021**, *132*, 930–941. [CrossRef]

90. Lim, E.; Ali, Z.; Ali, A.; Routledge, T.; Edmonds, L.; Altman, D.G.; Large, S. Indirect comparison meta-analysis of aspirin therapy after coronary surgery. *BMJ* **2003**, *327*, 1309. [CrossRef]
91. Gasecka, A.; Nieuwland, R.; Budnik, M.; Dignat-George, F.; Eyileten, C.; Harrison, P.; Lacroix, R.; Leroyer, A.; Opolski, G.; Pluta, K.; et al. Ticagrelor attenuates the increase of extracellular vesicle concentrations in plasma after acute myocardial infarction compared to clopidogrel. *J. Thromb. Haemost.* **2020**, *18*, 609–623. [CrossRef] [PubMed]
92. Zhu, Y.; Xue, Q.; Zhang, M.; Hu, J.; Liu, H.; Wang, R.; Wang, X.; Han, L.; Zhao, Q. Effect of ticagrelor with or without aspirin on vein graft outcome 1 year after on-pump and off-pump coronary artery bypass grafting. *J. Thorac. Dis.* **2020**, *12*, 4915–4923. [CrossRef]
93. Brouwer, J.; Nijenhuis, V.J.; Delewi, R.; Hermanides, R.S.; Holvoet, W.; Dubois, C.L.; Frambach, P.; De Bruyne, B.; Van Houwelingen, G.K.; Van Der Heyden, J.A.; et al. Aspirin with or without Clopidogrel after Transcatheter Aortic-Valve Implantation. *N. Engl. J. Med.* **2020**, *383*, 1447–1457. [CrossRef]
94. García Rodríguez, L.A.; Martín-Pérez, M.; Hennekens, C.H.; Rothwell, P.M.; Lanas, A. Bleeding Risk with Long-Term Low-Dose Aspirin: A Systematic Review of Observational Studies. *PLoS ONE* **2016**, *11*, e0160046. [CrossRef] [PubMed]

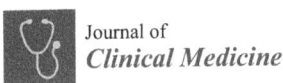

Systematic Review

Fractional Flow Reserve versus Angiography–Guided Management of Coronary Artery Disease: A Meta–Analysis of Contemporary Randomised Controlled Trials

Annette M. Maznyczka [1], Connor J. Matthews [1], Jonathan M. Blaxill [1,2], John P. Greenwood [1,2], Abdul M. Mozid [1,2], Jennifer A. Rossington [1,2], Murugapathy Veerasamy [1,2], Stephen B. Wheatcroft [1,2], Nick Curzen [3,4] and Heerajnarain Bulluck [1,2,*]

1. Yorkshire Heart Centre, Leeds General Infirmary, Leeds Teaching Hospitals NHS Trust, Leeds LS1 3EX, UK
2. Leeds Institute of Cardiovascular and Metabolic Medicine, University of Leeds, Leeds LS1 3EX, UK
3. Faculty of Medicine, University of Southampton, Southampton SO17 1BJ, UK
4. Coronary Research Group, University Hospital Southampton NHS Trust, Southampton SO17 1BJ, UK
* Correspondence: h.bulluck@leeds.ac.uk

Abstract: Background and Aims: Randomised controlled trials (RCTs) comparing outcomes after fractional flow reserve (FFR)-guided versus angiography-guided management for obstructive coronary artery disease (CAD) have produced conflicting results. We investigated the efficacy and safety of an FFR-guided versus angiography-guided management strategy among patients with obstructive CAD. Methods: A systematic electronic search of the major databases was performed from inception to September 2022. We included studies of patients presenting with angina or myocardial infarction (MI), managed with medications, percutaneous coronary intervention, or bypass graft surgery. A meta-analysis was performed by pooling the risk ratio (RR) using a random-effects model. The endpoints of interest were all-cause mortality, MI and unplanned revascularisation. Results: Eight RCTs, with outcome data from 5077 patients, were included. The weighted mean follow up was 22 months. When FFR-guided management was compared to angiography-guided management, there was no difference in all-cause mortality [3.5% vs. 3.7%, RR: 0.99 (95% confidence interval (CI) 0.62–1.60), p = 0.98, heterogeneity (I^2) 43%], MI [5.3% vs. 5.9%, RR: 0.93 (95%CI 0.66–1.32), p = 0.69, I^2 42%], or unplanned revascularisation [7.4% vs. 7.9%, RR: 0.92 (95%CI 0.76–1.11), p = 0.37, I^2 0%]. However, the number patients undergoing planned revascularisation by either stent or surgery was significantly lower with an FFR-guided strategy [weighted mean difference: 14 (95% CI 3 to 25)%, p =< 0.001]. Conclusion: In patients with obstructive CAD, an FFR-guided management strategy did not impact on all-cause mortality, MI and unplanned revascularisation, when compared to an angiography-guided management strategy, but led to up to a quarter less patients needing revascularisation.

Keywords: fractional flow reserve; angiography; coronary artery disease; percutaneous coronary intervention; coronary artery bypass graft surgery

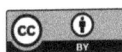

1. Introduction

Current guidelines recommend fractional flow reserve (FFR) to guide revascularisation for intermediate stenoses with no prior evidence of myocardial ischaemia on non-invasive testing and in the setting of multivessel coronary disease [1]. These recommendations are predominantly based on the FAME (Fractional Flow Reserve Versus Angiography for Multivessel Evaluation) trial, which demonstrated lower rates of major adverse cardiac events (MACE), predominantly driven by repeat revascularisation, in patients with multivessel disease who had FFR-guided revascularisation, compared to angiography-guidance [2].

Subsequent randomised controlled trials (RCTs), performed in a variety of clinical settings, comparing outcomes after FFR-guided versus angiography-guided revascularisation have produced conflicting results, but have, in general, failed to demonstrate the expected additional benefit from using FFR in addition to angiography to guide diagnosis, management and revascularization [2–8]. Most recently, the FRAME-AMI trial (FFR- vs. Angiography-guided PCI in AMI with multivessel disease) found lower MACE with FFR-guided complete revascularisation, compared to angiography-guided, among 562 patients with ST-segment elevation myocardial infarction (STEMI) who had been committed to complete revascularisation of non-culprit coronary disease [3]. Furthermore, RIPCORD-2 (Does Routine Pressure Wire Assessment Influence Management Strategy at Coronary Angiography for Diagnosis of Chest Pain?) randomised 1100 patients undergoing diagnostic angiography for stable angina or non-ST elevation MI (NSTEMI) to either angiographic diagnosis and management alone, of angiography plus FFR assessment of all major coronary arteries. It found no difference in MACE, cost, or quality of life between the groups [4].

Given the discrepant outcome data, the aim of this study was to perform a contemporary meta-analysis of RCTs (including patients with stable angina or AMI, managed with medications, percutaneous coronary intervention (PCI) or coronary artery bypass grafts surgery (CABG), to compare clinical outcomes after an FFR-guided versus an angiography-guided management strategy in patients with obstructive CAD.

2. Methods

This study was performed following the PRISMA (Preferred Reporting Items for systematic Reviews and Meta-Analyses) guidelines [9]. The protocol for this study was registered with the International Prospective Register of Systematic Reviews (PROSPERO ID: CRD42022356766).

2.1. Search Strategy

A systematic search of the online databases Medline and Embase via Ovid was performed, from inception to September 2022. Peer-reviewed RCTs were selected using combinations of the following keywords: 'fractional flow reserve'; 'pressure wire'; 'FFR'; 'coronary angiogram'; and 'coronary angiography'. The electronic database search was supplemented by using the clinical trial registry 'ClinicalTrials.gov', to identify other relevant studies. The reference lists of included trials were also reviewed, for other appropriate trials. For completeness, we searched conference abstracts from recent major cardiology meetings, specifically the European Society of Cardiology, EuroPCR, Transcatheter Cardiovascular Therapeutics, the American College of Cardiology and the American Heart Association. Two investigators (C.J.M and A.M) independently screened abstracts against eligibility criteria. In case of discrepancies among the two independent investigators, a third independent investigator (H.B) was available to review the data, to resolve discrepancies by consensus among the investigators.

2.2. Eligibility Criteria

We included all RCTs comparing an FFR-guided versus an angiography-guided management strategy in patients with obstructive CAD, and reporting outcomes on death, MI and unplanned revascularisation. For studies with multiple publications, we used data from the longest reported follow-up. We included RCTs in which patients presented with either stable coronary artery disease, or acute coronary syndrome (ACS), including RCTs assessing non-infarct related artery stenoses following revascularisation of the culprit vessel in STEMI. RCTs of patients undergoing revascularisation with either coronary artery bypass graft surgery or percutaneous coronary intervention were included. Non-randomised trials, publications not in English, and those not reporting clinical outcomes of interest were excluded. We also excluded studies that used an FFR cut-off other than ≤0.8 to define significant ischaemia, because 0.8 is the FFR threshold accepted by international clinical guidelines for defining haemodynamically significant lesions [1].

2.3. Data Extraction

Baseline demographic and clinical outcome data were extracted from the main study reports. Supplementary material was also reviewed. Clinical outcome data were extracted on an intension-to-treat basis. For RCTs including an all-comer population undergoing angiography, we only included outcomes on the subsets with obstructive CAD.

2.4. Quality Assessment

We assessed the risk of bias and the quality of included studies, according to the Cochrane risk of bias assessment tool [10] (Figure 1).

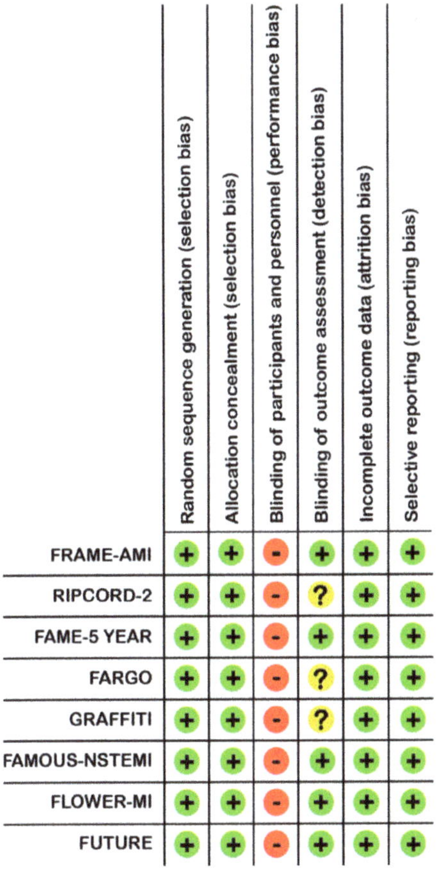

	Random sequence generation (selection bias)	Allocation concealment (selection bias)	Blinding of participants and personnel (performance bias)	Blinding of outcome assessment (detection bias)	Incomplete outcome data (attrition bias)	Selective reporting (reporting bias)
FRAME-AMI	+	+	−	+	+	+
RIPCORD-2	+	+	−	?	+	+
FAME-5 YEAR	+	+	−	+	+	+
FARGO	+	+	−	?	+	+
GRAFFITI	+	+	−	?	+	+
FAMOUS-NSTEMI	+	+	−	+	+	+
FLOWER-MI	+	+	−	+	+	+
FUTURE	+	+	−	+	+	+

Figure 1. Risk of bias summary for the individual studies, by Cochrane risk assessment tool. + = low risk of bias, − − = risk of bias, ? = unclear.

2.5. Outcomes

The main endpoints of interest were all-cause mortality, MI and unplanned revascularisation. We also investigated the number of stents implanted and number of patients proceeding to revascularisation in each group. We originally planned to stratify the results according to patients presenting with stable CAD or ACS, but outcome data for these individual endpoints were not available from the trial-level data. However, we were able to provide the pooled, trial-defined major composite endpoint analysis, stratified by stable CAD or ACS if available, from the selected RCTs.

2.6. Statistical Analysis

Weighted mean follow-up duration was calculated according to study size. We summarised the estimate of effect incorporating the clinical outcome as the risk ratio (RR) with 95% confidence intervals (CI). The pooled RR was calculated with a random-effects model, due to anticipated heterogeneity between included RCTs, using the Mantel-Haenszel method. We performed heterogeneity testing with Higgins I^2, with a threshold of >50% suggestive of significant heterogeneity [11]. The statistical analyses were performed using Review Manager (RevMan) [Computer program]. Version 5.4, The Cochrane Collaboration, 2020.

3. Results

Figure 2 shows the process of trial selection. Eight RCTs met the eligibility criteria [2–8,12], including a total of 5077 patients, with 1 of those [3] only recently presented in detail at the recent ESC 2022 conference and not yet published in full text. Among these, 2544 patients were in the FFR-guided group and 2533 were in angiography-guided group. Out of the included RCTs, five had follow-up of 1 year [4,6–8,12], one had follow up of 6 months [5], and two RCTs had longer follow-up of 3.5 [3] and 5 years [2]. The weighted mean follow-up was 22 months. Overall, the loss to follow-up of patients in this study was <1%.

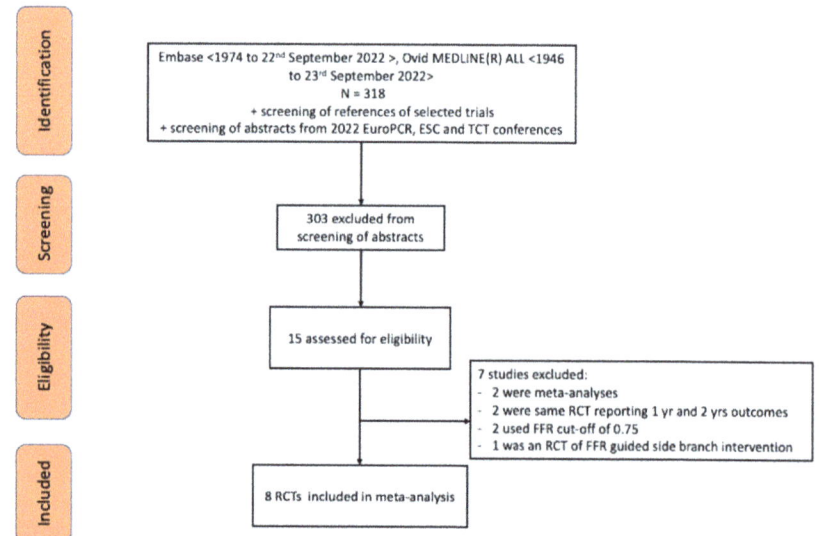

Figure 2. PRISMA diagram of the trial selection process.

3.1. Characteristics of Included RCTs

There was heterogeneity of clinical presentations included in the trials, endpoint definitions and treatment with CABG or PCI (Tables 1 and 2). The trial-defined composite endpoint was not uniform in the RCTs, as highlighted in bold in Table 1. Revascularisation was exclusively with CABG in two RCTs (FARGO [Fractional Flow Reserve Versus Angiography Randomization for Graft Optimization] and GRAFFITI [Graft Patency After FFR-Guided Versus Angio-Guided CABG]) [5,6]. By contrast, revascularisation was exclusively with PCI in three RCTs (FRAME-AMI, FAME, FLOWER-MI [Flow Evaluation to Guide Revascularisation in Multivessel ST-elevation Myocardial Infarction]) [2,3,7]. Revascularisation was predominantly with PCI in the remaining three included trials (RIPCORD-2, FAMOUS-NSTEMI [Fractional Flow Reserve Versus Angiographically Guided Management to Optimise Outcomes in Unstable Coronary Syndromes], FUTURE [Functional Testing Underlying Coronary Revascularisation]) [4,8,12]. In general, there was low risk of bias across the included RCTs (Figure 1).

Table 1. Characteristics of RCTs, comparing FFR with angiography, for guiding revascularisation.

Study	Year Published	Enrolment Centres	Participants and Presentation	Primary Endpoint	Follow-Up (Years)	Loss to Follow-Up, n (%)	Findings
FRAME-AMI [3] (NCT02715518)	2022	14 sites in Korea	562 patients (STEMI/NSTEMI)	MACE defined as the composite of death, MI, or unplanned revascularisation	3.5	0.4	Lower composite rates of death, MI, or unplanned revascularisation with FFR-guidance vs. angiography-guidance (7.4% vs. 19.7%, hazard ratio: 0.43 [95% CI: 0.25, 0.75] $p = 0.003$)
RIPCORD-2 [4] (NCT02892903)	2022	17 sites in United Kingdom	1100 patients (stable angina/NSTEMI)	Total hospital cost and quality of life	1	0.3	No difference in median hospital costs or quality of life for FFR-guidance vs. angiography-guidance. No difference in the composite of death, stroke, MI, or unplanned revascularisation for FFR-guidance vs. angiography-guidance (9.5% vs. 8.7%, $p = 0.064$).
FAME 5 year [2] (NCT00267774)	2015	20 sites in the United States and Europe	1005 patients (stable/unstable Angina)	MACE defined as the composite of death, MI, or unplanned revascularisation	5	7.5	At 5 years, no difference in the composite of death, MI, or unplanned revascularisation with FFR-guidance vs. angiography-guidance (28% vs. 31%, relative risk: 0.91 [95% CI: 0.75, 1.10] $p = 0.31$). At 2 years, MACE was lower with FFR-guidance vs. angiography-guidance. Number of stents implanted per patient was lower with FFR-guidance vs. angiography-guidance (mean 1.9 ± 1.3 vs. 2.7 ± 1.2, $p < 0.0001$).
FARGO [5] (NCT02477371)	2018	3 sites in Denmark	100 patients (stable angina/NSTEMI)	Graft failure in the percentage of all grafts	0.5	0.0 (for MACE) 25.0 (for angiogram follow-up at 6 months)	No difference in graft failure rates with FFR guidance vs. angiography-guidance (16% vs. 12%, $p = 0.97$). No difference in the composite of death, nonprocedural MI, unplanned revascularisation and stroke with FFR-guidance vs. angiography-guidance (12% vs. 12%, $p = 0.97$).
GRAFFITI [6] (NCT01810224)	2019	6 sites in Europe	172 patients (stable angina/NSTEMI)	Graft occlusion	1	1.7 (for MACE) 35.5 (for Coronary imaging follow-up at 6 months)	No difference in graft failure rates with FFR-guidance vs. angiography-guidance (19% vs. 20%, $p = 0.885$). No difference in the composite of death, MI, unplanned revascularisation and stroke with FFR-guidance vs. angiography-guidance (3.7% vs. 7.1%, hazard ratio: 1.28 [95% CI: 0.39, 4.16], $p = 0.687$).

Table 1. *Cont.*

Study	Year Published	Enrolment Centres	Participants and Presentation	Primary Endpoint	Follow-Up (Years)	Loss to Follow-Up, n (%)	Findings
FAMOUS-NSTEMI [12] (NCT01764334)	2014	6 sites in the United Kingdom	350 patients (NSTEMI)	Proportion of patients allocated to medical management	1	0.0	Higher proportion of patients initially treated by medical therapy with FFR-guidance vs. angiography guidance (22.7% vs. 13.2%, $p = 0.022$). No difference in the composite of cardiovascular death, MI, or unplanned hospitalisation for heart failure (8.0% vs. 8.6%, risk difference −0.7% [95% CI: −6.7, 5.3%] $p = 0.89$).
FLOWER-MI [7] (NCT02943954)	2021	41 sites in France	1163 patients (STEMI)	MACE defined as the composite of death, MI, and unplanned hospitalisation leading to urgent revascularisation	1	0.4	At 5 years, no difference in the composite of death, MI and urgent revascularisation with FFR-guidance vs. angiography-guidance (5.5% vs. 4.2%, hazard ratio: 1.32 [95% CI: 0.78, 2.23] $p = 0.31$).
FUTURE [8] (NCT01881555)	2021	31 sites in France	927 patients (stable angina/ACS/atypical chest pain/silent ischaemia)	Composite of death, MI, stroke or unplanned revascularisation	1	0.1	No difference in the composite of death, MI, stroke or unplanned revascularisation with FFR-guidance vs. angiography-guidance (14.6% vs. 14.4%, hazard ratio: 0.97 [95% CI: 0.69, 1.36], $p = 0.85$).

Abbreviations: CI = confidence interval; FAME = Fractional Flow Reserve Versus Angiography for Multivessel Evaluation; FAMOUS-NSTEMI = Fractional Flow Reserve Versus Angiographically Guided Management to Optimise Outcomes in Unstable Coronary Syndromes; FARGO = Fractional Flow Reserve Versus Angiography Randomisation for Graft Optimisation; FFR = fractional flow reserve; FLOWER-MI = FLOW Evaluation to Guide Revascularisation in multivessel ST-elevation Myocardial Infarction; FRAME-AMI = FFR vs. Angiography-guided PCI in AMI with multivessel disease; FUTURE = Functional Testing Underlying Coronary Revascularisation; GRAFFITI = Graft Patency After FFR-Guided Versus Angio-Guided CABG; MACE = major adverse cardiac events; NSTEMI = non-ST segment elevation myocardial infarction; RIPCORD-2 = Does Routine Pressure Wire Assessment Influence Management Strategy at Coronary Angiography for Diagnosis of Chest Pain?; STEMI = ST segment elevation myocardial infarction.

Table 2. Patient and procedural characteristics from RCTs, comparing FFR with angiography only, for guiding revascularisation.

Study	Strategy	Age, Years (Mean ± SD, or Median [IQR])	Male (%)	Diabetes Mellitus (%)	Smoker (%)	ACS Presentation (%)	Treatment with CABG (%)	Procedure Time for PCI, Mins (Mean ± SD, or Median [IQR])	FFR Cut-Off	Angiogram Visual Stenosis Threshold for PCI (%)
FRAME-AMI [3] (NCT02715518)	Angio (n = 278)	62.7 ± 11.5	84.2	30.9	37.8	100.0	0	Not reported	NA	>50
	FFR (n = 284)	63.9 ± 11.4	84.5	34.2	32.0	100.0	0	Not reported	≤0.8	NA
RIPCORD-2 [4] (NCT02892903)	Angio (n = 552)	64.3 ± 10.2	77.2	17.6	65.0	53.1	9.2	42.4 ± 27.0	NA	≥30
	FFR (n = 548)	64.3 ± 10.0	73.5	20.6	58.5	50.4	11.9	69.0 ± 27.0	≤0.8	NA
FAME 5 year [2] (NCT00267774)	Angio (n = 496)	63.9 ± 10.0	74.0	25.0	30.0	31.3	0	70.0 ± 44	NA	>50
	FFR (n = 509)	64.5 ± 10.4	75.0	22.0	25.0	25.1	0	71.0 ± 43	≤0.8	NA
FARGO [5] (NCT02477371)	Angio (n = 48)	65.3 ± 8.8	89.0	23.0	17.0	14.0	100.0	NA	NA	≥50
	FFR (n = 49)	66.4 ± 6.4	88.0	22.0	27.0	31.0	100.0	NA	≤0.8	NA
GRAFFITI [6] (NCT01810224)	Angio (n = 84)	67 (63, 72)	79.00	40.0	42.0	11.0 (for entire population)	100.0	NA	NA	≥30
	FFR (n = 88)	67 (62, 72)	83.0	35.0	53.0		100.0	NA	≤0.8	NA
FAMOUS- NSTEMI [2] (NCT01764334)	Angio (n = 174)	61.6 ± 11.1	73.0	14.9	40.8	100	6.9	70.5 ± 33.5	NA	≥30
	FFR (n = 176)	62.3 ± 11.0	75.6	14.8	40.9	100	6.2	66.5 ± 23.4	≤0.8	NA
FLOWER-MI [7] (NCT02943954)	Angio (n = 577)	61.9 ± 11.4	81.1	14.2	36.4	100	0	32.0 (20.0, 24.0)	NA	≥50
	FFR (n = 586)	62.5 ± 11.0	85.0	18.3	40.1	100	0	31.0 (21, 45)	≤0.8	NA
FUTURE [8] (NCT01881555)	Angio (n = 467)	66.0 ± 11.0	82.0	32.0	26.0	46.0	12.0	Not reported	NA	≥50
	FFR (n = 460)	65.0 ± 10.0	85.0	31.0	24.0	47.0	12.0	Not reported	≤0.8	NA

Abbreviations: ACS = acute coronary syndrome; CABG = coronary artery bypass graft surgery; FFR = fractional flow reserve; IVUS = intravascular ultrasound; IQR = interquartile range; NA = not applicable; OCT = optical coherence tomography; PCI = percutaneous coronary intervention; SD = standard dev.

3.2. Baseline Characteristics of the Population

Trial characteristics are displayed in Table 1. Population and procedural characteristics are displayed in Table 2. The mean age of the entire population was 64 years and 81% were men. Overall, 39% of patients presented with stable CAD, whereas 61% presented with ACS. Twenty five percent of the population had diabetes mellitus.

3.3. Clinical Endpoints

There was no difference in the trial-defined composite endpoint, when stratified according to either stable CAD [32% vs. 35%, RR: 0.95 (95%CI 0.83 to 1.09), p = 0.47, I^2, 0% or ACS 15% vs. 16%, RR: 0.89 (95%CI 0.67 to 1.19), p = 0.44, I^2 61%, between an FFR-guided group and the angiography-guided group (Figure 3).

Trial-defined major composite endpoint

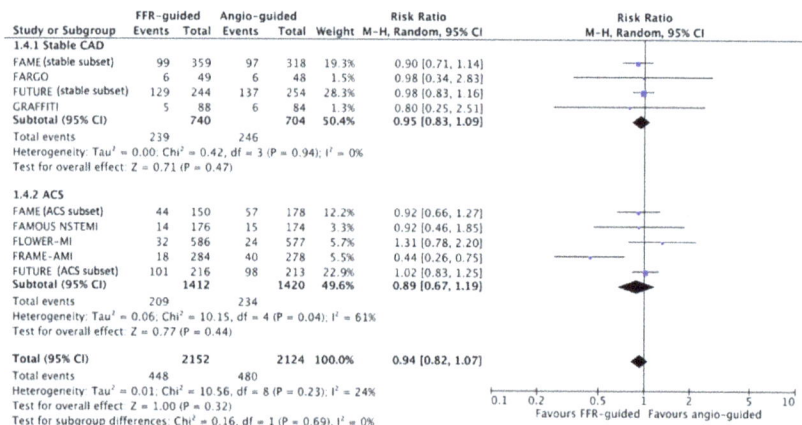

Figure 3. Forest plot of the trial-defined composite endpoint stratified by stable CAD and ACS.

There was no difference in all-cause mortality between the FFR-guided group and the angiography-guided group [3.5% vs. 3.7%, RR: 0.99 (95% confidence interval (CI) 0.62 to 1.60), p = 0.98, I^2 43%, Figure 4a.

There was also no difference in non-fatal MI [5.3% vs. 5.9%, RR: 0.93 (95%CI 0.66 to 1.32), p = 0.69, I^2 42%, Figure 4b] or unplanned revascularisation [7.4% vs. 7.9%, RR: 0.92 (95%CI 0.76 to 1.11), p = 0.37, I^2 0%, Figure 4c] between the FFR- versus angiography-guided groups.

Sensitivity analyses conducted via a leave-one-out meta-analysis did not change the statistical significance of the results.

3.4. Revascularisation and Stent Implanted per Allocated Strategy

The number patients undergoing planned revascularisation by either stent or surgery was significantly lower in the FFR-guided group [weighted mean difference: 14 (95% CI: 3 to 25)%, $p \leq 0.001$], Figure 5a, when compared to the angiography-guided revascularisation strategy.

The pooled average number of stents was significantly lower in the FFR-guided group compared to the angiography-guided group [mean difference −0.45 (95%CI −0.70 to −0.20), p = 0.004], Figure 5b.

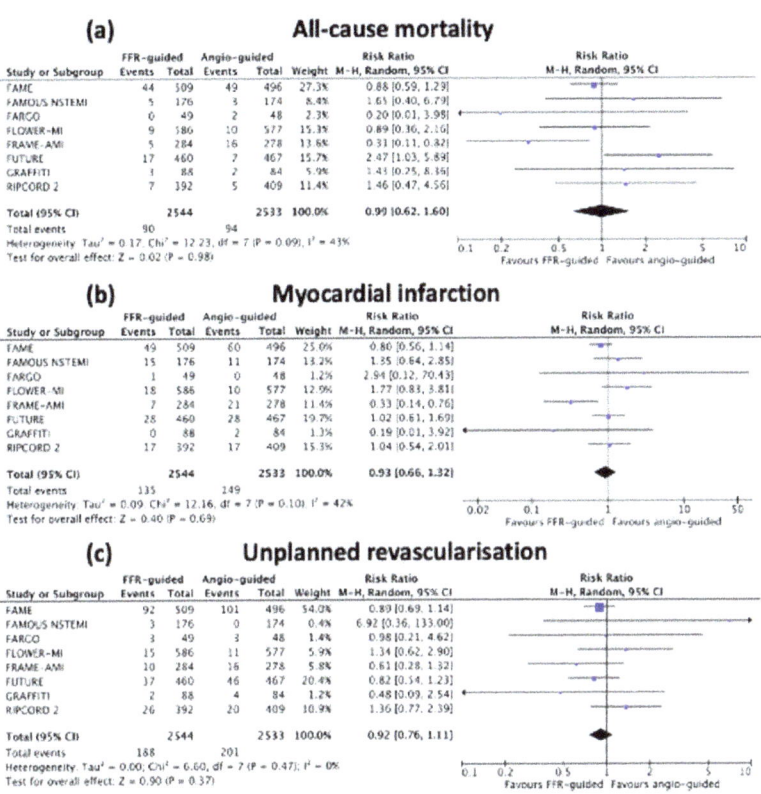

Figure 4. Forest plots of (**a**) all-cause mortality; (**b**) non-fatal myocardial infarction; and (**c**) unplanned revascularisation.

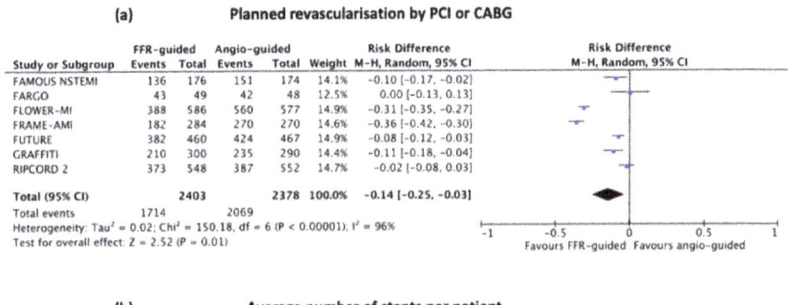

Figure 5. Forest plots of (**a**) average number of stented implanted; and (**b**) percentage of patients undergoing planned revascularisation as per their randomisation group.

4. Discussion

In this contemporary meta-analysis of RCTs comparing FFR-guided (using a cut-off of ≤0.80) to angiography-guided management strategy for obstructive CAD, we found no difference in mortality, MI, or unplanned revascularisation, between the 2 strategies. However, an FFR-guided approach was associated with a lower number of patients who underwent revascularisation by up to a quarter (upper limit of the 95% CI). The latter finding is of considerable importance, highlighting the benefit to patients and the local health resource of such an approach. In fact, our findings could be summarised as follows: despite reducing the number of patients requiring revascularisation by up to 25%, an FFR-guided management strategy has no penalty in terms of the rate of adverse clinical events.

Two previous meta-analyses included 5094 patients from 7 RCTs [13], and an analysis from 5 RCTs totalling 2288 patients [14]. Both of these meta-analyses [13,14] found no difference in mortality when FFR-guidance was compared to angiography-guidance for complete revascularisation. However, our study also includes FRAME-AMI [3], only recently reported. We also excluded the RCT by Quintella et al. [15] (n = 69), which was included in the previous meta-analysis [14], and the DEFER-DES trial [16] (Fractional Flow Reserve to Determine the Appropriateness of Angioplasty in Moderate Coronary Stenosis), which was included in the larger prior meta-analysis [13], as they used an FFR threshold of <0.75. Furthermore, we excluded the DK-CRUSH VI trial (Double Kissing Crush Versus Provisional Stenting Technique for Treatment of Coronary Bifurcation Lesions) [17], which was included in the larger prior meta-analysis [13], as only the side branch involved in a provisional bifurcation stenting strategy was randomised to either FFR-guided or angiography-guided revascularisation, rather than the lesion in the main vessel. Furthermore, we took care to only include patients with obstructive CAD from the RIPCORD-2 trial [4], to better reflect current clinical practice of when FFR use would be considered, which was not the case in the previous meta-analysis [13]. Lastly, we also included trials with CABG as the revascularisation strategy, which makes our findings more relevant to everyday clinical practice, and our meta-analysis builds on the previous work by Matthews et al. [18], which only included 3 trials [7,8,19] of patients undergoing PCI only and clinical outcomes were limited to 1 year.

The role of FFR in acute MI setting has been a subject of debate. FFR is usually performed in the non-infarct related artery in the setting of STEMI rather that the infarct related artery. Therefore, the impact of acute infarct and edema is minimal. However, STEMI patients may have caffeine or caffeine-containing product on board, and therefore FFR done during the index procedure would have a high false-negative rate. In NSTEMI, FFR can be done both in the infarct-related artery and the non-infarct related artery as shown in FAMOUS-NSTEMI but was not powered for clinical outcomes. One would expect that if a NSTEMI patient with a large infarct size or area of edema, FFR could be falsely negative in view of the inability of that infarct related territory to reach maximum hyperemia. We did attempt to stratify the trial-defined MACE by clinical presentation and in view of the inherent limitation of doing FFR in acute MI setting, although there was no difference in MACE between the 2 groups, the heterogeneity was high at 61%. Further studies are required to confirm the role of FFR in acute MI setting.

It is well known that discrepancy exists between angiographic visual estimates of stenosis severity, and physiologically significant flow limitation that causes downstream myocardial ischaemia [20]. The prevalence of a discordance between the visual estimate of stenosis significance and FFR measurement is between 20–30% of all lesions, and this mismatch involves lesions as little as 30% stenosis by eye and above 90% [4,21]. The absence of myocardial ischaemia is associated with excellent outcomes using optimal medical therapy [22] and FFR is regarded as the reference standard invasive method to define lesion-specific ischaemia [23]. It has been logically been suggested that judgements based on angiographic visual estimates of lesion severity are subjective, potentially leading to misdiagnosis and unnecessary stent implantation or even CABG, with the possibility of procedure-related complications, leading to worse outcomes [20]. In contrast, our findings demonstrate that guiding revascularisation in a range of clinical scenarios encountered in our daily practice based on angiography alone, without FFR, does not adversely impact on major adverse ischaemic events. One potential explanation for our findings might be the impact of vulnerable plaque characteristics, which have been shown to be associated with adverse outcomes [24] and could potentially exist in lesions without significant ischaemia. Most recently, this was demonstrated in the COMBINE OCT-FFR trial (Combined Optical Coherence Tomography Morphologic and Fractional Flow reserve Haemodynamic Assessment of Non-Culprit Lesions to Better Predict Adverse Event outcomes in Diabetes Mellitus patients) [25]. COMBINE OCT-FFR found that, among diabetic patients with ≥1 FFR-negative lesions, thin-cap fibroatheroma detected on optical coherence tomography was associated with a five-fold higher rate of MACE, despite the absence of ischaemia [25]. Therefore, there has recently been a paradigm shift in our understanding that plaque burden (the higher the plaque burden, the more likely for vulnerable plaques to develop), may impact on hard clinical outcomes irrespective of the physiological significance of lesions. Further studies are warranted to improve understanding of whether revascularization decisions could be improved by assessment using the combination of both plaque vulnerability with OCT and physiological lesion significant with FFR The INTERCLIMA trial (Interventional Strategy for Non-culprit Lesions with Major Vulnerability Criteria at OCT in Patients with ACS) (NCT05027984), PREVENT trial (The Preventive Coronary Intervention on Stenosis With Functionally Insignificant Vulnerable Plaque) (NCT02316886) and COMPARE STEMI ONE trial (Comparison Of Reduced DAPT Followed by P2Y12 Inhibitor Monotherapy With Prasugrel vs. standard Regimen in STEMI Patients Treated With OCT-guided vs. aNgio-guided complete Revascularisation) (NCT05491200), are currently ongoing, to assess whether an imaging-guided approach to identify vulnerable plaques, would improve clinical outcomes.

There are a number of limitations to our study. Firstly, it is an aggregate of trial-level data, rather than individual patient-level data. Therefore, we could not perform in-depth sub-group analyses, stratified by diabetes status, clinical presentation, or treatment with CABG. We cannot exclude the possibility that heterogeneity of the populations, for example the prevalence of diabetes, may have influenced the conclusions. Nonetheless, evidence suggests that robustly performed trial-level meta-analyses often produce similar conclusions to patient-level meta-analyses [26]. We did provide subgroup analysis for the trial-defined composite endpoint for patients presenting with stable CAD or ACS and our findings were similar to those observed for all the RCTs were pooled together. Secondly, there was heterogeneity across the included RCTs, with respect to inclusion criteria, primary endpoints, and follow up duration. Of note, RIPCORD-2 [4], GRAFFITI [6] and FAMOUS-NSTEMI [12] included lesions with 30% angiographic stenosis assessed visually, compared to 50% in the other studies included in our meta-analysis [2,3,5,7,8]. The percentage of patients with ACS was lowest in the GRAFFITI trial [6]. In contrast, FLOWER-MI [7] exclusively included STEMI patients with bystander disease, and FRAME-AMI [3] only included patients with STEMI or NSTEMI. FAMOUS-NSTEMI [12] exclusively included patients with NSTEMI. Approximately half of the patients included in RIPCORD-2 [4] and FUTURE [8] presented with ACS. However, these studies reflect the patient population we would encounter in our clinical practice for pressure wire use to guide treatment. It should also be noted that the indication for FFR use to guide PCI is more widely clinically applicable whereas the aim of FFR use in the 2 RCTs to guide CABG (FARGO and GRAFFITI trials) was to assess graft patency post-surgery. Therefore, FFR use in those already planned for CABG is less clinically applicable at present, pending further adequately powered RCTs for hard clinical outcomes in CABG patients and is a limitation of our study.

In conclusion, this contemporary meta-analysis shows that an FFR-guided management strategy did not impact on all-cause mortality, MI and unplanned revascularisation, when compared to an angiography-guided management strategy, after a weighted mean follow-up of 22 months. However, an FFR-guided approach led to up to 1 in 4 less patients needing revascularisation, which has important benefits to patients and the local provision of health resources.

Funding: This research received no external funding.

Institutional Review Board Statement: Not applicable.

Informed Consent Statement: Not applicable.

Data Availability Statement: The data underlying this article are available in the article.

Acknowledgments: All contributors have been acknowledged as co-authors.

Conflicts of Interest: NC reports receiving unrestricted research grants from Boston Scientific (RIP-CORD2) and HeartFlow (FORECAST).

References

1. Lawton, J.S.; Tamis-Holland, J.E.; Bangalore, S.; Bates, E.R.; Beckie, T.M.; Bischoff, J.M.; Bittl, J.A.; Cohen, M.G.; DiMaio, J.M.; Don, C.W.; et al. 2021 ACC/AHA/SCAI Guideline for Coronary Artery Revascularization: Executive Summary: A Report of the American College of Cardiology/American Heart Association Joint Committee on Clinical Practice Guidelines. *Circulation* **2022**, *145*, e4–e17. [CrossRef]
2. van Nunen, L.X.; Zimmermann, F.M.; Tonino, P.A.L.; Barbato, E.; Baumbach, A.; Engstrøm, T.; Klauss, V.; A MacCarthy, P.; Manoharan, G.; Oldroyd, K.G.; et al. Fractional flow reserve versus angiography for guidance of PCI in patients with multivessel coronary artery disease (FAME): 5-year follow-up of a randomised controlled trial. *Lancet* **2015**, *386*, 1853–1860. [CrossRef]
3. Hahn, J.Y. FFR vs. Angiography-guided PCI in AMI with multivessel disease—FRAME-AMI trial. In Proceedings of the European Society of Cardiology Conference, Barcelona, Spain, 27–31 August 2022.
4. Stables, R.H.; Mullen, L.J.; Elguindy, M.; Nicholas, Z.; Aboul-Enien, Y.H.; Kemp, I.; O'Kane, P.; Hobson, A.; Johnson, T.W.; Khan, S.Q.; et al. Routine Pressure Wire Assessment Versus Conventional Angiography in the Management of Patients with Coronary Artery Disease: The RIPCORD 2 Trial. *Circulation* **2022**, *146*, 687–698. [CrossRef]
5. Thuesen, A.L.; Riber, L.; Veien, K.T.; Christiansen, E.H.; Jensen, S.E.; Modrau, I.S.; Andreasen, J.J.; Junker, A.; Mortensen, P.E.; Jensen, L.O. Fractional Flow Reserve Versus Angiographically-Guided Coronary Artery Bypass Grafting. *J. Am. Coll. Cardiol.* **2018**, *72*, 2732–2743. [CrossRef]
6. Toth, G.G.; De Bruyne, B.; Kala, P.; Ribichini, F.L.; Casselman, F.; Ramos, R.; Piroth, Z.; Fournier, S.; Piccoli, A.; Van Mieghem, C.; et al. Graft patency after FFR-guided versus angiography-guided coronary artery bypass grafting: The GRAFFITI trial. *EuroIntervention* **2019**, *15*, e999–e1005. [CrossRef]
7. Puymirat, E.; Cayla, G.; Simon, T.; Steg, P.G.; Montalescot, G.; Durand-Zaleski, I.; le Bras, A.; Gallet, R.; Khalife, K.; Morelle, J.-F.; et al. Multivessel PCI Guided by FFR or Angiography for Myocardial Infarction. *N. Engl. J. Med.* **2021**, *385*, 297–308. [CrossRef]
8. Rioufol, G.; Dérimay, F.; Roubille, F.; Perret, T.; Motreff, P.; Angoulvant, D.; Cottin, Y.; Meunier, L.; Cetran, L.; Cayla, G.; et al. Fractional Flow Reserve to Guide Treatment of Patients with Multivessel Coronary Artery Disease. *J. Am. Coll. Cardiol.* **2021**, *78*, 1875–1885. [CrossRef]
9. Moher, D.; Shamseer, L.; Clarke, M.; Ghersi, D.; Liberati, A.; Petticrew, M.; Shekelle, P.; Stewart, L.A. Preferred reporting items for systematic review and meta-analysis protocols (prisma-p) 2015 statement. *Syst. Rev.* **2015**, *4*, 1. [CrossRef]
10. Higgins, J.P.T.; Altman, D.G.; Gøtzsche, P.C.; Jüni, P.; Moher, D.; Oxman, A.D.; Savović, J.; Schulz, K.F.; Weeks, L.; Sterne, J.A.C.; et al. The Cochrane Collaboration's tool for assessing risk of bias in randomised trials. *BMJ* **2011**, *343*, d5928. [CrossRef]
11. Higgins, J.P.T.; Thompson, S.G.; Deeks, J.J.; Altman, D.G. Measuring inconsistency in meta-analyses. *BMJ* **2003**, *327*, 557–560. [CrossRef]
12. Layland, J.; Oldroyd, K.G.; Curzen, N.; Sood, A.; Balachandran, K.; Das, R.; Junejo, S.; Ahmed, N.; Lee, M.M.; Shaukat, A.; et al. Fractional flow reserve vs. angiography in guiding management to optimize outcomes in non-ST-segment elevation myocardial infarction: The British Heart Foundation FAMOUS-NSTEMI randomized trial. *Eur. Heart J.* **2014**, *36*, 100–111. [CrossRef]
13. Elbadawi, A.; Sedhom, R.; Dang, A.T.; Gad, M.M.; Rahman, F.; Brilakis, E.S.; Elgendy, I.Y.; Jneid, H. Fractional flow reserve versus angiography alone in guiding myocardial revascularisation: A systematic review and meta-analysis of randomised trials. *Heart* **2022**, *108*, 1699–1706. [CrossRef]
14. Prasad, R.M.; Baloch, Z.Q.; Gumbita, R. Updated meta-analysis comparing FFR-guided and angiographic-guided intervention in patients with multivessel coronary artery disease. *Int. J. Heart Vasc. Syst.* **2022**, *2*, 6–10.
15. Quintella, E.F.; Ferreira, E.; Azevedo, V.M.P.; Araujo, D.V.; Sant'anna, F.M.; Amorim, B.; De Albuquerque, D.C. Clinical Outcomes and Cost-Effectiveness Analysis of FFR Compared with Angiography in Multivessel Disease Patient. *Arq. Bras. Cardiol.* **2018**, *112*, 40–47. [CrossRef]
16. Park, S.H.; Jeon, K.-H.; Lee, J.M.; Nam, C.-W.; Doh, J.-H.; Lee, B.-K.; Rha, S.-W.; Yoo, K.-D.; Jung, K.T.; Cho, Y.-S.; et al. Long-Term Clinical Outcomes of Fractional Flow Reserve–Guided Versus Routine Drug-Eluting Stent Implantation in Patients with

Intermediate Coronary Stenosis: Five-Year Clinical Outcomes of DEFER-DES Trial. *Circ. Cardiovasc. Interv.* **2015**, *8*, e002442. [CrossRef]
17. Chen, S.-L.; Ye, F.; Zhang, J.-J.; Xu, T.; Tian, N.-L.; Liu, Z.-Z.; Lin, S.; Shan, S.-J.; Ge, Z.; You, W.; et al. Randomized Comparison of FFR-Guided and Angiography-Guided Provisional Stenting of True Coronary Bifurcation Lesions: The DKCRUSH-VI Trial (Double Kissing Crush Versus Provisional Stenting Technique for Treatment of Coronary Bifurcation Lesions VI). *JACC Cardiovasc. Interv.* **2015**, *8*, 536–546. [CrossRef]
18. Matthews, C.J.; Naylor, K.; Blaxill, J.M.; Greenwood, J.P.; Mozid, A.M.; Rossington, J.A.; Veerasamy, M.; Wheatcroft, S.B.; Bulluck, H. Meta-Analysis Comparing Clinical Outcomes of Fractional-Flow-Reserve- and Angiography-Guided Multivessel Percutaneous Coronary Intervention. *Am. J. Cardiol.* **2022**, *184*, 160–162. [CrossRef]
19. Tonino, P.A.L.; De Bruyne, B.; Pijls, N.H.J.; Siebert, U.; Ikeno, F.; van't Veer, M.; Klauss, V.; Manoharan, G.; Engstrøm, T.; Oldroyd, K.G.; et al. Fractional flow reserve versus angiography for guiding percutaneous coronary intervention. *N. Engl. J. Med.* **2009**, *360*, 213–224. [CrossRef]
20. White, C.W.; Wright, C.B.; Doty, D.B.; Hiratza, L.F.; Eastham, C.L.; Harrison, D.G.; Marcus, M.L. Does Visual Interpretation of the Coronary Arteriogram Predict the Physiologic Importance of a Coronary Stenosis? *N. Engl. J. Med.* **1984**, *310*, 819–824. [CrossRef]
21. Curzen, N.; Rana, O.; Nicholas, Z.; Golledge, P.; Zaman, A.; Oldroyd, K.; Hanratty, C.; Banning, A.; Wheatcroft, S.; Hobson, A.; et al. Does Routine Pressure Wire Assessment Influence Management Strategy at Coronary Angiography for Diagnosis of Chest Pain? *Circ. Cardiovasc. Interv.* **2014**, *7*, 248–255. [CrossRef]
22. Shaw, L.J.; Berman, D.S.; Maron, D.J.; Mancini, G.B.J.; Hayes, S.W.; Hartigan, P.M.; Weintraub, W.S.; O'Rourke, R.A.; Dada, M.; Spertus, J.A.; et al. Optimal Medical Therapy with or Without Percutaneous Coronary Intervention to Reduce Ischemic Burden: Results from the Clinical Outcomes Utilizing Revascularization and Aggressive Drug Evaluation (COURAGE) trial nuclear substudy. *Circulation* **2008**, *117*, 1283–1291. [CrossRef]
23. Pijls, N.H.; A van Son, J.; Kirkeeide, R.L.; De Bruyne, B.; Gould, K.L. Experimental basis of determining maximum coronary, myocardial, and collateral blood flow by pressure measurements for assessing functional stenosis severity before and after percutaneous transluminal coronary angioplasty. *Circulation* **1993**, *87*, 1354–1367. [CrossRef]
24. Stone, G.W.; Maehara, A.; Lansky, A.J.; de Bruyne, B.; Cristea, E.; Mintz, G.S.; Mehran, R.; McPherson, J.; Farhat, N.; Marso, S.P.; et al. A Prospective Natural-History Study of Coronary Atherosclerosis. *N. Engl. J. Med.* **2011**, *364*, 226–235. [CrossRef]
25. Kedhi, E.; Berta, B.; Roleder, T.; Hermanides, R.S.; Fabris, E.; Ijsselmuiden, A.J.J.; Kauer, F.; Alfonso, F.; von Birgelen, C.; Escaned, J.; et al. Thin-cap fibroatheroma predicts clinical events in diabetic patients with normal fractional flow reserve: The COMBINE OCT–FFR trial. *Eur. Heart J.* **2021**, *42*, 4671–4679. [CrossRef]
26. Smith, C.T.; Marcucci, M.; Nolan, S.J.; Iorio, A.; Sudell, M.; Riley, R.; Rovers, M.M.; Williamson, P.R. Individual participant data meta-analyses compared with meta-analyses based on aggregate data. *Cochrane Database Syst. Rev.* **2016**, *2016*, MR000007. [CrossRef]

MDPI
St. Alban-Anlage 66
4052 Basel
Switzerland
www.mdpi.com

Journal of Clinical Medicine Editorial Office
E-mail: jcm@mdpi.com
www.mdpi.com/journal/jcm

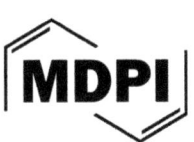

Disclaimer/Publisher's Note: The statements, opinions and data contained in all publications are solely those of the individual author(s) and contributor(s) and not of MDPI and/or the editor(s). MDPI and/or the editor(s) disclaim responsibility for any injury to people or property resulting from any ideas, methods, instructions or products referred to in the content.

www.ingramcontent.com/pod-product-compliance
Lightning Source LLC
LaVergne TN
LVHW070151100526
838202LV00015B/1932